Metabolic Syndrome: A Growing Concern

Metabolic Syndrome: A Growing Concern

Edited by Wade Chambers

hayle
medical

New York

Hayle Medical,
750 Third Avenue, 9th Floor,
New York, NY 10017, USA

Visit us on the World Wide Web at:
www.haylemedical.com

ISBN: 978-1-63241-604-9

Cataloging-in-Publication Data

Metabolic syndrome : a growing concern / edited by Wade Chambers.
        p. cm.
Includes bibliographical references and index.
ISBN 978-1-63241-604-9
1. Metabolic syndrome. 2. Metabolism--Disorders. 3. Syndromes.
4. Insulin resistance. I. Chambers, Wade.
RC662.4 .M48 2019
616.399--dc23

Table of Contents

Preface

Metabolic syndrome is the combination of three or more medical conditions, including high blood sugar, high blood pressure, high serum triglycerides, central obesity and low serum high-density lipoprotein. This condition increases the risk of developing type 2 diabetes and cardiovascular diseases. Nearly 20-25% of the world's adult population is afflicted by metabolic syndrome. Metabolic syndrome is an active area of medical research. The underlying cause is believed to be a disorder of energy storage and utilization. The commonly associated risk factors of metabolic disorders include sedentary behavior, genetics, diet, aging, etc. Recent research points to the contribution of prolonged chronic stress to metabolic syndrome. The objective of this book is to give a general view of the different aspects of metabolic syndrome. Different approaches, evaluations, methodologies and advanced studies on metabolic syndrome have been included herein. It is a vital tool for all researching or studying this disorder as it gives incredible insights into emerging trends and concepts.

This book unites the global concepts and researches in an organized manner for a comprehensive understanding of the subject. It is a ripe text for all researchers, students, scientists or anyone else who is interested in acquiring a better knowledge of this dynamic field.

I extend my sincere thanks to the contributors for such eloquent research chapters. Finally, I thank my family for being a source of support and help.

Editor

Treating Hyperinsulinemia with *Momordica charantia*

Frank Comhaire

Department of Endocrinology, Ghent University Hospital, Belgium

*Corresponding author:Prof. Frank Comhaire, Brakelmeersstraat, 18 B9830 Sint Martens-Latem, Belgium; E-mail: Frank@comhaire.com

Abstract

Objectives: To assess the efficacy of a novel nutraceutical mainly containing the extract of bitter gourd *(Momordica charantia)* and α-lipoic acid for the treatment of patients with hyperinsulinemia.

Methods: Pilot prospective open-label cohort trial including 11 patients with hyperinsulinemia due to insulin resistance. The concentrations of insulin, C-peptide, glucose, haemoglobin A1c, total cholesterol, triglycerids, gamma- glutamyltransferase, and C-reactive protein were measured in blood take between 3 and 4 hours after dinner.

Results: One and 4 months after initiation of treatment there was a significant decrease of the concentrations of insulin (to average 25% of initial value), C-peptide (to average 44% of initial value), glucose, hemoglobin A1c and gamma-glutamyl transpeptidase.

Clinical significance: Treatment of patients with hyperinsulinemia, with or without diabetes or metabolic syndrome, using a novel nutraceutical containing *Momordica charantia* and α-lipoic acid dramatically reduced insulin resistance and may have improved non-alcoholic fatty liver disease.

Keywords: Insulin resistance; Hyperinsulinemia; *Momordica charantia*; Bitter gourd; Alpha lopoic acid; Nutraceutical

Introduction

Insulin resistance is the common denominator of the metabolic syndrome and obesity, pre-diabetes, and type 2 diabetes. It induces compensatory insulin hypersecretion. Impaired insulin sensitivity is frequent during statin treatment [1]. Hyperinsulinemia has been associated with prostate- [2] and breast cancer [3,4], and with non-alcoholic fatty liver disease.

In addition to live style adjustment and appropriate diet, Metformin is considered the first-line treatment of hyperinsulinemia. As efficient as this treatment may be, it is not devoid of serious side effects such as lactic acidosis, renal toxicity, and gastro-intestinal discomfort.

There are several non-pharmaceutical agents that counteract insulin resistance and may decrease hyperinsulinemia, of which the extract of *Momordica charantia* (bitter gourd or bitter melon) is well-known. Its mechanisms of action include increased phosphorylation of acetyl-CoA carboxylase and AMP-activated protein kinase (AMPK) [5], reduction of lipogenesis, enhanced thermogenesis and lipolysis [6]. The extract down-regulates the expression of peroxisome proliferator-activated receptor (PPAR)-gamma, nuclear factor kappaB (NF-kB), and interferon-gamma in heart tissue, with cardio-protective effect thanks to reduction of inflammation [7]. In addition, Momordica exerts an interesting endocrine effect where it inhibits the enzyme 11β-hydroxysteroid dehydrogenase type 1, that metabolises the mineralocorticoid cortisone to the glucocorticoid cortisol [8]. There is evidence for increased activity of this enzyme in adipose cells [9], and that this may be an important aetiological factor in the pathogenesis of obesity-associated insulin resistance.

Alpha-lipoic acid is a water soluble anti-oxidant which has been proven to reduce insulin resistance [10] in patients with type 2 diabetes [11] or obese and overweight non-diabetic men [12] and women [13], and it may potentially be used in cardiovascular diseases [14]. Alpha-lipoic acid was shown to improve angiogenesis and bioenergetics in hyperglycemia [15], and to upregulate irisin secretion in adipocytes, protecting against deleterious effects of glucose impairment [16].

The combination of Momordica extract and alpha-lipoic acid was expected to act in synergism because these agents are effective along different molecular pathways.

Here we report the results of an open-label, pilot trial of the treatment of a cohort of patients suffering from hyperinsulinemia, using a novel nutraceutical that combines the extract of *Momordica charantia* with alpha-lipoic acid.

Materials and Methods

Eleven consecutive patients consulting at the private clinic of the author and presenting hyperinsulinemia were invited to participate in an open-label, prospective trial using a novel nutraceutical containing 350 mg of the 1:4 extract of *Momordica charantia* and 50 mg alpha-lipoic acid (Cambridge Commodities, UK) in vegicaps (Pharmacy Van Wambeke, Elversele, Belgium)(Belgian patent # 1021188). Patients were requested to take 1 capsule after breakfast and one after dinner. The cohort consisted of 7 women and 4 men aged between 56 to 76 years. One woman was under treatment for type 2 diabetes with Metformin and Glipizide, with insufficient result and elevated haemoglobin A1c concentration. The nutraceutical was added to her initial medication. Patients were already given "healthy diet" recommendations before the initiation of the trial, emphasizing the importance of reducing sugar and fructose intake. Two patients dropped out for personal reasons, though one patient resumed participation at a later date (data not included).

Before treatment was initiated, blood was taken, and this was repeated after 1 and 4 months of treatment. Blood was taken between 3 and 4 hours after lunch, and analysed for glycemia, haemoglobin A1c, insulin, C-peptide, triglycerids, total cholesterol, gamma glutamyl transpeptidase, and C-reactive protein (CRP) using well-established standard procedures (Anacura laboratory Ltd., Evergem, Belgium).

Results were plotted into the spreadsheet of the MedCalc statistical software (MedCalc Ltd, Ostend, Belgium) and described by means of parametrical (mean, standard deviation) and non-parametrical variables (median, 95% confidence intervals). Individual data of relevant biological markers are also presented in box-and-whisker plots with dots.

The significance of changes over time was assessed using the non-parametrical Wilcoxon's signed-rank test for paired observations, that is independent of the distribution of the data. The effective P-values of this test are listed.

Results

There was a highly significant correlation between the concentrations of insulin and C-peptide both before treatment (r=0.92, P= 0.009) and after 1 month of nutraceutical intake (r=0.80, P=0.029). The results of all measurements are listed in Table 1.

The concentrations of insulin, C-peptide, glycemia, gamma glutamyl transpeptidase and hemoglobin A1c presented a significant decrease ($P<0.05$) over the observation period (Table 2). Triglycerids, total cholesterol, and C-reactive protein did not change significantly. The individual values of insulin (Figure 1), C-peptide (Figure 2), and gamma glutamyl transpeptidase (Figure 3) are shown in box-and-whisker plots with dots.

Varaible	Time 0 (mean, SD)	Time 0 (median, 95% CI)	1 mth (mean, SD)	1 mth (median, 95% CI)	1 mth (median, 95% CI)	4 mth (median, 95% CI)
insulin	75,6 (50,2)	76,8 (39,3-107,4)	41,1 (23,1)	39,9 (18,9-54,9)	18,7 (7,2)	17,7 (10,8-17,8)
C-peptide	9,38 (2,85)	8,41 (7,00-11,91)	6,27 (1,72)	5,96 (4,85-7,59)	4,18 (1,27)	3,83 (3,45-4,88)
glycemia	129 (39,1)	127 (99,3-167,1)	105,5 (18,8)	97 (89,0-126,1)	99,0 (27,6)	91,0 (80,2-119,5)
hemoglobin A1c	6,77 (1,7)	6,30 (5,56-8,21)	6,42 (1,57)	6,00 (5,34-7,26)	6,08 (0,86)	5,9 (5,42-6,70)
trigyclicerids	245 (96,6)	241 (176-314)	238 (137)	248 (68-408)	270 (114)	218 (130-412)
total cholesterol	209 (47,0)	202 (157-242)	208 (40,9)	202 (166-245)	229,7 65,7)	210 (179-333)
gamma GT	42,3 (18,5)	41,5 (23,3-55,6)	36,4 (13,4)	37,0 (24,0-48,8)	31,8 (11,1)	34,0 (19,4-42,2)
C-reactive protein	3,67 (2,43)	3,70 (1,24-5,89)	2,67 (1,98)	2,1 (0,19-5,13)	4,72 (2,96)	4,65 (0,01-9,44)

Table 1: Time 0 lists the measurements before initiation of treatment. 1 month and 4 month list the measurements after respectively 1 and 4 months of intake of the nutraceutical. Gamma GT stands for gamma glutamyl transpeptidase. Values given are mean and standard deviation (SD), median and 95% confidence interval. Units: Insulin: µU/L; C-peptide: ng/mL; Glycemia: mg/mL; Hemoglobin A1c: %; Triglycerides: mg/dL; total cholestrerol: mg/dL, Gamma glutamyl transpeptidase: U/L; C-reactive protein: mg/L.

Variable	Time 0 vs. 1 month	1 month vs. 4 month	Time 0 vs. 4 month
insulin	0.004	0.008	0.008
C-peptide	0.0003	0.008	0.0003
glycemia	0.037	0.54	0.039
hemoglobin A1c	0.031	0.63	0.031
triglycerids	0.44	0.91	0.54
total cholesterol	0.64	0.31	0.44
gamma GT	0.016	0.62	0.031
C-reactive protein	0.63	0.41	0.87

Table 2: P-values of the comparison between values measured at different time intervals, using the non-parametrical Wilcoxon signed-rank test for paired observations.

The concentrations of insulin (Figure 1), C-peptide (Figure 2), glycemia, gamma glutamyl transpeptidase (Figure 3) and hemoglobin A1c presented a significant decrease (P<0.05) over the observation (Table 2). Triglycerids, total cholesterol, and C-reactive protein did not present significant changes.

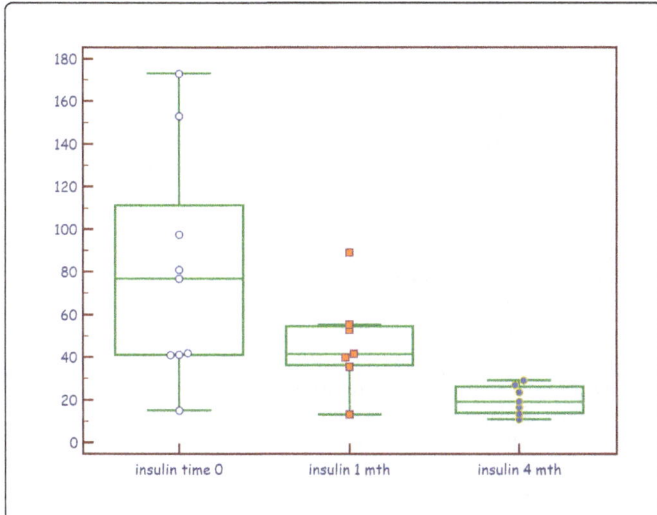

Figure 1: Box and whisker plots of Insulin concentration (in µU/L, on the vertical axis) at time 0, before initiation of treatment, after 1 month, and after 4 months of nutriceutical intake. The median is given, the boxes indicate the 25th and 75th percentile, and the whiskers correspond to the 5th and 95th percentile. Individual data are plotted.

Discussion

The benefit of *Momordica charantia* has been amply documented for the treatment of type 2 diabetes. It increases sensitivity of the insulin receptor [17], reduces insulin resistance and hyperinsulinemia, with favourably influence on the metabolic syndrome [18] and diabetes [19] in humans.

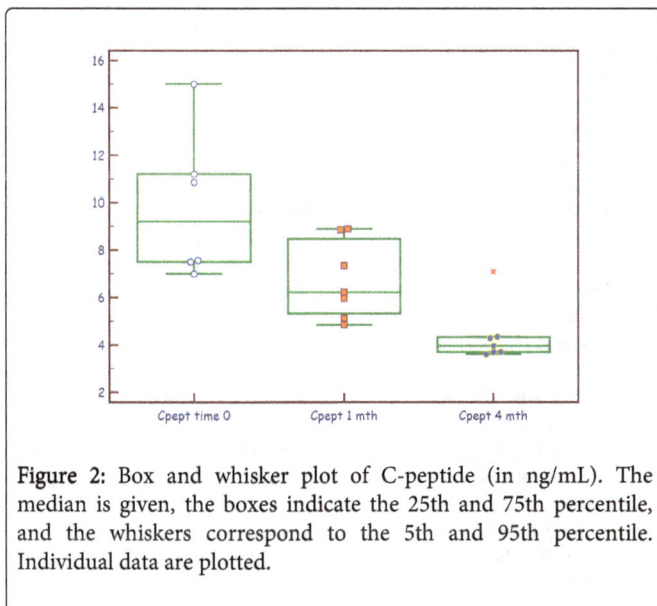

Figure 2: Box and whisker plot of C-peptide (in ng/mL). The median is given, the boxes indicate the 25th and 75th percentile, and the whiskers correspond to the 5th and 95th percentile. Individual data are plotted.

Obesity promotes prostate cancer [20] which has been related to hyperinsulinemia and insulin resistance [2, 21-23]. Momordica extract exerts chemo-protective effect against prostate cancer cells *in vitro* [24,25]. Its insulin-reducing effect may decrease neoplastic growth of the prostate in humans [26]. Also, insulin resistance has been found to impair cognitive function [27] and to promote Alzheimer disease [28]. The association between lower urinary tract symptoms (LUTS) and risk of dementia [29] may relate to hyperinsulinemia as common pathogenic factor. Therefore, decreasing insulin resistance may possibly contribute to the prevention of brain damage.

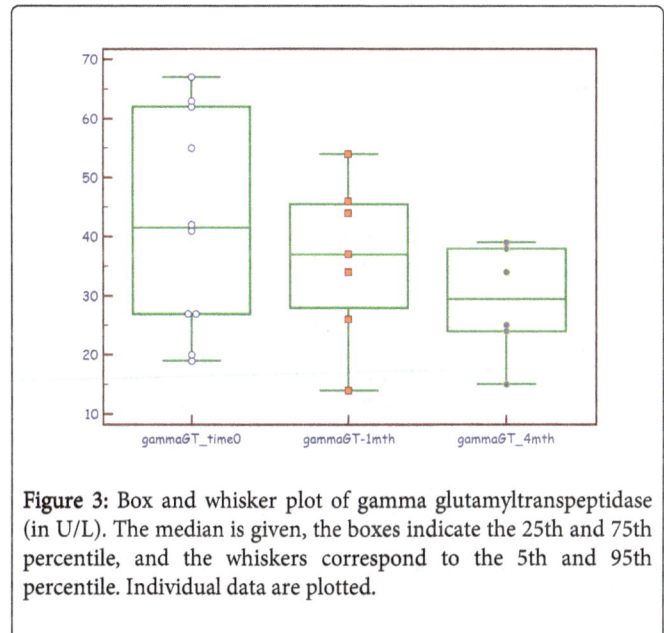

Figure 3: Box and whisker plot of gamma glutamyltranspeptidase (in U/L). The median is given, the boxes indicate the 25th and 75th percentile, and the whiskers correspond to the 5th and 95th percentile. Individual data are plotted.

Little is known about the efficiency of Momordica, associated with alpha-lipoic acid on hyperinsulinemia in patients, some of whom satisfy the criteria for the diagnosis of metabolic syndrome or with diabetes type 2. Clamp tests were not performed, but the recommendations of Jones and Hattersley [30] were implemented by measuring insulin and C-peptide in blood taken between 3 and 4 hours after dinner.

Under these circumstances all cases presented an important improvement of their metabolic status, with persistent reduction of the hyperinsulinemia and other biological markers. Serum gamma-glutamyl transpeptidase concentration was reported to distinguish non-alcoholic fatty liver disease at high risk [31,32] particularly in patients with the metabolic syndrome [33]. The decreased gamma-glutamyl transpeptidase activity observed during nutraceutical intake suggests a beneficial effect on non-alcoholic fatty liver disease [34,35], since this was shown to be associated with histologic improvement [36], and it may reduce the risk of developing type-2 diabetes [37].

There were no side effects, and gastro-intestinal tolerance was excellent. Vital signs and blood tests for renal function, and peripheral red and white blood cells count remained unchanged. Two cases mentioned weight loss over 10%, which they were unable to attain before initiation of treatment, even though adhering to the same diet.

Our findings underscore the benefit of nutraceutical treatment using the novel formulation in patients suffering from hyperinsulinemia, which should stimulate further research into its possible effectiveness for the prevention of diseases associated with this condition.

Conclusion

The treatment of patients suffering from hyperinsulinemia with a nutraceutical mainly composed of the extract of *Momordica charantia* and the antioxidant alpha lipoic acid may be considered as an alternative for the conventional pharmaceutical approach. In this preliminary trial, including a limited number of cases, the nutraceutical was found to be effective as for as biological markers were concerned. It was well tolerated and devoid of side effects.

References

1. Cederberg H, Stancakova A, Yaluri N, Modi S, Kuusisto J, et al. (2015) Increased risk of diabetes with statin treatment is associated with impaired insulin sensitivity and insulin secretion: a 6 year follow-up study of the METSIM cohort. Diabetologia 58: 1109-1117.

2. Grossmann M, Wittert G (2012) Androgens, diabetes and prostate cancer. Endocr Relat Cancer 19: F47-F62.

3. Gunter MJ, Xie X, Xue X, Kabat GC, Rohan TE, et al. (2015) Breast cancer risk in metabolically healthy but overweight postmenopausal women. Cancer Res 75: 270-274.

4. Wysocki PJ, Wierusz-Wysocka B (2010) Obesity, hyperinsulinemia and breast cancer: novel targets and a role for metformin. Expert Rev Mol Diagn.10: 509-519.

5. Tan, MJ, Ye JM, Turner N, Hohnen-Behrens C, Ke CQ, et al. (2008) Antidiabetic activities of triterpenoids isolated from bitter melon associated with activation of the AMPK pathway. Chem. Biol.15: 263-273.

6. Chen PH, Chen GC, Yang MF, Hsieh CH, Chuang SH, et al. (2012) Bitter melon seed oil-attenuated body fat accumulation in diet-induced obese mice is associated with cAMP-dependent protein kinase activation and cell death in white adipose tissue. J. Nutr. 142: 1197-1204.

7. Gadang V, Gilbert W, Hettiararchchy N, Horax R, Katwa L, et al. (2011) Dietary bitter melon seed increases peroxisome proliferator-activated receptor-gamma gene expression in adipose tissue, down-regulates the nuclear factor-kappaB expression, and alleviates the symptoms associated with metabolic syndrome. J. Med. Food 14: 86-93.

8. Blum A, Loerz C, Martin HJ, Staab-Weijnitz CA, Maser E (2012) Momordica charantia extract, a herbal remedy for type 2 diabetes, contains a specific 11beta-hydroxysteroid dehydrogenase type 1 inhibitor. J. Steroid Biochem. Mol. Biol. 128: 51-55.

9. Morton NM, Seckl JR (2008) 11beta-hydroxysteroid dehydrogenase type 1 and obesity. Front Horm. Res. 36: 146-164.

10. Jacob S, Ruus P, Hermann R, Tritschler HJ, Maerker E, et al. (1999) Oral administration of RAC-alpha-lipoic acid modulates insulin sensitivity in patients with type-2 diabetes mellitus: a placebo controlled pilot trial. Free Radic Biol Med 27: 309-314.

11. Hendriksen EJ, Diamond-Stanic MK, Marchionne EM (2011) Oxidative stress and the etiology of insulin resistance and type 2 diabetes Free Radic Biol Med 51: 993-999.

12. Xiao C, Giacca A, Lewis GF (2011) Short-term oral α-lipoic acid does not prevent lipid-induced dysregulation of glucose homeostasis in obese and overweight nondiabetic men. Am J Physiol Endocrinol Metabol 301: E736-741.

13. Capelli V, Di Sabatino A, Musacchio MC, De Leo V (2013) Evaluation of a new association between insulin-sensitizers and α-lipoic acid in obese women affected by PCOS. Minerva Ginecol 65: 425-433.

14. Ghibu S, Richard C, Delemasure S, Vergely C, Zeller M, (2008) An endogenous dithiol with antioxidant properties: alpha-lipoic acid, potential uses in cardiovascular diseases. Ann Cardiol Angeiol (Paris) 57: 161-165.

15. Coletta C, Modis K, Szczesny B, Brunyanszki A, Olah G, et al. (2015) Regulation of vascular tone, angiogenesis and cellular bioenergetics by the 3-mercaptopyruvate sulfurtrensferase/H2S pathway: functional impairment by hyperglycemia and restoration by DL-α-lipoic acid. Mol Med 21: 1–14.

16. Huerta AE, Prieto-Hontoria PL, Fernandez-Galilea M, Sainz N, Cuervo N, et al. (2015) Circulating irisin and glucose metabolism in overweight/obese women: effects of α-lipoic acid and eicosapentaenoic acid. J Physiol Biochem 28.

17. Shetty AK, Kumar GS, Sambaiah K, Salimath PV (2005) Effect of bitter gourd (Momordica charantia) on glycaemic status in streptozotocin induced diabetic rats. Plant Foods Hum. Nutr. 60: 109-112.

18. Tsai CH, Chen EC, Tsay HS, Huang CJ (2012) Wild bitter gourd improves metabolic syndrome: a preliminary dietary supplementation trial. Nutr. J. 11: 4.

19. Rizvi SI, Mishra N (2013) Traditional Indian medicines used for the management of diabetes mellitus. J. Diabetes Res. 712092.

20. Lee A, Chia SJ (2015) Prostate cancer detection; The impact of obesity on Asian men. Urol Oncol 9 pii: S1708-1439.

21. Allott EH, Masko EM, Freedland SJ (2013) Obesity and prostate cancer: weighing the evidence. Eur. Urol. 63: 800-809.

22. Arcidiacono B, Iiritano S, Nocera A, Possidente K, Nevolo MT, et al. (2012) Insulin resistance and cancer risk: an overview of the pathogenetic mechanisms. Exp. Diabetes Res.789174.

23. Vardhan SP, Krishnamma A, Naidu JN, Naidu MP (2014) Study of insulin resistance and antioxidant vitamin status in prostate cancer patients. Int. J. Res. Med. Sci. 2: 643-646.

24. Ru P, Steele R, Nerurkar PV, Phillips N, Ray RB (2011) Bitter melon extract impairs prostate cancer cell-cycle progression and delays prostatic intraepithelial neoplasia in TRAMP model. Cancer Prev. Res. (Phila) 4: 2122-2130.

25. Pitchakarn P, Suzuki S, Ogawa K, Pompimon W, Takahashi S, et al. (2012) Kuguacin J, a triterpeniod from Momordica charantia leaf, modulates the progression of androgen-independent human prostate cancer cell line, PC3. Food Chem. Toxicol. 50: 840-847.

26. Nandeesha H (2009) Insulin: a novel agent in the pathogenesis of prostate cancer. Int. Urol. Nephrol. 41: 267-272.

27. Sasaoka T, Wada T, Tsuneki H (2014) Insulin resistance and cognitive function. Nihon Rinsho 72: 633-640.

28. De Felice FG (2013) Alzheimer's disease and insulin resistance: translating basic science into clinical applications. J. Clin. Invest. 123: 531-539.

29. Janeczko LL (2015) Older adults with lower urinary tract symptoms have increased dementia risk. DGNews. 30th International Conference of Alzheimer Disease International (ADI) Perth, April 21.

30. Jones AG, Hattersley AT (2013) The clinical utility of C-peptide measurement in the care of patients with diabetes. Diabet Med 30: 803-807.

31. Tahan V, Cabakan B, Balci H, Dane F, Akin H, et al. (2008) Serum gamma-glutamyltranspeptidase distinguishes non-alcoholic fatty liver disease at high risk. Hepatogastroenterology 55: 1433-1438.

32. Frazini M, Fornaciari I, Fierabracci V, Elawadi HA, Bolognesi V, (2012). Accuracy of b-GGT fraction for the diagnosis of non-alcoholic fatty liver disease. Liver Int 32: 629-634.

33. Banderas DZ, Escobedo J, Gonzalez E, Liceaga MG, Ramirez JC, (2012) Y-glutamyl transferase: a marker of non-alcoholic fatty liver disease in patients with the metabolic syndrome. Eur J Gastroenterol Hepatol 24: 805-810.

34. Salgado W , dos Santos JS, Sankarankutty AK, De Castro e Silva O (2006) Nonalcoholic fatty liver disease and obesity. Acta Cir Bras 21 suppl. 1: 72-78.

35. Fabbrini E, Sullivan S, Klein S (2010) Obesity and nonalcoholic fatty liver disease: biochemical, metabolic and clinical implications. Hepatology 51: 679-689.

2

Magnitude of Obesity, Abdominal Adiposity and their Association with Hypertension and Diabetes- A Cross Sectional Study

Unyime Sunday Jasper*

Department of physiotherapy, Plateau State Specialist Hospital, Jos, Nigeria

*Corresponding author: Unyime Sunday Jasper, Department of physiotherapy, Plateau State Specialist Hospital, P.M.B 2113, Jos, Plateau State, Nigeria; E-mail: jaspersnd64@gmail.com

Abstract

Background: The transition from customary African lifestyles to a "western" standard has resulted in the increase of obesity, abdominal adiposity and diabetes known to contribute significantly to morbidity and mortality rates around the world. We therefore aimed to identify the magnitude of overweight, obesity, abdominal adiposity and hypertension among a sample of patients with type 2 diabetes.

Methods: A sample of convenience was utilized to recruit all Type 2 diabetes patients that attended the 2013 World Diabetes day celebration. Sociodemographic information along with anthropometric measurements was taken (BMI, WC, WHR). Furthermore, blood pressure and fasting blood sugar level was measured for each participant.

Result: Out of the 468 diabetics that participated in this study, majority 248 (53.0%) were males and 220 (47.0%) females. The mean age and FBS was 42.6 ± 11.3 years and 6.9 ± 3.2mm/dl respectively. Hypertension was reported in 226 (48.3%) diabetics; while 182 (38.9%) were within the normal weight range, 41.0% (192) were overweight and 20.1% (94) were obese. A high WC was reported in 51.7% (n=242) and a high WHR in 52.6% (n=246). Obesity was significantly associated with middle-age (40-64 years) (p=0.001, F=15.4) and females (p=0.000, F=15.8). Those who were hypertensive had a significantly higher BMI (p=0.000, F=12.4), WHR (p=0.000, F=2.1) and WC (p=0.000, F=5.2). High WHR and WC was associated with higher FBS (p=0.000).There was a tenuous but significant difference in WHR by gender (p<0.05), with females having a higher WHR than males (0.88 ± 0.1 vs. 0.87 ± 0.1). There was a relationship between BMI, WC and WHR.

Conclusion: The proportion of obesity, abdominal adiposity and hypertension among type 2 diabetics is worrisome. Early diagnosis of obesity and abdominal adiposity and advice on lifestyle modification is imperative. Furthermore, a coherent and multifaceted public health strategy aimed at systematically debunking unhealthy myths and encouraging adoption of healthy lifestyles is imperative.

Keywords: Body Mass Index (BMI), Abdominal adiposity, Obesity, Hypertension, Diabetes

Introduction

Developing countries of Africa are vulnerable to the predicted diabetes epidemic, projected to become one of the world's main disabler and killer within the next twenty-five years [1]. This can be attributed to increase in urbanization, which has resulted in a continuous generational paradigm shift of lifestyle from the customary African model to a more "western" standard. Many have abandoned the rural life characterized by agriculture based energy-intensive occupations in search of so-called "white collar" jobs characterized by sedentary lifestyle along with dependence on unhealthy or "junk" meals. Furthermore, as income and social development improves, lifestyles have become more sedentary due to internet communications, computer games, televised entertainment, academic study and private lessons and poor urban planning [2]. Also, healthier conventional lifestyles characterised by regular and vigorous physical activity accompanied by sustenance on high fibre whole grain-based diet rich in vegetables and fruits has been replaced by over-reliance on motorised transport and consumption of unhealthy diets rich in carbohydrates, fats, sugars, and salts [3]. The resultant effects of this "adopted" regime is a change in disease patterns with communicable diseases being replaced by non-communicable or life style related diseases like diabetes, obesity, cardiovascular disease and cancer [4].

Globally, the proportion of chronic, non-communicable diseases is increasing at an alarming rate. Propelling the upsurge in cases of diabetes and hypertension which are major predisposing factors for cardiovascular disease is the growing prevalence of overweight and obesity. The World Health Organization has estimated that by 2015, 2.3 billion adults will be overweight and 700 million adults will be obese [5]. Obesity has in the last decade joined underweight, malnutrition, and infectious diseases as major health problems threatening the developing world [6]. Overweight and obesity are risk factors for a number of non-communicable diseases including diabetes and as the prevalence rate rises, so does the rates of diabetes. Approximately 197 million people worldwide have impaired glucose tolerance, most commonly because of obesity and the associated metabolic syndrome. This number is expected to increase to 420 million by 2025 [7].

Except proactive measures are taken quickly, a non-communicable disease epidemic is expected with obesity and diabetes leading the way especially considering the intimate relationship they share. According to Wannamethee and Shaper [8], adult weight gain, the degree of obesity and the duration of obesity are all independently and strongly predicting the risk of type 2 diabetes. Furthermore, diabetes is by far the most important of the direct and indirect costs associated with obesity [9] and it is generally accepted that the increasing prevalence of diabetes is associated with increased rates of overweight and obesity [10], with an estimated 90% of Type 2 diabetes attributed to excess weight [7]. Lahti-Koski et al. [11] reported that an elevated waist to hip ratio (WHR) signifying abdominal obesity is shown to be a strong risk factor for Type 2 diabetes mellitus. Also, some prospective studies have supported the association of various anthropometric indices of abdominal adiposity and the future development of diabetes [12]. It has been suggested that abdominal adiposity is an independent predictor of alteration in the plasma lipid, lipoprotein and plasma glucose concentrations [13].

In a bid to curb the global rising trends of non-communicable the rising trends in morbidity and mortality related to chronic non-communicable diseases, the World Health Organization and other international and national organizations have devised strategies for chronic non-communicable disease prevention and control [14]. Nigeria is not left out of this campaign which aims to identify risk factors involved in these medical conditions so as to formulate a suitable and effective programme for prevention, early detection and effective control. However, anecdotal evidence suggests that clinicians fail to diagnose obesity and in essence obesity-related co-morbidities, thus passing up the opportunity to screen these patients for obesity-related morbidities and counsel them on lifestyle modification. This is possibly because obesity is accepted in some social and cultural classes as a sign of affluence and well-being. Early recognition of these disorders will lead to a reduction in the morbidity and mortality associated with non-communicable diseases. The aim of this study was to identify the magnitude of overweight, obesity, abdominal adiposity and hypertension among a sample of patients with Type 2 diabetes (Figure 1).

Material and Methods

This was a cross sectional descriptive study carried out during the world diabetes day celebration at a diabetes screening centre in Jos, Plateau State, Nigeria. Approval to carry out this study was sought and obtained from the management of the diabetes screening centre. A sample of convenience was utilized to recruit all the diabetic patients who attended the screening programme. The weight was measured in kilograms, with patients standing bare feet in their minimal clothing and with their pockets free of objects that might add to their weights such as mobile phones, wallets, keys, rings, etc. using a bathroom weighing scale (Hamson, China), which was validated daily using a known 10 kg weighted mass and measured to the nearest 0.1 kg.

The weighing scale was checked for zero error after each measurement. The patients' heights were taken from a measuring scale drawn against the wall. In measuring the height, the patient who was barefooted and without head-gear or cap stood against the marked wall with the Achilles, gluteus and occiput touching it. A pointer was firmly pressed against the scalp and the measurement was read off on the wall scale in meters.

Body Mass Index (BMI) was calculated using the formula, weight (in kg) divided by height (in m^2). The hip circumference was measured at the maximum circumference around the hips, and the waist circumference was obtained at the level of the umbilicus with the subject supine. The waist to hip ratio (WHR) was also calculated. Venous blood sample of all the subjects was collected after an overnight fast. Subjects were defined as having diabetes if they met the WHO criteria (fasting whole venous blood glucose $\geq$ 126 mg/dl or 2 h blood glucose after a 75 g oral glucose test $\geq$ 200 mg/dl) or if there was documented evidence of diabetes in the medical records (Figures 2 and 3).

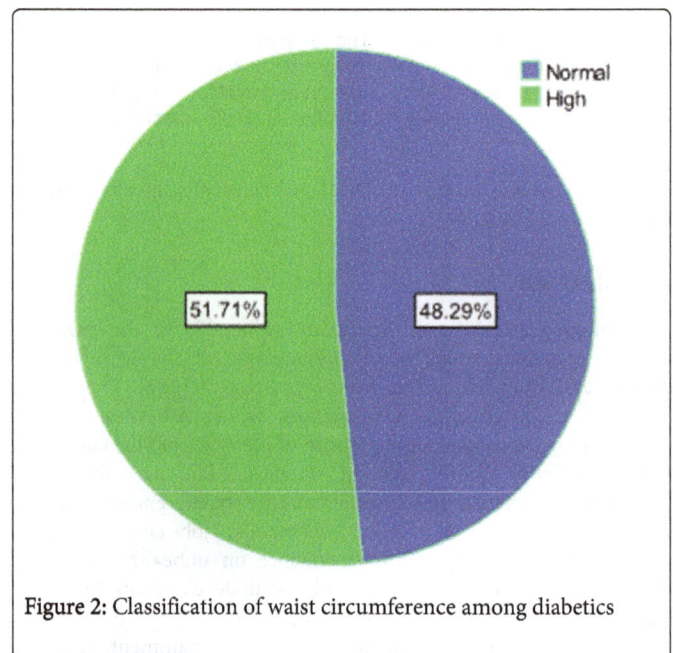
Figure 1: Proportion of hypertension among diabetics

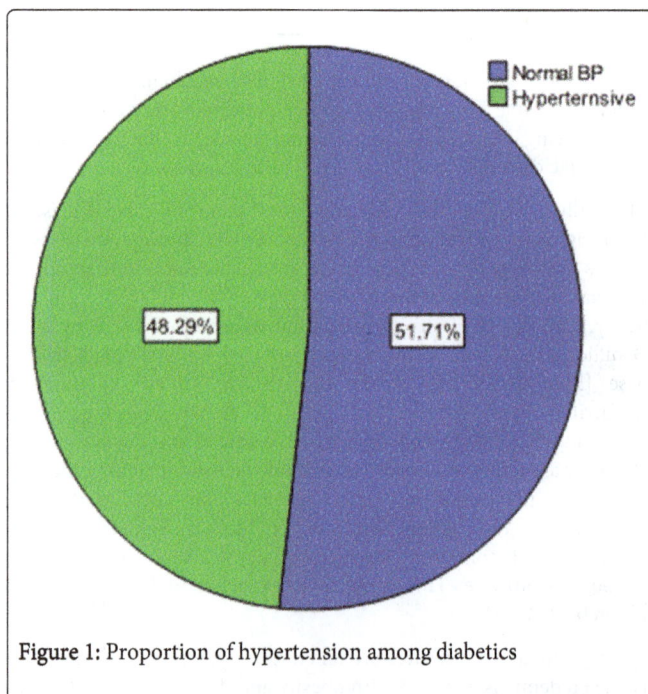
Figure 2: Classification of waist circumference among diabetics

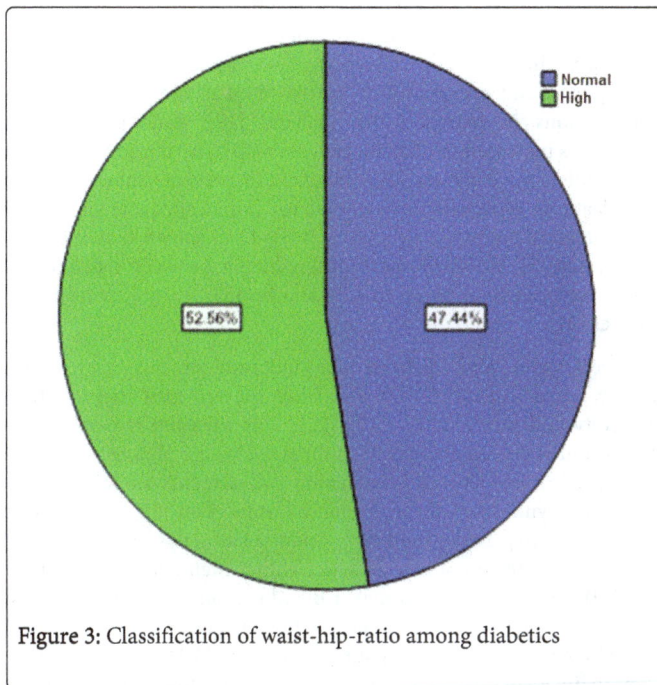

Figure 3: Classification of waist-hip-ratio among diabetics

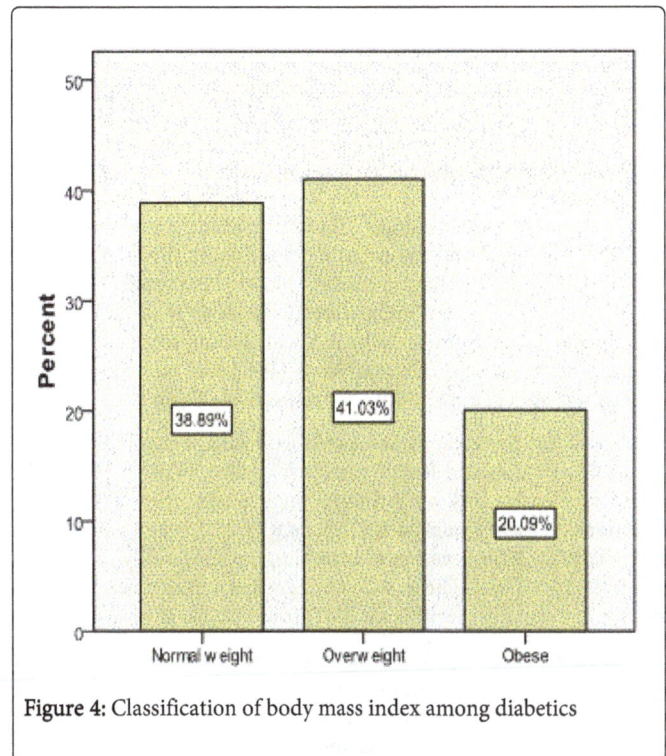

Figure 4: Classification of body mass index among diabetics

The blood pressure (BP) was measured using the auscultatory method with standard mercury in glass sphygmomanometer. Prior to the measurement, the patient was seated and rested for 5 min in a sitting position on a chair that supported the back comfortably. For each participant, the BP was measured every 2 minutes for three times and the average score was recorded.

Data was analysed using Statistical Package for Social Sciences (SPSS) version 17. Results were summarised as mean (SD), frequencies and percentages. Independent T-test and one-way Anova was used to compare differences in mean as appropriate, while spearman rank correlation was used to find relationships between variables. Values of $p < 0.05$ were considered statistically significant.

Results

A total of 468 diabetic patients participated in this study. There were 248 (53.0%) males and 220 (47.0%) females, with a male to female ratio of 1:1.3. A simple majority were not hypertensive (51.7%, n=242), while 226 (48.3%) were hypertensive. One hundred and eighty two (38.9%) were within the normal weight range, 41.0% (192) were overweight and 20.1% (94) were obese. A further classification of obesity revealed that 61.7% (58) had class one obesity, 27.7% (26) were in the class two obesity ranges, while 10.6% (10) were diagnosed as having class three obesity.

A simple majority of the patients had abdominal adiposity measured by WC (51.7%, n=242) and WHR (52.6%, n=246). This is shown in table 1 and Figure 4.

Variables	Mean (SD)	Frequency (n)	%
Age	42 (11.3) years		
Fasting blood sugar	6.9 (2.3) mm/dl		
Diastolic BP	91.9 (13.6) mmHg		
Systolic BP	142 (22.6) mmHg		
BMI	26.5 (4.7) kg/m2		
Waist circumference	90 ± 12 cm		
Waist-to-hip ratio	0.9 ± 0.1		
Gender			
Male		248	53.0
Female		220	47.0
Hypertensive			
Yes		226	48.3
No		242	51.7
BMI class			
Normal Weight		182	38.9
Overweight		192	41.0
Obese		94	20.1
Waist Circumference			
Normal		226	48.3
High		242	51.7

Waist-to-hip ratio			
Normal		222	47.4
High		246	52.6

Table 1: Clinical Characteristics of study subjects

The age of the patients ranged from 21 to 90 years, with a mean age of 42.6 ± 11.3 years and mean fasting blood sugar (FBS) of 6.9 ± 3.2 mm/dl. The mean systolic and diastolic blood pressure was 142 ± 22.6 mmHg and 91.9 ± 13.6 mmHg respectively. Body mass index of the participants ranged from 18-43 kg/m2, with a mean score of 26.5 ± 4.7 kg/m2. The mean waist circumference (WC) and waist-to-hip ratio (WHR) was 90 ± 12 cm and 0.9 ± 0.1 respectively Table 1.

Obesity was significantly associated with middle-age (40-64 years) (p=0.0001, F=15.4) and female gender (p=0.000, F=15.8). Those who were hypertensive had a significantly higher BMI (p=0.000, F=12.4) than normotensive participants (27.6 ± 4.6 vs. 25.4 ± 4.6), with systolic and diastolic blood pressure increasing exponentially as weight increases (p=0.000). There was no significant difference in blood glucose level among the different BMI groups (p>0.05).

Diabetics with a high WHR had significantly higher blood glucose level (p=0.000, F=28.2) than those with normal WHR (7.2 ± 3.9 vs. 6.5 ± 2.1). There was a tenuous but significant difference in WHR by gender (p<0.05), with females having a higher WHR than males (0.88 ± 0.1 vs. 0.87 ± 0.1). A high WHR was significantly associated with hypertension (p=0.000, F=2.1), systolic blood pressure (p=0.000, F=16.5) and diastolic blood pressure (p=0.000, F=18.0). Furthermore, there was a significant relationship between BMI and WHR (r=0.43, p=0.000).

Females had a significantly higher WC (p=0.001, F=10.6) than males (91.6 ± 13.0 vs. 86.6 ± 10.6). Hypertensive diabetics had a significantly higher WC (91.8 ± 12.0) than diabetics without hypertension (86.3 ± 11.5) (p=0.000, F=5.2). A higher FBS was associated with a high WC (7.1 ± 2.8 vs. 6.3 ± 2.0). Furthermore, a high WHR was significantly associated with systolic blood pressure (p=0.000, F=15.3) and diastolic blood pressure (p=0.000, F=13.9). There was a significant relationship among WC and BMI (r=0.78, p=0.000) and WC and WHR (r=0.54, p=0.000).

Discussion

Appropriate prevention and management strategies are delayed or non-existent because the health and economic burden from diabetes associated with obesity has probably been under estimated by governmental and non governmental agencies in Nigeria. This has increased the risk of developing and worsening the elements of metabolic syndrome. In an economic environment where it is difficult to access diabetes medication for the less privileged, emphasis should be on lifestyle modification in other to lessen the risk of developing metabolic syndrome. A major means of achieving this is to identify persons with diabetes who are at risk of developing obesity and abdominal adiposity or are already obese.

In this study, 48.3% (226) of diabetics are hypertensive or are currently on anti-hypertensive, a finding which is in line with earlier Nigerian studies which have reported a hypertension prevalence of between 30 to 55% among clinical patients with diabetes [15-17]. It is however lower than figures in western climes where more than 70% of

people with diabetes reportedly have high blood pressure or are being treated with medications for hypertension [18]. This is plausibly due to differences in geography. Hypertension in diabetes accelerates development and progression of micro vascular and macro vascular complications in patients with diabetes [19]. Among Nigerians, mortality is increased in diabetic patients with hypertension compared to normotensive diabetics [20]. In other to prevent diabetes related complications, especially those of vascular origin, adequate and timely blood pressure control is necessary. It has been shown that a 10 mm Hg decrease in blood pressure can reduce a person's risk for any diabetic complication by up to 12% and by 15% for deaths related to diabetes [21].

Hypertension and diabetes are independent risk factors for cardiovascular disease (CVD), and when they co-exist they multiply morbidity and mortality of CVD [22]. This situation is worse when obesity and abdominal adiposity is thrown into the picture because of the risk of developing and worsening the elements associated with metabolic syndrome through mechanisms that include insulin resistance, hypercoagulability, endothelial dysfunction, and inflammation. In our study, diabetics with a high abdominal obesity and BMI (48.3%) also had a higher blood pressure. Earlier, a study in Nigeria has reported the presence of both hypertension and obesity defined by BMI in 44.9% of patients with T2DM [17]. Obese people have an incidence of hypertension that is five times the incidence among people of normal weight [7]. Co-existence of adiposity, dyslipidemia and hypertension are risk factors for insulin resistance syndrome [23] and with diabetes, the risk of developing atherosclerosis increases [24]. To prevent the above complications in diabetics, physicians, dieticians and physical therapists should intensify efforts at educating diabetics on the need for proper blood glucose and blood pressure monitoring, well balanced diabetes diet and adequate physical activity. It has been shown that blood pressure reduction has been associated with a decreased risk of T2DM-related complications, stroke and the need for retinal photocoagulation [21], while weight loss through dieting or exercise helps correct insulin resistance and dyslipidemia found in patients with T2DM [25].

Majority of the diabetics in this study were either overweight or obese (61.1%). The mean weight score revealed that the study group was overweight, a finding which is in line with another study [26]. Furthermore, mean fasting blood glucose level revealed a not too effective but encouraging control of diabetes. A major means of reducing metabolic syndrome is to prevent or control the coexistence of obesity and diabetes, especially among those with poorly controlled diabetes because obesity worsens all the elements of metabolic syndrome. Since components of the syndrome synergistically increase vascular risk, the obvious corollary is that with increasing BMI, many Nigerians especially diabetics will be predisposed to cardiovascular events such as coronary heart disease and stroke. This places a huge economic burden on Nigeria since they are expensive to manage.

Abdominal obesity (high WHR and WC) was recorded in a simple majority of the participants, a finding consistent with other studies in Nigeria [27] and India [26]. Towards the middle of the 20th century, relative proportion of body fat in the upper body versus lower body was an important factor to consider while investigating obesity-related health problems. However, since the 1980-90s more attention has been focused on abdominal obesity, rather than obesity per se as an important correlates for various metabolic disturbance [28]. A common myth in some West African countries including Nigeria, pictures abdominal obesity and a "large" waist-to-hip ratio as a sign of good health, affluence, robustness and beauty. For example, a study in Cameroon found that heavy men were perceived as imposing and authoritative and thinness was antithetical to power [29]. This probably makes it difficult for diabetics to make adjustments even after thorough advice from health workers on the need to reduce weight, especially around the central area. A study emphasizes that a modest but achievable weight loss of 5% to 10% can be a realistic goal for improving glycemic control in patients with Type 2 diabetes [30].

Middle aged diabetics had a higher BMI than other age groups, a finding consistent with a Pakistani study which reported the highest prevalence of obesity and overweight among those aged 35–64 years [31]. Furthermore, females had a higher BMI than their male counterparts. Earlier studies in Nigeria [27], Pakistan [31] and Trinidad [32] have revealed a higher female to male obesity preponderance. Among the predisposing factors for obesity and overweight in Nigeria is female gender and age above 40 years [33,34]. Also across Sub-Saharan Africa, there is a universal preference for a curvy body shape among women and extra weight is seen as an indicator that her husband is caring for her well [35]. It is not surprising that in our study, women also had higher levels of abdominal adiposity (measured by WC and WHR) than men. In a bid to address this trend, it has been suggested that black females with DM should be considered a special subgroup at risk of obesity-related complications and be given a distinct focus of targeted therapies to reduce the prevalence and impact of obesity in DM [27]. Furthermore, to curb the rising levels of obesity and other non communicable diseases associated with it in Sub-Saharan Africa and Nigeria specifically, time tasted but unhealthy myths and practices has to be systematically discouraged among the general population and especially among those at risk of developing metabolic syndrome.

A high blood sugar level was associated with abdominal adiposity but not obesity. A study reported that abdominal adiposity (WHR) was a strong risk factor for Type 2 diabetes mellitus [11]. This is probably because a preponderance of enlarged fat cells in intra-abdominal fat depot increases the risk of glucose intolerance, hyperinsulinemia and hypertriglyceridemia [12,28]. This finding is a wake-up call for medical and health personnel and researchers in Africa to consider WHR and WC in people who may not necessarily be obese while assessing and advising for weight loss. It is also imperative to raise public health awareness of WHR and WC as an important measure of obesity-related health risk. There was a relationship between WC, WHR and BMI in our study; a finding previously reported by Fasanmade and Okubadejo [27]. This probably underscores the interdependence of each anthropometric measure in the diagnosis and management of adiposity, overweight and cardio metabolic risk factors.

Conclusion

This study brought to the fore the proportion of overweight, obesity and abdominal adiposity in a cohort of Type 2 diabetics. Obesity and abdominal adiposity was found in a majority of the study cohort. Even though a simple majority were not hypertensive, hypertension was associated with BMI and abdominal obesity (WHR and WC). Female diabetics were more likely to be obese and have a high WHR and WC compared to males. WHR and WC were associated with a high blood sugar level; and the three anthropometric measures utilized in this study were related to each other. Early diagnosis of obesity and abdominal obesity and advice on weight loss and other lifestyle modification along with good glycemic control is imperative to avoid

the development of metabolic syndrome and other complications associated with obesity, hypertension and diabetes. Furthermore, a coherent and multifaceted public health strategy aimed at systematically debunking unhealthy myths and encouraging adoption of healthy lifestyles is imperative.

Limitations

This study was carried out in a single center, thus limiting the generalization of its findings. However, being a population based study lends some power and eligibility to its outcome. Furthermore, we did not assess the serum biochemical profile of the study population, which would have further explored the risk of developing metabolic syndrome among diabetics with different measures of adiposity. Future studies should look at the relationship between serum biochemical profile of diabetes patients and their individual adiposity levels.

References

1. Ding CH, Teng CL, Koh CN (2006) Knowledge of diabetes mellitus among diabetic and non-diabetic patients in Klinik Kesihatan Seremban. Med J Malaysia 61: 399-404.

2. Bar-Or O, Foreyt J, Bouchard C, Brownell KD, Dietz WH, et al. (1998) Physical activity, genetic, and nutritional considerations in childhood weight management. Med Sci Sports Exerc 30: 2-10.

3. Mehta RS, Karki P, Sharma SK (2006) Risk factors, associated health problems, reasons for admission and knowledge profile of diabetes patients admitted in BPKIHS. Kathmandu Univ Med J (KUMJ) 4: 11-13.

4. International Diabetes Federation (IDF) (2006) Diabetes Atlas (3rd Edn), Brussels, Belgium.

5. World Health Organization (2010) Global strategy on diet, physical activity and health: obesity and overweight.

6. Haslam DW, James WP (2005) Obesity. Lancet 366: 1197-1209.

7. Hossain P, Kawar B, El Nahas M (2007) Obesity and diabetes in the developing world--a growing challenge. N Engl J Med 356: 213-215.

8. Wannamethee SG, Shaper AG (1999) Weight change and duration of overweight and obesity in the incidence of type 2 diabetes. Diabetes Care 22: 1266-1272.

9. Wolf AM, Colditz GA (1998) Current estimates of the economic cost of obesity in the United States. Obes Res 6: 97-106.

10. Lipscombe LL, Hux JE (2007) Trends in diabetes prevalence, incidence, and mortality in Ontario, Canada 1995-2005: a population-based study. Lancet 369: 750-756.

11. Lahti-Koski M, Pietinen P, Männistö S, Vartiainen E (2000) Trends in waist-to-hip ratio and its determinants in adults in Finland from 1987 to 1997. Am J Clin Nutr 72: 1436-1444.

12. Karter AJ, Mayer-Davis EJ, Selby JV, D'Agostino RB Jr, Haffner SM, et al. (1996) Insulin sensitivity and abdominal obesity in African-American, Hispanic, and non-Hispanic white men and women. The Insulin Resistance and Atherosclerosis Study. Diabetes 45: 1547-1555.

13. DeNino WF, Tchernof A, Dionne IJ, Toth MJ, Ades PA, et al. (2001) Contribution of abdominal adiposity to age-related differences in insulin sensitivity and plasma lipids in healthy nonobese women. Diabetes Care 24: 925-932.

14. WHO (2006) Global strategy on diet, physical activity and health. Bulletins of the WHO 5: 16-18.

15. Agaba IE, Anteyi EA, Puepet FH, Omudu PA, Idoko JA (2002) Hypertension in Type 2 diabetes in Jos Teaching Hospital, Jos Nigeria. Highland Med Research J 1: 22-24

16. Unadike BC, Eregie A, Ohwovoriole AE (2011) Prevalence of hypertension amongst persons with diabetes mellitus in Benin City, Nigeria. Niger J Clin Pract 14: 300-302.

17. Isezuo SA, Ezunu E (2005) Demographic and clinical correlates of metabolic syndrome in Native African type-2 diabetic patients. J Natl Med Assoc 97: 557-563.

18. Zimmet P, Alberti KG, Shaw J (2001) Global and societal implications of the diabetes epidemic. Nature 414: 782-787.

19. Adler AI, Stratton IM, Neil HA, Yudkin JS, Matthews DR, et al. (2000) Association of systolic blood pressure with macrovascular and microvascular complications of Type 2 diabetes (UKPDS 36): prospective observational study. BMJ 321: 412-419.

20. Kolawole BA, Ajayi AA (2000) Prognostic indices for intra-hospital mortality in Nigerian diabetic NIDDM patients. Role of gender and hypertension. J Diabetes Complications 14: 84-89.

21. [No authors listed] (1998) Tight blood pressure control and risk of macrovascular and microvascular complications in type 2 diabetes: UKPDS 38. UK Prospective Diabetes Study Group. BMJ 317: 703-713.

22. Gress TW, Nieto FJ, Shahar E, Wofford MR, Brancati FL (2000) Hypertension and antihypertensive therapy as risk factors for Type 2 diabetes mellitus. Atherosclerosis Risk in Communities Study. N Engl J Med 342: 905-912.

23. Ana SR (2002) Atherosclerosis and thrombosis in diabetic mellitus. J international fed clinical chemistry lab med 1: 1305-1308.

24. Siminialayi IM, Emem-Chioma PC (2004) Glucocorticoids and the insulin resistance syndrome. Niger J Med 13: 330-335.

25. American Diabetes Association (2013) Standards of medical care in diabetes--2013. Diabetes Care 36 Suppl 1: S11-66.

26. Sharma S, Jain S (2009) Prevalence of Obesity among Type-2 Diabetics. J Hum Ecol 25: 31-35

27. Fasanmade OA, Okubadejo NU (2007) Magnitude and gender distribution of obesity and abdominal adiposity in Nigerians with Type 2 diabetes mellitus. Niger J Clin Pract 10: 52-57.

28. Chandalia M, Abate N, Garg A, Stray-Gundersen J, Grundy SM (1999) Relationship between generalized and upper body obesity to insulin resistance in Asian Indian men. J Clin Endocrinol Metab 84: 2329-2335.

29. Kiawi E, Edwards R, Shu J, Unwin N, Kamadjeu R, et al. (2006) Knowledge, attitudes, and behavior relating to diabetes and its main risk factors among urban residents in Cameroon: a qualitative survey. Ethn Dis 16: 503-509.

30. Lau DC, Teoh H (2013) Benefits of modest weight loss on the management of Type 2 diabetes mellitus. Can J Diabetes 37: 128-134.

31. Jafar TH, Chaturvedi N, Pappas G (2006) Prevalence of overweight and obesity and their association with hypertension and diabetes mellitus in an Indo-Asian population. CMAJ 175: 1071-1077.

32. Ezenwaka CE, Offiah NV (2002) Abdominal obesity in type 2 diabetic patients visiting primary healthcare clinics in Trinidad, West Indies. Scand J Prim Health Care 20: 177-182.

33. Oyeyemi AL, Adegoke BO, Oyeyemi AY, Deforche B, De Bourdeaudhuij I, et al. (2012) Environmental factors associated with overweight among adults in Nigeria. Int J Behav Nutr Phys Act 9: 32.

34. Adedoyin RA, Mbada CE, Balogun MO, Adebayo RA, Martins T, et al. (2009) Obesity prevalence in adult residents of Ile-Ife, Nigeria. Nig Q J Hosp Med 19: 100-105.

35. Puoane T, Bradley H, Hughes G (2005) Obesity among black South African women. Human Ecology Special 13: 91-95.

3

Bioimpedance Evaluation of Body Fat Composition in Congolese HIV-Infected Patients under Antiretroviral Therapy Regimen Non-Containing Protease Inhibitors nor Stavudine

Jean-Robert Rissassy Makulo[1,2*], Djuma Lukonga[1], Augustin Luzayadio Longo[1,2], Jean De Dieu Manyebwa[1,3], Tresor Monsere[1,2], Ernest Kiswaya Sumaili[1,2], Hippolyte Nanituma Situakibanza[1,3], Jean Bosco Lasi Kasiam[1,4], Roger Mwimba Mbungu[1,5], Jean-Marie Ntumba Kayembe[1,6] and Francois Bompeka Lepira[1,2]

[1]Faculty of Medicine, University of Kinshasa, DR Congo

[2]Nephrology Unit, Department of Internal Medicine, University Clinics of Kinshasa, University of Kinshasa, DR Congo

[3]Infectious Diseases Unit, Department of Internal Medicine, University Clinics of Kinshasa, University of Kinshasa, DR Congo

[4]Endocrinology and Metabolic Diseases Unit, Department of Internal Medicine, University Clinics of Kinshasa, University of Kinshasa, DR Congo

[5]Department of Gynecology and Obstetrics, University Clinics of Kinshasa, University of Kinshasa, DR Congo

[6]Pneumology Unit, Department of Internal Medicine, University Clinics of Kinshasa, University of Kinshasa, DR Congo

*Corresponding author: Jean-Robert Rissassy Makulo, Nephrology Unit, University Clinics of Kinshasa, University of Kinshasa, DR Congo; E-mail: jrmakulo@yahoo.fr

Abstract

Background: Protease inhibitors (PI) and stavudine are frequently associated with abnormalities of the body composition. The present study aimed to evaluate the body fat composition of HIV-infected Congolese patients receiving antiretroviral other than PI or stavudine.

Patients and Methods: Anthropometric measures and body composition of 125 HIV-infected Congolese patients (average age 41 years, 76% women, 74% on antiretroviral therapy) attending a primary healthcare center was cross-sectionally evaluated. Patients receiving PI and/or stavudine were excluded. Subclinical abnormalities of body composition, evaluated by bioimpedance (BIA), were defined as elevated percentage of fat mass (FM) and perivisceral fat mass (PVF) and low percentage of total FM.

Results: Clinically evaluated abnormalities of fat distribution were rarely seen, with any case of obesity or lipodystrophy. Overweight (16%) and central obesity (6.3%) were present only in a few women. BIA parameters of body fat composition were similar among antiretroviral naive and treated patients. An average higher percentage of FM (28% vs. 12.1%; p<0.001) and PVF (4.0% vs. 2.3%; p=0.002) were observed in women, with as well as a higher proportion of subjects with high levels of FM (12.6%) and PVF (2.2%) in the same group. Thinness was observed only in 6% of patients of whom 83.3% of men and 68.4% of women (p=0.059) had low levels of FM.

Conclusion: Subclinical abnormalities of FM were present in these case series without clinically overt fat distribution abnormalities, highlighting the need for early detection of these FM abnormalities.

Keywords: Body composition; Bio-electric impedance; Antiretroviral therapy; HIV black patients

Introduction

HIV infection is a major public health problem worldwide, especially in sub-Saharan Africa (SSA) [1]. At the beginning of the pandemic, it was observed in approximately 60-90% of infected patients, severe malnutrition characterized by a significant unwanted excess weight loss of more than 10% of body weight [2]. The development of highly active antiretroviral therapy (HAART) has certainly improved the survival and quality of life of patients, but it exposed them to multiple metabolic disorders including lipid profile disorders and abnormalities of the body composition [3-5].

Protease inhibitors (PI) and nucleoside reverse transcriptase inhibitors (NRTI), specially the stavudine, are drugs that have been implicated [3,4]. PI are associated with alteration of the adipocyte differentiation as well as insulin resistance. *In vitro*, they also stimulate apoptosis in differentiated adipocytes.

The NRTI do not affect the process of adipocyte differentiation *in vitro*. However, there is some evidence for the hypothesis of mitochondrial toxicity as responsible for lipoatrophy induced by these drugs; this would also explain hyperlactatemia, fatty liver with hypertriglyceridemia, polyneuropathy or pancreatic damage sometimes associated with lipodystrophy.

Among the instrumental methods to assess the body composition, the bio-electrical impedance (BIA) is one of the simplest, fastest, more accessible thanks to its low cost and very easy to handle especially in the medical office [6]. Otherwise, a recent study showed that the results of the body composition assessed by the BIA in HIV infected patients had good sensitivity and good specificity compared to the method of dual-energy X-rays absorptiometry (DEXA), which is the gold standard [7].

In the Democratic Republic of the Congo (DRC), generic ARV program has been launched since 2002 using a first line regimen based on a combination of 2 NRTI (AZT, 3TC) and Nevirapine. Since 2006, a second line regimen containing PI has been introduced. Although body composition using BIA has been evaluated in non HIV-infected women [8], no study has yet evaluated the body composition of naive or antiretroviral treated HIV-infected patients. Thus, the aim of the present study was to evaluate the body composition of naive and antiretroviral treated HIV-infected patients seen at a primary healthcare centre of the outskirts of Kinshasa, the capital City and to identify the anthropometric parameter best correlated to perivisceral fat mass (PVF).

Methods

The present cross-sectional study included all consecutive HIV-infected patients aged ≥ 18 years who attended from September, 17 to November 6, 2013 the HIV-Outpatient Clinic of Kimbondo Hospital located at the outskirts of Kinshasa, the capital City. The parameters of interest included age, gender, marital status, duration of HIV infection, WHO clinical stage, opportunistic infections and comorbidities, type and duration of HAART, lifestyle habits, personal and family of obesity, height, weight, body mass (BMI), waist circumference (WC), blood pressure (BP), capillary blood glucose, CD4 cell count and body composition.

Weight was measured using the OMRON BF511 device [9]; with subject without shoes and heavy garments. WC was determined using a tape measure. Seated BP was measured on the left arm after 5 minutes of relaxation using an electronic OMRON M2 basic apparatus; the average of 3 measurements was used for statistical analyses.

Capillary blood glucose was measured by enzymatic method using a Brand One Touch Ultra Glucometer. The body composition was determined by the BIA using a body composition monitor OMRON BF511 [9]. This device determines the percentage of total fat mass (FM) and PVF. Patients on HAART were defined as those who are receiving at least 3 antiretroviral drugs for at least 3 months.

Thinness, normal weight, overweight and obesity were defined as BMI<18.5 Kg/m^2, 18.5-24.9 Kg/m^2, 25-29.9 Kg/m^2 and ≥ 30 Kg/m^2. Abdominal obesity was defined as WC>102 cm for men and >88 cm for women [10]. Lipodystrophy included lipoatrophy and lipohypertrophy defined on the basis of morphological criteria [11].

Percentage of FM and PVF was classified as low, normal, high or very high according to the classification of Gallagher et al. with reference to gender and age [12]. The study received the clearance of the institutional review board and was conducted in respect of Helsinki Declaration with reference to confidentiality and informed consent.

Statistical Analysis

Whereas the prevalence of lipodystrophy varies between 5 and 8% in HIV infected-patients not receiving protease inhibitors and stavudine [13], the minimum sample size was calculated at 113 (p=1.96x1.96x0.08x0.92/0.05x0.05). We used SPSS version 20 software for statistical analysis. The Student test and the U Mann-Whitney test were used to compare groups of patients according to the distribution of their variables or not followed the curve of Gauss.

The chi-square test of Pearson was used to compare the degree of association between categorical variables. The correlation between PVF (in %) and anthropometric parameters was studied using the Pearson correlation test. P<0.05 defined the level of statistical significance.

Results

A total of 125 patients (76% women) with a mean age of 41 ± 10 years were included in the present cross-sectional study; 92 of them (73.6%) were receiving a combination in one pill of zidovudine, lamivudine and nevirapine.

Variables of interest	Whole group (n 125)	on HAART (n 92)	Naive (n 33)	p
Female, %	76.0	79.4	66.6	0.112
Age (years)	41.3 ± 10.0	39.9 ± 12.4	47.1 ± 13.4	0.001
Family history of obesity, %	25.6	34.7	0	<0.001
Alcohol, %	8.0	5.4	15.2	0.087
Tobacco, %	3.2	1.1	9.1	0.056
Major OIs in the past, %	47.2	59.8	12.1	<0.001
Disease duration (months)	(0 - 216)*	14.5 (1-216)*	1 (0 -120)*	<0.001
Duration of HAART (months)	-	8 (3-216)*	-	-
HTA,%	37.6	36.9	33.4	0.481
Weight (kg)	57 ± 10	57 ± 9	53 ± 7	0.010
Size (cm)	162 ± 8	162 ± 7	162 ± 7	0.740
WC (cm)	76 ± 7	76 ± 7	74 ± 8	0.143
BMI (kg/m^2)	21 ± 3	22 ± 3	20 ± 2	0.014

Table 1: Clinical characteristics of patients. Data expressed as a percentage (%) or mean ± standard deviations (SD). *Data expressed as median (minimum and maximum). OIs = opportunistic infections, HAART = highly active antiretroviral therapy, WC = waist circumference, BMI = body mass index.

With reference to anthropometric measures, overweight (16%) and central obesity (6.3%) were observed only in women; thinness was present in 13% of patients without significant gender's differences. Clinical signs suggestive of lipodystrophy were not observed in the present case series.

Tables 1 and 2 summarize general characteristics, anthropometric and body composition parameters of the study population according to treatment status. Compared to naive patients (Table 1), those under ARV therapy were younger (39.9 ± 12.4 vs. 47.1 ± 13.4 years; p=0.001) and had in average significantly higher BMI levels (22 ± 3 vs. 20 ± 2 Kg/m^2; p=0.014) and proportion of subjects with family history of obesity (34.7 vs. 0%; p<0.001) and opportunistic infections (59.8 vs. 12.1%; p<0.001). With reference to measures of body composition (Table 2), ARV treated patients tended to have in average a higher percentage of total fat mass; however, the observed difference did not reach the level of statistical significance.

Compared to men, women had in average a significantly higher percentage of total FM (28 ± 8.1 vs. 12.1 ± 5%; p<0.001) and PVF (4 ±

2.3 vs. 3 ± 1.8%; p=0.002); they have, however, a significantly lower percentage of muscle mass (29.1 ± 3.1 vs. 41.1 ± 6.0%; p<0.001).

Variables of interest	Whole group (n 125)	on HAART (n 92)	Naive (n33)	p
CD4 (cells/mm^3)	303±184	263 ±166	414 ±188	<0.001
Glycemia (mg / dl)	107±23	105 ± 21	113 ± 24	0.108
% of muscle mass	32±6	31± 6	33 ± 6	0.192
% of total FM	25±10	25 ±10	22 ± 8	0.066
% of PVF	4±2	4 ±1	4 ± 2	0.530

Table 2: Biological Characteristics of patients. Data are expressed as mean ± standard deviations (SD). CD4=Cluster Differentiation; FM=Fat Mass.

Anthropometric correlates of total FM and PVF of the study population are given in Table 3. BMI emerged as the anthropometric

parameter best correlated with PVF (r = 0.56; p<0.001) and total FM (r=0.56; p<0.001).

Anthropometric parameters	Total fat mass		Perivisceral fat mass	
	r	p	r	p
Weight	0.420	<0.001	0.588	<0.001
Size	0.291	0.001	0.262	0.003
Waist	0.402	<0.001	0.527	<0.001
BMI	0.568	<0.001	0.731	<0.001

Table 3: Correlation between anthropometric parameters and fat mass

Discussion

The main findings of the present cross-sectional study are as follows: first, the absence of clinical signs of lipodystrophy and the presence of concomitant subclinical body composition abnormalities. Second, ARV treated patients were comparable to naive ones with reference to body composition parameters and proportion of subjects with subclinical body composition abnormalities. Third, BMI emerged as the anthropometric characteristic best correlated to perivisceral fat mass.

Although clinical signs of lipodystrophy were absent, subclinical abnormalities were present in the present case series. It has been reported that although HIV-infected patients with subclinical abnormalities of body fat distribution generally maintain a body mass index in normal or overweight range, they often experience cardio metabolic complications such as dyslipidemia and impaired glucose tolerance similar to those seen in frank obesity [14]. Another large cross-sectional study found more visceral adipose tissue among HIV-infected versus uninfected women, despite similar average BMI in both groups [15]. Previous studies also found that more than half of HIV-infected patients present with abnormal fat accumulation [14,16].

Subclinical body fat composition was similar between ARV-treated and naive patients. This finding in the present case series could have several potential explanations. First, 12 months have been reported to

be the average time period necessarily to the development and progression of body fat composition abnormalities in ART-treated HIV [17,18]; the average ART duration in the present case series was 8 months. Second, untreated HIV infection eventually results in wasting, including loss of adipose tissue. Fat gain, which is widely prevalent in the general population and increases with age, may in part be the result of effective ART reversing fat loss due to HIV infection [13]. Third, it has been reported that visceral fat is less influenced by ART than subcutaneous fat, relatively resistant to change in HIV-infected population and influenced by factors others than ART [16].

BMI was best correlated with perivisceral fat mass. This finding agrees with the report by Joy et al. [19]. These authors found that visceral adipose tissue was increased among HIV-infected men and women in the normal (18.5 to 24.9 Kg/m^2) and overweight (25 to 29.9 Kg/m^2) categories relative to controls but not among those in the obese category (≥ 30 Kg/m^2). In the present post-hoc analysis, the majority of patients were in the normal weight category and obesity was not found.

Difference observed between men and women can be explained by their hormonal profile. Woman undergoes during his sexual life, the influence of hormones to various effects that modulate its weight, either naturally (puberty, cycles, pregnancy, menopause) or due to their therapeutic use (contraception, hormone replacement therapy) [20]. The subclinical abnormalities of body composition associated with other antiretroviral therapy than PI and Stavudine corroborate some recent literature data. Is the case of Van Vonderen et al. who showed that Zidovudine/lamivudine + lopinavir/ritonavir, but not nevirapine + lopinavir/ ritonavir in antiretroviral therapy naive patients, is associated with lipoatrophy and greater relative intraabdominal lipohypertrophy, suggesting other nucleoside inhibitors contributes to lipodystrophy [21].

The interpretation of the results of the present analysis should take into account some limitations. The major limitation of the present analysis is its cross-sectional design precluding temporal and causal relationship of abnormalities of body fact composition with ART and HIV-infection. The use of BIA that is less sensitive than dual Y ray absorptiometry and computerized tomography in assessing body composition [22]. Additional limitations are the small sample size and the lack of repeat measurements of body fat composition which are recommended to increase specificity.

Conclusion

Subclinical abnormalities of body composition were common finding in the present case series without clinical signs of lipodystrophy. Body composition parameters were similar among ART-treated and naive patients. BMI emerged as the anthropometric parameter best correlated with perivisceral fat mass.

Acknowledgement

The authors thank the officials and both medical and paramedical staff of the hospital Kimbondo for all facilities granted.

References

1. Beyrer C, Abdool Karim Q (2013) The changing epidemiology of HIV in 2013. Curr Opin HIV AIDS 8: 306-310.

2. Mocroft A, Brettle R, Kirk O, Blaxhult A, Parkin JM, et al. (2002) Changes in the cause of death among HIV positive subjects across Europe: results from the Euro SIDA study. AIDS 16: 1663-1671.

3. Bedimo RJ (2008) Body-fat abnormalities in patients with HIV: progress and challenges. J Int Assoc Physicians AIDS Care 7: 292-305.

4. Calza L, Manfredi R, Chiodo F (2004) Dyslipidaemia associated with antiretroviral therapy in HIV-infected patients. J Antimicrob Chemother 53: 10-14.

5. Aghdassi E, Arendt B, Salit IE, Allard JP (2007) Estimation of body fat mass using dual-energy X-ray absorptiometry, bioelectric impedance analysis, and anthropometry in HIV-positive male subjects receiving highly active antiretroviral therapy. J Parenter Enteral Nutr 31: 135-141.

6. Baumgartner RN, Chumlea WC, Roche AF (1988) Bioelectric impedance phase angle and body composition. Am J Clin Nutr 48: 16-23.

7. Siqueira Vassimon H, Jordao AA, Albuquerque de Paula FJ, Artioli Machado A, Pontes Monteiro J (2011) Comparison of bioelectrical

8. Mbungu MR, Tandu-Umba NFB, Muls E (2005) Etude de la composition corporelle de la femme noire Congolaise par l'impedance bio-electrique. Congo Medical 4: 25-31.

9. Omron Health Care. Omron BF 511: Body composition monitor, Manual instruction. www.omron-healthcare.com.

10. WHO (2000) The problem of overweight and obesity. Obesity: preventing and managing the global epidemic. Report of a WHO Technical Report Series 894. Geneva: WHO, 537.

11. Mallon PWG (2007) Pathogenesis of lipodystrophy and lipid abnormalities in patients taking antiretroviral therapy. AIDS Rev 9: 3-15.

12. Gallagher D, Heymsfield SB, Heo M, Jebb SA, Murgatroyd PR, et al. (2000) Healthy percentage body fat ranges: an approach for developing guidelines based on body mass index. Am J Clin Nutr 72: 694-701.

13. De Waal R, Cohen K, Maartens G (2013) Systematic Review of Antiretroviral-Associated Lipodystrophy: Lipoatrophy, but Not Central Fat Gain, Is an Antiretroviral Adverse Drug Reaction. Plos One 8: e 63623.

14. Stanley TL, Grinspoon SK (2012) Body composition and metabolic changes in HIV-infected patients. JID 205 (Suppl 3): S383.

15. Brown TT, Xu X, John M, Singh J, Kingsley LA, et al. (2009) Fat distribution and longitudinal anthropometric changes in HIV-infected men with and without clinical evidence of lipodystrophy and HIV-uninfected controsl: a substudy of the multicenter AIDS control study. AIDS Research and Therapy 6: 8.

16. Martinez E, Visnegarwala F, Grund B, Thomas A, Gibert C, et al. (2010) The effects of intermittent, CD4-guided antiretroviral therapy on body composition and metabolic parameters. AIDS 24: 353-363.

17. Feleke Y, Felade D, Mezegebu Y (2012) Prevalence of highly active antiretroviral therapy associated metabolic abnormalities and lipodystrophy in HIV-infected patients. Ethiop Med J 50: 221-30.

18. Monnerat BZ, Cerutti Jr C, Canicali S, Motta RT (2008) Clinical and biochemical evaluation of HIV-related lipodystrophy in an ambulatory population from the Hospital Universitario Antonio de Morais, Vitoria, ES, Brazil. Br J infect Dis 12: 264-68.

19. Joy T, Keogh HM, Hadigan C, Dolan SE, Fitch K, et al. (2008) Relation of body mass index in HIV-infected patients with metabolic abnormalities. J Acquir Immune Defic Syndrome 47: 174-184.

20. Astrup A, Buemann B, Christensen NJ, Madsen J, Gluud C, et al. (1992) The contribution of body composition, substrates, and hormones to the variability in energy expenditure and substrate utilization in premenopausal women. J Clin Endocrinol Metab 74: 279-286.

21. Van Vonderen MG, Van Agtmael MA, Hassink EA, Milinkovic A, Brinkman K, et al. (2009) Zidovudine/lamivudine for HIV-1 infection contributes to limb fat loss. PLoS One 21; 4:5647.

22. Browning LM, Mugridge O, Chatfield M, Dixon A (2010) Validity of a new abdominal bioelectrical impedance device to measure abdominal and visceral fat: comparison with MRI. Obesity 18: 2385–2391.

impedance with skinfold thickness and x-rayabsorptiometry to measure body composition in HIV-infected with lipodistrophy. Nutr Hosp 26:458-464.

4

Improvement of Conception in Sheep Using Different Hormonal Treatments during Mating and their Influence on the Antioxidant Status

Derar Refaat[1*] and Hamdoun[2]

[1]Department of Theriogenology, Faculty of Veterinary Medicine, Assiut University, Assiut, Egypt

[2]Department of Animal & Poultry Production, Faculty of Agriculture, Sohag University, Sohag, Egypt

*Corresponding author: Derar Refaat, Assiut University, Faculty of Veterinary Medicine, Department of Theriogenology, Assiut, Egypt; E-mail: derar40@gmail.com and derar40@yahoo.com

Abstract

The objective of this study was to compare the effects of GnRH, prostaglandin F2α (PGF2α) and oxytocin treatments at the time of natural mating on the conception rate (CR) of non lactating pluriparous ewes. All ewes (n=61) were served naturally by fertile rams every 12 hours after the beginning of estrus. After natural mating, ewes were randomly assigned into four treatment groups; G1 received PGF2α (n=14); G2 received GnRH (n=12); G3received oxytocin (n=15) and G4 or control received placebo (n=20). Pregnancy diagnosis was performed 25 days post-insemination by transrectal ultrasonography. Ewes were bled at the day of mating and every 10 days till Day 50 post mating to determine the changes in the total antioxidants during the first third of pregnancy. Pregnancy rate was higher (P<0.05) for all the treatment groups (69.33%) compared with the control group (55.54%). Litter size did not differ between groups except for oxytocin group. Ewe lambs dominate male in this study and the sex ratio unexpectedly preferred them. Total antioxidants did not differ significantly between groups in the present study but they were at their lowest values during estrus in all the studied groups. Gestation length, birth weight, number of services, body weight did not affect the pregnancy rate. It could be concluded that treatments with GnRH and PGF and oxytocin at the time of service could improve conception rate in pluriparous ewes.

Keywords: Antioxidants; Conception; Ewe; Hormones

Introduction

Many trials have been attempted to increase fertility in ewes. Gonadotropin-releasing hormone (GnRH) and its analogues administered at the time of artificial insemination (AI) are the most common treatments in management programmers for sheep flocks [1,2]. Improvement of the conception following GnRH treatment has been attributed to the prevention of an ovulation failure or a reduced variation in the interval between the onset of estrus and ovulation [3]. However, the results are controversial after GnRH treatment of lactating cows. Many previous works reported that conception rate in cows was improved [3], while others reported no effect on pregnancy rate was obtained [1,4]. Oxytocin and PGF2α have been shown as essential parts of ovulation process [5,6] and has been known that the increase of uterine and oviduct contractility (Hawk, 1983) affects the sperm transport. There are few studies focused on the effect of PGF2α administration at the time of AI on pregnancy [6]. Oxytocin was used to increase conception rate by improving the sperm transport in the female reproductive tract of several species [7-9]. Clitoral massage which probably releases oxytocin following artificial insemination increased pregnancy in beef cows [10]. The administration of oxytocin following AI also increased CR in lactating dairy cows [9] but in another study it had hardly any effect on pregnancy in cows [11]. The objective of the present study was to study the effect of different hormonal treatments used to improve the reproductive efficiency in ewes on different reproductive parameters and antioxidant profiles after natural mating in subtropics.

Materials and Methods

This work was carried out in the Animal Production Experimental Farm, Animal and Poultry Production Department, Faculty of Agriculture, Sohag University, Egypt (latitude 28°07′N and 30°33′E)

Animals and management

Sixty one ewes Sohagi healthy, pluriparous, non parturient and non lactating ewes were used in this study. Ewes were kept away from rams before the beginning of the study and housed in semi-open pens. Ewes were fed on a concentrate mixture with wheat straw and green fodder, providing 14% crude protein and 70% total digestible nutrients during the experimental period (from September 15th till December 31st). Water was available all time. Estrus was detected using well trained teasers and personnel. Estrous ewes were mated with fertile rams every 12 hours till the end of estrus. Immediately after the last mating, animals were assigned into four groups: G1 (n=14) received 15 mg of Dinoprost IM (PGF2α. Lutalyse, Pharmacia & Upjohn, NY); G2 (n=12) received 25 µg Gonadorelin IM (Factrel, Fort Dodge, IA, USA); G3 (n=15) treated with 20 IU oxytocin IM (Biomeda-MTC Animal Health Inc., Cambridge, Ontario, Canada) and G4 (control group, n=20) received 5 ml normal saline IM. Doses and route of administration of each drug in the present study were administered according to the instructions of the manufacturers. Pregnancy was diagnosed on Day 25 post mating for all animals using a real-time, B-mode echocamera (EUB-405B, Hitachi, Tokyo, Japan) attached with a 5-7.5 MHz transducer. Visualization of a fluid-filled uterine horn with embryonic vesicles and the presence of an embryo were used as positive indicators for pregnancy. Pregnancy rate was calculated as the number of ewes diagnosed pregnant divided by the number of mated ewes.

Serum total antioxidants status

Blood samples were collected from animals beginning on day 0 (day of treatment) and every 10 days till day 50 post mating. Serum was separated and stored at -20°C till assayed for total antioxidants. The total antioxidant status was measured using Total Antioxidant Capacity (TAC) Assay Kit (K274-100 BioVision, Inc. Headquarters, 155 South Milpitas Blvd., Milpitas, California 95035).

Statistical analyses

All statistical procedures were performed using the computational software of SAS [12]. Chi-square analysis using the PROC FREQ procedure was used to compare the pregnancy rate among the treatment groups. A t-test was used to analyze the effect of treatments on pregnancy and antioxidants concentration in the studied ewes.

Results

Pregnancy rate detected on days 25 were higher (P<0.05) in all the treated groups compared with the control one. However, pregnancy rate and birth weight differed non significantly among G1, G2 and G3 (Table 1). The second group treated with GnRH possessed the longest gestation length, the heavier birth weight and the higher male birth percentage. Different treatment protocols did not improve the incidence of twinning but pregnancy rate was noticeably better than the control. Total antioxidants did not differ significantly between groups in the present study as affected by day of gestation (Table 2). Total antioxidants increased gradually from the day of mating till the 10th day postmating. A significant increase in the level of total antioxidants was observed in all studied groups by the 50th day of gestation.

Treatment	Gestation length	Ewe Body weight	Birth weight	Pregnancy rate%	Male births%	Twining %	Triplets %	litter size
PGF2α	154.1 ± 7.34	36.3 ± 3.42	3.5 ± 0.23	71[a]	21.42	14.28	----	1.2
GnRH	157.13 ± 8.79	36.12 ± 5.96	3.71 ± 0.41	66[a]	33.33	25.00	----	1.37
Oxytocin	153.7 ± 6.32	38 ± 9.54	3.29 ± 0.52	71[a]	13.33	26.66	6.66	1.66
Control	152.44 ± 0.84	38.29 ± 7.67	3.56 ± 0.43	55.54[b]	15.00	40.00	5.00	1.23

Table 1: Effect of different hormonal regimens on the reproductive performance of Sohagi ewes.

Days after mating	PGF2α	GnRH	Oxytocin	control
0	0.31 ± 0.01[a]	0.32 ± 0.01[a]	0.25 ± 0.01[a]	0.11 ± 0.02[a]
10	4.23 ± 0.01[b]	4.04 ± 0.91[b]	5.58 ± 0.6[b]	3.22 ± 0.12[b]
20	4.29 ± 0.45[b]	5.18 ± 0.37[b]	5.27 ± 0.59[b]	4.38 ± 1.09[b]
30	5.09 ± 0.56[b]	4.66 ± 0.45[b]	4.40 ± 0.51[b]	6.23 ± 0.87[b]
40	4.99 ± 0.36[b]	5.22 ± 0.31[b]	5.36 ± 0.75[b]	4.91 ± 1.20[b]
50	7.36 ± 0.42[c]	7.06 ± 0.93[c]	6.84 ± 0.74[c]	8.34 ± 1.65[c]

Table 2: The Serum concentration of total antioxidant (mmol) in Sohagi ewes treated with different hormonal regimens.

Discussion

With regard to pregnancy rate, the reproductive performance of sheep in the present study improved significantly in treated ewes compared with non treated control ones and notably oxytocin treatment had a positive effect on the litter size. However, birth weight, gestation length and sex ratio as well as total antioxidants were not changed.

The present results of lambing rate in treated groups come close to the results of Beck et al. [13] who found that treatment with GnRH analogue on Day 12 post-mating increased lambing rates and litter size in ewes. In cattle, GnRH improved pregnancy rate by 7-21% [3]. This comes in inconsistency with other studies indicating that pregnancy rate was not affected by GnRH treatment following AI [1,4].

Variability in pregnancy rate among the different studies might be associated with the potency of GnRH on gonadotropin release [14] or the timing of GnRH and mating relative to the onset of estrus. Earlier studies showed that the timing of GnRH injection according to the onset of estrus affected gonadotropin release. Although exogenous GnRH at the onset of estrus increased the pre-ovulatory LH surge [3,4], conception rate increased in one study [3] but not in others [4]. However, the administration of GnRH at the time of AI, approximately 12 hours after the initiation of standing estrus, did not result in a greater surge of LH [15]. In addition, the insufficient LH surge did not have any ovulatory effect [3,15] and did not improve pregnancy. The present results indicated that administration of PGF at the time of AI following spontaneous estrus have a beneficial effect on pregnancy rate. It was suggested that a rapid increase of PGF2α in the ovary may play some important role(s) in the ovulatory process [16,17]. Others reported that prostaglandins of the E series, and particularly PGE, play a crucial role in ovulation by determining the targeting of follicle rupture at the apex, thus allowing release of oocytes to the periovarian space [18]. A prostaglandin analogue, Cloprostenol, administration on the day of estrous of buffalo demonstrated to increase P4 levels on day 11, probably via ET-1 and Ang-II genes inhibition. It has been hypothesized that this phenomenon may be due to specific changes in genes expression, which prevent the intraluteal production of these molecules [6]. If this hypothesis is accepted, the higher pregnancy rates recorded in PG Group could be explained by the reduction of embryo mortality. Moreover, cloprostenol administration in our experiment may have helped ovary contraction and follicle rupture, improving ovulation synchrony. Furthermore, it has been proposed that PGF2a may exert a fertility effect, by causing LH release independent of progesterone withdrawal [19] and that PGF2a administration 30 h before GnRH, elevated the GnRH-induced LH release. It is still unclear if prostaglandin is able to act on LH release by a mechanism different from that induced by GnRH, or if it only enhances GnRH-induced LH release.

In sheep few studies showing the effect of oxytocin on pregnancy rate at the time of AI were published [9,11]. Bekeova et al. [20] indicated that oxytocin, GnRH treatments affected conception rate in post partum ewes through increasing the level of thyroxin, Triiodothyronin, oestradiol 17β and progesterone and suggested that the causes of depression of T4 and T3 levels after parturition in spring might be a lack of gonadotropins. Low concentration of T4 and T3 in certain phases of the post-partum period might be retroactively responsible for the decline in post-partum sexual activity in ewes. However, the study of Yildiz [9] indicated that pregnancy rate increased in lactating dairy cows after oxytocin administration just before AI, which agreed with the present findings. This could be due to changes in uterine contractility and possibly to the acceleration of sperm transport in the reproductive tract of ewes [7,8,21]. Oxytocin possibly exerted its influence by stimulating prostaglandin production [22,23]. In addition to involutory effects upon the uterus [24] prostaglandins may have acted as LH-stimulating [25] and estrogen-stimulating factors [26]. Although there was no significant differences among the experimental groups regarding the level of total antioxidant but it was worthy notable that the level of these elements was gradually increased throughout the early pregnancy period towards the end of the first trimester of the studied ewes. Changes in the antioxidant enzymatic defense could be a part of placentome adaptation to reactive oxygen species-induced oxidative stress at specific early developmental stages of pregnancy. Previous reports showed that the activities of antioxidant enzymes in the sheep corpus luteum (CL) are subject to major changes during early pregnancy, suggesting that the CL of early pregnancy may be rescued from luteolysis through increasing activities of key antioxidant enzymes and inhibition of apoptosis. Maintained levels of antioxidant enzymes in the CL throughout pregnancy may be linked to reactive oxygen species continuously generated in the steroidogenesis activity of luteal cells, and may be involved in the maintenance of luteal steroidogenic activity, cellular integrity and preventive to oxidative stress, improving pregnancy outcomes [27]. Even though the total antioxidant levels were not significantly different, some changes for single antioxidants such as vitamin E, as well as neuroendocrinology-related CART level [28].

Conclusion

In conclusion, the results suggest that the administration of GnRH, oxytocin and PGF at the time of natural mating increased pregnancy rate in subtropical ewes.

References

1. Chenault JR (1990) Effect of fertirelin acetate or buserelin on conception rate at first or second insemination in lactating dairy cows. J. Dairy Sci 73: 633-638.

2. Morgan WF, Lean IJ (1993) Gonadotrophin-releasing hormone treatment in cattle: a meta-analysis of the effects on conception at the time of insemination. Aust Vet J 70: 205-209.

3. Kaim M, Bloch A, Wolfenson D, Braw-Tal R, Rosenberg M, et al. (2003) Effects of GnRH administered to cows at the onset of estrus on timing of ovulation, endocrine responses, and conception. J Dairy Sci 86: 2012-2021.

4. Perry GA, Perry BL (2009) GnRH treatment at artificial insemination in beef cattle fails to increase plasma progesterone concentrations or pregnancy rates. Theriogenology 71: 775-779.

5. Algire JE, Srikandakumar A, Guilbault LA, Downey BR (1992) Preovulatory changes in follicular prostaglandins and their role in ovulation in cattle. Can J Vet Res 56: 67-69.

6. Neglia G, Natale A, Esposito G, Salzillo F, Adinolfi L, et al. (2008) Effect of prostaglandin F2alpha at the time of AI on progesterone levels and pregnancy rate in synchronized Italian Mediterranean buffaloes. Theriogenology 69: 953-960.

7. Sayre BL, Lewis GS (1997) Fertility and ovum fertilization rate after laparoscopic or transcervical intrauterine artificial insemination of oxytocin-treated ewes. Theriogenology 48: 267-275.

8. King ME, Mckelvey WAC, Dingwall WS, Matthews KP, Gebbie FE, et al. (2004) Lambing rates and litter sizes following intrauterine or cervical insemination or frozen/thawed semen with or without oxytocin administration. Theriogenology 62: 1236-1244.

9. Yildiz (2005) Effect of oxytocin on conception rate in cows. J. Firat Uni. Health. Sci 19: 75-78.

10. Cooper MD, Newman SK, Schermerhorn EC, Foote RH (1985) Uterine contractions and fertility following clitoral massage of dairy cattle in estrus. J Dairy Sci 68: 703-708.

11. Hays RL, Van Demark NL, Ormiston EE (1958) Effect of oxytocin and epinephrine on the conception rate of cows. J. Dairy Sci 41: 1376-1379.

12. SAS (2001) Statistical Analysis System: A user's Guide. Version 8.2. Institute Inc.Cary, NC.

13. Beck NFG, Peters AR, Williams SP (1994) The effect of GnRH agonist (buserelin) treatment on day 12 post mating on the reproductive performance of ewes. Anim, Prod. 58: 243-247.

14. Souza AH, Cunha AP, Silva EPB, Gümen A, Ayres H, et al. (2009) Comparison of gonadorelin products in lactating dairy cows: efficacy based on induction of ovulation of an accessory follicle and circulating luteinizing hormone profiles. Theriogenology. 72: 271-279.

15. Lucy MC, Stevenson JS (1986) Gonadotropin-releasing hormone at estrus: luteinizing hormone, estradiol, and progesterone during the periestrual and postinsemination periods in dairy cattle. Biol Reprod 35: 300-311.

16. Iesaka T, Sato T, Igarashi M (1975) Role of prostaglandin F2alpha in ovulation. Endocrinol Jpn 22: 279-285.

17. Armstrong DT (1981) Prostaglandins and follicular functions. J Reprod Fertil 62: 283-291.

18. Gaytán F, Tarradas E, Bellido C, Morales C, Sánchez-Criado JE (2002) Prostaglandin E(1) inhibits abnormal follicle rupture and restores ovulation in indomethacin-treated rats. Biol Reprod 67: 1140-1147.

19. Cruz LC, do Valle ER, Kesler DJ (1997) Effect of prostaglandin F2 alpha- and gonadotropin releasing hormone-induced luteinizing hormone

releases on ovulation and corpus luteum function of beef cows. Anim Reprod Sci 49: 135-142.

20. Bekeova E, Krajnicakova M, Hendrichovsky V, Maracek I (1995) The effects of long-acting oxytocin, GnRH and FSH administration on thyroxin, triiodothyronin, oestradiol 17-fl and progesterone levels as well as conception rates in post-partum ewes. Anim. Reprod. Sci 37: 311-323.

21. Hawk HW (1983) Sperm survival and transport in the female reproductive tract. J Dairy Sci 66: 2645-2660.

22. Kittok RJ, Britt JH (1977) Corpus luteum function in ewes given estradiol during the estrous cycle or early pregnancy. J Anim Sci 45: 336-341.

23. McCracken JA, Schramm W, Okulicz WC (1984) Hormone receptor control of pulsatile secretion of PGF2P from ovine uterus during luteolysis and its abrogation in early pregnancy. Anim Reprod Sci. 7: 31-55.

24. Fredriksson G (1985) Release of PGF(2alpha) during parturition and the postpartum period in the ewe. Theriogenology 24: 331-335.

25. Agmo A (1975) Effects of prostaglandins E-1 and F-2ALPHA on serum luteinizing hormone concentration and on some sexual functions in male rabbits. Prostaglandins 9: 451-457.

26. Dodson KS, Watson J (1980) Stimulatory action of prostaglandin F2 alpha on androgen aromatization in the pig follicle. Eur J Obstet Gynecol Reprod Biol 11: 49-56.

27. Al-Gubory KH, Bolifraud P, Germain G, Nicole A, Ceballos-Picot I (2004) Antioxidant enzymatic defence systems in sheep corpus luteum throughout pregnancy. Reproduction 128: 767-774.

28. Mao J, Ren X, Zhang L, Van Duin DM, Cohen RC, et al. (2012) Insights into hydroxyl measurements and atmospheric oxidation in a California forest. Atmos. Chem. Phys 12: 8009-8020.

5

Lipoprotein (a) Status and Effect of Laparoscopic Cholecystectomy on it in Bangladeshi Patients with Cholelithiasis

Giasuddin ASM[1*]**, Khadija Akther Jhuma**[2]**, Md Abdul Mobin Choudhury**[2]**, Mujibul Haq AM**[2]

[1]*Medical Research Unit (MRU), MHWT, Dhaka-1230, Bangladesh*

[2]*Medical College for Women and Hospital, Dhaka-1230, Bangladesh*

*****Corresponding author:** Dr. Giasuddin ASM, MSc PhD PGD CSciFIBMS MNYAS, Professor of Biochemistry and Immunology, Director, Medical Research Unit (MRU), MHWT, Uttara Model Town Dhaka-1230, Bangladesh; E-mail: mru.mhwt@gmail.com

Abstract

Objective: Although it was reported that cholecystectomy had complex impact on lipid profile in cholelithiasis, lipoprotein (a) [Lp(a)] was not studied. The present study was therefore conducted on serum Lp(a) status in Bangladeshi patients with cholelithiasis and effect of cholecystectomy on it.

Patients and Methods: Adult patients (n=44) with cholelithiasis and 30 normal controls (NC) were included in the study. The blood sample was taken from fasting patients before cholecystectomy (Serum-I^0), gall bladder bile sample during cholecystectomy (Bile-I^0) and blood sample again after 2-3 months at follow-up (Serum-II^0) and from fasting NC subjects. Lp(a) level was quantitated in serum and bile by immunoturbidimetric method using commercially available research kit. The results were compared statistically by ANOVA, Student's t-test and Chi-squared test using SPSS programme.

Results: The Lp(a) status (mg/dl, Mean ± SD) in controls and patients and their statistical analysis revealed that Lp(a) was much higher in patients compared to controls (NC: 29.07 ± 14.1, Patients Serum-I^0: 290.84 ± 110.93, Patients Bile-I^0 : 37.12 ± 28.61, Patients Serum-II^0: 203.70 ± 90.13) (P<0.001). Lp(a) was lowered after cholecystectomy, but remained elevated in patients Serum-II^0 compared to NC significantly (P<0.001). No significant difference was observed for Lp(a) levels between NC and patients Bile-I^0 (P=0.173). The proportions of patients for Serum-I^0, Bile-I^0 and Serum-II^0 with Lp(a) levels above and within normal limits and their statistical analyses showed significant associations (P<0.001).

Conclusions: Cholelithiasis had complex impact on Lp(a) status indicating a special function of gall bladder relevant to its metabolism. Further studies are warranted.

Keywords: Lipoprotein (a); Cholelithiasis; Cholecystectomy

Introduction

One of the common gastrointestinal disorders prevalent in about 10-15% of adults in the developing countries is Cholelithiasis (gallstone disease) [1,2]. Surgical removal of the gallbladder and gallstones, i.e. cholecystectomy is the treatment of choice currently [3,4]. Studies over 30 years ago showed that more than 50% of patients with gallstone would have lipid disorder [1,5].

The pathogenesis of cholesterol gallstone is widely accepted as an altered lipid metabolism, because of which there is a relative increase in the cholesterol levels compared to other lipids secreted by the liver into the bile [1,4,5]. Many factors including nucleation of cholesterol crystals, binding together of these crystals with mucin and hypomotility of the gallbladder play an important role in gallstone formation [6-8]. The molecular events that underlie these processes have not been understood completely, although association between gallstones and altered lipid profile has been shown in some studies [4,9,10].

Lipoprotein (a) [Lp(a)] has been implicated as a probable cause for atherosclerosis [3,4]. Since its identification by Norwegian geneticist

Kare Berg in 1963, Lp(a) has become a focus of research interest owing to the results of case-control and prospective studies linking elevated plasma levels of this lipoprotein with the development of coronary artery disease (CAD) [5,6]. Based on the similarity of Lp(a) to both low density lipoprotein (LDL) and plasminogen, it has been hypothesized that the function of this lipoprotein may represent a link between the fields of atherosclerosis and thrombosis [6-8].

Apolipoprotein A1 (Apo A1), ApoE, CETP and Mucin have been implicated with cholelithiasis In some studies [4,11-13]. HDL-C, VLDL and Lp(a) were implicated with coronary artery disease(CAD), diabetes mellitus, polycystic ovarian syndrome (POS) [3,14-17]. Higher levels of Lp(a), Leptin, ApoB and malondialdehyde (MDA) and lower levels of HDL-C and paraoxonase activity were reported to be associated in cholelithiasis [18,19].

The fact that plasma Lp(a) levels are largely genetically determined and vary widely among different ethnic groups adds scientific interest to the ongoing research on this enigmatic molecule. Only limited studies have been reported on serum levels of Lp(a) in some populations including Indian subcontinent [20,21]. Although determination of the function of Lp(a) in vivo remains elusive, serum Lp(a) levels were reported to be elevated in DM and an independent risk factor for CAD in DM, particularly non-insulin dependent DM

(NIDDM) patients [22-24]. However, these results were variable and need confirmation by further studies in cholelithiasis patients.

Literature review indicated that no study had been done or reported involving cholelithiasis patients from Bangladesh, although two studies reported not relevant to lipid metabolism were on day care laparoscopic cholecystectomy (LC) and intra-operative flexible choledochoscopy (IFC) in Bangladeshi patients [25,26]. We have therefore decided to investigate in phases the various aspects of lipid profile and their metabolism in cholelithiasis patients followed by cholecystectomy at Medical Research Unit (MRU), MHWT, Dhaka, Bangladesh. Previously, we reported the results on lipid profile i.e. triglyceride (TG), total cholesterol (TC), low density lipoprotein-cholesterol (LDL-C) and high density lipoprotein-cholesterol (HDL-C) levels in serum and bile of cholelithiasis patients before cholecystectomy (I⁰) and after cholecystectomy (II⁰) and in normal control subjects [27]. In the present article, we have reported results of the study on Lp(a) status in serum and bile of cholelithiasis patients preoperatively and postoperatively at MRU, MHWT Dhaka, Bangladesh.

Patients and Methods

Adult patients with cholelithiasis (Number: 44, Gender: 8 males, 36 females; Age range: 25-65 years, Mean age ± SD: 45.5 ± 12.2 years) with cholelithiasis (gall stone disease) and healthy adults as normal controls (Number: 30, Gender: 12 males, 18 females; Age range: 28-60 years; Mean age ± SD: 42.5 ± 10.5 years) were included in the present case-control prospective interventional study.

The patients with gallstone disease (cholelithiasis) were diagnosed as having cholelithiasis according to standard clinical and laboratory criteria as practiced in hospital and patients not fulfilling the criteria for our study on cholelithiasis were excluded [27-29]. The diagnostic algorithm for cholelithiasis were taking medical history, clinical examination, ultrasonogram (USG) of hepato-biliary system and pancreas and routine laboratory investigations including liver function tests (LFTs). After obtaining consent, patient's demographic details and clinical findings such as pain (severity, duration, location), Murphy's sign, USG, etc were recorded as per 'PROFORMA' at diagnosis.

The fasting blood samples were taken at diagnosis before laparoscopic cholecystectomy, and conducted routine laboratory tests. The serum separated was aliquoted and stored frozen at -300°C to -80°C as first degree serum sample (I°). At the time of laparoscopic cholecystectomy, gallbladder bile was also collected from the same patient, centrifuged, aliquoted and stored frozen at -300°C to -80°C as first degree bile sample (I°).

After Cholecystectomy, treatments/medications were given as required for the patients. After 2-3 months at follow-up, fasting blood samples were taken again from the same patient, serum separated, aliquoted and stored frozen at -300°C to -80°C as second degree serum samples (II°) until analyzed for the lipid profile (i.e. TG, TC, HDL-C, LDL-C) and Lp(a). All quantitative estimations in serum and bile were made by standard medical laboratory methods for lipid profile and Lp(a) using standard diagnostics kits from internationally reputed companies and LDL-C calculated by Friedwald formula [27,30].

The results of laboratory analyses in biological specimens of patients (I°, II°) and controls (NC) for Lp(a) were compared statistically by ANOVA, Student's t-test and Chi-squared test using SPSS programme in computer [31]. The results of our study on the other lipid profile, i.e.

TG, TC, HDL-C, LDL-C were reported previously [27]. In the present article, the results on Lp(a) status and effect of laparoscopic cholecystectomy on it in Bangladeshi Patients with Cholelithiasis are reported.

Results

The Lp(a) status in our study subjects and their statistical analyses are stated in Table 1. Lp(a) was much elevated in patients Serum-I0 compared to NC (P<0.001). This was lowered after laparoscopic cholecystectomy, but remained elevated in patients Serum-II⁰ compared to NC significantly (P<0.001).

No significant difference was observed for Lp(a) levels between NC and patients Bile-I⁰ (P=0.173). The proportion of patients for Serum-I⁰, Bile-I⁰ and Serum-II⁰ with Lp(a) levels above and within normal limits and their statistical analyses are stated in Tables 2 and 3 respectively.

Discussion

Our findings in Bangladeshi patients with cholelithiasis that serum Lp(a) level was significantly elevated and that significantly larger proportion of patients had higher serum Lp(a) levels were consistent with some reports in the literature from other countries [2,7,11]. However, it should be noted that cut off value of 30.0 mg/dl for the higher end of the 95% (normal) range reported in the literature is not absolute as it varied from study to study.

The probable factors responsible for variations in plasma/serum Lp(a) level could be that different studies used different plasma/serum storage temperatures (-200°C, -300°C, -800°C) for various time periods (up to 1 year, 7 years, 15-18 years) prior to analysis by assay methods as varied as radioimmunoassay, enzyme immunoassay, radial immunodiffusion, immunoturbidimetry, etc. [17-20]. Secondly, plasma/serum Lp(a) level is genetically determined and it varies according to populations, ethnic groups and geographical regions of the world [9,10].

The incidence of cholesterol gallstones, although less in our male population, was probably related to sedentary lifestyle and consumption of diet particularly rich in animal fats, refined sugars and poor in vegetable fats and fibers, all of which are significant risk factors for gallstone formation [32-34]. The consumption of a high calorie diet in the west is more common and is clearly an important factor in the formation of cholesterol gallstones. This trend has gradually spread to the East Asian countries, with dietary habits becoming unhealthier [34-36].

Elevated plasma/serum level of Lp(a) has been linked with CAD [5,6,17,18]. Another important aspect is that baseline Lp(a) levels were not measured in cases and controls in many follow-up studies with cholesterol lowering therapy. However, some studies showed that cholestyramine treatment was not effective in lowering Lp(a) levels, although cholesterol level was reported to be reduced [15,18,24].

In recent overviews on the management of primary hyperlipidemia by statins, serum Lp(a) level and its reduction were not mentioned and considered in the discussion [25-27]. Even the updated National Cholesterol Education Programme (NCEP) report, USA published in July 2004 discussed and debated LDL-C only and no consideration for Lp(a) level was suggested in the NCEP report [27,28].

Serum and Bile Lp(a) Level (mg/dl)*	Subjects and Biological Specimens			
	Normal Controls(NC)	Patients (Serum-I^0)	Patients (Bile-I^0)	Patients (Serum-II^0)
Observed Range	9.51-58.24	119.01-582.01	12.01-125.01	65.0-391.6
Mean ± SD	29.07±14.17	290.84±110.93	37.12±28.61	203.70±90.13
(SE)	(2.59)	(16.72)	(5.22)	(15.46)
95%CIM	23.78-34.36	257.12-324.57	26.43-47.80	172.25-235.14
Statistical Analysis* (Groups Compared)	Statistical Parameters			
ANOVA (NC, Serum -I^0, Bile-I^0, Serum- II^0)	df=3,134, F=96.41, p<0.001*			
Student's t-test				
NC vs Serum -I^0	df=72, t=-12.83, p<0.001*			
NC vs Serum-II^0	df=62, t=-10.49, p<0.001*			
NC vs Bile- I^0	df=58, t=-1.381, p=0.173 (NS)			
Bile- I^0 vs Serum -I^0	df=72, t=-12.23, p<0.001*			
Bile- I^0 vs Serum- II^0	df=62, t=-9.69, p<0.001*			
Serum -I^0 vs Serum- II^0	df=76, t=3.73, p<0.001*			

* Lp(a): Lipoprotein (a); SD: Standard Deviation; SE: Standard Error; 95%CIM: 95% Confidence Interval of Mean; NC: Normal Controls; Serum -I^0: Patients (Serum -I^0); Serum -II^0: Patients (Serum -II^0); Bile- I^0: Patients (Bile- I^0); df: Degree of Freedom; F: F-ratio; p ≤ 0.05: Significant; p>0.05: Not significant (NS).

Table 1: Lp(a) levels in Serum and bile before cholecystectomy (Serum-I^0, Bile-I^0) and after cholecystectomy (Serum-II^0) and their statistical analyses.

Lp(a) may compete with plasminogen, because of its sequence homology, for binding to fibrin and impair fibrinolysis. High levels of Lp(a) in serum may, therefore represent a potential source of antifibrinolytic activity [11,29]. In addition to this antifibrinolytic activity, high concentration of Lp(a) also suppresses the activity of transforming growth factor-β (TGF-β) which has the potential to inhibit the proliferation of endothelial cells and smooth muscle cells.

This probably causes increased proliferation of the vascular endothelial cells and smooth muscle cells resulting in the progression of atherosclerosis [11,30]. So, treatment of hypercholesterolemia with cholestyramine/statins may reduce but cannot abolish progression of atherogenesis and hence risk of long term complications in DM and CAD.

These clearly indicate that in the studies with cholesterol lowering drugs such as cholestyramine/ statins, serum Lp(a) levels should be followed up as well. In addition, recent reports suggested that TGF-β is involved in ultra structural tissue changes in patients with cholelithiasis and subsequently in gallbladder fibrosis leading to hypomotility which may be an important step in gallbladder dysfunction in this disorder [37,38].

The inhibition of TGF-β by higher levels of Lp(a), therefore, may be a probable protective mechanism against gallstone disease. Thus, it is equally important to investigate whether Lp(a) has any protective role against cholelithiasis contrary to atherosclerosis.

Apolipoprotein A1 (Apo A1), Apo E, CETP and mucin have been implicated with cholelithiasis in some studies [4,11-13]. In a recent study, it was reported that cholelithiasis patients have higher leptin levels and altered lipoprotein profile, with increased Lp(a) and Apo(B)levels and decreased ApoA-1 levels [19].

Another recent study showed that symptomatic cholelithiasis patients have increased malondialdehyde (MDA) levels indicating lipid peroxidation and decreased antioxidant capacity [18]. These changes in plasma lipids are, therefore, likely to have significant effect in the induction of gallstone disease and subsequently CAD postoperatively in patients with cholecystectomy. Abnormalities in lipids and apolipoproteins metabolism may, however, arise from a combination of various factors such as excess dietary cholesterol/fat, obesity, diabetes and genetic factors [4,39].

Some prominent facts known about Lp(a) are that it is a genetically determined particle containing a ApoB-100 linked to Apo(a), cholestyramine treatment is not effective in lowering serum Lp(a) level and Lp(a) has structural homology with plasminogen implicating in atherosclerosis and CADs.

In conclusion, however, it was evident from our results that changes in Lp(a) in cholelithiasis were significant and interesting, but a complex one and laparoscopic cholecystectomy did have significant impact on them.

These changes in Lp(a) is of crucial importance and the gallbladder may have a definitive role in it leading to development of gallstone disease i.e. cholelithiasis. Thus, incorporation of Lp(a) routinely in lipid profile analysis would be useful in identifying high risk patients and follow-up. Further studies are therefore warranted investigating several aspects of lipids, Lp(a), and apolipoproteins metabolism in cholelithiasis patients followed by cholecystectomy.

Lp(a) level (mg/L)	Subjects			Chi-squared (χ^2) test
	NCs	Serum-I^0	Total	
≤57.5	29	1	30	χ^2=62.08
>57.5	1	43	44	df=1
Total:	30	44	74	p<0.001*

NCs: Normal control subjects; Serum-I^0: Patients Serum-I^0

Lp(a) level (mg/L)	Subjects			Chi-squared (χ^2) test
	NCs	Bile-I^0	Total	
≤57.5	29	20	49	χ^2=7.124
>57.5	1	10	11	df=1
Total:	30	30	60	p=0.007*

NCs: Normal Control Subjects; Bile-I^0: Patients Bile-I^0

Lp(a) level (mg/L)	Subjects			Chi-squared (χ^2) test
	NCs	Serum-II^0	Total	
≤57.5	29	2	31	χ^2=49.02
>57.5	1	32	33	df=1
Total:	30	34	64	p<0.001*

NCs: Normal Control Subjects; Serum-II^0: Patients Serum-I^0

Table 2: Proportion of cholelithiasis patients with Lp(a) levels above and within normal limit and their statistical analysis by Chi-squared (χ^2) test.

Lp(a) level (mg/L)	Subjects				Chi-squared (χ^2) test
	Serum-I^0	Bile-I^0	Serum-II^0	Total	
≤57.5	1	20	2	23	χ^2=51.16
>57.5	43	10	32	85	df=2
Total:	44	30	34	108	p<0.001*

Serum-I^0: Patients Serum-I^0; Bile-I^0: Patients Bile-I^0; Serum-II^0: Patients Serum-II^0

Table 3: Proportion of cholelithiasis patients with Serum-I^0, Bile-I^0 and Serum-II^0 Lp(a) levels above and within normal limit and their statistical analysis by Chi squared (χ^2) test.

Funding Details

The work was supported by The Medical and Health Welfare Trust (MHWT), Plot-4 Road-9 Sector-1, Uttara Model Town, Dhaka-1230, Bangladesh.

Acknowledgements

The authors appreciate Mr. Taposh K Datta, Medical Technologist, for helping with laboratory analysis, Mr Shohag MN Ali for computer composing the manuscript and Mr. AHM Salman for statistical analysis. The authors gratefully acknowledge the generous financial support of The Medical and Health Welfare Trust (MHWT), Dhaka, Bangladesh for this research project.

References

1. James HG, Kenneth RM, Scot LF (1996) Current diagnosis and treatment in gastroenterology, Int. ed; Connecticut: Appletin and Lange.
2. Everhart JE, Khare M, Hill M, Maurer KR (1999) Prevalence and ethnic differences in gallbladder disease in the United States. Gastroenterology 117: 632-639.
3. Batajoo H, Hazra NK (2013) Analysis of serum lipid profile in cholelithiasis patients. J Nepal Health Res Counc 11: 53-55.
4. Rao PJ, Jarari A, E1 Awami H, Patil TN (2012) Lipid profile in bile and serum of cholelithiasis patients – A Comparative study. J Basic Med & Allied Sci 1: 15-21.
5. Apstein MD, Carey MC (1996) Pathogenesis of cholesterol gallstones: a parsimonious hypothesis. Eur J Clin Invest 26: 343-352.
6. Channa NA (2008) Gallstone disease: a review. Pak Arm Forces Med J 58: 197-208.
7. Tandon RK (1990) Current development in the pathogenesis of gallstones. Trop Gastroenterol 11: 130-139.
8. Portincasa P, Di Ciaula A, Vendemiale G, Palmieri V, Moschetta A, et al. (2000) Gallbladder motility and cholesterol crystallization in bile from patients with pigment and cholesterol gallstones. Eur J Clin Invest 30: 317-324.
9. Malik AA, Wani ML, Tak SI, Irshad I, Ul-Hassan N (2011) Association of dyslipidaemia with cholilithiasis and effect of cholecystectomy on the same. Int J Surg 9: 641-642.
10. Skill NJ, Scott RE, Wu J, Maluffio MA (2011) Hepatocellular carcinoma associated lipid metabolism reprogramming. J Surg Res 169: 51-56.
11. Hasegawa T, Makino I (1995) Measurement of apolipoprotein A1 in cholesterol gallstones and gallbladder bile of patients with gallstones. J Gastroenterol 30: 96-102.
12. Juvonen T, Kervinen K, Kairaluoma MI, Kesäniemi YA (1995) Effect of cholecystectomy on plasma lipid and lipoprotein levels. Hepatogastroenterology 42: 377-382.
13. Pinheiro-Júnior S, Pinhel MA, Nakazone MA, Pinheiro A, Amorim GF, et al. (2012) Effect of genetic variants related to lipid metabolism as risk factors for cholelithiasis after bariatric surgery in Brazilian population. Obes Surg 22: 623-633.
14. Danesh J, Collins R, Peto R (2000) Lipoprotein(a) and coronary heart disease. Meta-analysis of prospective studies. Circulation 102: 1082-1085.
15. Barghash NA, Elewa SM, Hamdi EA, Barghash AA, El Dine R (2004) Role of plasma homocysteine and lipoprotein (a) in coronary artery disease. Br J Biomed Sci 61: 78-83.
16. Giasuddin ASM, Jhuma KA, Mujibul Haq AM (2008) Lipoprotein (a) status in Bangladeshi patients with diabetes mellitus. J Med Coll Women Hosp 6: 74-82.
17. Haq AMM, Giasuddin ASM, Huque MM (2011) Serum total homocysteine and lipoprotein (a) levels in acute myocardial infarction and their response to treatment with vitamins. J Coll Physicians Surg Pak 21: 266-270.
18. Atamer A, Kurdas-Ovunc AO, Yesil A, Atamer Y (2014) Evaluation of paraoxonase, malondialdehyde, and lipoprotein levels in patients with asymptomatic cholelithiasis. Saudi J Gastroenterol 20: 66-73.
19. Saraç S, Atamer A, Atamer Y, Can AS, Bilici A, et al. (2015) Leptin levels and lipoprotein profiles in patients with cholelithiasis. J Int Med Res 43: 385-392.

20. Devanapalli B, Lee S, Mahajan D, Bermingham M (2002) Lipoprotein (a) in an immigrant Indian population sample in Australia. Br J Biomed Sci 59: 119-122.

21. Gaw A, Brown EA, Gourlay CW, Bell MA (2000) Analytical performance of the Genzyme LipoPro Lp(a) kit for plasma lipoprotein(a)-cholesterol assay. Br J Biomed Sci 57: 13-18.

22. Powers AC (2005) Diabetes mellitus. In: Kasper DL, Fauci AS, Longo DL, Braunwald E, Hauser SL, Jameson JL (Editors). Harrison's Principals of Internal Medicine (16th Edn) New York: McGraw-Hill.

23. Marcovina SM, Koschinsky ML (1998) Lipoprotein(a) as a risk factor for coronary artery disease. Am J Cardiol 82: 57U-66U.

24. Berg K (1963) A New serum type system in man--The LP system. Acta Pathol Microbiol Scand 59: 369-382.

25. Khan MH, Khan AW, Aziz MM, Rabbi MA (2012) Day case Laparoscopic Cholecystectomy: experience at the Bangabandhu Sheikh Mujib Medical University. Mymenshingh Med J 21: 485-489.

26. Ahmed T, Alam MT, Ahmed SU, Jahan M (2012) Role of intraoperative flexible Choledochoscopy in calculous biliary tract disease. Mymensingh Med J 21: 462-468.

27. Haq AMM, Giasuddin ASM, Jhuma KA, Choudhury MAM (2015) Effect of cholecystectomy on lipidprofile in Bangladeshi patients with cholelithiasis. J Metabolic Synd 5.

28. Anstee QM, Jones DEJ (2014) Liver and biliary tract disease. Davidson's Principles & Practice of Medicine (22nd Edn) Edinburgh: Churchill Livingstone (Elsevier) 2014: 921-88.

29. Cuschieri SA (2002) Disorders of the biliary tract. Essential Surgical Practice (4th Edn) London: Arnold.

30. Remaley AT, Rifai N, Warnick GR (2015) Lipids, Lipoprotein, apolipoproteins and other cardiac risk factors. In: Burtis CA, Bruns DE. (Editors). Tietz Fundamentals of Clinical Chemistry and Molecular Diagnostics (7th Edn), St. Louise, Missouri: Elsevier Inc (Saunders), USA.

31. Kirkwood BR, Sterne JAC (2008) Essential Medical Statistics, 2nd Edition (Reprinted); Oxford:Blackwell Science Ltd.

32. Cuevas A, Miquel JF, Reyes MS, Zanlungo S, Nervi F (2004) Diet as a risk factor for cholesterol gallstone disease. J Am Coll Nutr 23: 187-196.

33. Misciagna G, Centonze S, Leoci C, Guerra V, Cisternino AM, et al. (1999) Diet, physical activity, and gallstones--a population-based, case-control study in southern Italy. Am J Clin Nutr 69: 120-126.

34. Tsai CJ, Leitzmann MF, Willett WC, Giovannucci EL (2004) The effect of long-term intake of cis unsaturated fats on the risk for gallstone disease in men: a prospective cohort study. Ann Intern Med 141: 514-522.

35. Tsunoda K, Shirai Y, Hatakeyama K (2004) Prevalence of cholesterol gallstones positively correlates with per capita daily calorie intake. Hepatogastroenterology 51: 1271-1274.

36. Aulakh R, Mohan H, Attri AK, Kaur J, Punia RP (2007) A comparative study of serum lipid profile and gallstone disease. Indian J Pathol Microbiol 50: 308-312.

37. Köninger J, di Mola FF, Di Sebastiano P, Gardini A, Brigstock DR, et al. (2005) Transforming growth factor-beta pathway is activated in cholecystolithiasis. Langenbecks Arch Surg 390: 21-28.

38. Ebadi P, Daneshmandi S, Ghasemi A, Karimi MH (2013) Cytokine single nucleotide polymorphisms in patients' with gallstone: dose TGF-I^2 gene variants affect gallstone formation? Mol Biol Rep 40: 6256-6260.

39. Weiss KM, Ferrell RE, Hanis CL, Styne PN (1984) Genetics and epidemiology of gallbladder disease in New World native peoples. Am J Hum Genet 36: 1259-1278.

6

Anaesthetic Management of a Dwarf with Hypopituitarism Presenting for Epigastric Hernioplasty

Rajat Choudhuri, Sandeep Kr. Kar*, Dhiman Adhikari and Sabyasachi Sinha

Department of Anaesthesiology & Department of Cardiac Anaesthesiology, Institute of Post Graduate Medical Education &Research, Kolkata, India

*Corresponding author: Sandeep Kr. Kar, Department of Anaesthesiology & Department of Cardiac Anaesthesiology, Institute of Post Graduate Medical Education &Research, Kolkata, India; E-mail: sndpkar@yahoo.co.in

Abstract

Hypoplastic pituitary, a rare entity in itself and when presented to us requires a detailed evaluation and postoperative follow up. We are presenting a 48 year old lady who is short statured posted for epigastrichernioplasty. Detailed evaluation revealed secondary hypothyroidism, difficult airway, cardiomegaly, pericardial effusion, secondary adrenocortical insufficiency, growth hormone deficiency. CT scan of brain revealed cerebrospinal fluid filled sellar region and magnetic resonance imaging proved hypo plastic pituitary. After optimization with L-thyroxine she was planned for balanced general anaesthesia with epidural analgesia under steroid coverage. Peroperatively we faced resistant hypotension and due to inadequate reversal she was shifted to intensive care unit on ventilator. Subsequently we proved that her postoperative adrenocorticotropic hormone and cortisol level were low. However 24 hours later she could be extubated and finally she was discharged one week after the operation. However such cases are a challenge to the attending anaesthesiologist and as there is no strict protocol for anaesthetizing such a rare entity we have thought for detailing the case.

Keywords: Adrenocortical insufficiency; Balanced general anaesthesia; Epidural analgesia; Hypoplastic pituitary; Resistant hypotension

Introduction

The anterior pituitary often referred to as the 'master gland' orchestrating the complex regulatory functions of multiple other endocrine glands along with hypothalamus and the hormones produced by this gland elicit specific responses in peripheral target tissues [1]. Congenital hypoplastic pituitary is a very rare entity and the diagnosis is often elusive, emphasizing the importance of recognizing subtle clinical manifestations and performing the correct laboratory diagnostic tests. Hypopituitarism is not a common encounter that we as anaesthesiologists face in our day to day practice. Associated anomalies, short stature, difficult airway, secondary hypothyroidism and hypothalamo-pituitary-adrenal axis suppression require vigilant management and are a real challenge for anaesthesiologists.

Here we are presenting such a case of Hypopituitarism, who presented to our pre-anaesthetic check up clinic with a 5 year history of Epigastric hernia now posted for epigastrichernioplasty.

Case Report

A 48 year old lady presented to the preanaestheticcheck up clinic with congenital dwarfism, gradually progressive uncomplicated ventral hernia for 5 years and hoarseness of voice since several years. She had history of premature menopause (at 40 years) and cold intolerance. Her father was short statured and her birth and maternal history were unremarkable.

On examination, her weight was 20 kg and height was 98 cm. Proportionate shortening of limb and trunk, coarse skin, hoarse voice were noted. Airway assessment revealed small nostrils, interincisor distance-3 cm, Mallampati class-3, thyromental distance-4 cm, atlanto-occipital Extension >35°, short thick neck. Her heart rate was 86/min. and blood pressure was 110/72 mm. of Hg.

Examination of back revealed very short interspinous spaces without kyphoscoliosis.

The routine investigations: chest x-ray (CXR) postero-anterior view showed cardiomegaly, electrocardiogram (ECG) showed low voltage complex, Echocardiography findings were left ventricular ejection fraction (LVEF)-66%, Concentric left ventricular hypertrophy (LVH) and mild pericardial effusion.

Hormonal assays preoperatively revealed tri-iodothyronine (T3)-0.29ng/ml (Normal range: 0.8-2.0 ng/ml), thyroxine (T4)-3.29 µg/dl (Normal range: 4.6-12 µg/dl), thyroid stimulating hormone (TSH)-3.23 µIU/ml (Normal range: 0.27-4.2 µIU/ml), free T3-1.8 pg/ml (Normal range: 2.3-4.2 pg/ml), free T4-0.5 ng/L (Normal range: 0.8-1.8 ng/L), prolactin-8.3 ng/ml (Normal range: 1.9-25.9 ng/ml), luteinizing hormone (LH)-37.4 µIU/ml (Normal range: 8.2-40.8 µIU/ml), follicle stimulating hormone (FSH)-83.3 µIU/ml (Normal range: 35-151 µIU/ml), morning cortisol (7-9 A.M.)-17.14 µg/dl (Normal range: 4.3-22.4 µg/dl), adrenocorticotropic hormone (ACTH)-11.0 pg/ml (Normal range: 6-46 pg/ml), GH-0.2ng/ml (Normal range: 0.5-17.0 ng/ml).

Other routine investigation findings were haemoglobin (Hb)-9.7 gm%, total leukocyte count (TLC)-8600/cu.mm. (Normal range: 4000-11000/cu.mm.), differential leukocyte count (DLC)-$N_{72}L_{17}M_1E_8B_2$, fasting blood sugar (FBS)-68 mg/dl (Normal range: 80-110 mg/dl), postprandial blood sugar (PPBS)-96 mg/dl (Normal range:<140 mg/dl), urea-32 mg/dl (Normal range: 20-40 mg/dl), creatinine-0.46 mg/dl (Normal range: 0.5-1.5 mg/dl). So, the patient was also hypoglycemic, as it is not uncommon in hypopituitarism.

CT scan of brain showed physiological calcifications in globipallidi and dentate nuclei, cerebrospinal fluid (CSF) filled sellar region. Pituitary gland was not visualized. Magnetic resonance imaging (MRI) of brain revealed hypoplastic pituitary. There were bilateral small ovaries on ultrasonography (USG) of abdomen.

Preoperative Optimisation

L-thyroxine 12.5 μg once daily for 10 days followed by 25 μg for 10 days and then 37.5 μg for next 3 weeks. After 6 weeks of optimization thyroid hormone levels improved (T3: 0.56 ng/ml; T4: 4.82 μg/dl; TSH: 2.1 μIU/ml).

Clonidine (100 μg orally) stimulation test showed 60 minutes later GH value of 0.26 ng/ml and 90 minutes later GH level was 0.27 ng/ml. Pre-anaesthetic airway evaluation could not be done by indirect laryngoscopy. Hence it was done by fibreoptic bronchoscope which revealed edematous vocal cords, narrow glottic opening but no mass was obstructing the glottic aperture.

Anaesthetic Management

After adequate optimization, obtaining informed written consent, keeping the difficult airway cart and resuscitative drugs and equipments ready, the patient was taken for anaesthesia. Intra-venous (IV) access was done in both hands. Early in the morning patient was administered 37.5 μg of L-thyroxine. Airway anaesthesia was done by nebulisation with 4% xylocaine for 20 mins after injection glycopyrrolate (0.2 mg) in intra-muscular (IM) route. Superior laryngeal nerve and recurrent laryngeal nerve blocks were given by 2% xylocaine around 1 ml at each site. Monitors were attached. Besides routine monitoring, neuromuscular monitoring and bi-spectral index (BIS) monitoring were done in this case. Blood glucose was also monitored. Plan of anaesthesia was balanced general anaesthesia combined with thoracic epidural analgesia. After preloading the patient with 10ml/kg of balanced salt solution, thoracic epidural catheterization was done at T8-T9 intervertebral space using 18G Tuohy needle with patient in sitting posture followed by 2 ml of test dose of 2% Xylocaine with adrenaline. Premedication was with inj. hydrocortisone 50 mg (IV) 30 minutes before intubation, Ondansetron 2 mg. (IV) 30 minutes before intubation, metoclopramide 10 mg (IV) and glycopyrrolate 0.2mg (IM) 20 mins before intubation, fentanyl 50 μg (IV) 6 mins before intubation, midazolam 2 mg. (IV) 2 mins before intubation. Pre-oxygenation was done with 100% oxygen (O_2) for 5 mins.

Awake fibreoptic guided tracheal intubation was done by 5.5 mm. internal diameter (ID) poly vinyl chloride (PVC) cuffed endotracheal tube after adequate airway anaesthesia and preparation. Muscle relaxant atracurium (0.5mg/kg) administered after confirmation of tube placement, dose titrated as guided by neuromuscular monitors. Maintenance of anaesthesia was done with O_2:N_2O = 33:67 and isoflurane (0.4-0.6 minimum alveolar concentration). Intermittent positive pressure ventilation (IPPV) was provided with respiratory rate (RR)-12/min, tidal volume (TV)-160 ml, inspiration and expiration ratio=1:2.5. Epidural analgesia was maintained with 0.125% bupivacaine and fentanyl (2 mcg/ml) as infusion at a rate of 4ml/hr. IV fluid ringer lactate 700 ml was given in 1 hour. 20 mins after induction of anaesthesia there was sudden hypotension with bradycardia nonresponsive to IV fluids though heart rate was stabilized with atropine 0.3 mg (IV). The epidural infusion rate was then halved and another 150 ml of IV fluid was infused. Dopamine (200 mg/50 ml

normal saline) infusion was started at a rate of 2 ml/hr via infusion pump. Operation was done successfully and patient was sent to intensive care unit (ICU) with endotracheal tube in-situ after hemodynamic stabilization with inotrope. Urine output, capillary blood glucose (CBG), arterial blood gas (ABG) analysis were within normal limits in the immediate postoperative phase.

She regained consciousness almost after 4 hrs; reflexes were normal, hemodynamics adequately stabilized. She was extubated after a successful weaning trial 24 hrs later. Postoperative ACTH level was 8.0 pg/ml which was low and cortisol was also in the low normal range of 8.2 μg/dl, despite in a stressful scenario. Her haemoglobin did not alter significantly in the postoperative period.

The next day i.e. 2nd post-operative day she was transferred to surgical ward and was discharged with good health with the advice of tapering steroid dosage and continuation of thyroid hormone replacement therapy 7 days after the operation.

Discussion

Hypopituitarism, an underactive pituitary gland results from impaired production of one or more of the pituitary trophic hormones. Reduced pituitary function can result from inherited disorders, more commonly it is acquired and reflects mass effects of tumours or the consequence of trauma, infiltrative disorders, vascular and infectious aetiologies [1-3].

Our patient had a congenital inherited disorder, aetiology of which was unknown as evidenced by Low TSH and ACTH in the period of stress, a low GH with a secondary hypothyroid background, secondary adrenocortical insufficiency. MRI also suggested a hypoplastic pituitary. Pituitary gland development from rathkes pouch involves a complex interplay of lineage specific transcription factors expressed in pleuripotent stem cells and gradients of locally produced growth factors [1].

The clinical manifestations of hypopituitarism depend on which hormones are lost and the extent of hormone deficiency.GH deficiency causes growth disorders in children and leads to abnormal body composition in adults. Gonadotrophin deficiency causes menstrual disorders and infertility in women and decreased sexual function, infertility and loss of secondary sexual characters in men. Somatotrophin and gonadotrophin seem to be affected first. TSH and ACTH deficiency usually develop later in the course of pituitary failure [3].

TSH deficiency causes growth retardation in children and features of hypothyroidism in children and in adults. The secondary form of adrenal insufficiency caused by ACTH deficiency leads to decreased production of cortisol with relative preservation of mineralocorticoid production. Prolactin deficiency causes failure of lactation. When lesions involve posterior pituitary, features like polyuria and polydipsia reflect loss of vasopressin secretion. Epidemiological studies have documented an increased mortality rate in patients with long standing pituitary damage primarily due to increased cardiovascular and cerebrovascular disease.

Our patient had a low free T3 and free T4 with a low TSH indicating a secondary hypothyroid state. This was the laboratory finding along with clinical suspicion which prompted us to investigate further.

The diagnosis of ACTH deficiency is difficult [2]. Partial ACTH deficiency may be unmasked in the presence of an acute medical or surgical illness when clinically significant hypocortisolism reflects diminished ACTH reserve [1]. Under surgical and anaesthetic stress, the adrenal glands secrete 116-185 mg of cortisol daily [4]. Under maximum stress, they may secrete 200 to 500 mg/day [4]. Good correlation exists between the severity and duration of the operation and the response of the adrenal gland. Major surgery would be represented by procedures such as major vascular, skeletal, neurologic repairor major reconstruction of the gastrointestinal tract and minor surgery by procedures such as herniorrhaphy. In one study of 20 patients during major surgery, the mean maximal concentration of cortisol in plasma was 47 µg/dl (Range 22 to 75 µg/dl). During minor surgery, the mean maximal concentration of cortisol in plasma was 28 µg/dl (Range 10 to 44 µg/dl) [3].

In our case the hormonal assay of ACTH and cortisol postoperatively reflected a secondary adrenocortical insufficiency. Also preoperative ACTH level was in low normal range in a stressful situation, which depicted a pituitary pathology. The diagnoses of GH deficiency can be made by GH assays before and after stimulation tests such as clonidine test, Argenine test and insulin provoked hypoglycaemia test [2]. Our patient had a pre-existing hypoglycemia.

Glucocorticoid replacement therapy improves most features of ACTH deficiency [1].

Because these patients cannot respond to stressful situations, it was traditionally recommended that they may be given a stress dose of glucocorticoids preoperatively [5].

However, Symreng and colleagues gave 25 mg of hydrocortisone intravenously to adults at the start of the operative procedure followed by 100 mg intravenously over the next 24 hours and this regimen did not worsen the situation. As minimum dosage was required in our patient to avoid the side effects of steroid, this regimen became more attractive [6].

The total daily dose of hydrocortisone replacement should not exceed 300 mg divided into 2-3 doses. Prednisolone 5 mg (morning dose) and 2.5 mg (evening dose) having fewer mineralocorticoid action and long duration of action is preferred in patients who are orally allowed to intake. Doses are increased several folds during periods of acute illness or stress [1]. Hence our patient was administered a steroid dosage regimen i.e. 50mg hydrocortisone which might have been inadequate considering dosage and duration but is an issue of debate due to lack of strict guidelines.

In a well controlled study of glucocorticoid replacement in primates, the investigators clearly defined the life-threatening events that can be associated with inadequate perioperative corticosteroid replacement [7]. L-thyrorine is recommended in 0.075-0.15 mg daily dose till patient is euthyroid [1]. Replacement of GH is indicated only if the diagnosis of adult GH deficiency is unequivocally established. If evolved GH<0.3 ng/ml then, in adults somatotrophin 0.1-1.25 mg subcutaneously four times daily and in children 0.02-0.05 mg /kg/day administered for around 6 months [1]. In our case as adult growth hormone deficiency (AGHD) was not established, GH replacement was not considered. Difficult airway management, hypotension not responding to standard regimen, decrease in core body temperature in spite of active warming, very low concentration of anaesthetic drug requirement due to reduced metabolism, higher incidence of postoperative gastrointestinal and neuropsychiatric complications, electrolyte and coagulation disturbances, delayed emergence from

anaesthesia, perioperative stress management, steroid management are the main highlights of perioperative vigilant anesthetic care [8-11]. In patients with concurrent thyrotrophin and corticotrophin deficiency, thyroxin must not be given without cortisol as this may precipitate a pituitary crisis [2].

The response to surgical and traumatic stress is triggered by hypothalamic activation secondary to afferent neuronal input from an area of injury or emotional activity centered in the limbic system and humoral factors such as inflammatory cytokines (interleukins, tumour necrosis factor and interferon). This is characterized by an increase in plasma levels of cortisol, ACTH, antidiuretic hormone/ vasopressin (ADH), renin, catecholamines, endorphins and by metabolic changes such as hypoglycemia and negative nitrogen balance [12-14]. Regional anaesthesia and general anaesthesia appears to blunt the release of various stress hormones [15]. Hence in this case epidural analgesia was considered.

Since it was a predicted difficult airway with history of hoarseness and as indirect laryngoscopy by otorhinolaryngologists was inconclusive we planned to evaluate the airway preoperatively so that peroperative airway management can be planned accordingly [16-18].

After excluding any major upper airway problem, we decided to go for awake fibreoptic intubation as per difficult airway algorithm, keeping in mind all the required precautions and keeping all the resuscitation drugs and equipments ready [19,20]. Maximum secretion of ACTH occurs during reversal of anaesthesia, during extubation and in immediate postoperative period [21]. In the postoperative stressed state ACTH and cortisol increases 2-3 folds with circadian rhythm disruption more in women [3,22-24].

This lady postoperatively revealed a low normal cortisol and ACTH which showed that secondary adrenocortical insufficiency might have been one of the probable causes of intraoperative hypotension though epidural analgesia induced hypotension can't be negated or proved.

Conclusion

Hypo plastic pituitary, though a rare entity but when presents to us, requires thorough evaluation including step wise hormonal assays with close eye on clinical presentation. A planned optimization plan should be sought out and only after adequate optimization we should proceed with such patients anticipating the risks of cardiovascular and cerebrovascular instability. Further it requires a vigilant anaesthetic management even in the post operative period regarding ventilatory support and postoperative hormonal evaluation. Proper guideline is still lacking regarding hormone replacement therapy in perioperative phase and the use of regional analgesia. But a keen eye, proper preparation and anticipation of complications can help to overcome the difficulties. So we can conclude that perioperative anaesthetic care in patients with hypopituitarism requires careful preoperative assessment and meticulous perioperative management.

References

1. Melmed S, Jameson L (2009) Disorders of the anterior pituitary and hypothalamus, Harrison's Principles of Internal Medicine edited by Braunwald, Kasper (17th edn), Vol.II 333: 2195-2216.

2. http://www.endocrinesurgeon.co.uk/index.php/the-history-of-the-pituitary-gland

3. Prabhakar VK, Shalet SM (2006) Aetiology, diagnosis, and management of hypopituitarism in adult life. Postgrad Med J 82: 259-266.

4. Shaikh S, Verma H, Yadav N, Jauhari M and Bullangowda J (2012) Applications of Steroid in Clinical Practice: A Review. ISRN Anesthesiology 12:11-21.

5. Udelsman R, Ramp J, Gallucci WT, Gordon A, Lipford E, et al. (1986) Adaptation during surgical stress. A reevaluation of the role of glucocorticoids. J Clin Invest 77: 1377-1381.

6. Molitch ME, Clemmons DR, Malozowski S, Merriam GR, Shalet SM, et al. (2006) Evaluation and treatment of adult growth hormone deficiency: an Endocrine Society Clinical Practice Guideline. J Clin Endocrinol Metab 91: 1621-1634.

7. http://www.pituitary.org.uk

8. http://www.linkinghub.elsevier.com

9. Ladenson PW, Levin AA, Ridgway EC, Daniels GH (1984) Complications of surgery in hypothyroid patients. Am J Med 77: 261-266.

10. Weinberg AD, Brennan MD, Gorman CA, Marsh HM, O'Fallon WM (1983) Outcome of anesthesia and surgery in hypothyroid patients. Arch Intern Med 143: 893-897.

11. Hopkins SJ (2007) Central nervous system recognition of peripheral inflammation: a neural, hormonal collaboration. Acta Biomed 78 Suppl 1: 231-247.

12. Weissman C (1990) The metabolic response to stress: an overview and update. Anesthesiology 73: 308-327.

13. Langouche L, Van den Berghe G (2006) The dynamic neuroendocrine response to critical illness. Endocrinol Metab Clin North Am 35: 777-791, ix.

14. Jeffrey J, Schwartz S (2009) Endocrine function: Endocrine response to surgical stress. Clinical Aneasthesia edited by Barash 49:1302.

15. Benumof JL (1991) Management of the difficult adult airway. With special emphasis on awake tracheal intubation. Anesthesiology 75: 1087-1110.

16. Ovassapian A (1996) Fiberoptic endoscopy and the Difficult Airway, Philadelphia, Lippincott-Raven 47.

17. Rosenblatt WH, Wagner PJ, Ovassapian A, Kain ZN (1998) Practice patterns in managing the difficult airway by anesthesiologists in the United States. Anesth Analg 87: 153-157.

18. American Society of Anesthesiologists Task Force on Management of the Difficult Airway (2003) Practice guidelines for management of the difficult airway: an updated report by the American Society of Anesthesiologists Task Force on Management of the Difficult Airway. Anesthesiology 98: 1269-1277.

19. Popat M (2003) The airway. Anaesthesia 58: 1166-1171.

20. Stephen P, Fischer S (2009) Preoperative evaluation, Miller's Text Book of Anaesthesia edited by Ronald D. Miller 34:1023.

21. Otte C, Hart S, Neylan TC, Marmar CR, Yaffe K, et al. (2005) A meta-analysis of cortisol response to challenge in human aging: importance of gender. Psychoneuroendocrinology 30: 80-91.

22. Gögenur I, Ocak U, Altunpinar O, Middleton B, Skene DJ, et al. (2007) Disturbances in melatonin, cortisol and core body temperature rhythms after major surgery. World J Surg 31: 290-298.

23. Roizen MF, Fleisher LA (2009) Anaesthetic implications of concurrent diseases, (7thedn), Miller's Text book of Anaesthesia edited by Ronald D Miller 35: 1083.

24. Symreng T, Karlberg BE, Kågedal B, Schildt B (1981) Physiological cortisol substitution of long-term steroid-treated patients undergoing major surgery. Br J Anaesth 53: 949-954.

7

Metabolically Healthy Obesity and the Fit/Fat Phenotype: Associations with Mortality, Subclinical Cardiovascular Disease and Approach to Treatment

Ayesha Farooq[1], Sufian Sorathia[1], Sameer Shaharyar[1,2], Lara Roberson[2] and Hamid Feiz[1*]

[1]Aventura Hospital and Medical Center, Aventura, USA

[2]Center for Prevention and Wellness Research, Baptist Health South Florida, Miami, FL 33139, USA

[*]Corresponding author: Hamid Feiz, Aventura Hospital and Medical Center, Aventura, FL 33180, USA; E-mail: hamid.feiz@hcahealthcare.com

Abstract

Obesity is a global epidemic affecting over a third of the adult population. Within the obese, subgroups have been identified, including the metabolically healthy obese (MHO) and the fit/fat phenotypes. The MHO phenotype was traditionally thought to have lower cardiovascular risk than the 'typically obese', a notion that is being challenged by recent data. Similarly, the emerging fit/fat phenotype is raising questions about the impact of obesity on mortality and cardiovascular risk. The present narrative review provides an overview of these phenotypes and summarizes current evidence and viewpoints regarding the same. The review then incorporates this data into a format that can be utilized by clinicians and researchers to aid clinical decision-making.

Keywords: Obesity; Cardiovascular diseases; Cholesterol

Background

Since 1980, worldwide obesity has more than doubled and continues to increase in prevalence. According to the World Health Organization, in 2014, more than 1.9 billion adults were overweight, which equates to roughly 39% of the adult population1. According to the Centers for Disease Control and Prevention, in the United States between 2011 and 2012, approximately 3 out of every 5 adults were overweight and more than one-third were obese, which equates to 78.6 million adults [1,2]. Obesity is a preventable risk factor of all-cause mortality, cardiovascular related mortality and cancer related mortality [3]. However, a subset of obese patients have been identified who do not display the typical obesity related metabolic disorders, and are thought to have a risk in between healthy-normal weight individuals and those with metabolic syndrome.

In the 1940s, Dr. Jean Vague was the first to observe a constellation of risk factors for diabetes mellitus, dyslipidemia and atherosclerosis in obese patients [4]. His "vague" observations led to recognition of metabolic syndrome as a cluster of related conditions conferring increased cardiovascular risk and have since led to many debates regarding its diagnosis, with a consensus definition being achieved only recently (Table 1) [5].

Components	Values
Central Obesity**	Men Waist Circumference > 40 inches Women Waist Circumference > 35 inches
Hypertriglyceridemia***	Triglycerides > 150 mg/dL
Reduced HDL Cholesterol***	Men HDL cholesterol < 40 mg/dL Women HDL cholesterol < 50 mg/dL
Elevated Blood Pressure***	Blood Pressure > 130/85 mmHg
Fasting Hyperglycemia***	Blood Glucose > 100 mg/dL
* Criteria is based on components jointly agreed upon by International Diabetes Federation Task Force on Epidemiology and Prevention, National Heart, Lung, and Blood Institute, American Heart Association, World Heart Federation, International Atherosclerosis Society, and International Association for the Study of Obesity	
** Non-Europeans cut points (population and country-specific definitions)	

Table 1: Metabolic Syndrome Criteria (3 of the 5 must be present for diagnosis)[*5]

While originally associated with increased risk in all obese individuals, recent studies reveal that metabolic syndrome may not actually manifest in all with a high body mass index (BMI). In fact, studies have shown that up to 30% of the obese do not display the typical metabolic disorders of insulin resistance, dyslipidemia and hypertension [6-13] and actually display favorable inflammatory, hormonal, liver enzymes and immune profiles. This led to identification of a new subgroup within the obese population termed metabolically healthy obesity (MHO). MHO can be compared to the metabolically unhealthy but normal weight (MUNW), who have a normal BMI but display the typical metabolic disorders seen with obesity (Table 2) [7,10,12,14-19].

Metabolic Health*		Healthy	Unhealthy
WEIGHT**	Obese	Metabolically Healthy Obese (MHO)	Metabolically Unhealthy Obese (MUO)=Metabolic Syndrome
	Normal	Metabolically Healthy Normal Weight (MHNW)	Metabolically Unhealthy Normal Weight (MUNW)
* Varying definitions have been used in the literature			
** Based on BMI (Obese: BMI>30.0; Normal: BMI 18.5-24.9)			

Table 2: Different Metabolic Phenotypes.

The present narrative review provides an overview of the MHO phenotype in the context of all-cause mortality and cardiovascular disease risk. We further discuss the biological associations of the MHO phenotype, as well as discuss the interplay of physical fitness and obesity status in determining CVD risk. Finally, the review offers suggestions for incorporating these data into clinical practice and assisting future research.

One of the Many Faces of Obesity: The Mho Phenotype

For a given BMI category, patients can be classified into subgroups based on the presence of metabolic risk factors (Table 2). This divides patients into the metabolically healthy normal weight (MHNW), metabolically unhealthy normal weight (MUNW), metabolically healthy obese (MHO) and the metabolically unhealthy obese (MUO) - which, depending on the definition employed, can be synonymous with metabolic syndrome. Traditionally, obesity is graded into classes based on body mass index (BMI), either being classified as overweight (BMI>25 and <30) or obese (BMI>30). Some studies assessing metabolic risk in the context of overweight individuals categorize patients as metabolically healthy overweight (MH-Overweight) and metabolically healthy obese, whereas others merge these into the same category.

Metabolically healthy obesity was first identified in 2001 in terms of visceral adiposity and insulin resistance (IR) but since then, it has had various meanings. Most commonly, it has been defined as obesity with a range of 0, 1, or 2 features of metabolic syndrome [20], sometimes excluding patients with diabetes mellitus all together, but no standard definition for MHO has been established [12,21]. Other definitions of metabolic risk factors have included C reactive protein (CRP), white blood cell (WBC) count, insulin sensitivity, waist circumference, body fat percentage and combinations of the same. Although a consensus

was reached on the definition of metabolic syndrome in 2009, published literature continues to define it differently making it difficult to compare results on this topic [22]. Depending on the definition employed, the prevalence of the MHO phenotype is thought to range from 10-32% of obese individuals [11,13,23].

Is MHO a "Benign" Phenotype?

When the phenotype was first identified, MHO was thought to have a lower risk of cardiovascular disease and mortality than MUO and was interpreted as a 'benign' condition. Recent evidence [20,24], however, places MHO on a continuum with MHNW, MUNW, and MUO individuals as is demonstrated in Figure 1.

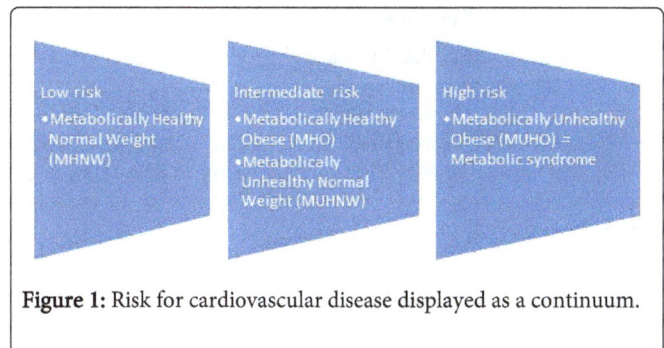

Figure 1: Risk for cardiovascular disease displayed as a continuum.

Kramer et al. [24] conducted a pooled analysis of unadjusted data from eight studies (n=61 386; 3988 events, follow-up range 3-30 years) and demonstrated that the MHO phenotype was associated with a 24% increased risk of all-cause mortality and CVD events as compared to the MHNW population (Table 3).

Groups	Pooled Risk Estimate	Pooled Risk Estimate >10y follow up
MHNW (referent)	1	1
MUNW	3.14 (2.36–3.93)	-
MH-Overweight	1.10 (0.90–1.24)	1.21 (0.91–1.61)
MH-Obese	1.19 (0.98–1.38)	1.24 (1.02–1.55)

| MU-Overweight | 2.70 (2.08–3.30) | - |
| MU-Obese | 2.65 (2.18–3.12) | - |

Table: 3a Pooled Risk Estimates for all-cause mortality and CVD events by metabolic and obesity category.

Groups	Pooled Risk Estimate	Pooled Risk Estimate >10y follow up
MUNW	1	-
MU-Obese	1.12 (0.92–1.37)	-
MU-Overweight	1.13 (0.93–1.37)	-
Ref: Kramer et al.24		

Table 3b: Pooled risk estimates for all-cause mortality and CVD events compared to metabolically unhealthy normal weight (MUNW) as referent.

However, this increased risk was not apparent in studies with follow-up durations of less than 10 years. This 10 year 'lag' period may explain the findings in initial published reports, which labeled MHO as a benign phenotype; since the risk increase is only evident after 10 years, studies with shorter follow-up durations would have yielded negative results despite the existence of a true association. Some studies suggest that metabolically healthy individuals may be younger than their metabolically unhealthy counter parts suggesting that over time, they too will develop CVD [25,26]. Additionally, the conversion of MHO to the higher risk MUO over time may explain this effect, as in 2 studies, MHO was seen to convert to MUO in 34.2% [27] and >50% of subjects over prolonged follow-up [28].

In contrast to these data, mortality risk in MHO individuals in NHANES III who were followed for approximately 15 years was determined to be similar to that of MHNW individuals [25]. However, the NHANES study had a relatively small number of subjects classified as MHO (A total of 40 MHO out of 1160 obese) as compared to the Kramer analysis, which may have limited their ability to exclude a relationship.

Interestingly, in the Kramer meta-analysis [24], those who were overweight and metabolically healthy (distinct from obese and metabolically healthy) did not seem to have a higher risk of mortality or CVD events. This again is in favor with the "delayed injury" hypothesis, as the overweight individuals may progress to obesity over time, gaining the risk profile of that population, which would require a longer follow-up to detect this difference.

Having established that the MHO was associated with increased all-cause mortality and/or CVD risk, Kramer et al. [24] further studied the effect of metabolic status across obesity groups by comparing the MUO and MU-overweight groups with the MUNW group. They noted no significant differences in mortality or CVD risk between these three groups. This is highly indicative of the relative importance of metabolic dysfunction and obesity in creating disease, in that it may be reasonable to consider metabolic dysfunction as the major contributor or primary risk factor for CVD, with obesity being a secondary or "enabling" risk factor, in that the absence of metabolic derangements seems to be more protective for mortality and CVD risk as compared to the absence of obesity (Figure 2).

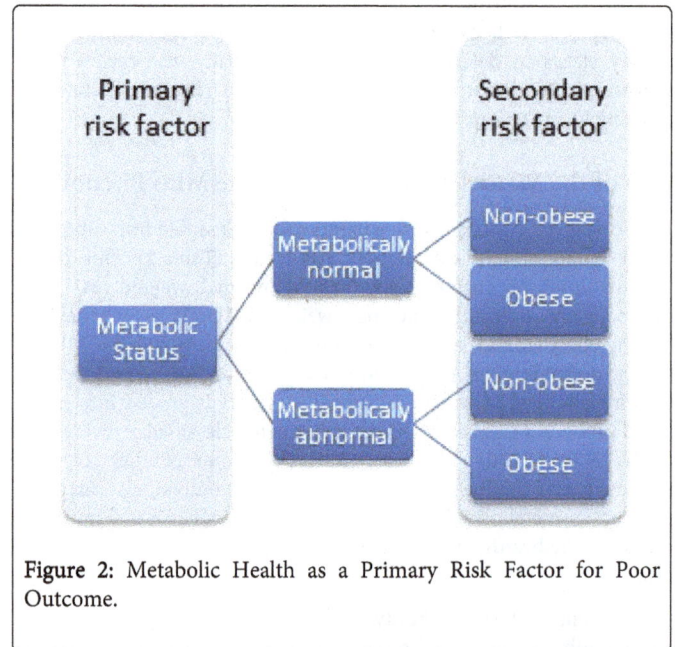

Figure 2: Metabolic Health as a Primary Risk Factor for Poor Outcome.

Alternatively, it may be reasonable to think of obesity as another "metabolic" risk factor rather than a means of primary stratification, a concept embraced in the unified diagnostic criteria for metabolic syndrome. This notion is supported by their observation that the MUNW group had a high overall risk (OR: 3.14), which was comparable to that of the MHO group. This is supported by data from the NHANES study [24], which documented an increased risk in MUNW individuals.

Regardless of the relative importance of metabolic status or obesity, the Kramer analysis and other data [20,29] demonstrate that the MHO phenotype is far from benign and does confer considerable increased risk for CVD and mortality, albeit possibly less than the risk conferred by the presence of both obesity and metabolic dysfunction.

MHO and Subclinical Atherosclerotic Disease

Although a consensus has not been reached in literature, a number of studies have demonstrated an increase in subclinical CVD in the MHO group (Table 4) [26,27,30-35].

Author, Year	N	Results
Marini et al., 2007 [34]	153	↑ CCA-IMT in MHO (0.79) vs MHNW (0.61), p<0.001
Lind et al. 2011 [33]	1016	↓vasoreactivity, ↑ echolucent carotid artery wall, ↑ left ventricular mass and function, impaired coagulation/fibrinolysis in MHO vs MHNW (P<0.05 to 0.001)
Wildman et al., 2011 [35]	1889	↑ CRP, IL-6 in MHO vs. MHNW
Khan et al., 2011 [32]	3302	↑ CCA-IMT, CAC, aPWV in MHO vs. MHNW
Heianza et al., 2014 [27]	29564	↑ odds of developing diabetes (OR: 2.32;1.50-3.59) in MHO vs MHNW over 5 years follow-up. This was attenuated after adjusting for fatty liver, however, MHO with fatty liver was associated with ↑ odds of incident diabetes.
Jung et al., 2014 [31]	4009	↑ abnormal MDCT findings (coronary artery stenosis, any plaque, calcified plaque, mixed plaque, CAC>0, and CAC>100) in MHO vs MHNW
Shaharyar et al., 2015 [26]	5519	↑ prevalence of hsCRP ≥ 3 and hepatic steatosis in MHO vs MHNW
Indulekha et al., 2015 [30]	1304	↑ CRP, TNF-α, IL-6, MCP in MHO vs MHNW.
MCP: Monocyte Chemoattractant Protein, CRP: C-Reactive Protein, Hscrp: High Sensitivity C: Reactive Protein, CCA-IMT: Common Carotid Artery Intima Media Thickness, CAC: Coronary Artery Calcification, Apwv: Aortic Pulse Wave Velocity, MDCT: Multiple Detector Computerized Tomograph		

Table 4: Biological and Clinical Associations of the MHO phenotype – Summary of Selected Literature.

Roberson et al. [20], in a review, examined four studies reporting a mean difference in common carotid artery intima media thickness (CCA-IMT) between MHO and MHNW individuals, of which two reported significantly higher levels in the MHO. However, in the two studies that did not attain statistical significance, the mean CCA-IMT tended to be higher in the MHO group as compared to the MHNW.

Heianza et al. [27] demonstrated that MHO phenotype had a higher prevalence of hepatic steatosis (47.8% vs 11.3%, p<0.01) as compared to MHNW participants. The MHO phenotype was associated with higher odds of hepatic steatosis in age and gender adjusted models (OR: 6.70; 95% CI 5.62-7.99). After development of hepatic steatosis (HS), MHO+ hepatic steatosis was associated with increased odds of incident diabetes. Similarly, Shaharyar et al. [26] documented an increased prevalence and odds of hepatic steatosis in the MHO group as compared to the MHNW group (40% vs 8%, p<0.001 and OR: 5.80; 95% CI 4.72–7.13, respectively).

Lind et al. [33] examined 1016 individuals and found an increased subclinical atherosclerotic disease burden as assessed by a variety of markers in MHO versus the MHNW groups. Wildman et al. [35], and Indulekha et al. [30] demonstrated an increased inflammatory burden in patients with MHO. Khan et al. [32], demonstrated that in a series of 3302 participants, the MHO phenotype was associated with significantly altered carotid intima media thickness, coronary artery calcification and aortic pulse wave velocity in MHO patients as compared to their normal weight counterparts.

Among the various subclinical disease markers used to determine CVD risk, coronary artery calcification is perhaps the most robust in terms of predicting future CVD risk. CAC scores have been shown to consistently provide prognostic information above and beyond traditional cardiovascular risk factors [36-39] and CAC scoring is now incorporated into the AHA/ACCF clinical guidelines [40] for risk stratification in patients with indeterminate risk. Khan et al. [32] demonstrated that women with MHO were twice as likely to have coronary calcification (OR: 2.30; 95% CI 1.20-4.70, p=0.013) compared to MHNW women. Jung et al. [31] examined 4009 individuals with multidetector CT scanning and found a significantly higher prevalence of coronary calcification (OR: 1.38; 95% CI 1.04-1.82), and significantly higher prevalence of severe coronary calcification (OR: 1.69; 95% CI 1.03-2.78) in MHO versus MHNW. Chang et al. [41] assessed CAC in a large sample (n=14828) of young Korean adults free from hypertension or diabetes. They demonstrated that MHO was associated with increased CAC scores in multivariate analysis (OR: 2.26; 95% CI 1.48–3.43), however adjustment for fasting blood glucose, systolic blood pressure, triglyceride levels, HDL-C, and HOMA-IR slightly reduced the associations, but they remained statistically significant. Further adjustment for LDL-C markedly attenuated the association between MHO and CAC, so that it was no longer statistically significant. The authors concluded that although MHO was associated with CAC, the relationship was mediated by metabolic risk factors, which is in line with our proposed distinction of primary and secondary risk factors in the previous section.

In summary, the MHO phenotype seems to be associated with a variety of markers of subclinical atherosclerotic disease, ranging from inflammatory "risk factors" to imaging techniques assessing subclinical atherosclerotic burden. However, the studies on carotid intima media thickness and MHO remain inconclusive, with some in favor, while others finding no association. Therefore we caution the reader against assuming this association to be evident in all cases, especially regarding carotid intima media thickness and the MHO phenotype. However, to the best of our knowledge, only three studies assessing coronary calcification have been reported in the literature, of which two demonstrated a significant association between MHO and CAC, whereas the third demonstrated an association only in unadjusted and partially adjusted models. This, coupled with the variety of markers that have been linked with MHO and CVD, offer reasonable evidence of increased subclinical disease burden in this population.

The Role of Physical Fitness: The Fit/Fat Phenotype

A wealth of evidence has linked decreased cardiorespiratory fitness (CRF) with increased all-cause mortality and worse health outcomes [42-44]. Interestingly, two systematic reviews [42,43] examined the association of cardiorespiratory fitness with cardiovascular and all-cause mortality, and both demonstrated that CRF was associated with a reduction in mortality, independently of BMI status. A recent meta-

analysis performed by Barry et al. [44] lends further support to these findings. Barry et al. [44] pooled data from 10 studies (N=92,986), and demonstrated that those who were overweight but fit, did not have a statistically significant increased mortality risk (OR: 1.13; 95% CI 1.00–1.27) as compared to normal weight, fit individuals. Similarly, obese but fit individuals did not have an increased risk of mortality as compared to their normal weight, fit counterparts (OR: 1.21; 95% CI 0.95–1.52). In agreement with these findings, Ortega et al. [45] noted that MHO (after accounting for physical fitness levels) was not associated with increased mortality as compared to the MHNW.

A little reflection on these results yields the following points of interest. Firstly, these findings fit with the model that obesity per se may not be a primary risk factor for the development of CVD, but may instead have a secondary or permissive role (Figure 3).

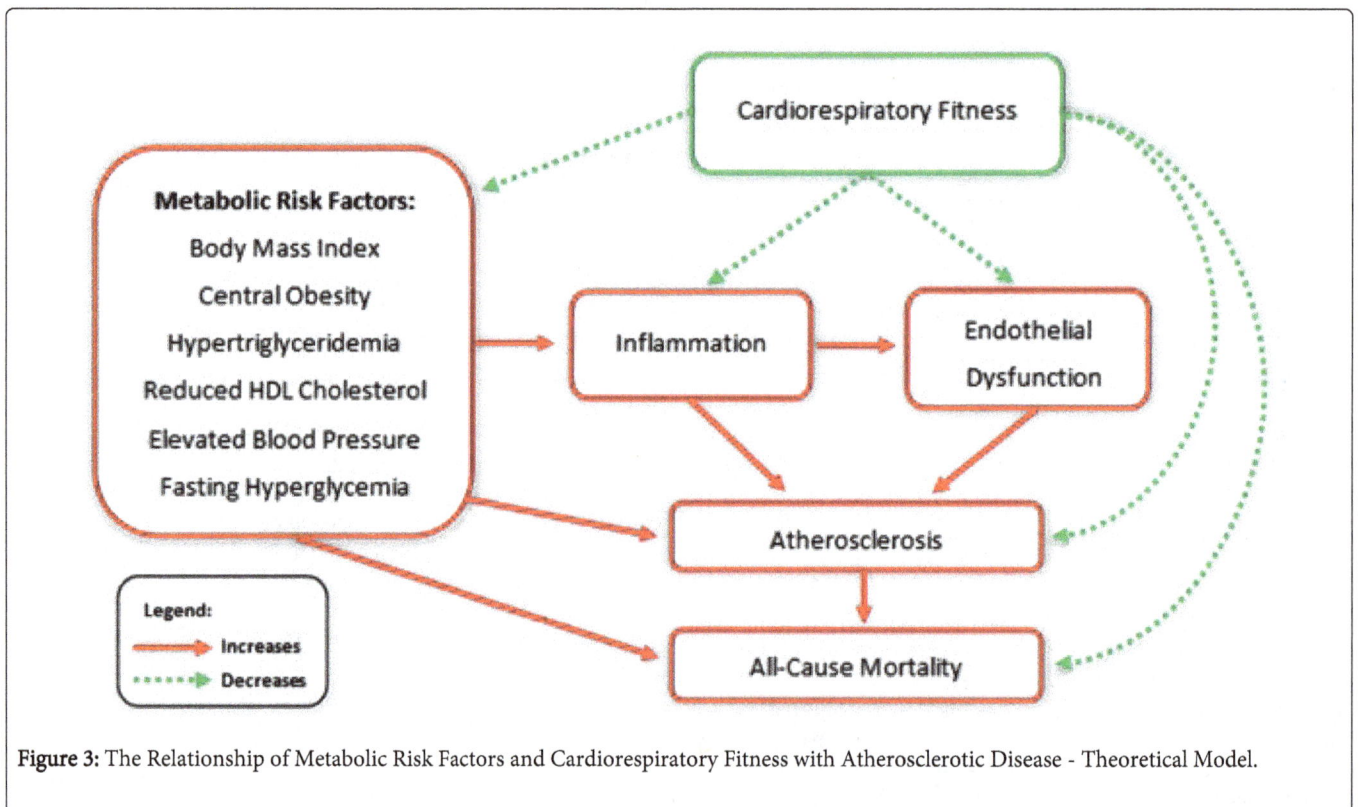

Figure 3: The Relationship of Metabolic Risk Factors and Cardiorespiratory Fitness with Atherosclerotic Disease - Theoretical Model.

Indeed, the finding that CRF completely mitigates the increased mortality risk in this population lends support to this claim. Secondly, this raises important considerations for the utility of physical activity and physical fitness levels – i.e., does adoption of increased physical activity levels impact mortality, obesity and metabolic health?

Of these questions, perhaps the easiest to answer is the relationship of physical activity with mortality. The notion that improved physical activity levels are associated with decreased mortality and improved health outcomes is self-evident and well documented [46-48]. Regarding the second question, achieving sustained significant weight loss by lifestyle changes is a highly variable intervention with a wide range of results. Although initially accompanied with a significant reduction in weight, most participants tend to regain lost weight over the subsequent years. A meta-analysis by Dombrowski et al. [49] demonstrated that lifestyle changes with or without drug therapy was associated with small, but significant sustained weight reduction over a 24-month period. This was in line with a previous analysis by Galani et

al. [50]. Similarly, a meta-analysis by Baillot et al. [51] demonstrated that long-term lifestyle interventions achieved a weight loss of 11.3 kg in those with Class II or III obesity. All three of these analyses further demonstrated that physical activity lifestyle changes were associated with improvements in metabolic risk profiles (waist circumference, fasting glucose, serum lipids, blood pressure) to varying degrees.

However, an analysis by Harrington et al. [52] demonstrated that intentional weight loss in the MHO was not associated with reductions in risk of mortality. A re-analysis of the Framingham Heart Study and the Tecumseh Community Study suggested that weight loss due to reduction in body fat may reduce all-cause mortality whereas weight loss as a result of a reduction in lean body mass may increase it [53]. These data underscore the fallacy of chasing weight goals while ignoring the method used to achieve it. Given this and the preceding data, the importance of including physical activity and fitness-based strategies in weight reduction cannot be understated.

Although the meta-analysis by Kramer et al. [24] noted an increased CVD risk in MHO individuals, that analysis was conducted on unadjusted data, which did not account for the impact of physical activity. The analysis by Barry et al. [44] and by Kramer et al. [24] cannot therefore be directly compared. Synthesis of these disparate viewpoints into a unified message for clinical practice remains an area of active research. In summary, current data suggests, with caveats, that improved physical activity and fitness is associated with

a) Reductions in weight,

b) Reductions in nearly all metabolic risk factors and

c) Reduction in all-cause mortality.

Putting it all Together – Conclusions

The present review demonstrates that the MHO phenotype may not be a benign condition, as it is associated with increased mortality and with measures of subclinical cardiovascular disease. However, the issue of physical fitness and its impact on MHO risk has not yet been conclusively settled. At the same time, the MHO phenotype is noted to be associated with increased physical activity/fitness levels as compared to the MUO, lending support to the claim that physical activity/fitness is involved in the risk in these groups. Furthermore, given the demonstrated utility of physical fitness/activity in reducing obesity, metabolic derangements and mortality, improving physical activity levels should be an essential component of any therapeutic or prevention efforts.

Implications for research

We reiterate the findings of previous reports emphasizing the need for adherence to uniform criteria for defining metabolic syndrome and its associated phenotypes in order to facilitate direct comparison of results. Secondly, we note the relative lack of literature assessing the relationship of MHO with subclinical disease parameters in the context of physical activity/fitness levels and we advocate inclusion of a physical fitness model into the definition of the metabolic syndrome. Thirdly, we note the need for longitudinal studies assessing both metabolic status and physical activity according to unified criteria to reconcile the differences observed in the meta-analyses cited in our commentary.

Implications for clinical practice

The absence of metabolic abnormalities should not reassure physicians regarding the CVD risk of their patients; instead efforts should be directed to reverse this condition. The authors recommend "chasing labs and weight" rather than "chasing weight" when setting goals for patients, since the benefits of improved physical activity and fitness extend beyond those of simple weight reduction. Bearing in mind that individuals with MHO may commonly have one metabolic abnormality, preventive goals should be aimed at both reducing weight and reducing metabolic derangements, for which physical activity seems ideally suited. The authors advise against setting treatment goals solely on weight, since elimination of obesity without elimination of corresponding metabolic risk factors would reclassify patients into the MUNW group, which has a mortality risk which is comparable to that of the MHO.

References

1. World Health Statistics by World Health Organization. 2014; http://apps.who.int/iris/bitstream/10665/112738/1/9789240692671_eng.pdf

2. Ogden CL, Carroll MD, Kit BK, Flegal KM (2014) Prevalence of childhood and adult obesity in the United States, 2011-2012. JAMA 311: 806-814.

3. Flegal KM, Kit BK, Orpana H, Graubard BI (2013) Association of all-cause mortality with overweight and obesity using standard body mass index categories: a systematic review and meta-analysis. JAMA 309: 71-82.

4. Vague J (1947) La différenciation sexuelle, facteur determinant des formes de l'obésité. (Sexual differentiation as a factor determining the forms of obesity). Presse Med 30: 339-340.

5. Alberti KG, Eckel RH, Grundy SM, (2009) Harmonizing the metabolic syndrome: a joint interim statement of the International Diabetes Federation Task Force on Epidemiology and Prevention; National Heart, Lung, and Blood Institute; American Heart Association; World Heart Federation; International Atherosclerosis Society; and International Association for the Study of Obesity. Circulation 120: 1640-1645.

6. Sims EA (2001) Are there persons who are obese, but metabolically healthy? Metabolism 50: 1499-1504.

7. Karelis AD, St-Pierre DH, Conus F, Rabasa-Lhoret R, Poehlman ET (2004) Metabolic and body composition factors in subgroups of obesity: what do we know? J Clin Endocrinol Metab 89: 2569-2575.

8. Karelis AD, Faraj M, Bastard JP, St-Pierre DH, Brochu M, et al. (2005) The metabolically healthy but obese individual presents a favorable inflammation profile. J Clin Endocrinol Metab 90: 4145-4150.

9. Meigs JB, Wilson PW, Fox CS, Vasan RS, Nathan DM, et al. (2006) Body mass index, metabolic syndrome, and risk of type 2 diabetes or cardiovascular disease. J Clin Endocrinol Metab 91: 2906-2912.

10. Karelis AD (2008) Metabolically healthy but obese individuals. Lancet 372: 1281-1283.

11. Blüher M (2010) The distinction of metabolically 'healthy' from 'unhealthy' obese individuals. Curr Opin Lipidol 21: 38-43.

12. Primeau V, Coderre L, Karelis AD, Brochu M, Lavoie ME, et al. (2011) Characterizing the profile of obese patients who are metabolically healthy. Int J Obes (Lond) 35: 971-981.

13. Karelis AD (2011) To be obese--does it matter if you are metabolically healthy? Nat Rev Endocrinol 7: 699-700.

14. Ruderman N, Chisholm D, Pi-Sunyer X, Schneider S (1998) The metabolically obese, normal-weight individual revisited. Diabetes 47: 699-713.

15. Conus F, Allison DB, Rabasa-Lhoret R, St-Onge M, St-Pierre DH, et al. (2004) Metabolic and behavioral characteristics of metabolically obese but normal-weight women. J Clin Endocrinol Metab 89: 5013-5020.

16. Succurro E, Marini MA, Frontoni S, Hribal ML, Andreozzi F, et al. (2008) Insulin secretion in metabolically obese, but normal weight, and in metabolically healthy but obese individuals. Obesity (Silver Spring) 16: 1881-1886.

17. Lee K (2009) Metabolically obese but normal weight (MONW) and metabolically healthy but obese (MHO) phenotypes in Koreans: characteristics and health behaviors. Asia Pac J Clin Nutr 18: 280-284.

18. Lee SH, Han K, Yang HK, Kim MK, Yoon KH, et al. (2015) Identifying subgroups of obesity using the product of triglycerides and glucose: the Korea National Health and Nutrition Examination Survey, 2008-2010. Clin Endocrinol (Oxf) 82: 213-220.

19. Du T, Yu X, Zhang J, Sun X (2015) Lipid accumulation product and visceral adiposity index are effective markers for identifying the metabolically obese normal-weight phenotype. Acta Diabetol.

20. Roberson LL, Aneni EC, Maziak W (2014) Beyond BMI: The "Metabolically healthy obese" phenotype & its association with clinical/subclinical cardiovascular disease and all-cause mortality -- a systematic review. BMC Public Health.

21. Pataky Z, Bobbioni-Harsch E, Golay A (2010) Open questions about metabolically normal obesity. Int J Obes (Lond) 34 Suppl 2: S18-23.

22. Seo MH, Rhee EJ (2014) Metabolic and cardiovascular implications of a metabolically healthy obesity phenotype. Endocrinol Metab (Seoul) 29: 427-434.

23. Wildman RP, Muntner P, Reynolds K (2008) The obese without cardiometabolic risk factor clustering and the normal weight with cardiometabolic risk factor clustering: prevalence and correlates of 2 phenotypes among the US population. Arch Intern Med 168: 1617-1624.

24. Kramer CK, Zinman B, Retnakaran R (2013) Are metabolically healthy overweight and obesity benign conditions?: A systematic review and meta-analysis. Ann Intern Med 159: 758-769.

25. Durward CM, Hartman TJ, Nickols-Richardson SM (2012) All-cause mortality risk of metabolically healthy obese individuals in NHANES III. J Obes 2012: 460321.

26. Shaharyar S, Roberson L, Jamal O (2015) Obesity and Metabolic Phenotypes (Metabolically Healthy and Unhealthy Variants) Are Significantly Associated with Prevalence of Elevated C-Reactive Protein and Hepatic Steatosis in a Large Healthy Brazilian Population. Journal of Obesity.

27. Heianza Y, Kato K, Kodama S (2014) Risk of the development of Type 2 diabetes in relation to overall obesity, abdominal obesity and the clustering of metabolic abnormalities in Japanese individuals: does metabolically healthy overweight really exist? The Niigata Wellness Study. Diabet Med.

28. Eshtiaghi R, Keihani S, Hosseinpanah F, Barzin M, Azizi F (2015) Natural course of metabolically healthy abdominal obese adults after 10 years of follow-up: the Tehran Lipid and Glucose Study. Int J Obes (Lond) 39: 514-519.

29. Kuk JL, Ardern CI (2009) Are metabolically normal but obese individuals at lower risk for all-cause mortality? Diabetes Care 32: 2297-2299.

30. Indulekha K, Surendar J, Anjana RM, Geetha L, Gokulakrishnan K, et al. (2015) Metabolic obesity, adipocytokines, and inflammatory markers in Asian Indians--CURES-124. Diabetes Technol Ther 17: 134-141.

31. Jung CH, Lee MJ, Hwang JY, Jang JE, Leem J, et al. (2014) Association of metabolically healthy obesity with subclinical coronary atherosclerosis in a Korean population. Obesity (Silver Spring) 22: 2613-2620.

32. Khan UI, Wang D, Thurston RC, Sowers M, Sutton-Tyrrell K, et al. (2011) Burden of subclinical cardiovascular disease in "metabolically benign" and "at-risk" overweight and obese women: the Study of Women's Health Across the Nation (SWAN). Atherosclerosis 217: 179-186.

33. Lind L, Siegbahn A, Ingelsson E, Sundström J, Arnlöv J (2011) A detailed cardiovascular characterization of obesity without the metabolic syndrome. Arterioscler Thromb Vasc Biol 31: e27-34.

34. Marini MA, Succurro E, Frontoni S (2007) Metabolically healthy but obese women have an intermediate cardiovascular risk profile between healthy nonobese women and obese insulin-resistant women. Diabetes Care: 2145-2147.

35. Wildman RP, Kaplan R, Manson JE, Rajkovic A, Connelly SA, et al. (2011) Body size phenotypes and inflammation in the Women's Health Initiative Observational Study. Obesity (Silver Spring) 19: 1482-1491.

36. Detrano R, Guerci AD, Carr JJ, Bild DE, Burke G, et al. (2008) Coronary calcium as a predictor of coronary events in four racial or ethnic groups. N Engl J Med 358: 1336-1345.

37. Erbel R, Mohlenkamp S, Moebus S (2010) Coronary risk stratification, discrimination, and reclassification improvement based on quantification of subclinical coronary atherosclerosis: the Heinz Nixdorf Recall study. J Am Coll Cardiol 56: 1397-1406.

38. Polonsky TS, McClelland RL, Jorgensen NW, Bild DE, Burke GL, et al. (2010) Coronary artery calcium score and risk classification for coronary heart disease prediction. JAMA 303: 1610-1616.

39. Nasir K, Shaw LJ, Budoff MJ, Ridker PM, Peña JM (2012) Coronary artery calcium scanning should be used for primary prevention: pros and cons. JACC Cardiovasc Imaging 5: 111-118.

40. Greenland P, Alpert JS, Beller GA (2010) ACCF/AHA guideline for assessment of cardiovascular risk in asymptomatic adults: a report of the American College of Cardiology Foundation/American Heart Association Task Force on Practice Guidelines. Circulation.122: e584-636.

41. Chang Y, Kim BK, Yun KE, Cho J, Zhang Y, et al. (2014) Metabolically-healthy obesity and coronary artery calcification. J Am Coll Cardiol 63: 2679-2686.

42. Fogelholm M (2010) Physical activity, fitness and fatness: relations to mortality, morbidity and disease risk factors. A systematic review. Obes Rev 11: 202-221.

43. Pedersen BK (2007) Body mass index-independent effect of fitness and physical activity for all-cause mortality. Scand J Med Sci Sports 17: 196-204.

44. Barry V, Baruth M, Beets MW, Durstine JL, Liu J, et al. (2014) Fitness vs. fatness on all-cause mortality: a meta-analysis. Prog Cardiovasc Dis 56: 382-390.

45. Ortega FB, Lee DC, Katzmarzyk PT, Ruiz JR, Sui X, et al. (2013) The intriguing metabolically healthy but obese phenotype: cardiovascular prognosis and role of fitness. Eur Heart J 34: 389-397.

46. Samitz G, Egger M, Zwahlen M (2011) Domains of physical activity and all-cause mortality: systematic review and dose-response meta-analysis of cohort studies. Int J Epidemiol 40: 1382-1400.

47. Woodcock J, Franco OH, Orsini N, Roberts I (2011) Non-vigorous physical activity and all-cause mortality: systematic review and meta-analysis of cohort studies. Int J Epidemiol 40: 121-138.

48. Löllgen H, Böckenhoff A, Knapp G (2009) Physical activity and all-cause mortality: an updated meta-analysis with different intensity categories. Int J Sports Med 30: 213-224.

49. Dombrowski SU, Knittle K, Avenell A, Araújo-Soares V, Sniehotta FF (2014) Long term maintenance of weight loss with non-surgical interventions in obese adults: systematic review and meta-analyses of randomised controlled trials. BMJ 348: g2646.

50. Galani C, Schneider H (2007) Prevention and treatment of obesity with lifestyle interventions: review and meta-analysis. Int J Public Health 52: 348-359.

51. Baillot AO, Romain AJ, Boisvert-Vigneault K, Audet M, Baillargeon JP, et al. (2015) Effects of Lifestyle Interventions That Include a Physical Activity Component in Class II and III Obese Individuals: A Systematic Review and Meta-Analysis. PLoS One 10: e0119017.

52. Harrington M, Gibson S, Cottrell RC (2009) A review and meta-analysis of the effect of weight loss on all-cause mortality risk. Nutr Res Rev 22: 93-108.

53. Allison DB, Zannolli R, Faith MS, Heo M, Pietrobelli A, et al. (1999) Weight loss increases and fat loss decreases all-cause mortality rate: results from two independent cohort studies. Int J Obes Relat Metab Disord 23: 603-611.

8

Leptin Inhibits Preproinsulin mRNA Expression Induced by Suppression of Cytokine Signalling 3 in Beta-Cells

Jiaqiang Zhou[1]*, Jiahua Wu[1], Fengqin Dong[2], Zhe Zhang[2], Fang Wu[1] and Hong Li[1]

[1]Department of Endocrinology, Sir Run Run Shaw Hospital, Zhejiang University School of Medicine, Hangzhou, 310016, China

[2]Department of Endocrinology, The First Affiliated Hospital, Zhejiang University School of Medicine, Hangzhou, 310003, China

*Corresponding author: Jiaqiang Zhou, Department of Endocrinology, Sir Run Run Shaw Hospital, Zhejiang University, School of Medicine, 3 East Qingchun Road, Hangzhou, 310016, Zhejiang, China; E-mail: zhoujq27@foxmail.com

Abstract

Aim: To study the role of crosstalk between SOCS3 and leptin on insulin expression in rat insulinoma (RIN-5AH) cells that inducibly express SOCS3 mRNA.

Materials and Methods: SOCS3 and preproinsulin mRNA expression induced by 5 µM ponasterone A, and the effects of leptin on SOCS3 and preproinsulin mRNA levels were detected by RT-PCR and quantitative PCR, respectively. The effects of SOCS3 on STAT3 phosphorylation were investigated by Western blot analysis.

Results: We discovered that SOCS3 regulates preproinsulin mRNA levels in a dose-dependent and time-dependent manner. The insulin-suppressing effect of leptin appears to be mediated through reducing the suppressive effects of SOCS3 on STAT3 phosphorylation.

Conclusion: Our findings suggest that leptin inhibits preproinsulin mRNA expression induced by SOCS3 in RIN-5AH beta-cells.

Keywords: Leptin; Insulin; SOCS3; Beta-cells

Introduction

Obesity is a major cause of the increasing morbidity and mortality associated with diseases such as type-2 diabetes and cardiovascular disease. Leptin and insulin, which are key hormones involved in the regulation of energy production and glucose homeostasis, play roles in the pathogenesis of type-2 diabetes. On binding to the long form of the leptin receptor (LRb), leptin induces STAT3 phosphorylation, which subsequently regulates the expression of certain genes [1]. Dysfunctional mutations in leptin or its receptor in rodents and humans result in severe obesity, insulin resistance, and endocrine dysfunction [2-4].

Suppressor of cytokine signaling (SOCS) proteins are key negative regulators of cytokine signaling that inhibit the JAK/STAT signal transduction pathway [5]. SOCS3 negatively regulates the expression of multiple hormones and cytokines including TNF-α and IL-6 [6,7]. SOCS3 has also been reported to affect the signaling of both leptin and insulin. SOCS3 does not alter the levels of the leptin receptor but binds to Tyr985 on the receptor to suppress STAT3 signaling [8,9]. Heterozygous SOCS3 knockout mice (SOCS3+/-) display higher leptin sensitivity than wild-type mice. In response to leptin administration, these mice lose weight and exhibit hypothalamic leptin receptor signaling [10]. SOCS3 has also been shown to regulate insulin signaling. SOCS3 binds to Tyr960 on the insulin receptor and prevents STAT5b activation in adipocytes [11]. Using an adipocyte model derived from fibroblasts of wild-type and SOCS3-deficient mouse embryos, Shi et al. investigated the role of endogenous SOCS3 in insulin signaling. SOCS3 deficiency leads to increased insulin-

stimulated glucose uptake in adipocytes [12]. Shi et al. also established a transgenic mouse model in which SOCS3 was overexpressed in adipocytes. Overexpression of SOCS3 results in reduced glucose uptake and lipogenesis in adipocytes [13]. Thus, given its regulatory effects in both the leptin and insulin pathways, SOCS3 is likely to be a key node in the crosstalk between the leptin and insulin signaling cascades.

In this study, we investigated the role of crosstalk between SOCS3 and leptin in insulin expression. We discovered that SOCS3 regulates preproinsulin mRNA levels in a dose- and time-dependent manner. Leptin has been shown to suppress insulin expression by inhibiting the expression of SOCS3. Thus, these findings imply that SOCS3 plays a key role in mediating the interaction between the leptin and insulin pathways.

Materials and methods

Antibodies and reagents

Zeocin and ponasterone A were purchased from Invitrogen (Carlsbad, CA, USA). G418 was purchased from Calbiochem (Darmstadt, Germany). The anti-STAT3 and anti-pSTAT3 antibodies were both purchased from Upstate (Lake Placid, NY, USA). Leptin was purchased from R&D Systems (Minneapolis, MN, USA). Taq DNA polymerase was purchased from Promega (Madison, WI, USA). TRIzol reagent was purchased from Sigma (St. Louis, MO, USA). Cell lysis buffer (RIPA) was purchased from Beyotime (Jiangsu, China).

Beta-cell-derived stable cell line

RIN-5AH cells stably transfected with inducible SOCS3 (gift from Prof. Billestrup) [14] were cultured in RPMI-1640 medium supplemented with 10% heat-inactivated fetal calf serum, glutamax, 100 U/ml penicillin, 100 μg/ml streptomycin, 400 μg/ml zeocin, and 150 μg/ml G418 at 37°C in a humidified atmosphere containing 5% CO2. The cells were tested for ponasterone A-induced SOCS3 expression by RT-PCR.

Reverse-transcription PCR

Cells were cultured in a 6-well plate to 80% confluence and then treated with 5 μM ponasterone A for 48 h. Total RNA was isolated with TRIzol reagent. SOCS3 mRNA was amplified by reverse-transcription PCR. The 40 μl DNA amplification reactions contains 4 μl 10 x reaction buffer, 25 mM $MgCl_2$, 10 mM dNTP, 5 unit Taq DNA polymerase, 4 μlc DNA and 0.5 ul each of the primers. The reaction was denatured for 3 min at 94°C and subjected to 3-step amplification cycles with denaturation at 94°C for 15 sec, annealing at 57°C for 20 sec and extend at 60°C for 1 min. To amplify GAPDH gene, PCR program was cycled for 35 times. To amplify SOCS3 gene, PCR program was cycled for 30 times. The primer sequences were: SOCS3 forward, 5'-GGGCCCCTTCCTTTTCTTTAC-3'; SOCS3 reverse, 5'-GTCCAGGAACTCCCGAATG-3'; GAPDH forward, 5'-GTCGGTGTGAACGGATTT-3'; GAPDH reverse, 5'-ACTCCACGACGTACTCAGC-3'. PCR products were resolved on agarose gels, and bands were quantified using the BioSens Gel Imaging System.

Quantitative PCR

Cells were cultured in 6-well plates to 80% confluence and treated with 5 μM ponasterone A and the indicated agents. Total RNA was isolated using the TRIzol reagent. The level of preproinsulinm RNA was quantified by real-time PCR. The GAPDH mRNA level was used as an internal control. Real-time PCR was performed using the ABI 7000 system (Applied Biosystems, Foster City, CA, USA) according to the manufacturer's protocol. The primer sequences were: preproinsulin forward, 5'-CAACATGGCCCTGTGGATGC-3'; preproinsulin reverse, 5'-TACAGAGCCTCCACCAGGTG-3'; preproinsulin probe, 5'-FAM-CCTGCTGGCCCTGCTCGTCCTCT-TAMRA-3'; GAPDH forward, 5'-GACAGCCGCATCTTCTTG-3'; GAPDH reverse, 5'-GGCAACAATGTCCACTTTG-3'; GAPDH probe, 5'-FAM-CAGTGCCAGCCTCG-BHQ1-3'.

Western blotting

Cells were grown in 10-cm dishes to 80% confluence and then cultured in the presence of 5 μM ponasterone A for 46 h. The cells were washed twice with Krebs-Ringer buffer (140 mM NaCl, 3.6 mM KCl, 0.5 mM NaH_2PO_4, 0.5 mM $MgSO_4$, 1.5 mM $CaCl_2$, 10 mM HEPES, 2 mM $NaHCO_3$, and 0.1% BSA [pH 7.4]) and incubated in the same buffer for 2 h. The cells were then stimulated by treatment with 10 nM leptin for 30 min. To prepare protein extracts, cells were washed with cold PBS twice and lysed in RIPA. After centrifugation at 13,000 rpm for 10 min, the supernatants were collected. Protein concentration was measured using the BCA Protein Assay Kit from Pierce. Proteins were separated by electrophoresis in an 8% PAGE gel. Bands were visualized using the Super Signal West Femto Maximum Sensitivity Substrate from Pierce and a Kodak X-ray film.

Statistical analysis

Data are presented as mean ± SEM. Statistical differences between the various groups were determined using Student's t-test or ANOVA. P-values less than 0.05 were considered to indicate statistical significance.

Results

Ponasterone A induces SOCS3 expression in RIN-5AH cells

The RIN-5AH beta-cell line was used to establish cells that inducible express the SOCS3 protein [14]. To validate this inducible expression system, cells were incubated with various concentrations of ponasterone A, and the expression of SOCS3 mRNA was measured by RT-PCR as a function of time. As shown in Figure 1, the SOCS3 induction was dose- and time- dependent. The maximum expression of SOCS3 mRNA was observed in the presence of 5 μM ponasteroneA after 24 h of stimulation. Under these conditions, the levels of SOCS3 mRNA were 4.4-fold higher than those in untreated cells (p<0.05).

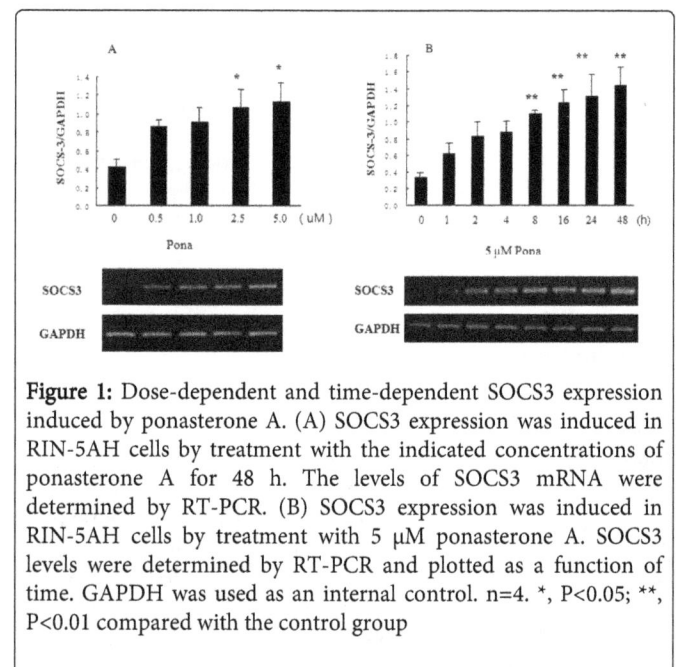

Figure 1: Dose-dependent and time-dependent SOCS3 expression induced by ponasterone A. (A) SOCS3 expression was induced in RIN-5AH cells by treatment with the indicated concentrations of ponasterone A for 48 h. The levels of SOCS3 mRNA were determined by RT-PCR. (B) SOCS3 expression was induced in RIN-5AH cells by treatment with 5 μM ponasterone A. SOCS3 levels were determined by RT-PCR and plotted as a function of time. GAPDH was used as an internal control. n=4. *, P<0.05; **, P<0.01 compared with the control group

SOCS3 expression enhances preproinsulin mRNA levels

Ponasterone A treatment also enhanced preproinsulin expression in the stable cell line. As shown in Figure 2, the expression of preproinsulin mRNA was dose- and time-dependent. After 8 h of treatment with 5 μM ponasterone A, we observed a significant increase in the preproinsulin mRNA levels, and the maximum effect was observed between 24 and 48 h (p<0.05). The maximum preproinsulin level was 4.4-fold higher than that of untreated cells (p<0.05). The expression of preproinsulin was strongly correlated with the expression of SOCS3.

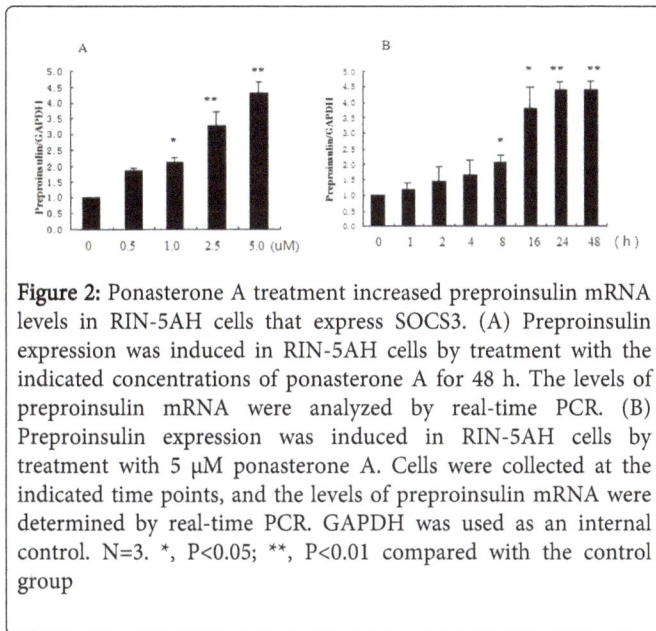

Figure 2: Ponasterone A treatment increased preproinsulin mRNA levels in RIN-5AH cells that express SOCS3. (A) Preproinsulin expression was induced in RIN-5AH cells by treatment with the indicated concentrations of ponasterone A for 48 h. The levels of preproinsulin mRNA were analyzed by real-time PCR. (B) Preproinsulin expression was induced in RIN-5AH cells by treatment with 5 μM ponasterone A. Cells were collected at the indicated time points, and the levels of preproinsulin mRNA were determined by real-time PCR. GAPDH was used as an internal control. N=3. *, $P<0.05$; **, $P<0.01$ compared with the control group

Leptin treatment inhibits the SOCS3 and preproinsulin mRNA levels

SOCS3 has been proposed to be a mediator of leptin resistance [15,16]. To further study the correlations between SOCS3, leptin, and insulin levels, the stable cell line was stimulated with ponasterone A and leptin. The SOCS3 and preproinsulin mRNA levels were measured using RT-PCR or quantitative PCR. As shown in Figure 3, in the absence of ponasterone A, under which condition SOCS3 induction was not triggered, addition of leptin did not change the preproinsulin levels.

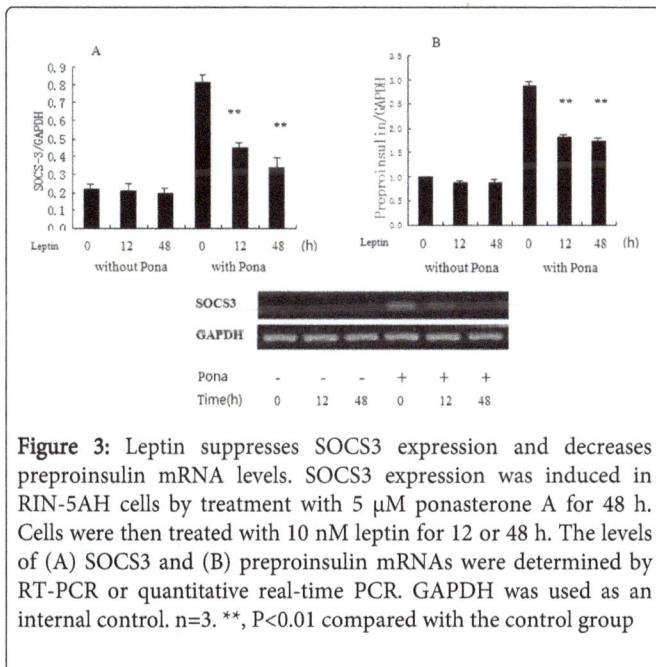

Figure 3: Leptin suppresses SOCS3 expression and decreases preproinsulin mRNA levels. SOCS3 expression was induced in RIN-5AH cells by treatment with 5 μM ponasterone A for 48 h. Cells were then treated with 10 nM leptin for 12 or 48 h. The levels of (A) SOCS3 and (B) preproinsulin mRNAs were determined by RT-PCR or quantitative real-time PCR. GAPDH was used as an internal control. n=3. **, $P<0.01$ compared with the control group

However, in the presence of ponasterone A, treatment with leptin suppressed SOCS3 as well as preproinsulin mRNA expression. The suppressive effect was time-dependent. After 10 μM leptin treatment

for 48 h, the SOCS3 mRNA level decreased by 58% and the preproinsulin mRNA level decreased by 40% relative to the levels in cells not treated with leptin ($p<0.01$). These data suggest that the suppressive effects of leptin on insulin are related to SOCS3.

Leptin reduces the suppressive effects of SOCS3 on STAT3 phosphorylation

SOCS3 has been reported to inhibit STAT3 phosphorylation [17]. As shown in Figure 4, ponasteroneA treatment of cells to induce SOCS3 expression decreased STAT3 phosphorylation. When cells induced to express SOCS3 were also treated with leptin, the STAT3 phosphorylation levels were similar to the levels in cells not treated with ponasterone A.

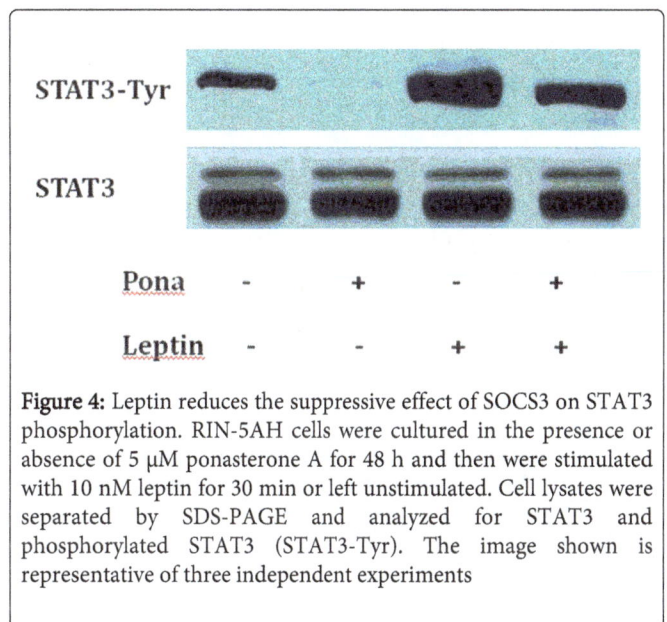

Figure 4: Leptin reduces the suppressive effect of SOCS3 on STAT3 phosphorylation. RIN-5AH cells were cultured in the presence or absence of 5 μM ponasterone A for 48 h and then were stimulated with 10 nM leptin for 30 min or left unstimulated. Cell lysates were separated by SDS-PAGE and analyzed for STAT3 and phosphorylated STAT3 (STAT3-Tyr). The image shown is representative of three independent experiments

Discussion

In this study, we used an insulin-producing beta-cell line to create an ecdysone-inducible system to mimic the interactions among leptin, SOCS3, and insulin. After incubation with ponasteroneA, exogenous SOCS3 was expressed in the beta-cell line in a dose- and time-dependent manner. The effect of ponasteroneA treatment on mRNA transcription and protein expression in these cells is well established [14]. Using this system, we investigated the effects of SOCS3 expression and leptin treatment on insulin expression. We found that SOCS3 affected the preproinsulin mRNA expression, and that treatment with leptin suppressed SOCS3 mRNA expression and decreased the preproinsulin mRNA levels.

STAT protein, which is key mediator in leptin signal transduction, is also suppressed by SOCS3 [17]. STATs have mainly been shown to transcriptionally enhance gene expression. However, Seufert et al. found that leptin increases the binding of STAT5b to the upstream sequences of the rat preproinsulin 1 promoter and inhibits insulin biosynthesis via transcriptional repression [18]. Furthermore, fructose increased SOCS3 expression, decreased STAT3 phosphorylation, increased Pdx1 and insulin gene expression, and induced hyperinsulinemia both in rats and in INS-1 cells [19]. Quercetin treatment suppressed the increased SOCS3 level, elevated the reduced STAT3 level, and improved leptin signalling, thereby protecting beta-cell function under high-fructose conditions [19]. In accordance with the previous studies, in our study, over expression of SOCS3 inhibited STAT3 phosphorylation and then increased preproinsulin mRNA expression. However, leptin decreased the SOCS3-induced preproinsulin expression through enhancement of STAT3 phosphorylation. As previously reported, SOCS3 expression reverses the stimulatory effect of growth hormones on pancreatic beta-cell proliferation and insulin secretion. Furthermore, SOCS3 protects pancreatic beta-cells from IL-1β- and IFN-γ-mediated cytotoxicity but does not alter insulin levels [14,20]. Based on these results, we propose that SOCS3 plays multiple roles in pancreatic beta-cells and that it might be an important mediator of crosstalk between the insulin and leptin pathways. As the RIN-5AH β-cell line did not induce a significant amount of insulin release with glucose, we could not investigate the effect of SOCS3 on glucose-stimulated insulin release. Further investigations that use islets from SOCS3 transgenic mice will be conducted to investigate the effect of SOCS3 on preproinsulin mRNA expression and glucose-stimulated insulin release.

Funding

This work was supported by a grant from the National Natural Science Foundation of China (No. 30400221).

References

1. Hübschle T, Thom E, Watson A, Roth J, Klaus S, et al. (2001) Leptin-induced nuclear translocation of STAT3 immunoreactivity in hypothalamic nuclei involved in body weight regulation. J Neurosci 21: 2413-2424.

2. Fischer-Posovszky P, von Schnurbein J, Moepps B, Lahr G, Strauss G, et al. (2010) A new missense mutation in the leptin gene causes mild obesity and hypogonadism without affecting T cell responsiveness. J Clin Endocrinol Metab 95: 2836-2840.

3. Mantzoros CS (1999) The role of leptin in human obesity and disease: a review of current evidence. Ann Intern Med 130: 671-680.

4. Cheung WW, Mao P (2012) Recent advances in obesity: genetics and beyond. ISRN Endocrinol 2012: 536905.

5. Murray PJ (2007) The JAK-STAT signaling pathway: input and output integration. J Immunol 178: 2623-2629.

6. Bruun C, Heding PE, Rønn SG, Frobøse H, Rhodes CJ, et al. (2009) Suppressor of cytokine signalling-3 inhibits Tumor necrosis factor-alpha induced apoptosis and signalling in beta cells. Mol Cell Endocrinol 311: 32-38.

7. Johnston JA (2004) Are SOCS suppressors, regulators, and degraders? J Leukoc Biol 75: 743-748.

8. Bjorbak C, Lavery HJ, Bates SH, Olson RK, Davis SM, et al. (2000) SOCS3 mediates feedback inhibition of the leptin receptor via Tyr985. J Biol Chem 275: 40649-40657.

9. Myers MG Jr (2004) Leptin receptor signaling and the regulation of mammalian physiology. Recent Prog Horm Res 59: 287-304.

10. Morton GJ, Schwartz MW (2011) Leptin and the central nervous system control of glucose metabolism. Physiol Rev 91: 389-411.

11. Emanuelli B, Peraldi P, Filloux C, Sawka-Verhelle D, Hilton D, et al. (2000) SOCS-3 is an insulin-induced negative regulator of insulin signaling. J Biol Chem 275: 15985-15991.

12. Shi H, Tzameli I, Bjørbaek C, Flier JS (2004) Suppressor of cytokine signaling 3 is a physiological regulator of adipocyte insulin signaling. J Biol Chem 279: 34733-34740.

13. Shi H, Cave B, Inouye K, Bjørbaek C, Flier JS (2006) Overexpression of suppressor of cytokine signaling 3 in adipose tissue causes local but not systemic insulin resistance. Diabetes 55: 699-707.

14. Rønn SG, Hansen JA, Lindberg K, Karlsen AE, Billestrup N (2002) The effect of suppressor of cytokine signaling 3 on GH signaling in beta-cells. Mol Endocrinol 16: 2124-2134.

15. Bjørbaek C, Elmquist JK, Frantz JD, Shoelson SE, Flier JS (1998) Identification of SOCS-3 as a potential mediator of central leptin resistance. Mol Cell 1: 619-625.

16. Król E, Speakman JR (2007) Regulation of body mass and adiposity in the field vole, Microtusagrestis: a model of leptin resistance. J Endocrinol 192: 271-278.

17. Dominguez E, Mauborgne A, Mallet J, Desclaux M, Pohl M (2010) SOCS3-mediated blockade of JAK/STAT3 signaling pathway reveals its major contribution to spinal cord neuroinflammation and mechanical allodynia after peripheral nerve injury. J Neurosci 30: 5754-5766.

18. Seufert J, Kieffer TJ, Habener JF (1999) Leptin inhibits insulin gene transcription and reverses hyperinsulinemia in leptin-deficient ob/ob mice. Proc Natl Acad Sci U S A 96: 674-679.

19. Li JM, Wang W, Fan CY, Wang MX, Zhang X, et al. (2013) Quercetin Preserves β-Cell Mass and Function in Fructose-Induced Hyperinsulinemia through Modulating Pancreatic Akt/FoxO1 Activation. Evid Based Complement Alternat Med 2013: 303902.

20. Karlsen AE, Rønn SG, Lindberg K, Johannesen J, Galsgaard ED, et al. (2001) Suppressor of cytokine signaling 3 (SOCS-3) protects beta -cells against interleukin-1beta - and interferon-gamma -mediated toxicity. Proc Natl Acad Sci U S A 98: 12191-12196.

9

Metabolic Disorders in HIV-infected Children Metabolic Disorders in HIV-infected Children

Spagnuolo MI[*], Liguoro I and Guarino A
Department of Translation Science of Medicine University, Federico II, Naples, Italy

[*]**Corresponding author:** Spagnuolo MI, Department of Translation Science of Medicine University, Federico II, Naples, Italy; E-mail: mispagnu@unina.it

Abstract

The introduction of highly active antiretroviral therapy (HAART) for the treatment of acquired immunodeficiency syndrome (AIDS) has resulted in greater survival of patients infected with the human immunodeficiency virus (HIV). However, the use of these drugs has been associated with lipodystrophic syndrome (LS), which is characterized by metabolic alterations (dyslipidemia, insulin resistance, diabetes, and lactic acidosis) and abnormal corporal fat distribution. Clinically, LS may manifest as three different forms: lipohypertrophy (accumulation of fat in the central part of the body), lipoatrophy (loss of fat in the extremities, face and buttocks) and mixed (lipohypertrophy + lipoatrophy). Although its physiopathology has not been elucidated, some mechanisms have been described, including leptin and adiponectin deficiency, mitochondrial dysfunction and use of antiretroviral drugs. The type, dose and duration of the antiretroviral treatment, as well as age and puberty are the main risk factors. LS are also associated with increased incidence of cardiovascular illnesses, atherosclerosis and diabetes mellitus. Follow up must be periodic, consisting of measurement of body fat distribution, evaluation of the lipid profile and insulin resistance.

Keywords: Hiv; Lipodystrophy; Highly active antiretroviral treatment; Children and adolescents

Introduction

Highly active antiretroviral therapy (HAART) has significantly improved the clinical outcome of HIV infection. However, HAART has been associated with potentially severe side effects in HIV-infected adults as well as in children. HIV-1-infected patients on HAART frequently develop a metabolic syndrome - in particular lipodystrophy syndrome (LS), which is characterised by peripheral lipoatrophy and visceral fat redistribution and is associated with metabolic alterations including dyslipidaemia, insulin resistance and cardiovascular risk [1-10]. The atherogenic profile of this syndrome may increase the risk of cardiovascular disease (CVD) even in young HIV-infected patients.

The pathophysiology of HAART-related lipodystrophy is still unknown, but the protease inhibitors (PIs) and nucleoside reverse transcriptase inhibitors (NRTIs), that are considered the mainstay of therapy, probably play a major role in this process [11-19]. It is also known that some antiretroviral molecules can inhibit differentiation and induce insulin resistance and apoptosis in adipose cells [20-26]. PIs are responsible for a decrease in cytoplasmic retinoic-acid protein-1, low-density lipoprotein receptor-related protein (LRP) and peroxisome proliferator activated receptor type-gamma (PPAR-γ) [27-32]. Instead, NRTIs and thymidine analogues cause mitochondrial dysfunction, as demonstrated by a decrease in subcutaneous adipose tissue mitochondrial DNA content. Both phenomena are responsible for a decreased differentiation of adiposities, increased levels of free fatty acids and lipoatrophy [33-41]. Even if it is now clear that the type and duration of NRTIs therapy is the dominant risk factor for the pathological changes of adipose tissue that underlie lipodystrophy [42-50], the pathogenesis of HAART-associated metabolic syndrome is complex and several other factors may be involved, such as adipocytokines leptin, adiponectin and resistin [51-109].

A better understanding of the molecular mechanisms responsible for this syndrome will lead to the discovery of new drugs that will reduce the incidence of lipodystrophy and related metabolic complications in HIV-infected patients receiving HAART.

HIV and metabolic syndrome

Evidence for the increased prevalence of disorders of glucose metabolism in HIV-infected patients was initially derived from patient cohorts with HAART-associated lipodystrophy [44-50]. One such study reported the prevalence of diabetes at 2% in PIs recipients with lipodystrophy, rising to 7% after 14 months of further observation. Other previous studies also reported high rates of disorders of glucose metabolism in HAART-associated lipodystrophy, with diabetes in 7% and impaired glucose tolerance in 35% of HIV-infected patients [110-118]. A more recent study reported a prevalence of 17% using National Cholesterol Education Program Adult Treatment Panel Three (ATP-III) criteria in 710 patients in Spain, considering several risk factors such as BMI and past or current exposure to PIs [119-125]. Prospective reports showed that 10% of HIV-infected HAART recipients developed diabetes during a four-year follow-up period. After adjusting for age and body mass index (BMI) and comparing to controls, the resulting difference represented a greater than four-fold increase in the relative risk of developing diabetes [1,126]. Potentially related complications are also represented by hypertension, nephrotic syndrome, acanthosis nigricans and polycystic ovary syndrome [127].

The effect of initiation of HAART on diabetes incidence in treatment-naive patients has been recently reported by the Data Collection on Adverse Metabolic Syndrome, with referral to the constellation of the phenotypes of abdominal obesity, hyperlipidaemia, elevated fasting glucose and hypertension [128-134]. Hyperinsulinaemia and insulin resistance can occur as a result of therapy with a PIs or as a consequence of the HIV infection. Initially, it was believed that PIs do not influence carbohydrate metabolism in pre-pubertal children due to the higher insulin sensitivity observed in this phase [135]. Nonetheless, recent studies have shown that these drugs lead to insulin resistance, both by decreasing the pancreatic beta cell response and through interference with the glucose transportation promoted by the GLUT-4 transport protein [125,135]. Therefore, treatment of HIV-infected children with PIs leads to the development of insulin resistance, similar to the situation observed in adults; the difference between the age groups is the difficulty in detecting this alteration.

The debate surrounding the predictive value of metabolic syndrome pivots around whether, as a composite, it predicts a multiplicative or additive increase in the risk of these conditions [136-139].

HIV and lipodystrophy

Lipodystrophy is observed with increasing frequency in HIV-infected adults and is considered a major public health problem because of its long-term cardiac and metabolic complications. However, there is limited information about abnormal fat distribution and complications in children. As yet, there are no well-defined criteria for the diagnosis of lipodystrophy in children [126].

The prevalence of lipodystrophy in HIV-infected children varies from 1 to 10% in the retrospective questionnaire-based surveys [129-134] and from 12 to 33% in studies conducted using anthropometry [50-110]. The frequency of lipodystrophy was determined by the sum of the three equally represented phenotypes (central lipohypertrophy, peripheral lipoatrophy and a combined pattern) and according to the European Paediatric HIV and Lipodystrophy Study Group, 46.7% of all children had clinical signs of fat redistribution [117,140].

Anthropometry can assess subcutaneous fat by measurement of skin-fold thickness in the biceps, triceps, subscapula and abdomen over the crest iliac, as well as by measurement of the circumference of the arm, leg, waist and hips. There is consensus that waist circumference is a good surrogate marker for visceral adipose tissue [1]. Jacquet defined peripheral fat wasting as facial, buttock or limb atrophy associated with arm skin-fold thickness below the third percentile of the reference values for sex and age, and truncal adiposity as breast enlargement or relative abdominal obesity with the skin-fold ratio at the trunk >2 standard deviations (SD) from the reference mean for sex and age [128-131].

The assessment of fat redistribution in HIV-infected children is also complicated by the normal dynamic alterations in body composition that occur during childhood and adolescence, therefore imaging could be considered more reliable than anthropometrics in diagnosing such modifications. Both dual-energy X-ray absorptiometry (DEXA) and abdominal magnetic resonance imaging (MRI) have been also validated to assess fat distribution in children [132-134]. DEXA provides information about regional fat distribution, but cannot be used on the face, while computed tomography (CT) and MRI scanning discriminate between subcutaneous and visceral fat and may be useful techniques for detecting facial fat changes [136,137]. Furthermore, a recent study using DEXA and MRI showed that peripheral lipoatrophy is detectable in childhood even in the absence of clinical signs of lipodystrophy and that true central obesity is present only in children with body-shape changes [129]. Although anthropometric measurements are easily obtained in children, CT represents the gold standard method for evaluation of fat distribution. However, it has several drawbacks, namely exposure to X-rays and need for sedation in infants and younger children that limit its use as a routine diagnostic tool. Therefore, it is preferable to evaluate body fat distribution in children using ultrasound rather than CT because of the lack of side effects, feasibility and lower costs [141].

The European Paediatric Lipodystrophy Group identified the following risk factors for lipodystrophy: severe clinical disease (US Centres for Disease Control and Prevention [CDS] stage C), female gender, older age, use of PIs, didehydrodeoxythymidine (d4T – stavudine) and efavirenz (belonging to Non-Nucleoside Reverse Transcriptase Inhibitors – NNRTIs – class) [142]. Besides, McComsey identified the puberty as the time in which HIV-infected children on HAART most likely develop lipodystrophy [43].

Pathogenesis of HIV lipodystrophy

Although the most compelling risk factor identified thus far has been HAART, genetic predisposition, virally mediated mechanisms involving HIV-1 accessory proteins, altered hormonal milieu and levels of inflammatory cytokines may also contribute to this syndrome and are currently under investigation

Drugs

Lipodystrophy has been closely linked to the use of PIs and, more recently, other antiretrovirals, including NRTIs and NNRTIs. Several mechanisms have been postulated to explain these adverse effects. PIs have the capacity to: inhibit the intrinsic activity of glucose transporter 4 (GLUT4) [34-41] alter degradation of sterol-regulatory-element-binding protein 1 (SREBP-1) and apolipoprotein B, resulting in lipodystrophy and increased lipid production; inhibit the function of LRP, leading to reduced TG clearance from the circulation [83]. NRTIs inhibit DNA polymerase gamma, an enzyme essential for mitochondrial DNA replication, resulting in mitochondrial DNA depletion, adipocyte death and lipoatrophy [143]. It has been also demonstrated that treatment with a NRTI-containing regimen of lamivudine or zidovudine in the absence of significant changes in body fat distribution, led to a 25% decrease in insulin-mediated peripheral glucose disposal and a 22% increase in fasting lipolysis [144]. However, a very recent study showed that substitution of stavudine with zidovudine could result in decreased severity or resolution of lipodystrophy among HIV-infected children and adolescents [145].

Pro-inflammatory cytokines

The increased levels of pro-inflammatory cytokines such as tumour necrosis factor (TNF)-α and interleukin (IL)-6 may further contribute to the development of lipodystrophy. TNF-α stimulates 11-β-hydroxysteroid dehydrogenase type-1, which converts inactive cortisone to active cortisol, resulting in increased lipid accumulation in adipocytes and insulin resistance. HAART drugs and inflammatory cytokines are also associated with a decrease in adiponectin levels [117-125] and this positively correlate with insulin resistance in HIV-infected patients with lipodystrophy.

Adipokines

Adipose tissue, previously seen as an inert energy storage organ, is now considered to be an endocrine organ in its own right. The hormonal changes caused by increases (in lipohypertrophy) or reduced subcutaneous fat (in lipoatrophy) may be central to the metabolic abnormalities observed in HIV-infected patients with lipodystrophy.

Adiponectin levels are significantly lower in patients with fat redistribution and inversely correlate with serum TGs and insulin resistance [120-125]. These findings are independent of age, leptin levels, HIV medication and severity of disease. Low adiponectin levels may reflect a direct toxic effect of HAART on subcutaneous adipose tissue, but may also simply reflect the accumulation of visceral adipose tissue. Decreased adiponectin (as well as leptin expression) due to decreased adipocyte differentiation could be involved in the whole-body insulin resistance and metabolic manifestations observed in HIV lipodystrophy [126-131].

Recently, several experimental and clinical observations have implicated resistin, a 12.5 kDa polypeptide hormone produced by adipocytes and immunocompetent cells, in the development of insulin resistance [18,19,132,133].

The administration of resistin to animals resulted in impaired glucose and lipid metabolism in some studies [132] but these findings were challenged by subsequent reports of no association between adipose tissue resistin expression and insulin resistance [134]. Findings in humans have also been highly variable. Elevated resistin levels have been noted in obese and diabetic subjects, and increased resistin has been associated with insulin resistance in lean and obese subjects [135,136]. In a recent study of patients with HAART-induced metabolic syndrome, resistin levels decreased after administration of rosiglitazone, an insulin sensitiser, but no correlation between resistin and insulin resistance or markers of inflammation and coagulation was found [137-159]. The study by Spagnuolo et al. in agreement with another report, confirmed that circulating resistin levels are related to adiposity, but are unlikely to play a major role in the Homeostasis Model Assessment—Insulin Resistance (HOMA-IR) and metabolic abnormalities associated with HAART-induced metabolic syndrome [159].

It is noteworthy that serum resist in levels were below the mean in a child without ultrasound signs of fat redistribution and on restricted caloric intake. In fact, this suggests that a dietary approach may be beneficial in HIV-related LS.

Lipoatrophy has been associated with low circulating leptin levels through loss of subcutaneous adipose tissue, in which leptin is predominantly expressed. Observational studies in adults have demonstrated that also in HIV lipodystrophy leptin levels are positively correlated with adipose tissue mass [138-140]. Lipoatrophy is associated with relative hypoleptinaemia, but it is now evident that the metabolic, neuroendocrine and immunological effects of leptin deficiency may become manifest only once leptin falls below a threshold level [141,143]. The clinical cut-off for hypoleptinaemia remains to be clearly defined and may vary depending on the assay used. However, several studies including subjects with mixed patterns of fat redistribution at enrolment have failed to find significantly lower leptin levels than in controls [150].

In addition to its metabolic effects, it is clear that leptin has an important role in immune regulation. Leptin affects both cell-mediated and humoral immunity [150-153]. Leptin has been shown to have direct effects on cells of the innate immune system, upregulating phagocytic function in macrophages, stimulating pro-inflammatory cytokine secretion and stimulating chemotaxis in polymorphonuclear cells. The presence of the leptin receptor ObRb on these immune cells indicates that the role of leptin is likely to be direct and not mediated

by other hormonal changes, through activation of the JAK-STAT3 pathway in lymphocytes; other pathways such as MAPK and PI3K may also be involved [154-159].

Genetics

The genetic basis of HIV lipodystrophy (HIVLD) is also unclear. Some studies have implicated nucleotide variation in apolipoprotein CIII (ApoCIII), the β3 adrenergic receptor or TNF-α. However, these studies focused on only one trait (e.g. triglycerides [TGs] or insulin resistance) and examined selected single nucleotide polymorphisms (SNPs) in a single gene [119].

HIV and dyslipidaemia

The main metabolic disorders presenting in lipodystrophy are dyslipidaemia, insulin resistance and lactic acidosis. It is usually of the mixed type, characterized by a decrease in high-density lipoprotein (HDL) cholesterol and increases in total cholesterol, LDL cholesterol and TGs. According to the European Paediatric Lipodystrophy Group, in 2004, 51% of children with lipodystrophy presented dyslipidaemia, 37% hypercholesterolaemia and 34% hypertriglyceridaemia [160]. Although dyslipidaemia can occur in children not treated with antiretroviral drugs, their usage, especially the PIs, favours the development of dyslipidaemia [161]. Among the PIs, ritonavir is the most commonly associated with dyslipidaemia [162-165].

Hyperlipidaemia has been described in HIV-positive children; HIV infection itself can modify the lipid profile, causing hyper-trigliceridaemia and hypocholesterolaemia, stimulating a chronic inflammatory response by the inflammatory cells [165-168]. Moreover, many studies conducted on both adults and children with HIV infection have demonstrated that the introduction of an antiretroviral drug can induce dyslipidemia when it is not yet present or may worsen an already existing lipid disorder [169].

In the last few years, several studies on HIV-infected children have found an association between the use of PIs and increased levels of cholesterol and TG. In these studies, the prevalence of elevated total cholesterol ranged from 15 to 68%, while the prevalence of elevated TG ranged from 11 to 79% [163]. Tassiopoulos and colleagues conducted a longitudinal evaluation of cholesterolaemia on 2,122 peri-natally HIV-infected children (Pediatric AIDS Clinical Trials Group 219C). The authors observed that a total of 277 of 2,122 children (13%) developed hypercholesterolaemia during a median follow-up of 50.4 months for an incidence rate of 3.4 cases per 100 person-years (95% confidence interval [CI] 3.0–3.9). After adjustment for age, boosted PIs use, PIs and NNRTIs use were associated with an increased risk of hypercholesterolaemia [164]. More recently, Chantry and colleagues observed that initiation or change in HAART was associated with significant increases in mean fasting total and LDL cholesterol during the 48 weeks of study observation. At week 48, the proportion of children with an abnormally high total cholesterol concentration significantly increased from 6% at entry to 21% (p=0.001) [165].

Management of dyslipidaemia in HIV-infected adults includes lifestyle changes, switching strategies and administration of lipid-lowering drugs. In terms of lifestyle changes, diet therapy is the primary approach to treating children and adolescents without HIV infection and with elevated blood cholesterol levels [170]. Although recent observational studies suggest that diet and physical exercise could improve lipid profile in HIV-infected patients [171,172], some RCTs did not corroborate this hypothesis [173,174]. However, a very recent randomized study evaluated patients who had just begun HAART and prescribed a hypocaloric diet and were strictly followed, while controls had no diet and no nutritional follow-up [175]. This kind of approach resulted to prevent HAART-related dyslipidemia and lipodystrophy.

Modification of HAART – switching from a PI or to a PI-sparing regimen – is one strategy for managing dyslipidaemia in HIV-infected adults, but scant data exist about the efficacy of these strategies in children. McComsey and colleagues [166] published a prospective, open-label, multicentre trial conducted on 17 children who were switched from a PI-containing regimen to efavirenz. After 48 weeks, the switch to efavirenz resulted in significant improvements in total cholesterol, LDL and TG, while maintaining excellent virological control. Vigano et al. [167] published a 48-week randomised, prospective study in 28 HIV infected children. Individuals were randomized to switch from PI to efavirenz and from stavudine to tenofovir at baseline (group 1) or at week 24 (group 2). This study showed a significant improvement in lipid profile after replacing a PI (nelfinavir, lopinavir and ritonavir) with efavirenz and replacing stavudine with tenofovir.

There are currently no published data regarding the pharmacological treatment of dyslipidaemia in HIV-infected children. From the studies on HIV-positive adults with dyslipidaemia, statins should be used cautiously due to the potential for significant drug interactions when used with PIs (rhabdomyolysis and hepatitis) [169].

HIV and Cardiovascular Disease (CVD)

CVD is the prevalent cause of mortality in the general population and a relevant factor among HIV-infected adults [176]. Subjects who develop CVD usually have multiple risk factors (lack of exercise, obesity, smoking, diabetes, dyslipidaemia, etc.). HIV replication may increase cardiovascular risk, since it is an independent risk factor for lipid changes similar to those associated with increased risk of CVD in the general population [167]. The Strategies for Management of Antiretroviral Therapy (SMART) study showed that interruption of HAART is associated with increased cardiovascular risk in HIV-infected patients [168]. The Data Collection on Adverse events of Anti-HIV Drugs (DAD) study showed a relative increase in the incidence of myocardial infarction (MI) of 26% per year of exposure to HAART [177-181].

Few studies have looked at CVD risk factors and early manifestations of atherosclerosis in HIV-infected children and adolescents [177-186]. Bonnet et al. performed a cross-sectional study to evaluate vascular dysfunction in 49 HIV-infected children compared with 24 age- and sex-matched healthy controls. Among the HIV-infected children, 32 were receiving HAART and 15 were naive to therapy. HIV-infected subjects showed cross-sectional compliance, less distended carotid arteries and higher diastolic wall stress than controls, while the intima-media thickness (IMT) of common carotid arteries was similar in cases and controls [181]. Charakida et al. showed that HIV infection in childhood is associated with adverse structural (increased IMT) and functional changes in the vasculature, and, among HIV-infected children, age and treatment were significantly associated with increased IMT. In particular, vascular abnormalities were more pronounced in children exposed to PI therapy. These findings support a role for both HIV infection itself and antiretrovirals, especially PIs, in the pathogenesis of early vascular disease, in particular atherosclerosis [178].

McComsey et al. found greater values of carotid IMT and higher levels of some cardiac biomarkers in antiretroviral-treated HIV-infected children compared with age-, sex-, race- and BMI-matched healthy controls. On regression analysis, only duration of ART predicted IMT measurements, while traditional atherosclerosis risk factors, HIV disease factors and duration of PI did not [164].

Vigano et al. evaluated a cohort of 23 adolescents and young adults vertically infected with HIV compared with age-, sex- and BMI-matched healthy controls. Common carotid IMT (CCIMT) was higher in HIV-infected than in control children (p<0.001). Predictors of CCIMT were HIV infection, male gender and vitamin B12 supplementation. Among the HIV-infected subjects, CCIMT was associated with the duration of exposure to a PI-based and NNRTI-based regimen plus single or double NRTI (treatment duration 11–20 years). The authors concluded that HIV infection and long duration of HAART are risk factors for higher CCIMT in adolescents and young adults [165].

HIV and bone

Many factors may negatively affect bone metabolism: direct interaction of HIV with cells of the bone, chronic T-cell activation, abnormal cytokine production affecting osteoblast and osteoclast function, disturbances of calcium homeostasis, parathyroid hormone function, vitamin D metabolism and adverse effects of HAART, especially PIs. Several studies on bone mineral measurements in HIV-infected children indicate a significant reduction of bone mineral content and bone mineral density (BMD).

Bone mineral accrual of HAART-treated children is impaired in comparison to healthy children [187,188]. In a prospective 12-month study, the BMD accrual of HAART-treated patients was comparable to that of healthy control patients at the vertebral site, but was lower than controls in the whole skeleton [187]. In another study, 60% of the patients had no change or decreased BMD SD-scores [188]. However, the use of tenofovir (one of the new molecules) has been linked to a reduction of bone mineral measurements in primates [189] and adult patients [190]. The available data in children are still poor and conflicting. Larger studies are needed to understand the effect of new drugs on bone mineral accrual in children.

HAART-treated children showed higher levels of markers of bone formation (bone alkaline phosphatase [BALP] and pro-collagen type 1 N-terminal pro-peptide [PINP]) and of bone resorption (N-telopeptide cross-links [NTx]) compared with antiretroviral-naive children and controls [191]. Children not receiving PIs showed reduced serum concentrations of osteocalcin and high levels of urinary NTx [187].

Serum concentrations of insulin-like growth factor-I (IGF-I) and insulin-like growth factor binding protein-3 (IGFBP3) in these patients were comparable to those of healthy controls. In another study, HIV-infected patients with severe symptoms showed significantly lower osteocalcin concentrations compared with patients with mild symptoms and healthy controls [192].

An open issue is the role of ART or HIV infection per se in the genesis of poor bone health in HIV-infected youths. Most studies have been performed in children who were receiving different antiretroviral drugs; the cohorts studied are heterogeneous in terms of treatment regimens employed, and thus it is not possible to reach definitive conclusions on the role of different classes of drug on skeletal health.

Few studies have reported results on untreated HIV-infected children [192,193]. In the first trial, 5 vertically infected patients were examined, and their DEXA measurements were compared with those of treated patients and healthy controls [192]. Vertebral and whole-body BMD values were found to be significantly higher than those of HAART-treated patients, and comparable to those of healthy children.

These results seem to indicate that HIV infection per se may not play an important role in the alteration of bone health in children, but more data are needed to clarify this issue.

Conclusion

Research should be undertaken into the metabolic risk.

References

1. McComsey GA, Leonard E (2004) Metabolic complications of HIV therapy in children. AIDS 18: 1753-1768.

2. Gallant JE, Staszewski S, Pozniak AL, DeJesus E, Suleiman JM, et al. (2004) Efficacy and safety of tenofovir DF vs stavudine in combination therapy in antiretroviral-naive patients: a 3-year randomized trial. JAMA 292: 191-201.

3. Leonard EG, McComsey GA (2003) Metabolic complications of antiretroviral therapy in children. Pediatr Infect Dis J 22: 77-84.

4. Brambilla P, Bricalli D, Sala N, Renzetti F, Manzoni P, et al. (2001) Highly active antiretroviral-treated HIV-infected children show fat distribution changes even in absence of lipodystrophy. AIDS 15: 2415-2422.

5. Beregszaszi M, Dollfus C, Levine M, Faye A, Deghmoun S, et al. (2005) Longitudinal evaluation and risk factors of lipodystrophy and associated metabolic changes in HIV-infected children. J Acquir Immune Defic Syndr 40: 161-168.

6. Farley J, Gona P, Crain M, Cervia J, , et al. (2005) Pediatric AIDS Clinical Trials Group Study 219C Team. Prevalence of elevated cholesterol and associated risk factors among perinatally HIV-infected children (4-19 years old) in Pediatric AIDS Clinical Trials Group 219C. J Acquir Immune Defic Syndr 38: 480-7.

7. Taylor P, Worrel C, Stainberg SM, Hazra R, Jankelevich S, et al. (2004) Natural history of lipid abnormalities and fat redistribution among human immunodeficiency virus -infected children receiving long term protease inhibitor-conteining, highly active antiretroviral regimens. Pediatrics 114e: 235-242.

8. Tong Q, Sankalé JL, Hadigan CM, Tan G, Rosenberg ES, et al. (2003) Regulation of adiponectin in human immunodeficiency virus-infected patients: relationship to body composition and metabolic indices. J Clin Endocrinol Metab 88: 1559-1564.

9. Gan SK, Samaras K, Thompson CH, Kraegen EW, Carr A, et al. (2002) Altered myocellular and abdominal fat partitioning predict disturbance in insulin action in HIV protease inhibitor-related lipodystrophy. Diabetes 51: 3163-3169.

10. Kosmiski L, Kuritzkes D, Lichtenstein K, Eckel R (2003) Adipocyte-derived hormone levels in HIV lipodystrophy. Antivir Ther 8: 9-15.

11. Mynarcik DC, Combs T, McNurlan MA, Scherer PE, Komaroff E, et al. (2002) Adiponectin and leptin levels in HIV-infected subjects with insulin resistance and body fat redistribution. J Acquir Immune Defic Syndr 31: 514-520.

12. Jan V, Cervera P, Maachi M, Baudrimont M, Kim M, et al. (2004) Altered fat differentiation and adipocytokine expression are inter-related and linked to morphological changes and insulin resistance in HIV-1-infected lipodystrophic patients. Antivir Ther. 9:555–564.

13. Samaras K, Gan SK, Peake PW, Carr A, Campbell LV (2009) Proinflammatory markers, insulin sensitivity, and cardiometabolic risk factors in treated HIV infection. Obesity (Silver Spring) 17: 53-59.

14. Samaras K (2009) Prevalence and pathogenesis of diabetes mellitus in HIV-1 infection treated with combined antiretroviral therapy. J Acquir Immune Defic Syndr. V50: 499-505.

15. Purnell JQ, Zambon A, Knopp RH, Pizzuti DJ, Achari R, et al. (2000) Effect of ritonavir on lipids and post-heparin lipase activities in normal subjects. AIDS 14: 51-57.

16. Jemsek JG, Arathoon E, Arlotti M, Perez C, Sosa N, et al. (2006) Body fat and other metabolic effects of atazanavir and efavirenz, each administered in combination with zidovudine plus lamivudine, in antiretroviral-naive HIV-infected patients. Clin Infect Dis 42: 273-280.

17. Vonkeman HE, ten Napel CH, van Oeveren-Dybicz AM, Vermes I (2000) Beta3-adrenergic receptor polymorphism and the antiretroviral therapy-related lipodystrophy syndrome. AIDS 14: 1463-1464.

18. Maher B, Alfirevic A, Vilar FJ, Wilkins EG, Park BK, et al. (2002) TNF-alpha promoter region gene polymorphisms in HIV-positive patients with lipodystrophy. AIDS 16: 2013-2018.

19. Foulkes AS, Wohl DA, Frank I, Puleo E, Restine S, et al. (2006) Associations among race/ethnicity, ApoC-III genotypes, and lipids in HIV-1-infected individuals on antiretroviral therapy. PLoS Med 3: e52.

20. Perou CM, Sorlie T, Eisen MB, van de Rijn M, Jeffrey SS, et al. (2000) Molecular portraits of human breast tumours. Nature 406: 747-752.

21. Ramaswamy S, Ross KN, Lander ES, Golub TR (2003) A molecular signature of metastasis in primary solid tumors. Nat Genet 33: 49-54.

22. Steppan CM, Bailey ST, Bhat S, Brown EJ, Banerjee RR, et al. (2001) The hormone resistin links obesity to diabetes. Nature 409: 307-312.

23. Dubé MP, Parker RA, Tebas P, Grinspoon SK, Zackin RA, et al. (2005) Glucose metabolism, lipid, and body fat changes in antiretroviral-naive subjects randomized to nelfinavir or efavirenz plus dual nucleosides. AIDS 19: 1807-1818.

24. Robbins GK, De Gruttola V, Shafer RW, Smeaton LM, Snyder SW, et al. (2003) Comparison of sequential three-drug regimens as initial therapy for HIV-1 infection. N Engl J Med 349: 2293–2303.

25. Arking DE, Pfeufer A, Post W, Kao WH, Newton-Cheh C, et al. (2006) A common genetic variant in the NOS1 regulator NOS1AP modulates cardiac repolarization. Nat Genet 38: 644-651.

26. Mallon PW, Miller J, Cooper DA, Carr A (2003) Prospective evaluation of the effects of antiretroviral therapy on body composition in HIV-1-infected men starting therapy. AIDS 17: 971-979.

27. Parker RA, Flint OP, Mulvey R, Elosua C, Wang F, et al. (2005) Endoplasmic reticulum stress links dyslipidemia to inhibition of proteasome activity and glucose transport by HIV protease inhibitors. Mol Pharmacol 67:1909–1919. Bibliographic Links.

28. International HapMap Consortium (2005) A haplotype map of the human genome. Nature 437: 1299-1320.

29. Botstein D, Risch N (2003) Discovering genotypes underlying human phenotypes: past successes for mendelian disease, future approaches for complex disease. Nat Genet (Suppl): 228–237.

30. Slonim N, Atwal GS, Tkacik G, Bialek W (2005) Information-based clustering. Proc Natl Acad Sci U S A 102: 18297-18302.

31. Banerjee RR, Rangwala SM, Shapiro JS, Rich AS, Rhoades B, et al. (2004) Regulation of fasted blood glucose by resistin. Science 303: 1195-1198.

32. Engert JC, Vohl MC, Williams SM, Lepage P, Loredo-Osti JC, et al. (2002) 5' flanking variants of resistin are associated with obesity. Diabetes 51: 1629-1634.

33. Wang H, Chu WS, Hemphill C, Elbein SC (2002) Human resistin gene: molecular scanning and evaluation of association with insulin sensitivity and type 2 diabetes in Caucasians. J Clin Endocrinol Metab 87: 2520-2524.

34. Sentinelli F, Romeo S, Arca M, Filippi E, Leonetti F, et al. (2002) Human resistin gene, obesity, and type 2 diabetes: mutation analysis and population study. Diabetes 51: 860-862.

35. Conneely KN, Silander K, Scott LJ, Mohlke KL, Lazaridis KN, et al. (2004) Variation in the resistin gene is associated with obesity and insulin-related phenotypes in Finnish subjects. Diabetologia 47: 1782-1788.

36. Osawa H, Yamada K, Onuma H, Murakami A, Ochi M, et al. (2004) The G/G genotype of resistin single-nucleotide polymorphism at -420 increases type 2 diabetes mellitus susceptibility by inducing promoter activity through specific binding of Sp1/3. Am J Hum Genet 75: 678–686.

37. Osawa H, Tabara Y, Kawamoto R, Ohashi J, Ochi M, et al. (2007) Plasma resistin, associated with single nucleotide polymorphism -420, is correlated with insulin resistance, lower HDL cholesterol, and high-sensitivity C-reactive protein in the Japanese general population. Diabetes Care 30: 1501–1506.

38. Grant SF, Thorleifsson G, Reynisdottir I, Benediktsson R, Manolescu A, et al. (2006) Variant of transcription factor 7-like 2 (TCF7L2) gene confers risk of type 2 diabetes. Nat Genet 38: 320-323.

39. Ledru E, Christeff N, Patey O, de Truchis P, Melchior JC, et al. (2000) Alteration of tumor necrosis factor-a T cell homeostasis following potent antiretroviral therapy: contribution to the development of human immunodeficiency virus-associated lipodystrophy syndrome. Blood 95: 3191–3198.

40. Lehrke M, Reilly MP, Millington SC, Iqbal N, Rader DJ, et al. (2004) An inflammatory cascade leading to hyperresistinemia in humans. PLoS Med 1: e45.

41. Reilly MP, Lehrke M, Wolfe ML, Rohatgi A, Lazar MA, et al. (2005) Resistin is an inflammatory marker of atherosclerosis in humans. Circulation 111: 932-939.

42. Ene L, Goetghebuer T, Hainaut M, Peltier A, Toppet V, et al. (2007) Prevalence of lipodystrophy in HIV-infected children: a cross-sectional study. Eur J Pediatr 166: 13-21.

43. Jaquet D, Lévine M, Ortega-Rodriguez E, Faye A, Polak M, et al. (2000) Clinical and metabolic presentation of the lipodystrophic syndrome in HIV-infected children. AIDS 14: 2123-2128.

44. Hartman K, Verweel G, de Groot R, Hartwig NG (2006) Detection of lipoatrophy in human immunodeficiency virus-1-infected children treated with highly active antiretroviral therapy. Pediatr Infect Dis J 25: 427-431.

45. European Paediatric Lipodystrophy Group (2004) Antiretroviral therapy, fat redistribution and hyperlipidaemia in HIV-infected children in Europe. AIDS 18: 1443-1451.

46. Paton NI, Yang Y, Tha NO, Sitoh YY (2007) Changes in facial fat in HIV-related lipoatrophy, wasting, and weight gain measured by magnetic resonance imaging. HIV Clin Trials 8: 227-234.

47. Vigano A, Mora S, Testolin C, Beccio S, Schneider L, et al. (2003) Increased lipodystrophy is associated with increased exposure to highly active antiretroviral therapy in HIV-infected children. J Acquir Immune Defic Syndr 32: 482-489.

48. Eley B (2008) Metabolic complications of antiretroviral therapy in HIV-infected children. Expert Opin Drug Metab Toxicol 4: 37-49.

49. Amaya RA, Kozinetz CA, McMeans A, Schwarzwald H, Kline MW (2002) Lipodystrophy syndrome in human immunodeficiency virus-infected children. Pediatr Infect Dis J 21: 405-410.

50. Sanchez Torres AM, Munoz Muniz R, Madero R, Borque C, Garcia-Miguel MJ, et al. (2005) Prevalence of fat redistribution and metabolic disorders in human immunodeficiency virus-infected children. Eur J Pediatr 164: 271-276.

51. Berg AH, Combs TP, Du X, Brownlee M, Scherer PE (2001) The adipocyte-secreted protein Acrp30 enhances hepatic insulin action. Nat Med 7: 947-953.

52. Yamauchi T, Kamon J, Waki H, Terauchi Y, Kubota N, et al. (2001) The fat-derived hormone adiponectin reverses insulin resistance associated with both lipoatrophy and obesity. Nat Med 7: 941-946.

53. Kubota N, Terauchi Y, Yamauchi T, Kubota T, Moroi M, et al. (2002) Disruption of adiponectin causes insulin resistance and neointimal formation. J Biol Chem 277: 25863-25866.

54. Okamoto Y, Kihara S, Ouchi N, Nishida M, Arita Y, et al. (2002) Adiponectin reduces atherosclerosis in apolipoprotein E-deficient mice. Circulation 106: 2767-2770.

55. Fain JN, Madan AK, Hiler ML, Cheema P, Bahouth SW (2004) Comparison of the release of adipokines by adipose tissue, adipose tissue matrix, and adipocytes from visceral and subcutaneous abdominal adipose tissues of obese humans. Endocrinology 145: 2273-2282.

56. Combs TP, Pajvani UB, Berg AH, Lin Y, Jelicks LA, et al. (2004) A transgenic mouse with a deletion in the collagenous domain of adiponectin displays elevated circulating adiponectin and improved insulin sensitivity. Endocrinology 145: 367-383.

57. Yki-Järvinen H (2004) Thiazolidinediones. N Engl J Med 351: 1106-1118.

58. Yu JG, Javorschi S, Hevener AL, Kruszynska YT, Norman RA, et al. (2002) The effect of thiazolidinediones on plasma adiponectin levels in normal, obese, and type 2 diabetic subjects. Diabetes 51: 2968-2974.

59. Phillips SA, Ciaraldi TP, Kong AP, Bandukwala R, Aroda V, et al. (2003) Modulation of circulating and adipose tissue adiponectin levels by antidiabetic therapy. Diabetes 52: 667-674.

60. Gavrila A, Hsu W, Tsiodras S, Doweiko J, Gautam S, et al. (2005) Improvement in highly active antiretroviral therapy-induced metabolic syndrome by treatment with pioglitazone but not with fenofibrate: a 2 x 2 factorial, randomized, double-blinded, placebo-controlled trial. Clin Infect Dis 40: 745-749.

61. van Wijk JP, de Koning EJ, Cabezas MC, op't Roodt J, Joven J, et al. (2005) Comparison of rosiglitazone and metformin for treating HIV lipodystrophy: a randomized trial. Ann Intern Med 143: 337-346.

62. Steppan CM, Lazar MA (2004) The current biology of resistin. J Intern Med 255: 439-447.

63. Degawa-Yamauchi M, Bovenkerk JE, Juliar BE, Watson W, Kerr K, et al. (2003) Serum resistin (FIZZ3) protein is increased in obese humans. J Clin Endocrinol Metab 88: 5452-5455.

64. Satoh H, Nguyen MT, Miles PD, Imamura T, Usui I, et al. (2004) Adenovirus-mediated chronic "hyper-resistinemia" leads to in vivo insulin resistance in normal rats. J Clin Invest 114: 224-231.

65. Lee JH, Chan JL, Yiannakouris N, Kontogianni M, Estrada E, et al. (2003) Circulating resistin levels are not associated with obesity or insulin resistance in humans and are not regulated by fasting or leptin administration: cross-sectional and interventional studies in normal, insulin-resistant, and diabetic subjects. J Clin Endocrinol Metab 88: 4848-4856.

66. Way JM, Gorgun CZ, Tong Q, Uysal KT, Brown KK, et al. (2001) Adipose tissue resistin expression is severely suppressed in obesity and stimulated by peroxisome proliferator-activated receptor gamma agonists. J Biol Chem 276: 25651-25653.

67. Youn BS, Yu KY, Park HJ, Lee NS, Min SS, et al. (2004) Plasma resistin concentrations measured by enzyme-linked immunosorbent assay using a newly developed monoclonal antibody are elevated in individuals with type 2 diabetes mellitus. J Clin Endocrinol Metab 89: 150-156.

68. Silha JV, Krsek M, Skrha JV, Sucharda P, Nyomba BL, et al. (2003) Plasma resistin, adiponectin and leptin levels in lean and obese subjects: correlations with insulin resistance. Eur J Endocrinol 149: 331-335.

69. Zhang B, MacNaul K, Szalkowski D, Li Z, Berger J, et al. (1999) Inhibition of adipocyte differentiation by HIV protease inhibitors. J Clin Endocrinol Metab 84: 4274-4277.

70. Heymsfield SB, Greenberg AS, Fujioka K, Dixon RM, Kushner R, et al. (1999) Recombinant leptin for weight loss in obese and lean adults: a randomized, controlled, dose-escalation trial. JAMA 282: 1568-1575.

71. Chan JL, Heist K, DePaoli AM, Veldhuis JD, Mantzoros CS (2003) The role of falling leptin levels in the neuroendocrine and metabolic adaptation to short-term starvation in healthy men. J Clin Invest 111: 1409-1421.

72. Chan JL, Mantzoros CS (2005) Role of leptin in energy-deprivation states: normal human physiology and clinical implications for hypothalamic amenorrhoea and anorexia nervosa. Lancet 366: 74-85.

73. Chan JL, Matarese G, Shetty GK, Raciti P, Kelesidis I, et al. (2006) Differential regulation of metabolic, neuroendocrine, and immune function by leptin in humans. Proc Natl Acad Sci U S A 103: 8481-8486.

74. Welt CK, Chan JL, Bullen J, Murphy R, Smith P, et al. (2004) Recombinant human leptin in women with hypothalamic amenorrhea. N Engl J Med 351: 987-997.

75. Brennan AM, Mantzoros CS (2006) Drug Insight: the role of leptin in human physiology and pathophysiology--emerging clinical applications. Nat Clin Pract Endocrinol Metab 2: 318-327.

76. Considine RV, Sinha MK, Heiman ML, Kriauciunas A, Stephens TW, et al. (1996) Serum immunoreactive-leptin concentrations in normal-weight and obese humans. N Engl J Med 334: 292-295.

77. Martini G, Valenti R, Giovani S, Campagna S, Franci B, et al. (2001) Leptin and body composition in healthy postmenopausal women. Panminerva Med 43: 149–154.

78. Yarasheski KE, Zachwieja JJ, Horgan MM, Powderly WG, Santiago JV, et al. (1997) Serum leptin concentrations in human immunodeficiency virus-infected men with low adiposity. Metabolism 46: 303-305.

79. Wunder D, Bersinger NA, Fux C, Weber R, Bernasconi E, et al. (2005) Plasma leptin levels in men are not related to the development of lipoatrophy during antiretroviral therapy. AIDS 19: 1837-1842.

80. Lee JH, Chan JL, Sourlas E, Raptopoulos V, Mantzoros CS (2006) Recombinant methionyl human leptin therapy in replacement doses improves insulin resistance and metabolic profile in patients with lipoatrophy and metabolic syndrome induced by the highly active antiretroviral therapy. J Clin Endocrinol Metab 91: 2605-2611.

81. Koutkia P, Canavan B, Breu J, Johnson ML, Depaoli A, et al. (2004) Relation of leptin pulse dynamics to fat distribution in HIV-infected patients. Am J Clin Nutr 79: 1103-1109.

82. Harris RB (1998) Acute and chronic effects of leptin on glucose utilization in lean mice. Biochem Biophys Res Commun 245: 502-509.

83. Ebihara K, Ogawa Y, Masuzaki H, Shintani M, Miyanaga F, et al. (2001) Transgenic overexpression of leptin rescues insulin resistance and diabetes in a mouse model of lipoatrophic diabetes. Diabetes 50: 1440-1448.

84. Shimomura I, Hammer RE, Ikemoto S, Brown MS, Goldstein JL (1999) Leptin reverses insulin resistance and diabetes mellitus in mice with congenital lipodystrophy. Nature 401: 73-76.

85. Petersen KF, Oral EA, Dufour S, Befroy D, Ariyan C, et al. (2002) Leptin reverses insulin resistance and hepatic steatosis in patients with severe lipodystrophy. J Clin Invest 109: 1345-1350.

86. Oral EA, Simha V, Ruiz E, Andewelt A, Premkumar A, et al. (2002) Leptin-replacement therapy for lipodystrophy. N Engl J Med 346: 570-578.

87. Mandel MA, Mahmoud AA (1978) Impairment of cell-mediated immunity in mutation diabetic mice (db/db). J Immunol 120: 1375-1377.

88. Matarese G, Moschos S, Mantzoros CS (2005) Leptin in immunology. J Immunol 174: 3137-3142.

89. Mancuso P, Gottschalk A, Phare SM, Peters-Golden M, Lukacs NW, et al. (2002) Leptin-deficient mice exhibit impaired host defense in Gram-negative pneumonia. J Immunol 168: 4018-4024.

90. Loffreda S, Yang SQ, Lin HZ, Karp CL, Brengman ML, et al. (1998) Leptin regulates proinflammatory immune responses. FASEB J 12: 57-65.

91. Caldefie-Chezet F, Poulin A, Vasson MP (2003) Leptin regulates functional capacities of polymorphonuclear neutrophils. Free Radic Res 37: 809-814.

92. Lord GM, Matarese G, Howard JK, Baker RJ, Bloom SR, et al. (1998) Leptin modulates the T-cell immune response and reverses starvation-induced immunosuppression. Nature 394: 897-901.

93. Baumann H, Morella KK, White DW, Dembski M, Bailon PS, et al. (1996) The full-length leptin receptor has signaling capabilities of interleukin 6-type cytokine receptors. Proc Natl Acad Sci U S A 93: 8374-8378.

94. Martin-Romero C, Sanchez-Margalet V (2001) Human leptin activates PI3K and MAPK pathways in human peripheral blood mononuclear cells: possible role of Sam68. Cell Immunol 212: 83-91.

95. Sanchez-Margalet V, Martin-Romero C (2001) Human leptin signaling in human peripheral blood mononuclear cells: activation of the JAK-STAT pathway. Cell Immunol 211: 30-36.

96. Howard JK, Lord GM, Matarese G, Vendetti S, Ghatei MA, et al. (1999) Leptin protects mice from starvation-induced lymphoid atrophy and increases thymic cellularity in ob/ob mice. J Clin Invest 104: 1051-1059.

97. Ozata M, Ozdemir IC, Licinio J (1999) Human leptin deficiency caused by a missense mutation: multiple endocrine defects, decreased sympathetic tone, and immune system dysfunction indicate new targets for leptin action, greater central than peripheral resistance to the effects of leptin, and spontaneous correction of leptin-mediated defects. J Clin Endocrinol Metab 84: 3686–3695.

98. Farooqi IS, Matarese G, Lord GM, Keogh JM, Lawrence E, et al. (2002) Beneficial effects of leptin on obesity, T cell hyporesponsiveness, and neuroendocrine/metabolic dysfunction of human congenital leptin deficiency. J Clin Invest 110: 1093-1103.

99. Chan JL, Stoyneva V, Kelesidis T, Raciti P, Mantzoros CS (2006) Peptide YY levels are decreased by fasting and elevated following caloric intake but are not regulated by leptin. Diabetologia 49: 169-173.

100. Canavan B, Salem RO, Schurgin S, Koutkia P, Lipinska I, et al. (2005) Effects of physiological leptin administration on markers of inflammation, platelet activation, and platelet aggregation during caloric deprivation. J Clin Endocrinol Metab 90: 5779-5785.

101. Mantzoros CS, Flier JS, Rogol AD (1997) A longitudinal assessment of hormonal and physical alterations during normal puberty in boys. V. Rising leptin levels may signal the onset of puberty. J Clin Endocrinol Metab 82: 1066-1070.

102. Licinio J, Caglayan S, Ozata M, Yildiz BO, de Miranda PB, et al. (2004) Phenotypic effects of leptin replacement on morbid obesity, diabetes mellitus, hypogonadism, and behavior in leptin-deficient adults. Proc Natl Acad Sci U S A 101: 4531-4536.

103. Musso C, Cochran E, Javor E, Young J, Depaoli AM, et al. (2005) The long-term effect of recombinant methionyl human leptin therapy on hyperandrogenism and menstrual function in female and pituitary function in male and female hypoleptinemic lipodystrophic patients. Metabolism 54: 255-263.

104. Clément K, Vaisse C, Lahlou N, Cabrol S, Pelloux V, et al. (1998) A mutation in the human leptin receptor gene causes obesity and pituitary dysfunction. Nature 392: 398-401.

105. LaPaglia N, Steiner J, Kirsteins L, Emanuele M, Emanuele N (1998) Leptin alters the response of the growth hormone releasing factor-growth hormone--insulin-like growth factor-I axis to fasting. J Endocrinol 159: 79-83.

106. Koutkia P, Eaton K, You SM, Breu J, Grinspoon S (2006) Growth hormone secretion among HIV infected patients: effects of gender, race and fat distribution. AIDS 20: 855-862.

107. Johannsson G, Marin P, Lonn L, Ottosson M, Stenlof K, et al. (1997) Growth hormone treatment of abdominally obese men reduces abdominal fat mass, improves glucose and lipoprotein metabolism, and reduces diastolic blood pressure. J Clin Endocrinol Metab 82: 727–734.

108. Wanke C, Gerrior J, Kantaros J, Coakley E, Albrecht M (1999) Recombinant human growth hormone improves the fat redistribution syndrome (lipodystrophy) in patients with HIV. AIDS 13: 2099-2103.

109. Spagnuolo MI, Bruzzese E, Vallone GF, Fasano N, De Marco G, et al. (2008) Is resistin a link between highly active antiretroviral therapy and fat redistribution in HIV-infected children? J Endocrinol Invest 31: 592-596.

110. Martinez E, Mocroft A, Garcia-Viejo MA, Pérez-Cuevas JB, Blanco JL, et al. (2001) Risk of lipodystrophy in HIV-1-infected patients treated with protease inhibitors: a prospective cohort study. Lancet 357: 592-598.

111. Chen D, Misra A, Garg A (2002) Clinical review 153: Lipodystrophy in human immunodeficiency virus-infected patients. J Clin Endocrinol Metab 87: 4845-4856.

112. Krause JC, Toye MP, Stechenberg BW, Reiter EO, Allen HF (2005) HIV--associated lipodystrophy in children. Pediatr Endocrinol Rev 3: 45-51.

113. Vigano A, Giacomet V (2005) Nucleoside analogues toxicities related to mitochondrial dysfunction: focus on HIV-infected children. In: Proceedings from the 1st Meeting on mithochondrial toxicity & HIV infection: understanding the pathogenesis for a therapeutic approach. 10 Suppl 2: M53-64.

114. Fredriks AM, van Buuren S, Fekkes M, Verloove-Vanhorick SP, Wit JM (2005) Are age references for waist circumference, hip circumference and waist-hip ratio in Dutch children useful in clinical practice? Eur J Pediatr 164: 216-222.

115. Scherzer R, Shen W, Bacchetti P, Kotler D, Lewis CE, et al. (2008) Comparison of dual-energy X-ray absorptiometry and magnetic resonance imaging-measured adipose tissue depots in HIV-infected and control subjects. Am J Clin Nutr 88: 1088-1096.

116. Janssen I, Katzmarzyk PT, Ross R (2002) Body mass index, waist circumference, and health risk: evidence in support of current National Institutes of Health guidelines. Arch Intern Med 162: 2074-2079.

117. Fernandez JR, Redden DT, Pietrobelli A, Allison DB (2004) Waist circumference percentiles in nationally representative samples of African-American, European-American, and Mexican-American children and adolescents. J Pediatr 145: 439-444.

118. Yoon C, Gulick RM, Hoover DR, Vaamonde CM, Glesby MJ (2004) Case-control study of diabetes mellitus in HIV-infected patients. J Acquir Immune Defic Syndr 37: 1464-1469.

119. Jerico C, Knobel H, Montero M, Ordonez-Llanos J, Guelar A, et al. (2005) Metabolic syndrome among HIV-infected patients: prevalence, characteristics, and related factors. Diabetes Care 28: 132-137.

120. Jacobson DL, Tang AM, Spiegelman D, Thomas AM, Skinner S, et al. (2006) Incidence of metabolic syndrome in a cohort of HIV-infected adults and prevalence relative to the US population (National Health and Nutrition Examination Survey). J Acquir Immune Defic Syndr 43: 458-466.

121. Palacios R, Santos J, Gonzalez M, Ruiz J, Marquez M (2007) Incidence and prevalence of the metabolic syndrome in a cohort of naive HIV-infected patients: prospective analysis at 48 weeks of highly active antiretroviral therapy. Int J STD AIDS 18: 184-187.

122. Wand H, Calmy A, Carey DL, Samaras K, Carr A, et al. (2007) Metabolic syndrome, cardiovascular disease and type 2 diabetes mellitus after initiation of antiretroviral therapy in HIV infection. AIDS 21: 2445-2453.

123. Samaras K (2008) Metabolic consequences and therapeutic options in highly active antiretroviral therapy in human immunodeficiency virus-1 infection. J Antimicrob Chemother 61: 238-245.

124. McGarry JD (2002) Banting lecture 2001: dysregulation of fatty acid metabolism in the etiology of type 2 diabetes. Diabetes 51: 7–18.

125. Lainka E, Oezbek S, Falck M, Ndagijimana J, Niehues T (2002) Marked dyslipidemia in human immunodeficiency virus-infected children on protease inhibitor-containing antiretroviral therapy. Pediatrics 110: e56.

126. Samaras K, Wand H, Law M, Emery S, Cooper D, et al. (2007) Prevalence of metabolic syndrome in HIV-infected patients receiving highly active antiretroviral therapy using international diabetes foundation and adult treatment Panel III criteria: associations with insulin resistance, disturbed body fat compartmentalization, elevated C-reactive peptide, and hypoadiponectinemia. Diabetes Care 30: 113–119.

127. Singhania R, Kotler DP (2011) Lipodystrophy in HIV patients: its challenges and management approaches. HIV AIDS (Auckl) 3: 135-143.

128. Salehian B, Bilas J, Bazargan M, Abbasian M (2005) Prevalence and incidence of diabetes in HIV-infected minority patients on protease inhibitors. J Natl Med Assoc 97: 1088-1092.

129. Amorosa V, Synnestvedt M, Gross R, Friedman H, MacGregor RR, et al. (2005) A tale of 2 epidemics: the intersection between obesity and HIV infection in Philadelphia. J Acquir Immune Defic Syndr 39: 557-561.

130. Howard AA, Floris-Moore M, Arnsten JH, Santoro N, Fleischer N, et al. (2005) Disorders of glucose metabolism among HIV-infected women. Clin Infect Dis 40: 1492-1499.

131. Justman JE, Benning L, Danoff A, Minkoff H, Levine A, et al. (2003) Protease inhibitor use and the incidence of diabetes mellitus in a large cohort of HIV-infected women. J Acquir Immune Defic Syndr 32: 298-302.

132. Tien PC, Schneider MF, Cole SR, Levine AM, Cohen M, et al. (2007) Antiretroviral therapy exposure and incidence of diabetes mellitus in the Women's Interagency HIV Study. AIDS 21: 1739-1745.

133. Yazicioglu G, Isitan F, Altunbas H, Suleymanlar I, Ozdogan M, et al. (2004) Insulin resistance in chronic hepatitis C. Int J Clin Pract 58: 1020-1022.

134. Ledergerber B, Furrer H, Rickenbach M, Lehmann R, Elzi L, et al. (2007) Factors associated with the incidence of type 2 diabetes mellitus in HIV-infected participants in the Swiss HIV Cohort Study. Clin Infect Dis 45: 111-119.

135. Grinspoon S, Carr A (2005) Cardiovascular risk and body-fat abnormalities in HIV-infected adults. N Engl J Med 352: 48-62.

136. Panz VR, Joffe BI (1999) Impact of HIV infection and AIDS on prevalence of type 2 diabetes in South Africa in 2010. BMJ 318: 1351A.

137. Levitt NS, Bradshaw D (2006) The impact of HIV/AIDS on Type 2 diabetes prevalence and diabetes healthcare needs in South Africa: projections for 2010. Diabet Med 23: 103-104.

138. Grundy SM, Brewer B, Cleeman JI, Smith SC, Lenfant C (2004) Definition of metabolic syndrome. Report of the National Heart, Lung, and Blood Institute/ American Heart Association Conference on Scientific Issues related to definition. Circulation 109: 433-438.

139. Alberti KG, Zimmet P, Shaw J; IDF Epidemiology Task Force Consensus Group (2005) The metabolic syndrome--a new worldwide definition. Lancet 366: 1059-1062.

140. Alam N, Cortina-Borja M, Goetghebuer T, Marczynska M, Vigano A, et al. (2012) for the European Paediatric HIV and Lipodystrophy Study Group in EuroCoord. Body Fat Abnormality in HIV-Infected Children and Adolescents Living in Europe: Prevalence and Risk Factors. J Acquir Immune Defic Syndr 59: 314-24.

141. Bockhorst JL, Ksseiry I, Toye M, Chipkin SR, Stechenberg BW, et al. (2003) Evidence of human immunodeficiency virus-associated lipodystrophy syndrome in children treated with protease inhibitors. Pediatr Infect Dis J 22: 463-465.

142. Arpadi S, Shiau S, Strehlau R, Martens L, Patel F, et al. (2013) Metabolic abnormalities and body composition of HIV-infected children on Lopinavir or Nevirapine-based antiretroviral therapy. Arch Dis Child 98: 258-264.

143. Morén C, Noguera-Julian A, Rovira N, Corrales E, Garrabou G, et al. (2011) Mitochondrial impact of human immunodeficiency virus and antiretrovirals on infected pediatric patients with or without lipodystrophy. Pediatr Infect Dis J 30: 992-995.

144. Blumer RM, van Vonderen MG, Sutinen J, Hassink E, Ackermans M, et al. (2008) Zidovudine/lamivudine contributes to insulin resistance within 3 months of starting combination antiretroviral therapy. AIDS 22: 227-236.

145. Aurpibul L, Puthanakit T, Taejaroenkul S, Sirisanthana T, Sirisanthana V (2012) Recovery from lipodystrophy in HIV-infected children after substitution of stavudine with zidovudine in a non-nucleoside reverse transcriptase inhibitor-based antiretroviral therapy. Pediatr Infect Dis J 31: 384-388.

146. Kamin D, Hadigan C, Lehrke M, Mazza S, Lazar MA, et al. (2005) Resistin levels in human immunodeficiency virus-infected patients with lipoatrophy decrease in response to rosiglitazone. J Clin Endocrinol Metab 90: 3423-3426.

147. Barb D, Wadhwa SG, Kratzsch J, Gavrila A, Chan JL, et al. (2005) Circulating resistin levels are not associated with fat redistribution, insulin resistance, or metabolic profile in patients with the highly active antiretroviral therapy-induced metabolic syndrome. J Clin Endocrinol Metab 90: 5324-5328.

148. Garg A (2004) Acquired and inherited lipodystrophies. N Engl J Med 350: 1220-1234.

149. Addy CL, Gavrila A, Tsiodras S, Brodovicz K, Karchmer AW, et al. (2003) Hypoadiponectinemia is associated with insulin resistance, hypertriglyceridemia, and fat redistribution in human immunodeficiency

virus-infected patients treated with highly active antiretroviral therapy. J Clin Endocrinol Metab 88: 627–636.

150. Nagy GS, Tsiodras S, Martin LD, Avihingsanon A, Gavrila A, et al. (2003) Human immunodeficiency virus type 1-related lipoatrophy and lipohypertrophy are associated with serum concentrations of leptin. Clin Infect Dis 36: 795-802.

151. Miller KK, Daly PA, Sentochnik D, Doweiko J, Samore M, et al. (1998) Pseudo-Cushing's syndrome in human immunodeficiency virus-infected patients. Clin Infect Dis 27: 68-72.

152. Carter VM, Hoy JF, Bailey M, Colman PG, Nyulasi I, et al. (2001) The prevalence of lipodystrophy in an ambulant HIV-infected population: it all depends on the definition. HIV Med 2: 174-180.

153. Santos CP, Felipe YX, Braga PE, Ramos D, Lima RO, et al. (2005) Self-perception of body changes in persons living with HIV/AIDS: prevalence and associated factors. AIDS 19 Suppl 4: S14-21.

154. Lichtenstein KA, Ward DJ, Moorman AC, Delaney KM, Young B, et al. (2001) Clinical assessment of HIV-associated lipodystrophy in an ambulatory population. AIDS 15: 1389-1398.

155. Thiebaut R, Daucourt V, Mercie P, Ekouevi DK, Malvy D, et al. (2000) Lipodystrophy, metabolic disorders, and human immunodeficiency virus infection: Aquitaine Cohort, France, 1999. Groupe d'Epidemiologie Clinique du Syndrome d'Immunodeficience Acquise en Aquitaine. Clin Infect Dis 31: 1482–1487.

156. Ranganathan S, Kern PA (2002) The HIV protease inhibitor saquinavir impairs lipid metabolism and glucose transport in cultured adipocytes. J Endocrinol 172: 155-162.

157. Imami N, Antonopoulos C, Hardy GA, Gazzard B, Gotch FM (1999) Assessment of type 1 and type 2 cytokines in HIV type 1-infected individuals: impact of highly active antiretroviral therapy. AIDS Res Hum Retroviruses 15: 1499-1508.

158. Maeda K, Okubo K, Shimomura I, Funahashi T, Matsuzawa Y, et al. (1996) cDNA cloning and expression of a novel adipose specific collagen-like factor, apM1 (AdiPose Most abundant Gene transcript 1). Biochem Biophys Res Commun 221: 286–289.

159. Fruebis J, Tsao TS, Javorschi S, Ebbets-Reed D, Erickson MR, et al. (2001) Proteolytic cleavage product of 30-kDa adipocyte complement-related protein increases fatty acid oxidation in muscle and causes weight loss in mice. Proc Natl Acad Sci U S A 98: 2005-2010.

160. Solorzano Santos F, Gochicoa Rangel LG, Palacios Saucedo G, Vazquez Rosales G, Miranda Novales MG (2006) Hypertriglyceridemia and hypercholesterolemia in human immunodeficiency virus-1-infected children treated with protease inhibitors. Arch Med Res 37: 129-132.

161. Tassiopoulos K, Williams P, George R, Marilyn c, James O, John F, et al. (2008) for the International Maternal Pediatric Adolescent AIDS Clinical Trials 219C Team Epidemiology and Social Science Association of Hypercholesterolemia Incidence With Antiretroviral Treatment, Including Protease Inhibitors, Among Perinatally HIV-Infected Children JAIDS 47: 607-614.

162. Chantry CJ, Hughes MD, Alvero C, Cervia JS, Meyer WA 3rd, et al. (2008) Lipid and glucose alterations in HIV-infected children beginning or changing antiretroviral therapy. Pediatrics 122: e129-138.

163. McComsey G, Bhumbra N, Ma JF, Rathore M, Alvarez A; First Pediatric Switch Study (2003) Impact of protease inhibitor substitution with efavirenz in HIV-infected children: results of the First Pediatric Switch Study. Pediatrics 111: e275-281.

164. Vigano A, Aldrovandi GM, Giacomet V, Merlo M, Martelli L, et al. (2005) Improvement in dyslipidaemia after switching stavudine to tenofovir and replacing protease inhibitors with efavirenz in HIV-infected children. Antivir Ther 10: 917-924.

165. Bitnun A, Sochett E, Babyn P, Holowka S, Stephens D, et al. (2003) Serum lipids, glucose homeostasis and abdominal adipose tissue distribution in protease inhibitor-treated and naive HIV-infected children. AIDS 17: 1319-27.

166. Expert Panel on Detection, Evaluation, and Treatment of High Blood Cholesterol in Adults (2001) Executive Summary of The Third Report of The National Cholesterol Education Program (NCEP) Expert Panel on

Detection, Evaluation, And Treatment of High Blood Cholesterol In Adults (Adult Treatment Panel III). JAMA 285: 2486-2497.

167. Bitnun A, Sochett E, Dick PT, To T, Jefferies C, et al. (2005) Insulin sensitivity and beta-cell function in protease inhibitor-treated and -naive human immunodeficiency virus-infected children. J Clin Endocrinol Metab 90: 168-174.

168. Brandao AP, Brandao AA, Berenson GS, Fuster V (2005) [Metabolic syndrome in children and adolescents]. Arq Bras Cardiol 85: 79-81.

169. Berenson GS, Srinivasan SR, Bao W, Newman WP 3rd, Tracy RE, et al. (1998) Association between multiple cardiovascular risk factors and atherosclerosis in children and young adults. The Bogalusa Heart Study. N Engl J Med 338: 1650-1656.

170. Dube MP, Stein JH, Aberg JA, Fichtenbaum CJ, Gerber JG, et al. (2003) Adult AIDS Clinical Trials Group Cardiovascular Subcommittee; HIV Medical Association of the Infectious Disease Society of America. Guidelines for the evaluation and management of dyslipidemia in human immunodeficiency virus (HIV)-infected adults receiving antiretroviral therapy: recommendations of the HIV Medical Association of the Infectious Disease Society of America and the Adult AIDS Clinical Trials Group. Clin Infect Dis 37: 613–27.

171. Thöni GJ, Fedou C, Brun JF, Fabre J, Renard E, et al. (2002) Reduction of fat accumulation and lipid disorders by individualized light aerobic training in human immunodeficiency virus infected patients with lipodystrophy and/or dyslipidemia. Diabetes Metab 28: 397-404.

172. Terry L, Sprinz E, Stein R, Medeiros NB, Oliveira J, et al. (2006) Exercise training in HIV-1-infected individuals with dyslipidemia and lipodystrophy. Med Sci Sports Exerc 38: 411-417.

173. Fitch KV, Anderson EJ, Hubbard JL, Carpenter SJ, Waddell WR, et al. (2006) Effects of a lifestyle modification program in HIV-infected patients with the metabolic syndrome. AIDS 20: 1843-1850.

174. Turcinov D, Stanley C, Canchola JA, Rutherford GW, Novotny TE, et al. (2009) Dyslipidemia and adherence to the Mediterranean diet in Croatian HIV-infected patients during the first year of highly active antiretroviral therapy. Coll Antropol 33: 423-430.

175. Lazzaretti RK, Kuhmmer R, Sprinz E, Polanczyk CA, Ribeiro JP (2012) Dietary Intervention Prevents Dyslipidemia Associated With Highly Active Antiretroviral Therapy in Human Immunodeficiency Virus Type 1–Infected Individuals. A Randomized Trial. JACC 59: 979–88.

176. Post WS (2011) Predicting and preventing cardiovascular disease in HIV-infected patients. Top Antivir Med 19: 169-173.

177. Charakida M, Donald AE, Green H, Storry C, Clapson M, et al. (2005) Early structural and functional changes of the vasculature in HIV-infected children: impact of disease and antiretroviral therapy. Circulation 112: 103-109.

178. d'Arminio A, Sabin CA, Phillips AN, Reiss P, Weber R, et al. (2004) Cardio- and cerebrovascular events in HIV-infected persons. Writing Committee of the D:A:D: Study Group. AIDS 18: 1811-1817.

179. Friis-Moller N, Sabin CA, Weber R, d'Arminio Monforte A, El-Sadr WM, et al. (2003) Combination antiretroviral therapy and the risk of myocardial infarction. N Engl J Med 349: 1993-2003.

180. Bonnet D, Aggoun Y, Szezepanski I, Bellal N, Blanche S (2004) Arterial stiffness and endothelial dysfunction in HIV-infected children. AIDS 18: 1037-1041.

181. Mary-Krause M, Cotte L, Simon A, Partisani M, Costagliola D; Clinical Epidemiology Group from the French Hospital Database (2003) Increased risk of myocardial infarction with duration of protease inhibitor therapy in HIV-infected men. AIDS 17: 2479-2486.

182. Bozzette SA, Ake CF, Tam HK, Chang SW, Louis TA (2003) Cardiovascular and cerebrovascular events in patients treated for human immunodeficiency virus infection. N Engl J Med 348: 702-710.

183. Lipshultz SE, Easley KA, Orav EJ, Kaplan S, Starc TJ, et al. (2000) Absence of cardiac toxicity of zidovudine in infants. Pediatric Pulmonary and Cardiac Complications of Vertically Transmitted HIV Infection Study Group. N Engl J Med 343: 759-766.

184. van der Valk M, Gisolf EH, Reiss P, Wit FW, Japour A, et al. (2001) and the Prometheus Study Group. Increased risk of lipodystrophy when

nucleoside analogue reverse transcriptase inhibitors are included with protease inhibitors in the treatment of HIV-1 infection. AIDS 15: 847–855.

185. Dolan SE, Hadigan C, Killilea KM, Sullivan MP, Hemphill L, et al. (2005) Increased cardiovascular disease risk indices in HIV-infected women. J Acquir Immune Defic Syndr 39: 44-54.

186. Mora S, Sala N, Bricalli D, Zuin G, Chiumello G, et al. (2001) Bone mineral loss through increased bone turnover in HIV-infected children treated with highly active antiretroviral therapy. AIDS 15: 1823-1829.

187. Mora S, Zamproni I, Beccio S, Bianchi R, Giacomet V, et al. (2004) Longitudinal changes of bone mineral density and metabolism in antiretroviral-treated human immunodeficiency virus-infected children. J Clin Endocrinol Metab 89: 24–28.

188. Jacobson DL, Spiegelman D, Duggan C, Weinberg GA, Bechard L, et al. (2005) Predictors of bone mineral density in human immunodeficiency virus-1 infected children. J Pediatr Gastroenterol Nutr 41: 339-346.

189. Castillo AB, Tarantal AF, Watnik MR, Martin RB (2002) Tenofovir treatment at 30 mg/kg/day can inhibit cortical bone mineralization in growing rhesus monkeys (Macaca mulatta). J Orthop Res 20: 1185-1189.

190. O'Brien KO, Razavi M, Henderson RA, Caballero B, Ellis KJ (2001) Bone mineral content in girls perinatally infected with HIV. Am J Clin Nutr 73: 821-826.

191. Zamboni G, Antoniazzi F, Bertoldo F, Lauriola S, Antozzi L, et al. (2003) Altered bone metabolism in children infected with human immunodeficiency virus. Acta Paediatr 92: 12-16.

192. Stagi S, Bindi G, Galluzzi F, Galli L, Salti L, et al. (2004) Changed bone status in human immunodeficiency virus type 1 (HIV-1) perinatally infected children is related to low serum free IGF-I. Clin Endocrinol 61: 692-699.

193. Mora S, Zamproni I, Giacomet V, Cafarelli L, Figini C, et al. (2005) Analysis of bone mineral content in horizontally HIV-infected children naive to antiretroviral treatment. Calcif Tissue Int 76: 336-340.

10

Effects of Lifestyle Modifications on Improvement in the Blood Lipid Profiles in Patients with Dyslipidemia

Ryoma Michishita[1*], Hiroaki Tanaka[1,2], Hideaki Kumahara[3], Makoto Ayabe[4], Takuro Tobina[5], Eiichi Yoshimura[6], Takuro Matsuda[2,7], Yasuki Higaki[1,2] and Akira Kiyonaga[1,2]

[1]Laboratory of Exercise Physiology, Faculty of Health and Sports Science, Fukuoka University, Fukuoka, Japan

[2]Institute for Physical Activity, Fukuoka University, Fukuoka, Japan

[3]Faculty of Nutritional Sciences, Nakamura Gakuen University, Fukuoka, Japan

[4]Faculty of Computer Science and Systems Engineering, Okayama Prefectural University, Okayama, Japan

[5]Faculty of Nursing and Nutrition, Laboratory of Exercise Physiology, University of Nagasaki, Nagasaki, Japan

[6]Department of Food and Health Science, Prefectural University of Kumamoto, Kumamoto, Japan

[7]Department of Physical Medicine and Rehabilitation, Fukuoka University Hospital, Fukuoka, Japan

*Corresponding author: Michishita R, Laboratory of Exercise Physiology, Faculty of Health and Sports Science, Fukuoka University, Fukuoka, Japan; E-mail: rmichishita@fukuoka-u.ac.jp

Abstract

Aim: This study was designed to clarify the difference in the effects of aerobic exercise training and diet on the improvement in the blood lipid profiles in patients with dyslipidemia.

Subjects and Methods: The study enrolled 86 patients with dyslipidemia [34 males and 52 females; age, 55 ± 10 years (33 to 71 years); low-density lipoprotein cholesterol (LDL-C), 150 ± 33 mg/dl (74 to 206 mg/dl); high-density lipoprotein cholesterol (HDL-C), 54 ± 12 mg/dl (35 to 87 mg/dl) and triglycerides, 165 ± 65 mg/dl (68 to 318 mg/dl)]. The subjects were randomly allocated to exercise training (n=42) or diet (n=44) group. These patients in the exercise training group were instructed to exercise for more than 300 min per week at the lactate threshold intensity. In the diet group, the target caloric intake was 25 kcal/kg of ideal body weight [height $(m)^2 \times 22$] according to the guideline of the Japan Society for the Study of Obesity.

Results: After the 12-week intervention, the LDL-C, triglyceride level and body weight decreased in both the exercise training and diet groups (p<0.05). There was no significant interaction effect for group × time on the LDL-C, fasting triglyceride level or body weight between the groups. The HDL-C increased only in the exercise training group, and a significant interaction effect for group × time was seen between the exercise training and diet groups for the HDL-C levels (p<0.05).

Conclusions: Based on our results, an improvement in the HDL-C level was observed in the exercise training group, but not in the diet group, despite the fact that the reductions in the LDL-C, triglycerides and body weight were not significantly different between the two groups. Therefore, these results suggest that lifestyle modification, especially exercise training, is considered to be important to reduce the risk of cardiovascular disease through by increasing the HDL-C.

Keywords: High-density lipoprotein cholesterol; Aerobic exercise training; Diet; Dyslipidemia

Introduction

A low high-density lipoprotein cholesterol (HDL-C) level is an important independent risk factor for coronary artery disease (CAD) [1]. The Japan Lipid Intervention Trial (J-LIT) observed that the risk of coronary events increased by 18% in males and 21% in females with each 10 mg/dl elevation in the low-density lipoprotein cholesterol (LDL-C), and decreased by 39% in males and 33% in females with each 10 mg/dl elevation of the HDL-C [2].

Lifestyle modifications, such as increases in the daily physical activity and changes in diet are an initial step for the prevention of CAD [3]. It has been well known that physical inactivity and decreased aerobic capacity are associated with significantly lower levels of HDL-C [4-6]. Conversely, habitual exercise training may be able to increase the HDL-C level [7]. On the other hand, it is well known that a low-fat diet has been considered to be an effective method for weight loss, and improvements in the blood lipid profiles by weight loss have been demonstrated [8,9].

Moreover, the weight loss is also effective for improving the HDL-C level. Dattilo et al. observed that a 1.0 kg reduction in body weight was associated with a significant increase in the HDL-C by 0.009 mmol/l (about 0.35 mg/dl) [10]. In prior reports, the National Cholesterol Education Program (NCEP) adult treatment panel published data the emphasizing the impact of weight control by implementing lifestyle modifications combined with exercise training and diet on the level of blood lipids [11]. However, at present, it is still unknown whether exercise training or diet is more important to improve the HDL-C, despite the observation that weight loss influences the increase in the HDL-C level. Furthermore, the differences in the effects and the mechanisms underlying the improvements in the HDL-C by both exercise training and diet have yet to been elucidated.

This study was designed to clarify the difference in the effects of exercise training and diet on improving the HDL-C level in patients with dyslipidemia. We hypothesized that the effects of exercise training and diet on the improvement in the HDL-C level may be different, because the increase in HDL-C occurs via different mechanisms for the two treatments. If the differences between the effects of exercise training and diet on HDL-C can be clarified, it may contribute to demonstrating which lifestyle modifications can good help to prevent dyslipidemia and CAD. Therefore, we focused on patients with dyslipidemia to clarify the differences in the effects of exercise training and diet on the improvement in the HDL-C level, because dyslipidemia is a major risk factor for future CAD.

Subjects and Methods

Subjects

The subjects were recruited by advertisements in newspaper, on the website and on public transportation. Among the 319 subjects who participated in our Metabolic Syndrome Intervention Program (Fukuoka University Randomized Controlled Trial; FURCT), 98 patients with dyslipidemia (41 males and 57 females, age; 55 ± 9 years) were enrolled in this study. The protocol for this program was described in a previous study [12]. Dyslipidemia was defined according to the criteria of the Japan Atherosclerosis Society (LDL-C ≥ 140 mg/dl and/or HDL-C < 40mg/dl and/or triglycerides ≥ 150 mg/dl) [13]. Patients taking anti-hyperlipidemic agents, such as statins or fibrates, were included in this study (statins use, five patients; fibrates use, two patients). Patients with a history of CAD, cerebrovascular diseases or dialysis treatment were excluded.

The patients were randomly allocated to an exercise training (n=50) or diet (n=48) groups using a random number table. Of the 12 patients who did not complete this program (exercise training group: n=8, diet group: n=4), three left for employment-related reasons, three were lost to follow-up, four were in poor physical condition during the 12-week intervention and two left for family reasons. Thus, 86 patients [34 males and 52 females; age, 55 ± 10 years (33 to 71 years); LDL-C, 150 ± 33 mg/dl (74 to 206 mg/dl); HDL-C, 54 ± 12 mg/dl (35 to 87 mg/dl) and triglycerides, 164.9 ± 65.2 mg/dl (68 to 318 mg/dl)] completed the 12-week intervention, with 42 in the exercise training group (17 males and 25 females; age, 55 ± 11 years; LDL-C, 149 ± 29 mg/dl; HDL-C, 55 ± 12 mg/dl and triglycerides, 154 ± 59 mg/dl) and 44 in the diet group (17 males and 27 females; age, 55 ± 9 years; LDL-C, 151 ± 36 mg/dl; HDL-C, 52 ± 11 mg/dl and triglycerides, 176 ± 70 mg/dl).

The flow of participants through the study is shown in Figure 1. All patients gave their informed consent after agreeing with the purpose, methods and significance of the study. This study was approved by the Ethics Committee of Fukuoka University (No. 09-05-01).

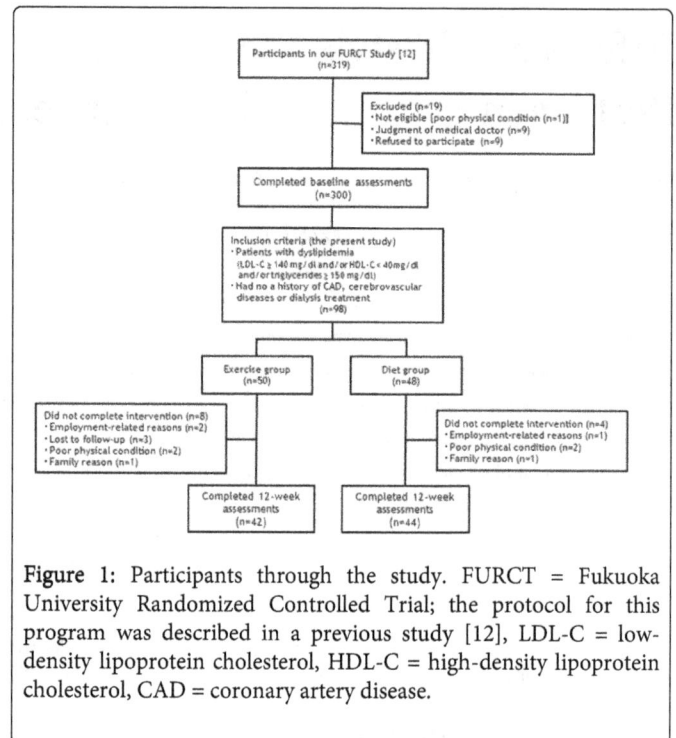

Figure 1: Participants through the study. FURCT = Fukuoka University Randomized Controlled Trial; the protocol for this program was described in a previous study [12], LDL-C = low-density lipoprotein cholesterol, HDL-C = high-density lipoprotein cholesterol, CAD = coronary artery disease.

Blood sampling

Blood samples were collected early in the morning by venipuncture from an antecubital vein after at least 12 hours of fasting. A blood biochemistry analysis was conducted by Special Reference Laboratories (SRL Inc., Tokyo, Japan). The fasting blood samples were used to measure the following parameters: the HDL-C and LDL-C levels by the direct method, the triglyceride levels by the enzyme method, the high-sensitivity C-reactive protein (hs-CRP) level by a nephelometry method, the plasma glucose by an ultraviolet/hexokinase method and the hemoglobin A1c (HbA1c; National Glycohemoglobin Standardization Program value) by high performance liquid chromatography. The insulin resistance was assessed using Matthews's homeostasis model assessment (HOMA-IR) [14] based on the following formula: fasting glucose (mg/dl) × fasting insulin (μIU/ml)/405.

Anthropometry measurement and body composition

The anthropometric measurement and body composition studies were conducted after 12 hours of fasting. The height and body weight were measured, and the body mass index (BMI) was calculated as the ratio of the body weight (kg) to the height squared (m^2). The waist circumference was measured at the level of the umbilicus. The body composition was measured using the underwater weighing method, and the body density was estimated after correction for residual air by the O2 re-breathing method during underwater weighing [15]. The percentage of body fat was calculated using the formula proposed by Brozek et al. [16]. The body fat mass and lean body mass (LBM) were respectively calculated using the following formula: "body weight × percentage of body fat/100" and "body weight – fat mass".

Computed tomography (CT) measurements

The visceral fat area (VFA), subcutaneous fat area (SFA) and middle-thigh muscle area were measured using computed tomography (CT; Toshiba Multi-CT Aquilion TSX-101A Scanner, Toshiba Medical Systems, Tokyo, Japan). For the CT measurements, the examination was conducted after a three-hour fast with only water intake. Images were captured with a maximum voltage of 135 kVp, at 400 mm or 500 mm, to adapt to the anthropometry of each patient. The VFA and SFA were measured at the level of the umbilicus, which were calculated using an image analysis software program (M900PRIMAL, Ziosoft Inc., Tokyo, Japan). The thigh muscle area was measured at the level of the middle thigh circumference, which was divided into low and normal-density muscle. The low- and normal-density muscle areas, markers of lipid-rich skeletal muscle and the contractile component of skeletal muscle were quantified. The data from six images, each 2 mm thick, from the intermediate position between the ends of the anterior iliac crest and patella, were superimposed to create volume data of 10 mm. The low- and normal-density muscle areas were determined based on the calculation of the Hounsfield units (HU) values, using a CT image analysis software program on a Macintosh computer (OsiriX ver 3.3; OsiriX Foundation, Geneva, Switzerland). The low- and normal-density muscle areas were quantified within a 0-29 HU and 30-100 HU attenuation value [17].

Exercise stress test

A ramp submaximal exercise stress test was performed on each subject using an electric bicycle ergometer (REhcor, Lode, Groningen, and The Netherlands) to determine the aerobic capacity and optimal exercise intensity. The work rate was initially set to 60 rpm and 10 watts for the first four minutes as a warm-up, after which it was increased by 15, 10 or 8 watts per minute during the exercise stress test. The increase in the work rate was determined based on the subjects' sex and age (<65-years-old males, 15 watts; ≥65-years-old males, 10 watts; <65-years-old females, 10 watts and ≥65-years-old females 8 watts) or based on the rate decided to be optimal for medical supervision. An exercise stress test was continued until subjective exhaustion was achieved and the oxygen uptake (VO_2) at the peak effort (peak VO_2) was calculated. A respiratory gas analysis was conducted using the mixing chamber method to evaluate the volume of expired air, and the O_2 and CO_2 fractions were analyzed by mass spectrometry (ARCO-2000, ARCO System, Chiba, Japan). Earlobe blood samples were obtained every 30 seconds to measure the lactate acid levels. These 20 μl blood samples were collected in blood collection tubes and evaluated using a lactate analyzer (Biosen 5040, EKF Diagnostik, Barleban, Germany). The workload at the first breaking point of the blood lactate level was used to determine the lactate threshold (LT), and five skilled staff members visually checked the results using log-log (work rate–lactate acid levels) graph paper, and the approximate mean value from three members out of the five members was taken. In this study, the peak VO_2 and metabolic equivalents (METs) at the LT intensity were used as the index for the aerobic capacity.

Exercise training

In the exercise training group, the patients were instructed to perform the bench stepping exercise, bicycle ergometry and walking or running for 60 minutes per session, three times per week under the supervision of exercise trainers, and for a further 120 minutes per week on their own at home to perform a total of at least 300 minutes of moderate exercise per week. The exercise intensity was set at the LT [18]. The difficulty of the training, including exercise at home, was controlled by heart rate at the LT intensity, which was determined by an exercise stress test. Polar FT1 monitors (Polar Electro, Kempele, Finland) were used to measure the heart rate.

Dietary record and diet intervention

Each patient's individual dietary intake was evaluated for three days using a self-record (two weekdays and either Saturday or Sunday) at baseline and during the post-intervention period. All of the meals were photographed to increase the accuracy of the measurement. In the diet group, the target calorie intake was 25 kcal/kg of ideal body weight [height $(m)^2 \times 22$] according to the guideline of the Japan Society for the Study of Obesity [19]. These data analyses and the nutritional guidance were carried out by skilled dieticians.

Statistical Analysis

The data were expressed as the means ± SD. The statistical analyses were performed using the SPSS version 18.0 software package (SPSS Inc., Chicago, IL, USA). The differences in the improvements in the coronary risk factors between the exercise training and diet groups were determined using a two-way repeated-measures analysis of variance for the intervention and groups × time interactions. Comparisons of the data at the baseline and after the intervention were performed using a one way repeated-measure analysis of variance for continuous variables. The inter-group comparisons were performed using the unpaired t-test for continuous variables and chi-square test for categorical variables. Simple linear regression and a partial correlation analysis were performed to determine the associations between the continuous variables. A probability value <0.05 was considered to be statistically significant.

Results

Table 1 shows comparisons of the patients' characteristics at the baseline in both the exercise training and diet groups. There were no significant differences in the age, sex, drinking habits, smoking habits and prevalence of medications used between two groups.

	Exercise training group (n=42)	Diet group (n=44)	p value
Age (years)	55 ± 11	55 ± 9	0.795
Sex (males/females)	17 (40.5)/25 (59.5)	17 (38.6)/27 (61.4)	0.853
Hypercholesterolemia (n,%)	30 (71.4)	29 (65.9)	0.767
Low-HDL cholesterolemia (n,%)	4 (9.5)	5 (11.3)	0.637
Hypertriglyceridemia (n,%)	22 (52.4)	25 (56.8)	0.289
Drinking habit (n,%)	16 (38.1)	12 (27.3)	0.489
Smoking habit (n,%)	3 (7.1)	5 (11.4)	0.737
Taking medications			
Statins (n,%)	2 (4.8)	3 (6.8)	0.584
Fibrates (n,%)	1 (2.4)	1 (2.3)	0.958

Anti-hypertensive drugs (n,%)	8 (19.0)	10 (22.7)	0.476
Hypoglycemic drugs (n,%)	1 (2.4)	2 (4.5)	0.513

Table 1: Characteristics of patient's at the baseline in the exercise training and diet groups

Table 2 shows comparisons of the coronary risk factors before and after the 12-week intervention in both the exercise training and diet groups. There were no significant differences in any of the risk factors between the groups before the intervention. At the baseline, low-HDL cholesterolemia (HDL-C<40mg/dl) was observed in 4/42 patients (9.5%) in the exercise training group and 5/44 patients (11.3%) in the diet group. After the 12-week intervention, the number of patients with low-HDL cholesterolemia decreased from four to one (75% reduction) in the exercise training group and from five to four patients (20% reduction) in the diet group.

	Exercise training group (n=42)		Diet group (n=44)		Group × time Interaction (p value)
	Baseline	12 weeks	Baseline	12 weeks	
Body weight (kg)	70.5 ± 13.6	68.3 ± 12.2 *	72.0 ± 13.1	68.8 ± 13.4 **	0.104
BMI (kg/m2)	27.4 ± 4.6	26.4 ± 4.4 *	27.7 ± 3.5	26.4 ± 3.5 **	0.147
Waist circumference (cm)	95.9 ± 10.2	92.9 ± 9.9 **	96.5 ± 9.6	93.5 ± 7.7 **	0.631
Body fat mass (kg)	21.7 ± 8.0	19.6 ± 7.7 *	23.0 ± 6.6	20.2 ± 5.5 **	0.147
LBM (kg)	48.9 ± 8.4	48.6 ± 7.7	49.3 ± 10.2	49.1 ± 10.1 *	0.562
VFA (cm2)	173.3 ± 60.5	146.1 ± 551 **	191.7 ± 62.0	163.6 ± 49.4 **	0.729
SFA (cm2)	293.7 ± 114.4	268.6 ± 119.6 **	295.7 ± 102.9	266.3 ± 97.4 **	0.462
Low-density muscle area (cm2)	32.8 ± 11.6	32.9 ± 11.9	35.8 ± 12.3	34.7 ± 13.0	0.967
Normal-density muscle area (cm2)	209.6 ± 50.8	216.4 ± 49.0 **	199.6 ± 53.7	192.7 ± 48.2 *	<0.0001
LDL-C (mg/dl)	149 ± 29	143 ± 33 *	151 ± 36	141 ± 25 *	0.49
HDL-C (mg/dl)	55 ± 12	59 ± 15 *	52 ± 11	51 ± 10	0.002
Triglycerides (mg/dl)	154 ± 59	123 ± 45 *	176 ± 70	134 ± 60 *	0.39
HbA1c (%; NGSP value)	5.8 ± 0.6	5.7 ± 0.4	5.7 ± 0.4	5.6 ± 0.3	0.401
Glucose (mg/dl)	103 ± 17	102 ± 14	101 ± 14	100 ± 10	0.354
Insulin (µIU/ml)	8.6 ± 5.1	7.0 ± 4.1 *	8.9 ± 3.9	7.5 ± 3.4 *	0.97
HOMA-IR	2.3 ± 1.5	1.8 ± 1.1 *	2.3 ± 1.2	1.9 ± 0.9 *	0.891
hs-CRP (ng/ml)	1776.1 ± 2260.4	1292.2 ± 1965.2	1789.7 ± 4766.9	743.3 ± 929.8	0.865
Systolic blood pressure (mmHg)	138 ± 16	131 ± 17 *	142 ± 19	135 ± 18 *	0.552
Diastolic blood pressure (mmHg)	87.0 ± 10.3	82.5 ± 10.4 *	87.0 ± 9.7	83.2 ± 7.6 *	0.616
Peak VO2 (ml/min/kg)	23.4 ± 5.2	27.7 ± 7.0 *	21.7 ± 5.3	23.7 ± 8.4	0.001
METs at LT intensity	3.6 ± 0.7	3.9 ± 1.0	3.4 ± 0.7	3.7 ± 1.4	0.496
Energy intake (kcal/day)	2059 ± 326	1993 ± 391	2033 ± 452	1578 ± 321 **	<0.0001
Protein intake (% of energy)	14.9 ± 1.9	15.4 ± 2.5	14.6 ± 2.0	15.4 ± 1.9 *	0.516
Fat intake (% of energy)	28.7 ± 4.0	28.2 ± 5.8	27.6 ± 4.8	26.4 ± 4.8	0.61
Carbohydrate intake (% of energy)	52.9 ± 5.4	53.2 ± 6.7	54.9 ± 6.1	56.0 ± 5.3	0.519

Table 2: Comparisons of the coronary risk factors at baseline and after the 12-week intervention between the exercise training and diet groups

Data are expressed as the means ± SD. *; p<0.05, **; p<0.01, compared to the values before intervention in each group. BMI: Body Mass Index; LBM: Lean Body Mass; VFA: Visceral Fat Area; SFA: Subcutaneous Fat Area: LDL-C: Low-Density Lipoprotein Cholesterol; HDL-C: High-Density Lipoprotein Cholesterol; Hba1c: Haemoglobin A1c; NGSP: National Glycohemoglobin Standardization Program;

HOMA-IR: Insulin Resistance Index By Homeostasis Model Assessment; Hs-CRP: High Sensitivity C-Reactive Protein; Peak VO2: Peak Oxygen Uptake; Mets At LT Intensity: Metabolic Equivalents At Lactate Threshold Intensity; NS: Not Significant.

After the 12-week of intervention, the LDL-C, triglyceride and insulin levels, as well as the HOMA-IR, body weight, BMI, waist circumference, body fat mass, VFA, SFA, systolic and diastolic blood pressure all decreased in both the exercise training and diet groups ($p<0.05$, respectively). The HDL-C, normal density muscle area (30-100 HU) and peak VO2 increased only in the exercise training group ($p<0.05$, respectively). The LBM and normal-density middle thigh muscle area (30-100 HU) decreased only in the diet intervention group ($p<0.05$, respectively).

A significant interaction effect for group × time was seen in the HDL-C, normal density muscle area (30-100 HU) and peak VO2 ($p<0.05$, respectively) between the exercise training and diet groups. There was no significant interaction effect for group × time in the other risk factors between the two groups.

Figure 2 shows the association between the changes in the HDL-C level and the amount of exercise duration per week, as determined by a simple regression analysis in the exercise training group. The mean exercise duration per week was 319 ± 76 minutes. The change in the HDL-C level was positively correlated with the amount of exercise duration per week ($r=0.398$, $p=0.009$).

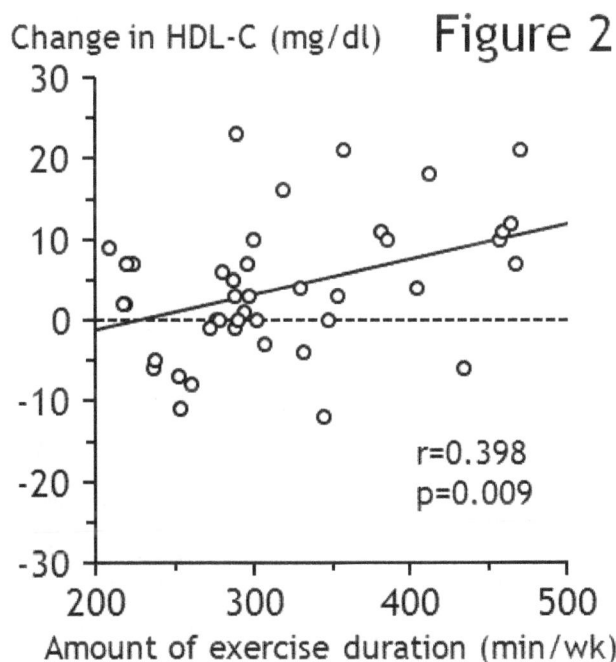

Figure 2: The association between the changes in the HDL-C level and the amount of exercise duration per week in the exercise training group.

Figure 3 shows the association between the changes in the HDL-C level and the changes in the normal-density muscle area (30-100 HU), as determined by a simple regression analysis in both the exercise training and diet groups. The change in the HDL-C level was positively correlated with the change in normal-density muscle area

(30-100 HU) only in the exercise training group ($r=0.382$, $p=0.016$). However, there were no significant relationships between the change in the HDL-C level and the changes in the peak VO2, METs at LT intensity, body weight, BMI, waist circumference, body fat mass, LBM, VFA or SFA in either of the groups.

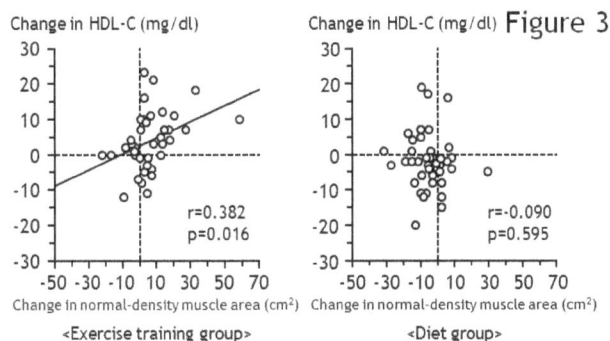

Figure 3: The association between the changes in the HDL-C level and the changes in the normal-density muscle area (30-100 HU) in the exercise training (left) and diet (right) groups.

In the partial correlation analysis, which was after adjusted for the amount of exercise duration per week, there was no significant correlation found between the changes in the HDL-C level and the normal density muscle area (30-100 HU, partial correlation coefficient=0.251, $p=0.128$).

Discussion

The major findings of our study were that the HDL-C level increased only in exercise training group, and a significant interaction effect for group × time was seen between the exercise training and diet groups. Furthermore, the number of patients with low-HDL cholesterolemia decreased from four to one (75% reduction) in the exercise training group and from five to four (20% reduction) in the diet group. Interestingly, in the diet group, there was no significant change in the HDL-C level, despite the observation that there was no significant interaction effect for group × time on the LDL-C, triglyceride levels and body weight between the groups.

It has recently been demonstrated that the combination of exercise training and diet can effectively improve the blood lipid profiles [20-23]. However, the differences in the effects of exercise training and diet on the improvement in the blood lipid profiles have been unknown. There have been many studies [24,25] that showing diet or improvement in the LDL-C and triglyceride levels. However, it has not been elucidated whether the HDL-C level increases following changes in diet. Mensink et al. [26] observed that the HDL-C level was increased by replacing carbohydrates with lipids at the same energy intake. Conversely, an excessive intake of saturated fatty acids has been thought to raise the LDL-C level and to increase the risk of CAD [25]. On the other hand, weight loss is also effective for improving the HDL-C level. Moreover, it is well known that a low-fat diet has been considered to be an effective method to lose weight, and an improvement in the HDL-C level by weight loss has been demonstrated [9,10]. Dattilo et al. observed that a 1.0 kg reduction in body weight was associated with a significant increase in HDL-C by 0.009 mmol/l (about 0.35 mg/dl) [8]. Conversely, Yu-Poth et al. [24]

showed that a low-fat diet using the NCEP Step I and Step II dietary programs decreased the total cholesterol and LDL-C levels, although a reduction in the HDL-C level was also observed. In the present study, the HDL-C level increased only in the exercise training group, while demonstrating no relationship with the change in body weight. Therefore, the improvement in the HDL-C by exercise training may be considered to occur via a mechanism that does not require weight loss.

In our study, the changes in HDL-C level were positively correlated with amount of exercise duration per week in the exercise training group. However, after adjusting for the amount of exercise duration per week, there was no significant correlation between the changes in the HDL-C level and the normal-density muscle area (30-100 HU). At the present, the possible mechanisms underlying the improvement in the HDL-C level by aerobic exercise training have been regarded to include that there is a reduction of the portal free fatty acid level by the decreased amount of visceral fat, that there is an acceleration of lipoprotein lipase (LPL) activity in the muscle and adipose tissue and that the production of HDL-C increases after VLDL decomposition [7]. However, in our study, the change in the normal-density muscle area was not an independent predictive factor for the improvement of the HDL-C level.

According to our data, the change in the HDL-C level was positively correlated with amount of exercise duration per week. We previously evaluated the effects of aerobic exercise training on the HDL-C level in elderly healthy subjects. Our researches suggested that an aerobic exercise training program can result in increases in the HDL-C level, and we have found at the first time, that the increase in HDL-C level was dependent on the total exercise volume [27]. Thus, our present results support the previous study showing that increase in the HDL-C induced by exercise training is dependent on the exercise volume. Recently, Kodama et al. [28] also showed that the increase in the HDL-C dependent on the exercise volume, and the minimum weekly exercise volume necessary to increase the HDL-C level was estimated to be 900 kcal of energy expenditure per week, or 120 minutes of exercise per week. In our exercise training program, the patients were instructed to perform the bench stepping exercise, exercise on a bicycle ergometer and walking or running for 60 minutes per session, and to engage in a further 120 minutes per week on their own at home to perform a total of at least 300 minutes of moderate exercise per week. Therefore, the HDL-C level may have increased only in the exercise training group, because only these subjects engaged in a sufficient volume of exercise.

There are several limitations associated with in this study. First, the limited study population resulted in a small number of subjects, all of whom were free of complications, and in whom there was a predominance of hypercholesterolemia and hypertriglyceridemia. Therefore, it remains unclear whether our findings are consistent with CAD patients and those with other complications. Second, the present study could not measure the LPL activity and apolipoprotein A-I, so we were unable to clarify whether these were involved in the mechanisms underlying the improvement of the HDL-C by aerobic exercise training. Finally, our study period was, only 12-week, which did not provide a sufficient follow-up period to evaluate the influences of diet and exercise training on the longer-term blood lipid profiles. A longer-term additional study including control group should be required to more precisely clarify the effects and mechanisms of lifestyle modifications such as exercise training and diet on the improvement in HDL-C level.

However, in recent several studies, it has been clearly demonstrated that lifestyle modifications can control the development of dyslipidemia and CAD [3, 20-23]. Moreover, aerobic exercise training is an initial step for the prevention of dyslipidemia and CAD. Therefore, we believe our study provides a paradigm, habitual exercise, to prevent CAD in high-risk patients, and might be the good treatment to increase the HDL-C in patients with dyslipidemia.

Conclusions

We found that an improvement in the HDL-C level was observed in the exercise training group, but not in the diet group, despite the fact that the reductions in the LDL-C, triglycerides and body weight were not significantly different between the two groups. These results suggest that lifestyle modification, especially exercise training, are considered to be important to reduce the risk of cardiovascular disease through increasing the HDL-C level, and also suggest that exercise training may be more effective than dieting.

Acknowledgments

We thank all of the members of the Laboratory of Exercise Physiology, Fukuoka University for help with the data analysis. We thank Fukuseikai Hospital, Fukuoka, Japan, for the excellent technical staffs and for their help with the CT examinations. We are also grateful all of to the participants in this study. This work was supported by Grants-in-Aid from The Ministry of Education, Science, Sports and Culture of Japan (No. 15300339 and No. 25242065) and The Fukuoka University Institute for Physical Activity, as well as a Fukuoka University Global FU Program grant.

References

1. Roger VL, Go AS, Lloyd-Jones DM, Benjamin EJ, Berry JD, et al. (2012) Heart disease and stroke statistics--2012 update: a report from the American Heart Association. Circulation 125: e2-2e220.

2. Sasaki J, Kita T, Mabuchi H, Matsuzaki M, Matsuzawa Y, et al. (2006) Gender difference in coronary events in relation to risk factors in Japanese hypercholesterolemic patients treated with low-dose simvastatin. Circ J 70: 810-814.

3. Ornish D, Scherwitz LW, Billings JH, Brown SE, Gould KL, et al. (1998) Intensive lifestyle changes for reversal of coronary heart disease. JAMA 280: 2001-2007.

4. Koba S, Tanaka H, Maruyama C, Tada N, Birou S, et al. (2011) Physical activity in the Japan population: association with blood lipid levels and effects in reducing cardiovascular and all-cause mortality. J Atheroscler Thromb 18: 833-845.

5. Naito M, Nakayama T, Okamura T, Miura K, Yanagita M, et al. (2008) Effect of a 4-year workplace-based physical activity intervention program on the blood lipid profiles of participating employees: the high-risk and population strategy for occupational health promotion (HIPOP-OHP) study. Atherosclerosis 197: 784-790.

6. Kokkinos PF, Holland JC, Narayan P, Colleran JA, Dotson CO, et al. (1995) Miles run per week and high-density lipoprotein cholesterol levels in healthy, middle-aged men. A dose-response relationship. Arch Intern Med 155: 415-420.

7. Slentz CA, Houmard JA, Johnson JL, Bateman LA, Tanner CJ, et al. (2007) Inactivity, exercise training and detraining, and plasma lipoproteins. STRRIDE: a randomized, controlled study of exercise intensity and amount. J Appl Physiol (1985) 103: 432-442.

8. Astrup A, Grunwald GK, Melanson EL, Saris WH, Hill JO (2000) The role of low-fat diets in body weight control: a meta-analysis of ad libitum dietary intervention studies. Int J Obes Relat Metab Disord 24: 1545-1552.

9. Lundgren JD, Malcolm R, Binks M, O'Neil PM (2009) Remission of metabolic syndrome following a 15-week low-calorie lifestyle change program for weight loss. Int J Obes (Lond) 33: 144-150.

10. Dattilo AM, Kris-Etherton PM (1992) Effects of weight reduction on blood lipids and lipoproteins: a meta-analysis. Am J Clin Nutr 56: 320-328.

11. Third Report of the National Cholesterol Education Program (NCEP) Expert Panel on Detection, Evaluation, and Treatment of High Blood Cholesterol in Adults (Adult Treatment Panel III). Circulation 106: 3143-3421.

12. Yoshimura E, Kumahara H, Tobina T, Matsuda T, Watabe K, et al. (2014) Aerobic exercise attenuates the loss of skeletal muscle during energy restriction in adults with visceral adiposity. Obes Facts 7: 26-35.

13. Teramoto T, Sasaki J, Ishibashi S, Birou S, Daida H, et al (2013) Executive summary of the Japan Atherosclerosis Society (JAS) guidelines for the diagnosis and prevention of atherosclerotic cardiovascular diseases for Japanese. J Atheroscler Thromb 14: 267-277

14. Matthews DR, Hosker JP, Rudenski AS, Naylor BA, Treacher DF, et al. (1985) Homeostasis model assessment: insulin resistance and beta-cell function from fasting plasma glucose and insulin concentrations in man. Diabetologia 28: 412-419.

15. Goldman R, Buskirk ER (1961) A method for underwater weighing and the determination of body density. Techniques for measuring body composition. Washington, DC: National Research Council 78-89.

16. BROZEK J, GRANDE F, ANDERSON JT, KEYS A (1963) DENSITOMETRIC ANALYSIS OF BODY COMPOSITION: REVISION OF SOME QUANTITATIVE ASSUMPTIONS. Ann N Y Acad Sci 110: 113-140.

17. Goodpaster BH, Kelley DE, Thaete FL, He J, Ross R (2000) Skeletal muscle attenuation determined by computed tomography is associated with skeletal muscle lipid content. J Appl Physiol (1985) 89: 104-110.

18. Ayabe M, Yahiro T, Mori Y, Takashima K, Tobina T, et al (2002) Simple assessment of lactate threshold by means of the bench stepping in older population. Int J Sports Health Sci 1: 207-215.

19. Japan Society for the Study of Obesity (2006) Japan Society for the Study of Obesity guideline for the treatment of obesity in Japan. Kyowa-Kikaku, Tokyo, 30-45.

20. Hellénius ML, de Faire U, Berglund B, Hamsten A, Krakau I (1993) Diet and exercise are equally effective in reducing risk for cardiovascular disease. Results of a randomized controlled study in men with slightly to moderately raised cardiovascular risk factors. Atherosclerosis 103: 81-91.

21. Stefanick ML, Mackey S, Sheehan M, Ellsworth N, Haskell WL, et al. (1998) Effects of diet and exercise in men and postmenopausal women with low levels of HDL cholesterol and high levels of LDL cholesterol. N Engl J Med 339: 12-20.

22. Nieman DC, Brock DW, Butterworth D, Utter AC, Nieman CC (2002) Reducing diet and/or exercise training decreases the lipid and lipoprotein risk factors of moderately obese women. J Am Coll Nutr 21: 344-350.

23. Kelley GA, Kelley KS, Roberts S, Haskell W (2012) Comparison of aerobic exercise, diet or both on lipids and lipoproteins in adults: a meta-analysis of randomized controlled trials. Clin Nutr 31: 156-167.

24. Yu-Poth S, Zhao G, Etherton T, Naglak M, Jonnalagadda S, et al. (1999) Effects of the National Cholesterol Education Program's Step I and Step II dietary intervention programs on cardiovascular disease risk factors: a meta-analysis. Am J Clin Nutr 69: 632-646.

25. Esposito K, Marfella R, Ciotola M, Di Palo C, Giugliano F, et al. (2004) Effect of a mediterranean-style diet on endothelial dysfunction and markers of vascular inflammation in the metabolic syndrome: a randomized trial. JAMA 292: 1440-1446.

26. Mensink RP, Katan MB (1992) Effect of dietary fatty acids on serum lipids and lipoproteins. A meta-analysis of 27 trials. Arterioscler Thromb 12: 911-919.

27. Sunami Y, Motoyama M, Kinoshita F, Mizooka Y, Sueta K, et al. (1999) Effects of low-intensity aerobic training on the high-density lipoprotein cholesterol concentration in healthy elderly subjects. Metabolism 48: 984-988.

28. Kodama S, Tanaka S, Saito K, Shu M, Sone Y, et al. (2007) Effect of aerobic exercise training on serum levels of high-density lipoprotein cholesterol: a meta-analysis. Arch Intern Med 167: 999-1008.

11

Alcoholic Liver Disease and Alcohol in Non-Alcoholic Liver Disease: Does it Matter?

Lesmana CRA*

Department of Internal Medicine, Hepatology Division, Cipto Mangunkusumo Hospital, Digestive Disease & GI Oncology Center, Medistra Hospital, Jakarta, Indonesia

***Corresponding author:** Lesmana CRA, Department of Internal Medicine, Cipto Mangunkusumo Hospital, Digestive Disease & GI Oncology Center, Medistra Hospital, Jakarta, Indonesia; E-mail: medicaldr2001id@yahoo.com

Abstract

Alcoholic Liver Disease (ALD) is still a major problem in Western and Asian countries. The long-term impact of ALD might further lead to liver disease complications, such as liver cirrhosis and liver cancer. The safe limit amount of alcohol might be different between Western and Asian countries as the genetic factor might also become an important role in the liver disease progression.

It is well-known that alcohol consumption would have synergistic liver injury effect together with chronic viral hepatitis infection. However, in non-alcoholic fatty liver disease (NAFLD), mild to moderate alcohol consumption might have a beneficial effect as it might protect the liver.

Further studies will be needed to confirm the beneficial effect of mild to moderate alcohol consumption for protecting the liver as the liver disease progression in many countries might have different influenced factors, especially in chronic viral hepatitis infection due to different genetic polymorphism and different virus genotype distribution. Obesity, which is now becoming one of the biggest problems in NAFLD patients, it would also give a different prognosis in liver disease progression between Western and Asian countries because of different type of food habits and lifestyle.

Alcohol consumption issue would become the emerging controversies issue in the near future as NAFLD is now becoming an emerging disease despite chronic viral hepatitis infection.

Keywords: Alcoholic liver disease; Liver cancer; Alcohol consumption; Viral hepatitis

Introduction

Alcoholism is still become a major problem either in Western countries or Asian countries, which responsible for 493.300 deaths and 14.544.000 disability adjusted life years (DALYs). Based on studies, mortality rate is higher in men compared to women, which the range of age between 35 to 64 years old. Alcoholic liver disease (ALD) is a spectrum from alcoholic steatosis, steatohepatitis, and liver cirrhosis which also can further lead to the liver cancer development. There are several limit of alcohol amount intake and the length of the consumption itself that can lead to the development of alcohol steatohepatitis until the development of liver cirrhosis based on literatures. Its prevalence around 20% among subjects who undergo liver biopsy and probably higher in hospitalized alcoholic liver patients [1-3].

The change of the lifestyle among young generation might be one of the important factors for the development of alcoholic liver disease. Based on an epidemiological study, looking at male-female differences in drinking and drinking related problems, the sociocultural influence also can be an important role in alcoholic liver disease development [4].

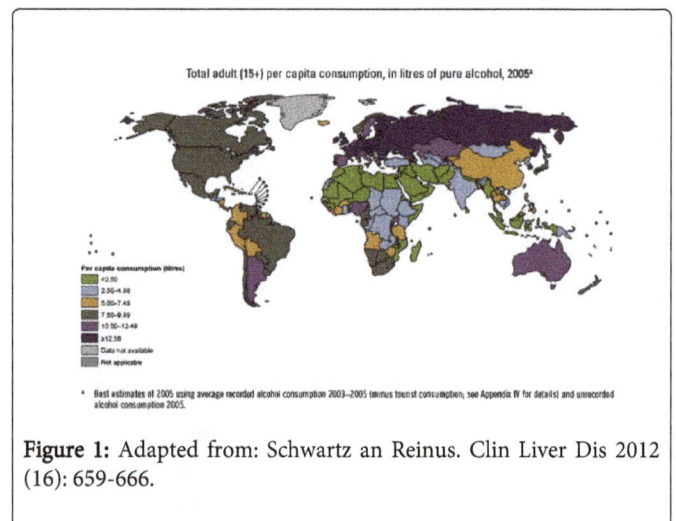

Figure 1: Adapted from: Schwartz an Reinus. Clin Liver Dis 2012 (16): 659-666.

Recently, there has been new paradigm about mild to moderate amount of alcohol consumption, where it is postulated that there might be an advantage for protecting the liver from liver disease progression. However, the impact of mild and moderate drinking in patients with chronic hepatitis viral infection is still become a controversy issue. On the other side, the liver condition improvement in the spectrum of the disease like Non-Alcoholic Fatty Liver Disease

(NAFLD) has been shown with mild to moderate alcohol consumption [5].

Alcohol content in beverages in the United States
14 g of alcohol is the equivalent to:
1 12-oz (350 mL) beer or cooler (~5% alcohol)
1 5-oz (148 mL) glass of wine (~12% alcohol)
1.5 oz (44 mL) of hard liquor (40% alcohol)
Maximal daily quantities:
28 g/d for men
14 g/d for women

Figure 2: Adapted from: Schwartz an Reinus. Clin Liver Dis 2012 (16): 659-666.

Pathogenesis of ALD

Based on previous studies, it has been well-known that alcohol intake will disrupt or injured the mitochondria by increasing the ratio of reduced nicotinamide adenine dinucleotide/oxidized nicotinamide adenine dinucleotide in hepatocytes, even though this pathogenesis is still not clear enough to be understood. As we know that alcohol is metabolized in the liver through the pathways: 1. by the enzyme alcohol dehydrogenase (ADH), 2. by cytohrome P-4502E1 (CYP2E1); and 3. by mitochondrial catalase. ADH is the most important factor which is also present in gastric mucosa; therefore the lower ADH activity will lead to the development of alcoholic liver disease. The first two enzymes will convert alcohol to acetaldehyde, which has role in the progression of liver injury. Acetaldehyde is thought to have a direct toxic effect on cells by the formation of protein adducts by binding to cysteine residue. These modified proteins may then evoke an immune response and the production of autoantibodies perpetuating an inflammatory response. Alcohol exposure also will stimulate lipogenesis and inhibits fatty acid oxidation. The increase of fatty acid synthesis will lead to the steatosis condition. Through its metabolite, acetaldehyde, alcohol consumption also could directly increase transcription of sterol regulatory element-binding protein 1c (SREBP-1c), a transcription factor that promotes fatty acid synthesis via up-regulation of lipogenic genes. The hepatic steatosis itself will further lead to steatohepatitis, where the reactive oxygen species generated and liver injury will progress. Alcohol consumption also increases gut permeability and the bacterial translocation which will contribute to the increase of LPS levels. The LPS will interact with TLR-4 which lead to production of oxidative stress and proinflammatory cytokines that cause hepatocellular damage [2,6].

Some evidence showed that alcoholism is a complex genetic disease where there have been two genes identified such as ADH1B and ALDH2 that play important role in alcohol metabolism in the liver [7].

Diagnosis of ALD

The diagnosis of ALD can be made based on the appropriate history of amount alcohol intake, physical examination and laboratory data [8].

Physical examination usually reveals a malnourished patient with fever, low blood pressure and tachycardia. The stigmata of advanced chronic liver disease might be easily found such as jaundice and ascites and a significant number of patients have hepatic encephalopathy. The liver is usually enlarged and tender. A minority patients will have an audible bruit in the right upper quadrant [8,9].

Laboratory tests are important for the diagnosis. The AST is greater than the ALT, and the total and direct bilirubin levels are usually elevated, with bilirubin level can be more than 15 mg/dL in severe cases. Other markers such as carbohydrate deficient transferring (CDT) and gamma glutamyl transpeptidase (GGT) are more reliable markers to detect previous alcohol consumption. The sensitivity for detection of daily ethanol consumption >50g of CDT (69%), and GGT (73%) are higher than those of AST (50%) and ALT (35%). However, the level of GGT can be influenced also by body mass index (BMI) and sex. Serum sodium and albumin are low, while INR is elevated. White blood cell (WBC) count is elevated, occasionally to >15.000/mm^3 [8,9].

Ultrasound examination of the abdomen is reliable to exclude biliary tract obstruction. Other examination such as liver biopsy provides a sensitive method of evaluating the severity and the degree of liver fibrosis. Whether liver biopsy is needed to be performed in all patients is still controversial. However, liver biopsy might be very useful to confirm the diagnosis, to evaluate the impact of co-existing disease (viral hepatitis), and to rule out other diagnosis. In more advanced disease, liver biopsy should be probably be performed by transjugular route to avoid the risk of hemorrhage [8,9].

Most of non-invasive markers showed a good correlation with the severity of liver damage or injury but good performance is only when it comes to the advanced stage of liver damage. Transient elastography also has a good performance to detect the severity of liver fibrosis, however it should be interpreted with other clinical and laboratory data as there are many factors might influenced the results itself [9].

Alcohol and Chronic Hepatitis B Virus (HBV) Infection

There is still lack of data about interaction between alcohol consumption and chronic HBV infection, especially in Asia. Until now, HBV infection is still become a major problem in developing countries. There are many different prognoses in CHB patients since they will be detected in different stages as well as different liver disease condition. Alcohol consumption might give synergistic injury and will further lead to the development of liver fibrosis and cirrhosis. Study in mice showed that chronic alcohol consumption led to increased levels of HBV surface antigen and viral replication compared with control that did not consume alcohol. Nomura et al found that the prevalence of abnormal liver function test in HBV carriers was increased in patients with light (<59 g/d) and heavy (≥ 60 g/d) alcohol consumption compared with non-drinkers. Another study also showed that alcohol consumption rapidly accelerated fibrosis and the development of cirrhosis in 777 patients with HBV infection [5,10].

Alcohol and Chronic Hepatitis C Virus (HCV) Infection

Chronic HCV infection is the leading cause of advanced liver disease in Western countries. Studies have shown that alcohol consumption results in synergistic liver injury. The liver fibrosis progression has been postulated by several mechanisms such as alcohol's effect on HCV viral replication, HCV-related cytotoxicity, hepatic oxidative stress, and immune modulation. Perlemuter et al found that alcohol consumption increased lipid peroxidation and enhanced production of the cytokines tumor necrosis factor-α and hepatic transforming growth factor-β, which are associated with increased reactive oxidative species generation and further lead to liver fibrosis stimulation [5,10].

There have been many studies showing that different limit amount of alcohol intake can lead to liver fibrosis, cirrhosis and even hepatocellular carcinoma. It has been well-understood that even small amount of alcohol intake (<30 g/d) can promote liver fibrogenesis. The problem with average daily alcohol consumption was not significantly associated with the liver disease progression, so it can be concluded that there was no safe limit amount of alcohol consumption in HCV patients. However, a multivariate study looking at liver fibrosis model found that alcohol consumption was not an independent predictor of fibrosis, and it showed that factors such as age, serum alanine aminotransferase, and histologic inflammation were independent predictors of fibrosis. This model suggested the possible of immunologic or genetic variable are more important than the alcohol intake itself [5,10].

Alcohol and Non-Alcoholic Fatty Liver Disease (NAFLD)

Non-alcoholic fatty liver disease (NAFLD) is an emerging spectrum of disease which is range from simple steatosis, steatohepatitis, and liver cirrhosis. The metabolic syndrome which is the risk factor for the development of NAFLD has also become one part of the disease together with NAFLD. The absence of alcohol intake or minimal alcohol intake has become necessary to confirm the diagnosis of NAFLD [10].

The different amount of alcohol intake in NAFLD patients might have different impact compared to patients with chronic viral hepatitis infection. Even though alcohol intake seems to be an important risk factor for liver fibrosis progression in non-alcoholic steatohepatitis (NASH), there was evidence that alcohol consumption impact is really dose-dependent in NAFLD patients. Alcohol consumption has been shown to be an additive risk factor for liver disease progression in obese fatty liver patients. However, recent studies have shown that light to moderate drinking (<20 g/d and 40 g/d) did not have any impact on the severity of steatosis and steatohepatitis and it might become a protective factor against NAFLD progression. This protective effect has been showed from most of Japanese studies with odds ratio 0.47, 0.824, and 0.754 [5]. Recent study from NASH Clinical Research Network (CRN) group showed that modest alcohol consumption was associated with lesser degree of severity in NAFLD patients (OR 0.56, 95% CI 0.39-0.84, p=0.002) [11].

Alcohol, Viral Hepatitis Infection, Metabolic Syndrome and Liver Cancer

There have been evidence showing that a synergistic interaction on hepatocellular carcinoma (HCC)/liver cancer was observed between alcohol consumption and diabetes (OR 4.2; 95% CI, 2.6-5.8), and between heavy alcohol consumption and viral hepatitis (OR 5.5; 95% CI, 3.9-7.0). It was concluded that heavy alcohol consumption, diabetes, and viral hepatitis were found to exert independent and synergistic effects on risk of HCC. A prospective control-study found that the risk of HCC increased 6-fold for patients with lifetime alcohol exposure, 5-fold with greater than 20 pack-years of smoking, and 4-fold with body mass index (BMI) greater than 30. Another study showed the significant synergy between heavy alcohol consumption, hepatitis virus infection, and diabetes mellitus. Synergistic interactions

on additive model were observed between heavy alcohol consumption and chronic hepatitis virus infection (OR 53.9; 95% CI, 7.0-415.7), and diabetes mellitus (OR 9.9; 95% CI, 2.5-39.3) [5,10,12,13].

Update on Management and Alcohol Issue As A Protective Agent

The main management of alcoholism and ALD is the abstinence, and the malnutrition evaluation. Based on studies, there are specific medications that have been used for alcoholic steatohepatitis treatment such as corticosteroids, pentoxifylline, anti-TNF agents, and N-acetylcysteine. However, despite the standard care management, the assessment of the progression of liver disease itself is more important than just giving medication as the patients might develop acute liver failure and liver transplantation might become a better choice. The problem with the donor and the waitlisted make majority of the patients would have died prior to this goal [3,14].

The recent paradigm showing that alcohol intake might be a protective agent to the liver. There have been studies about a constituent of the red wine which is well known as resveratrol suspected to have a beneficial effect for cardiovascular and cancer prevention. Resveratrol (3,5,4'-trihydroxystillbene) was first isolated from the roots of white hellebore in 1940, and later in 1963, from the roots of Polygonum cuspidatum, a plant used in traditional Chinese and Japanese medicine. Resveratrol was shown to inhibit the deposition of cholesterol and triglycerides in the livers of rats, and to decrease the rate of hepatic triglyceride synthesis. However, some recent studies failed to detect a significant effect on serum cholesterol or triglyceride concentrations [15,16].

When we learn from cardiovascular study, there was evidence that alcohol has beneficial effects on insulin and triglyceride levels, and also gives experimental cardio protection against ischemic-reperfusion injury in isolated hearts. Western studies have concluded that those who take no alcohol might be disadvantaging themselves by lack of beneficial lifestyle. Another study has shown that the men who are fairly heavy drinkers (≥ 3 drinks per day) had lower blood pressure as compared to those who were not had drink red wine. A meta-analysis showed that consumption of wine but not beer was protective to the cardiovascular diseases. In a randomized animal study, resveratrol significantly lowered serum lipid, hepatic cholesterol and triglyceride levels compared to the control. The overall potential of the antioxidant system was significantly enhanced by the resveratrol as plasma and hepatic thiobarbituric acid relative substances (TBARS) levels were significantly lowered while serum superoxide dismutase (SOD), glutathione peroxidase (GSH-Px) and catalase (CAT) activities were significantly increased in the cholesterol-fed rats. These findings suggest that resveratrol maintains an antioxidant efficacy as well as its anti-hyperlipidemic effect [17-20].

Future Perspective

In the future, further studies will be needed as there are different factors between Asian and Western Countries. Alcohol issue would still become an emerging issue as many studies have given new paradigm and controversies. Despite the alcohol itself, of course, it is more important to focus on viral hepatitis management when it is found incidentally with alcohol history. Light to moderate alcohol consumption with the right management of viral hepatitis infection might be a new cornerstone in the near future.

References

1. Rehm J, Samokhvalov AV, Shield KD (2013) Global burden of alcoholic liver diseases. J Hepatol 59: 160-168.

2. Radan Bruha, Karel Dvorak, Jaromir Petrtyl (2012) Alcoholic liver disease. World J Hepatol 4: 81-90.

3. Stickel F, Seitz HK (2013) Update on the management of alcoholic steatohepatitis. J Gastrointestin Liver Dis 22: 189-197.

4. Cheng HG, McBride O (2013) An epidemiological investigation of male-female differences in drinking and drinking-related problems between US-born and Foreign-born Latino and Asian Americans. J Addict.

5. Lee M, Kowdley KV (2012) Alcohol's effect on other chronic liver diseases. Clin Liver Dis 16: 827-837.

6. Gao B, Bataller R (2011) Alcoholic liver disease: pathogenesis and new therapeutic targets. Gastroenterology 141: 1572-1585.

7. Edenberg HJ, Foroud T (2013) Genetics and alcoholism. Nat Rev Gastroenterol Hepatol 10: 487-494.

8. Cohen SM, Ahn J (2009) Review article: the diagnosis and management of alcoholic hepatitis. Aliment Pharmacol Ther 30: 3-13.

9. European Association for the Study of Liver (2012) EASL clinical practical guidelines: management of alcoholic liver disease. J Hepatol 57: 399-420.

10. Altamirano J, Michelena J (2013) Alcohol consumption as a cofactor for other liver diseases. Clin Liver Dis 2.

11. Dunn W, Sanyal AJ, Brunt EM, Unalp-Arida A, Donohue M, et al. (2012) Modest alcohol consumption is associated with decreased prevalence of steatohepatitis in patients with non-alcoholic fatty liver disease (NAFLD). J Hepatol 57: 384-391.

12. Grewal P, Viswanathen VA (2012) Liver cancer and alcohol. Clin Liver Dis 16: 839-850.

13. Hassan MM, Hwang LY, Hatten CJ, Swaim M, Li D, et al. (2002) Risk factors for hepatocellular carcinoma: synergism of alcohol with viral hepatitis and diabetes mellitus. Hepatology 36: 1206-1213.

14. Tilg H, Day CP (2007) Management strategies in alcoholic liver disease. Nat Clin Pract Gastroenterol Hepatol 4: 24-34.

15. Baur JA, Sinclair DA (2006) Therapeutic potential of resveratrol: the in vivo evidence. Nat Rev Drug Discov 5: 493-506.

16. Cal C, Garban H, Jazirehi A, Yeh C, Mizutani Y, et al. (2003) Resveratrol and cancer: chemoprevention, apoptosis, and chemo-immunosensitizing activities. Curr Med Chem Anticancer Agents 3: 77-93.

17. Opie LH, Lecour S (2007) The red wine hypothesis: from concepts to protective signalling molecules. Eur Heart J 28: 1683-1693.

18. Di Castelnuovo A, Rotondo S, Iacoviello L, Donati MB, De Gaetano G (2002) Meta-analysis of wine and beer consumption in relation to vascular risk. Circulation 105: 2836-2844.

19. Zhu L, Luo X, Jin Z (2008) Effect of Resveratrol on serum and liver lipid profile and antioxidant activity in Hyperlipidemia rats. Asian-Aust J Anim Sci 21: 890-895.

20. Bishayee A, Darvesh AS, Politis T, McGory R (2010) Resveratrol and liver disease: from bench to bedside and community. Liver Int 30: 1103-1114.

12

Metabolic Profile of Persons with Newly Diagnosed Diabetes Using either Glycoslated Haemoglobin or Oral Glucose Tolerance Test in Primary Prevention Trials in Asian Indians

Arun Raghavan, Nanditha Arun, Snehalatha Chamukuttan, Priscilla Susairaj, Vijaya Lakshminarayanan and Ramachandran Ambady[*]

India Diabetes Research Foundation and Dr. A. Ramachandran's Diabetes Hospitals, Chennai, India

[*]**Corresponding author:** Dr. Ramachandran Ambady, President, India Diabetes Research Foundation and Chairman of Dr. A. Ramachandran's Diabetes Hospitals 28, Marshalls Road, Egmore, Chennai – 600 008, India; E-mail: ramachandran@vsnl.com

Abstract

Background: To compare cardio metabolic characteristics of Asian Indians with incident type 2 diabetes diagnosed by Oral Glucose Tolerance Test (OGTT) or by Glycosylated Haemoglobin (HbA1c).

Research Design and Methods: Data from two Indian Diabetes Prevention Studies in persons with Impaired Glucose Tolerance (IGT) was used. In 314 persons, diabetes was diagnosed by OGTT and another 67 persons had only HbA1c values ≥ 6.5% (≥48 mmol/mol). Cardiometabolic characteristics were compared in 3 sub-groups-1: Persons with positive OGTT only (HbA1c<6.5% (<48 mmol/mol) (n=125), 2: Persons with positive HbA1c but negative OGTT (n=67), 3: Those with both HbA1c and OGTT positive (n=189).

Results: Diagnostic sensitivity of HbA1c was 67.2% when compared with OGTT criteria. Prevalence of obesity, abdominal obesity, hypertension, insulin resistance and lipid abnormalities were similar in all groups. Persons in groups-1 and 2 had similar metabolic characteristics, but for higher plasma glucose in the former group and higher HbA1c in the latter group. Prevalence of abnormalities was similar in both groups. Group with both the tests positive, had higher levels of insulin resistance.

Conclusion: Metabolic characteristics of incident diabetic cases identified either by OGTT or by HbA1c were similar, except for a higher prevalence of insulin resistance among those who had both tests positive.

Keywords: Diagnosis of diabetes; Glycoslated haemoglobin; Incident diabetes; Metabolic profile; Oral glucose tolerance test; Dyslipidaemia; Cardiometabolic abnormalities

Abbreviations

2hrPG: 2hr Plasma Glucose; ADA : American Diabetes Association; BMI: Body Mass Index; EASD: European Association for Study of Diabetes; FPG: Fasting Plasma Glucose; HbA1c: Glycosylated Haemoglobin; HDL-Chol: High Density Lipoprotein Cholesterol; IDF: International Diabetes Federation; IGT: Impaired Glucose Tolerance; LDL-Chol: Low Density Lipoprotein Cholesterol; LSM: Lifestyle Modification; OGTT: Oral Glucose Tolerance Test; T-Chol: Total Cholesterol; TG: Triglycerides; WC: Waist Circumference; WHO: World Health Organization

Introduction

The debate over an ideal robust biochemical test for diagnosing diabetes continues. Blood glucose estimations, either a fasting glucose or an oral glucose tolerance test (OGTT) was considered as "the gold standard" measurement until 2010. Measurement of blood glucose levels are indices of acute changes in relation to food ingestion. Measurement of glycosylated haemoglobin (HbA1c) equals to assessments of multiple blood glucose (fasting and post prandial) values over a period of 2 to 3 months and therefore is a more robust estimation of average glycaemic status. A diagnostic tool gauging chronic rather than spot hyperglycaemia is certainly preferable [1].

It was only in 2008 an International Committee convened by the American Diabetes Association (ADA), the European Association for Study of Diabetes (EASD) and the International Diabetes Federation (IDF) evaluated the pros and cons of using HbA1c as an a diagnostic tool for diabetes [2] and the ADA [3] and the World Health Organization (WHO) [4] recommended its use for the diagnosis. Sensitivity of HbA1c with a diagnostic cutoff of ≥6.5% (≥48 mmol/mol) is considered to be significantly lower than that of an OGTT [5-16]. In Asian Indians, the sensitivity of HbA1c to identify incident diabetes was found to be only 51% when the results were compared with the OGTT [17]. Another study in Chennai, India showed a sensitivity of 78.2% to identify new cases of diabetes in a cross-sectional population survey [18]. However, whether a HbA1c or an OGTT test is superior in identifying persons with diabetes depends on the definition of diabetes. Variations in laboratory measurements and in rate of glycation of proteins can influence HbA1c values. HbA1c values could also be normal in cases with short duration of hyperglycaemia. If diabetes is considered to be a disease only of the glucose metabolism, an OGTT would appear to be an ideal test. Considering the high degree of non reproducibility of OGTT, HbA1c would be a better glycaemic index of the long term presence of hyperglycaemic values. HbA1c also shows strong correlations with diabetic complications [19].

In this analysis we compared the cardiometabolic characteristics of Asian Indian persons with incident diabetes, and the diagnosis had been made based on the OGTT criteria [20] or by the HbA1c criteria.

Research Design and Methods

The study samples were derived from two Indian Diabetes Prevention Studies; the Indian Diabetes Prevention Program-1 (IDPP-1) and the Indian Diabetes Prevention Program-2 (IDPP-2), the primary results of both were published [21,22]. The studies were approved by the Institutional Ethics Committee. All participants gave written informed consent. In these studies a total of 845 participants with persistant Impaired Glucose Tolerance (IGT) on 2 OGTTs, were followed up for a period of 3 years with assessment of the glycaemic status of all participants at 6 monthly intervals. In these randomized controlled trials, the impact of lifestyle modification (LSM) or use of metformin [21] or LSM and pioglitazone [22] for primary prevention of diabetes was compared with a control group which received standard lifestyle advice only at baseline. All cases included in the analysis (n=381, men:women 314:67) had OGTT and also HbA1c measurements. In the original studies [21,22] the diagnosis of diabetes was made based on the WHO criteria [20]. In this analysis, cases of incident diabetes diagnosed using the WHO criteria for OGTT [20] irrespective of the HbA1c values (Fasting Plasma Glucose (FPG) was ≥126 mg/dl and /or the 2hr plasma glucose (2 hr PG) value was ≥200 mg/dl (n=314)), and another group of 67 persons who had non-diabetic range of glycaemia on GTT, but had HbA1c values diagnostic of diabetes ≥ 6.5% (≥48 mmol/mol[3]) were included for the comparisons. Therefore a total of 381 participants were included in the analysis.

Measurements of height, weight, body mass index (BMI) (kg/m^2), waist circumference (WC) and measurement of blood pressure were done by standard methods.

Fasting and 120 minutes plasma glucose values were measured (glucose oxidase method using auto analyzer, Roche 911, Germany) and corresponding plasma insulin was measured using a radioimmunoassay kit from DiaSorin (Saluggia, Italy). Insulin

resistance was calculated using the homeostasis model assessment (HOMA-IR). A value ≥ 4.1 was considered abnormal for our population [23]. Fasting lipid profile consisting of total cholesterol (T-Chol), LDL-cholesterol (LDL-Chol), HDL-cholesterol (HDL-Chol) and triglycerides (TG) were measured by enzymatic procedures (Reagents of Roche Diagnostics, Germany). HbA1c was analyzed using the immunoturbidimetric method (Tina-Quant Reagents; Roche Diagnostics GmbH, Mannheim, Germany). This method shows good correlation with the high performance liquid chromatography method (r = 0.9937) and is an approved procedure by the International Federation of Clinical Chemistry, certified by the National Glycohemoglobin Standardization Procedure and traceable to the Diabetes Control and Complications Trial assay procedure. The intra-batch coefficient variation of HbA1c was <5% (<31 mmol/mol) and inter-batch variation was <7% (<53 mmol/mol).

Presence of hypertension (≥130/85 mmHg), newly diagnosed or known cases on medication were recorded. T-Chol of ≥200.8 mg/dl, HDL-Chol ≤ 40.2 mg/dl, LDL-Chol ≥ 100.4 mg/dl, and TG ≥ 150.4 mg/dl were considered as abnormal. BMI ≥ 25 kg/m^2 was indicative of obesity and WC ≥ 90 cm for men and ≥80 cm for women indicated abdominal obesity. A comparative assessment of abnormal anthropometric and metabolic parameters was made in persons categorized as shown below.

Group-1: Persons with diabetes who had positive OGTT but with HbA1c<6.5% (48 mmol/mol) (n=125)

Group-2: Person with negative OGTT but with HbA1c ≥ 6.5% (≥48 mmol/mol) (n=67)

Group-3: Persons satisfying both OGTT and HbA1c criteria for diabetes (n=189)

There was no overlap of persons in any group. The median follow up period until diagnosis of diabetes were 24 months, 30 months, and 18 months for groups 1,2 and 3 respectively. Figure 1 shows the total number of participants in each group and also the numbers available from IDPP-1 and IDPP-2 trials.

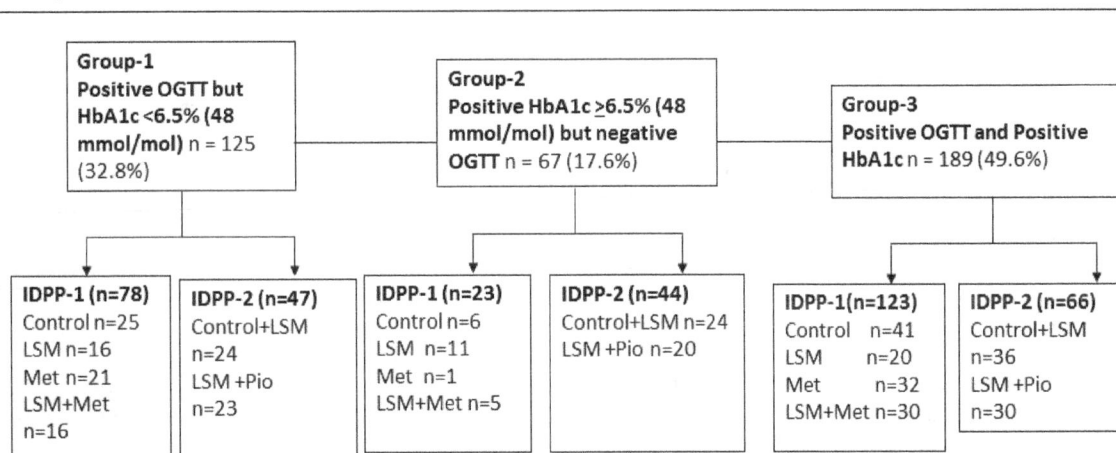

*OGTT – Oral glucose tolerance test, HbA1c - Glycosylated Haemoglobin, IDPP -1 & 2 - Indian Diabetes Prevention Programmes -1 & 2, LSM = Lifestyle Modification, MET – Metformin, LSM+MET - Lifestyle Modificaiton +Metformin

Figure 1: Description of the study groups, number of participants selected from IDPP-1 and IDPP-2 trials.

Statistical Analysis

Mean + SD are reported for normally distributed variables. Median values are shown for TG as it showed skewed distribution variables. One way ANOVA was used for group comparison of normally distributed variables. Intergroup comparisons were done by student's unpaired 't' test. For TG, the Kruskal-Wallis non-parametric test was applied for group comparison. Chi-square test was used to compare the proportions of abnormalities between groups. Prevalence of metabolic abnormalities were compared between men and women. Homeostatis model assessment (HOMA-IR) was used for deriving insulin resistance). HOMA-IR was calculated using the formula: ((fasting insulin(mU/L) × fasting glucose(mmol/L)) / 22.5)). HOMA-IR values were measured only in a subsample in which blood samples were available [24].

Results

The distribution of persons with diabetes in the three study groups is shown in Table 1. Among the total of 381 persons, 256 (67.2%) had the diagnostic HbA1c value also. Therefore, considering OGTT as the standard criteria, the sensitivity of HbA1c in this study cohort was 67.2%. Of the total 381, 189 participants (49.6%) had satisfied both diagnostic criteria. Among the total 381 persons, 314 had 2h glucose values ≥ 200 mg/dl and 98 persons had fasting plasma glucose ≥ 126 mg/dl.

Variables	Group-1	Group-2	Group-3	p value			
	Only Positive OGTT (n=125)	Only Positive HbA1c (n=67)	OGTT and HbA1c Positive (n=189)	(One-Way ANOVA)	Group 1 Vs 2	Group 2 Vs 3	Group 1 Vs 3
	Mean ± SD						
Age (baseline) (years)	46.1 + 5.8	46.2 + 5.7	45.8 + 5.5	0.859	0.834	0.602	0.723
Body Mass Index (Kg/m²)	26.1 + 3.3	26.4+ 3.9	26.7 + 3.6	0.352	0.652	0.512	0.144
Waist Circumference (cm)	91.0 + 7.8	89.1+ 7.0	92.2 + 9.0	0.036	0.094	0.013	0.258
Blood Pressure (mmHg) Systolic	118.6 + 11.1	121.0 + 11.7	122.8 + 12.0	0.008	0.157	0.301	0.002
Diastolic	80.2 + 9.3	78.7 + 8.7	77.6 + 9.0	0.043	0.267	0.389	0.013
Plasma Glucose (mg/dl) Fasting	110.8 + 15.2	107.8 + 9.6	126.0 + 28.3	<0.0001	0.142	<0.0001	<0.0001
120 min	223.6 + 26.1	154.9 + 31.2	247.2 + 42.9	<0.0001	<0.0001	<0.0001	<0.0001
HbA1c % (mmol/mol)	6.0+0.3 (41.6+ 3.4)	6.8 + 0.3 (50.4 + 3.3)	7.4 + 0.8 (57.1 + 8.9)	<0.0001	<0.0001	<0.0001	<0.0001
HOMA-IR†	5.8 (n=114)	4.3 (n=28)	6.3 (n=154)	0.003	0.044	<0.0001	0.059
Lipid Profile (mg/dl) Cholesterol	199.7 + 39.5	188.0 + 32.9	200.5 + 37.2	0.054	0.040	0.016	0.864
Triglycerides†	146	133	150	0.713	0.700	0.395	0.703
HDL-Cholesterol	42.8 + 8.9	40.5 + 9.8	41.8+ 8.5	0.207	0.094	0.311	0.280
LDL-cholesterol	122.5 + 37.1	114.7 + 31.1	122.0+ 37.6	0.306	0.141	0.156	0.892
†Median test; OGTT- Oral Glucose Tolerance Test; HbA1c – Glycoslated Haemoglobin							

Table 1: Metabolic characteristics of persons with diabetes diagnosed based only on OGTT (Group-1), those with only positive HbA1c (Group-2) and those satisfying both criteria (Group-3).

Use of OGTT or HbA1c criteria identified different people with diabetes. The metabolic characteristics of group-1: (only OGTT Positive), group-2: (HbA1c Positive) and group-3: (Both OGTT and HbA1c positive) are shown in Table 1. It was noted that BMI and the lipid profile values were similar in all categories of persons. As expected the glycaemic parameters were significantly higher in people who satisfied both the criteria. Persons in group-2 had significantly lower (P<0.05) values for WC, glycaemic parameters, HOMA-IR, HbA1c and cholesterol values than group-3. Table 2 shows the metabolic characteristics and percentage of abnormal cardiometabolic variables in the study groups. Prevalence of obesity, abdominal obesity, new and known hypertension and lipid abnormalities were similar in these groups. Prevalence of increased HOMA-IR was higher in group-3 than the other groups.

Variables	Group-1		Group-2		Group-3		p value
	Only Positive OGTT (n=125)		Only Positive HbA1c (n=67)		OGTT and HbA1c Positive (n=189)		
	n	%	n	%	n	%	
Body Mass Index ≥ 25 (kg/m^2)	72	57.6	43	64.2	127	67.2	0.223
Waist Circumference	59	53.2	27	60.0	95	60.1	0.492
Men ≥ 90 (cm)	12	85.7	19	86.4	24	77.4	0.651
Women ≥ 80 (cm)							
Cholesterol ≥ 200 (mg/dl)	57	45.6	23	34.3	90	47.6	0.165
Triglycerides ≥ 150 (mg/dl)	60	48.0	28	41.8	96	50.8	0.447
HDL-Cholesterol ≤ 40 (mg/dl)	53	42.4	37	55.2	96	51.1	0.178
LDL-cholesterol ≥ 100 (mg/dl)	99	79.2	50	74.6	145	77.1	0.756
Hypertension							
New	17	13.6	10	14.9	26	13.8	0.965
Known	14	11.2	8	11.9	22	11.6	0.987
HOMA-IR ≥ 4.1	78	68.4	16	57.1	124	80.5	0.010
OGTT- Oral Glucose Tolerance Test; HbA1c - Glycoslated Haemoglobin							

Table 2: Prevalence of cardiometabolic abnormalities among the study groups.

The comparative assessment of the abnormalities among men and women showed that prevalence of obesity was increased among females in group-1 (men 61%, women 77.8%, χ^2=4.0, p=0.046) and presence of higher WC was more among women in groups 2 and 3 (men 57.2%, women 84.4% (χ^2=10.9, p<0.0001). Prevalence of dyslipidaemia and hypertension were similar among men and women.

Discussion

This analysis in a fairly large number of incident diabetic cases available from prospective analysis of persons with IGT showed that the metabolic characteristics of the persons identified either by OGTT or by HbA1c were largely similar. Among the 381 persons diagnosed with diabetes by one of the two criteria, only 189 (49.6%) satisfied both the criteria. Sensitivity of HbA1c for diagnosing OGTT positive cases was 67.2% (256/381 cases). Several studies in populations of varied ethnicity and races had reported significantly lower sensitivity for HbA1c to detect diabetes when compared with OGTT [5-16]. OGTT and HbA1c categorized different persons with diabetes. The discordance between OGTT and HbA1c results occurred because the latter was compared with the OGTT results used as a gold standard.

The persons identified by the two diagnostic criteria will remain discordant to some extent as OGTT indicates acute changes in blood glucose levels while HbA1c is an index of long-term process of glycosylation and therefore they hallmark different physiological processes. Many cases with recent hyperglycaemia are unlikely to have the diagnostic levels of HbA1c for diabetes. Moreover ethnic variations in the rate of glycosylation might also affect the sensitivity of HbA1c as a diagnostic tool for diabetes [10,25,26].

We noted that the metabolic characteristics and cardiovascular risk profile of the incident diabetic cases diagnosed by either the OGTT or by the HbA1c criteria were similar in the Asian Indian population. Presence of insulin resistance was more common in persons positive for both diagnostic criteria. This could be related to the higher levels of fasting and postprandial plasma glucose values. Prevalence of obesity was also more in this group although the difference from the other two groups were not statistically significant.

Several studies [10,11,13,27-29] in varied ethnic populations had reported that diabetes diagnosed by HbA1c had higher age, BMI, lipid levels and insulin resistance than those diagnosed by OGTT. A study in Chinese population had reported more unfavourable cardiovascular and metabolic profile among those who had HbA1c ≥ 6.5% (≥48 mmol/mol) especially among the OGTT negative population [27]. The diagnostic sensitivity of HbA1c was reported to be 66.8% in this population, a value similar to that in our study. Vlaar et al. [11] screened 944 south Asians in Hague, Netherland (18-60 year old), with OGTT and HbA1c for diabetes and prediabetes. The overlap between the two criteria was partial both for diabetes and prediabetes. However the metabolic risk profiles were identical in the group identified by the different criteria.

Borg et al. [12] noted that the HbA1c and OGTT criteria identified similar prevalence of risk profiles in the Danish population. They reported HbA1c identified higher proportion (6.6%) of undiagnosed diabetes than OGTT (4.1%) in the population of the Danish Inter 99 Study. This was contrary to the observation of several other studies which reported lower sensitivity for HbA1c to diagnose diabetic cases [10,11,13,27-29]. Major population-based epidemiological studies have demonstrated a lower prevalence of diabetes by HbA1c criteria compared with OGTT [5,6,16].

Our cohort of persons with diabetes were collected from prospective studies and were newly diagnosed with not more than 6 months of duration. The participants underwent diagnostic tests for diabetes at 6 monthly intervals as all of them had IGT at the baseline. Cross sectional studies have the disadvantage that some may have undetected diabetes of varied durations with consequent metabolic changes.

High prevalence of metabolic abnormalities including overweight/obesity and insulin resistance was due to selection of persons with persistent IGT and also due to the selection of persons with other risk factors for diabetes.

This analysis in Asian Indian persons with type 2 diabetes (n=381), identified during the three year prospective analysis of IGT indicated that, although there was discordance among the diabetic groups diagnosed by the OGTT or HbA1c criteria, most of the cardiometabolic characteristics were similar. It was a limitation that there was a male predominance of (82.4%) in this study. However, a comparison of the metabolic characteristics of men and women in group-1 and 2 did not show significant gender differences. It was also noted that the prevalence of cardiometabolic abnormalities other than abdominal obesity was similar among men and women. It is well known that among middle aged men and women, abdominal obesity is higher in women [30].

As observed in many studies among varied populations, we also noted that OGTT and HbA1c identified different groups of persons with diabetes, with an overlap of about 50-60%.

As we had selected persons with IGT, prevalence of metabolic abnormalities was high. Although we had selected persons with risk factors for diabetes, the prevalence of cardiometabolic abnormalities were similar among persons diagnosed with diabetes either by using HbA1c or by glucose values. Diagnostic sensitivity of HbA1c appeared to be lower when compared with OGTT.

Acknowledgements

We gratefully acknowledge the help rendered by S. Selvam, Mary Simon, C.K. Sathish Kumar and A. Catherin Seeli in the conduct of the studies. No funding was received for this study.

References

1. Bonora E, Tuomilehto J (2011) The pros and cons of diagnosing diabetes with A1C. Diabetes Care 34: S184-S190.

2. The International Expert Committee (2009) Report on the role of the A1c assay in the diagnosis of diabetes. Diabetes Care 32: 1327-1334.

3. American Diabetes Association (2010) Diagnosis and classification of diabetes mellitus. Diabetes Care 33: S62-S69.

4. World Health Organization Consultation (2011) Use of glycated haemoglobin (HbA1c) in the diagnosis of diabetes mellitus. Diabetes Res Clin Pract 93: 299-309.

5. Cowie CC, Rust KF, Byrd-Holt DD, Gregg EW, Ford ES, et al. (2010) Prevalence of diabetes and high risk for diabetes using A1C criteria in the U.S. population in 1988-2006. Diabetes Care 33: 562-568.

6. Rathmann W, Kowall B, Tamayo T, Giani G, Holle R, et al. (2012) Hemoglobin A1c and glucose criteria identify different subjects as having type 2 diabetes in middle-aged and older populations: the KORA S4/F4 Study. Ann Med 44: 170-177.

7. Christensen DL, Witte DR, Kaduka L, Jørgensen ME, Borch-Johnsen K, et al. (2010) Moving to an A1C-based diagnosis of diabetes has a different impact on prevalence in different ethnic groups. Diabetes Care 33: 580-582.

8. Lorenzo C, Haffner SM (2010) Performance characteristics of the new definition of diabetes: the insulin resistance atherosclerosis study. Diabetes Care 33: 335-337

9. Olson DE, Rhee MK, Herrick K, Ziemer DC, Twombly JG, et al. (2010) Screening for diabetes and pre-diabetes with proposed A1C-based diagnostic criteria. Diabetes Care 33: 2184-2189.

10. Mostafa SA, Khunti K, Kilpatrick ES, Webb D, Srinivasan BT, et al. (2013) Diagnostic performance of using one- or two-HbA1c cut-point strategies to detect undiagnosed type 2 diabetes and impaired glucose regulation within a multi-ethnic population. Diab Vasc Dis Res 10: 84-92.

11. Vlaar EM, Admiraal WM, Busschers WB, Holleman F, Nierkens V, et al. (2013) Screening South Asians for type 2 diabetes and prediabetes: (1) comparing oral glucose tolerance and haemoglobin A1c test results and (2) comparing the two sets of metabolic profiles of individuals diagnosed with these two tests. BMC Endocr Disord 13: 8.

12. Borg R, Vistisen D, Witte DR, Borch-Johnsen K (2010) Comparing risk profiles of individuals diagnosed with diabetes by OGTT and HbA1c The Danish Inter99 study. Diabet Med 27: 906-910.

13. Boronat M, Saavedra P, Lopez-Rios L, Riano M, Wagner AM, et al. (2010) Differences in cardiovascular risk profile of diabetic subjects discordantly classified by diagnostic criteria based on glycated hemoglobin and oral glucose tolerance test. Diabetes Care 33: 2671-2673.

14. Xu N, Wu H, Li D, Wang J (2014) Diagnostic accuracy of glycated hemoglobin compared with oral glucose tolerance test for diagnosing diabetes mellitus in Chinese adults: A meta-analysis. Diabetes Res Clin Pract 106: 11-18.

15. Zhou X, Pang Z, Gao W, Wang S, Zhang L, et al. (2010) Performance of an A1C and fasting capillary blood glucose test for screening newly diagnosed diabetes and pre-diabetes defined by an oral glucose tolerance test in Qingdao, China. Diabetes Care 33: 545-550.

16. Borch-Johnsen K, Tuomilehto J, Balkau B (1998) Will new diagnostic criteria for diabetes mellitus change phenotype of patients with diabetes? Reanalysis of European epidemiological data. Br Med J 317: 371-375.

17. Ramachandran A, Snehalatha C, Shetty AS, Nanditha A (2011) Predictive value of HbA1c for incident diabetes among subjects with impaired glucose tolerance—analysis of the Indian Diabetes Prevention Programmes. Diabet Med 29: 94-98.

18. Mohan V, Vijayachandrika V, Gokulakrishnan K, Anjana RM, Ganesan A, et al. (2010) A1C cut points to define various glucose intolerance groups in Asian Indians. Diabetes Care 33: 515-519.

19. McCance DR, Hanson RL, Charles MA, Jacobsson LT, Pettitt DJ, et al. (1994) Comparison of tests for glycated haemoglobin and fasting and two hour plasma glucose concentrations as diagnostic methods for diabetes. BMJ 308: 1323-1328.

20. World Health Organization (1999) Definition, Diagnosis and Classification of Diabetes Mellitus and its Complications. Report of a WHO Consultation. Part 1: Diagnosis and Classification of Diabetes Mellitus, World Health Organization, Geneva.

21. Ramachandran A, Snehalatha C, Mary S, Mukesh B, Bhaskar AD, et al. (2006) The Indian Diabetes Prevention Programme shows that lifestyle modification and metformin prevent type 2 diabetes in Asian Indian subjects with impaired glucose tolerance (IDPP-1). Diabetologia 49: 289-297.

22. Ramachandran A, Snehalatha C, Mary S, Selvam S, Kumar CK, et al. (2009) Pioglitazone does not enhance effectiveness of lifestyle modification in preventing conversion of impaired glucose tolerance to diabetes in Asian Indians: results of the Indian Diabetes Prevention Programme-2 (IDPP-2). Diabetologia 52: 1019-1026.

23. Snehalatha C, Satyavani K, Sivasankari S, Vijay V, Ramachandran A (1999) Insulin secretion and action in different stages of glucose tolerance in Asian Indians. Diabet Med 16: 408-414.

24. Matthews DR, Hosker JP, Rudenski AS, Naylor BA, Treacher DF, et al. (1985) Homeostatis model assessment: insulin resistance and β-cell function from fasting plasma glucose and insulin concentrations in man. Diabetologia 28: 412-419.

25. Sacks DB (2011) A1c versus glucose testing: A comparison. Diabetes Care 34: 518-523.

26. Wisdom K, Fryzek JP, Havstad SL, Anderson RM, Dreiling MC, et al. (1997) Comparison of laboratory test frequency and test results between African-Americans and Caucasians with diabetes: opportunity for improvement. Findings from a large urban health maintenance organization. Diabetes Care 20: 971-977.

27. Peng G, Lin M, Zhang K, Chen J, Wang Y, et al. (2013) Hemoglobin A1c can identify more cardiovascular and metabolic risk profile in OGTT-negative Chinese population. Int J Med Sci 10: 1028-1034.

28. Zhang YH, Ma WJ, Thomas GN, Xu YJ, Lao XQ, et al. (2012) Diabetes and pre-diabetes as determined by glycated haemoglobin a1c and glucose levels in a developing southern Chinese population. PLoS one 7:e37260.

29. Kim CH, Kim HK, Bae SJ, Park JY, Lee KU (2011) Discordance between fasting glucose-based and hemoglobin A1c-based diagnosis of diabetes mellitus in Koreans. Diabetes Res Clin Pract 91: e8-e10.

30. Ramachandran A, Snehalatha C (2010) Rising burden of obesity in Asia. J Obes pii: 868573.

13

Impact of Metabolic Syndrome on Fibrosis Progression in Chronic Viral Hepatitis B Infection

Cem Aygun[*]

Department of Gastroenterology and Hepatology, Istanbul Medipol University, Istanbul, Turkey

[*]**Corresponding author:** Cem Aygun, Department of Gastroenterology and Hepatology, Istanbul Medipol University, School of Medicine, Istanbul, Turkey; E-mail: caygun1@yahoo.com

Abstract

Many factors may increase the risk of fibrosis development in chronic viral hepatitis infections. As the burden of obesity and metabolic syndrome has been increasing in recent years, there is growing concern regarding the association between metabolic factors and chronic viral hepatitis cases. However data regarding the influence of metabolic syndrome on progression of fibrosis in chronic hepatitis B virus (HBV) infection is limited. Metabolic syndrome is a constellation of problems that includes insulin resistance, obesity, hypertension, and hyperlipidemia. Initially, epidemiologic data demonstrated that HBsAg-positive serostatus was positively correlated with a high risk of metabolic syndrome; later on, HBV was considered as a "metabolovirus" because the gene expression of HBV and key metabolic genes in hepatocytes was found to be similarly regulated. Metabolic syndrome is not only found to accelerate the progression of liver disease in patients with chronic HBV infection but also found to induce cirrhosis or even hepatocellular carcinoma development. This review article it is aimed to highlight the association of metabolic syndrome with chronic HBV infection.

Introduction

Chronic hepatitis B virus (HBV) infection is well-known as a major risk factor for liver fibrosis, cirrhosis and hepatocellular carcinoma (HCC) [1-4]. Liver fibrosis may be represented by variable clinical manifestations, which are determined by the type and extent of liver damage, the underlying liver disease and the capacity of the whole body to respond. Cirrhosis is the end stage of liver fibrosis which is characterized by architectural disruption, aberrant hepatocyte regeneration, nodule formation and vascular changes [2]. It is important to accurately predict the rate of liver fibrosis progression in patients with chronic viral hepatitis, which has important clinical significance in terms of prognostic and treatment implications [5].

Metabolic syndrome (MS) is defined as a syndrome that involves three of the following characteristics: dyslipidemia (high levels of apoB lipoproteins and triglycerides, and/or low high density lipoprotein cholesterol), an impaired fasting glucose metabolism, hypertension or central obesity [5-6]. Metabolic syndrome is directly involved in the increased prevalence of coronary heart disease, atherosclerotic diseases, and diabetes mellitus type 2 [6-8]. Other metabolic abnormalities such as liver disease, proinflammatory and prothrombotic states and sleep apnea have also been frequently reported in patients with metabolic syndrome [6-8]. The data about the influence of MS on the prognosis of patients with HBV infection remains limited. Here we tried to investigate the impact of MS on the prognosis of this special patient group.

Epidemiologic link between metabolic syndrome and chronic hepatitis B infection

The association between hepatitis C virus (HCV) infection with lipid and glucose metabolism was demonstrated in many studies [9-10]. Similarly, in time HBV infection was suspected to be related to

dyslipidemia and metabolic syndrome. A study by Su *et al.* reported an association between asymptomatic chronic HBV infection and lower serum levels of total cholesterol (TC) and high-density lipoprotein cholesterol (HDL-C) [11]. In another campus-based study and with a transcriptional animal model, androgen production in HBV carriers with a low BMI (< 23 kg/m^2) was found to be more triggered and up-regulated HBV replication [12,13]. Several other studies reported a positive association between HBV infection and development of dyslipidemia and MS [14-16]. MS was also shown to cause worsening of cirrhosis in chronic HBV patients, suggesting a relationship between MS and progression of HBV infection. In a population based study chronic HBV patients diagnosed with MS had a higher HBV DNA load than patients without MS [17,18].

Hyperglycemia, insulin resistance and the consequent cellular shift to an increased oxidative stress carry a higher risk of progression in chronic liver diseases. Glycated Albumin (GA) is a marker of the glycemic control during the past three weeks which is the turnover time of albumin. The GA/HbA1c ratio is predicted to be high in patients with chronic liver diseases. Indeed, the GA/HbA1c ratio has been reported to be associated with the histological stage of liver fibrosis and portal hypertension in HCV-positive patients and nonalcoholic steatohepatitis. The GA/HbA1c ratio is also found to be increased in association with the stage of liver fibrosis in HBV-positive patients. However, the differences among the fibrosis stages were found to be relatively small [19].

The potential link between diabetes mellitus and metabolic factors with HBV-related HCC has also aroused increasing concern. A long-term community-based cohort revealed that diabetes mellitus was associated with HBV-related HCC. Extreme obesity (body mass index >or=30 kg/m^2) was independently associated with a 4-fold risk of HCC and there was more than 100-fold increased risk in HBV or HCV carriers with both obesity and diabetes, indicating synergistic effects of metabolic factors and chronic hepatitis [20].

This evidence suggested metabolic profiles and subsequent development of MS might be associated with chronic HBV infection. It seems vital to explore the relationship between chronic HBV and MS to inform better prevention and control strategies.

Mechanisms of metabolic syndrome in chronic hepatitis B infection

In the liver glucose, lipid and energy homeostasis is mainly regulated by peroxisome proliferator-activated receptor-γ coactivator 1 (PGC-1α). The elevated expression of PGC-1α may alter the metabolic properties of tissues and lead to various diseases with an underlying dysregulation of metabolism, such as obesity, diabetes, neurodegeneration, and cardiomyopathy [21-24]. Several reports have suggested that HBV adopts a mode of regulation similar to major gluconeogenesis genes in the liver, such as gluconeogenic enzyme phosphoenolpyruvate carboxykinase (PEPCK) and glucose-6-phosphatase (G6Pase), which are co-regulated by PGC-1α, HNF4α and FOXO1 [25,26]. Interestingly, PGC-1α induces oxidative phosphorylation, and the expression of tricarboxylic acid cycle genes —such as SLC25A1 and ACLY—also increases the expression of the de novo fatty acid synthesis enzymes, acetyl CoA carboxylase (ACC) and fatty acid synthase (FASN) [27]. The genes involved in the biosynthesis of lipids, such as FASN and SREBP-2, are up-regulated in HBV-transgenic mouse liver [28]. In HCC, the extent of aberrant lipogenesis correlates with clinical aggressiveness, activation of the AKT-mTOR signaling pathway, and suppression of Adenosine 5'-monophosphate-activated protein kinase (AMPK). In addition, the protein expression of FASN, a key enzyme of lipogenesis that is overexpressed in HCC, is known to be negatively regulated by AMPK [29]. These findings imply that aberrations of glucose and lipid metabolism are closely associated with chronic HBV infection.

Effects of metabolic syndrome on fibrosis in chronic viral hepatitis B

The total prognosis of HBV infected patients is directly dependent on the extent and rate of progression of fibrosis. Therefore prediction of liver fibrosis progression has a key role in the management of chronic viral hepatitis, as it will be translated into the future risk of cirrhosis and its various complications including hepatocellular carcinoma. Both hepatitis B and C viruses mainly lead to fibrogenesis induced by chronic inflammation and a continuous wound healing response. At the same time direct and indirect profibrogenic responses are also elicited by the viral infection. There are a handful of well-established risk factors for fibrosis progression including older age, male gender, alcohol use, high viral load and co-infection with other viruses. Metabolic syndrome is an evolving important risk factor of fibrosis progression (Table-1) [30]. In a study including 850 HBV patients, the prevalance of MS was found to be 5%. Among the components of metabolic syndrome, fasting glucose >100 mg/dL was more frequent and MS was related to older age and higher BMI. The extent of liver fibrosis was found more serious in patients accompanying metabolic syndrome. In the study group, old age, body mass index (BMI), increased aspartate aminotransferase/alanin aminotransferase (AST/ALT), and metabolic syndrome showed association with advanced fibrosis (fibrosis stages 3 to 4). In multivariate analysis metabolic syndrome was found to be independently associated with liver fibrosis [31].

Host related factors	Virus related factors	Additional factors
Older age (>40 years)	High HBV DNA levels	Heavy alcohol consumption
Male gender	HBV genotype(C worse than B, D worse than A)	Steatosis
Genetic diversity	HBV variant (core promoter, pre-S)	Diabetes
	HBV/HCV/HDV co-infection	Obesity
	HIV co-infection	Metabolic syndrome
HBV, hepatitis B virus infection; HCV, hepatitis C virus infection; HDV, hepatitis D virus; HIV, human immunodeficiency virus		

Table1: Factors associated with increased risk of progression to cirrhosis [30].

Another study including 179 cases of HBV-related HCC, who were surgically treated and pathologically confirmed, showed that the higher the BMI, the higher level of insulin and homeostasis model assessment for insulin resistance (HOMA-IR) were significant risk factors for HCC development. Authors concluded that metabolic abnormalities were closely associated with the occurrence and development of HBV-related HCC [32].

A large population based study in the United States investigated the association between metabolic syndrome and risk for both primary liver cancers, hepatocellular carcinoma (HCC) and intrahepatic cholangiocarcinoma (ICC). The results indicated that pre-existing metabolic syndrome, as defined by the 2001 US NCEP-ATP III criteria, confered a statistically significant 2.13 and 1.56 fold increased risk for terminal liver diseases as HCC and ICC which was independent of other risk factors [33]. Recent data from Chinese and Korean cohorts established that MS is a risk factor of advanced liver fibrosis and cirrhosis independent of viral factors in chronic HBV infection [34,35]. In a recent prospective cohort study of 663 CHB patients, new-onset metabolic syndrome and some of its components (namely central obesity and low high-density lipoprotein cholesterol) were found associated with liver fibrosis progression (Figure-1) [36,37]. Even the effect of such coincident metabolic syndrome was most apparent in the immune tolerant phase; its effect was independent of change in viral load and ALT level [36]. This is supported by the observation from a survey in general population that CHB is associated with a lower prevalence of fatty liver, hypertriglyceridemia and metabolic syndrome [37].

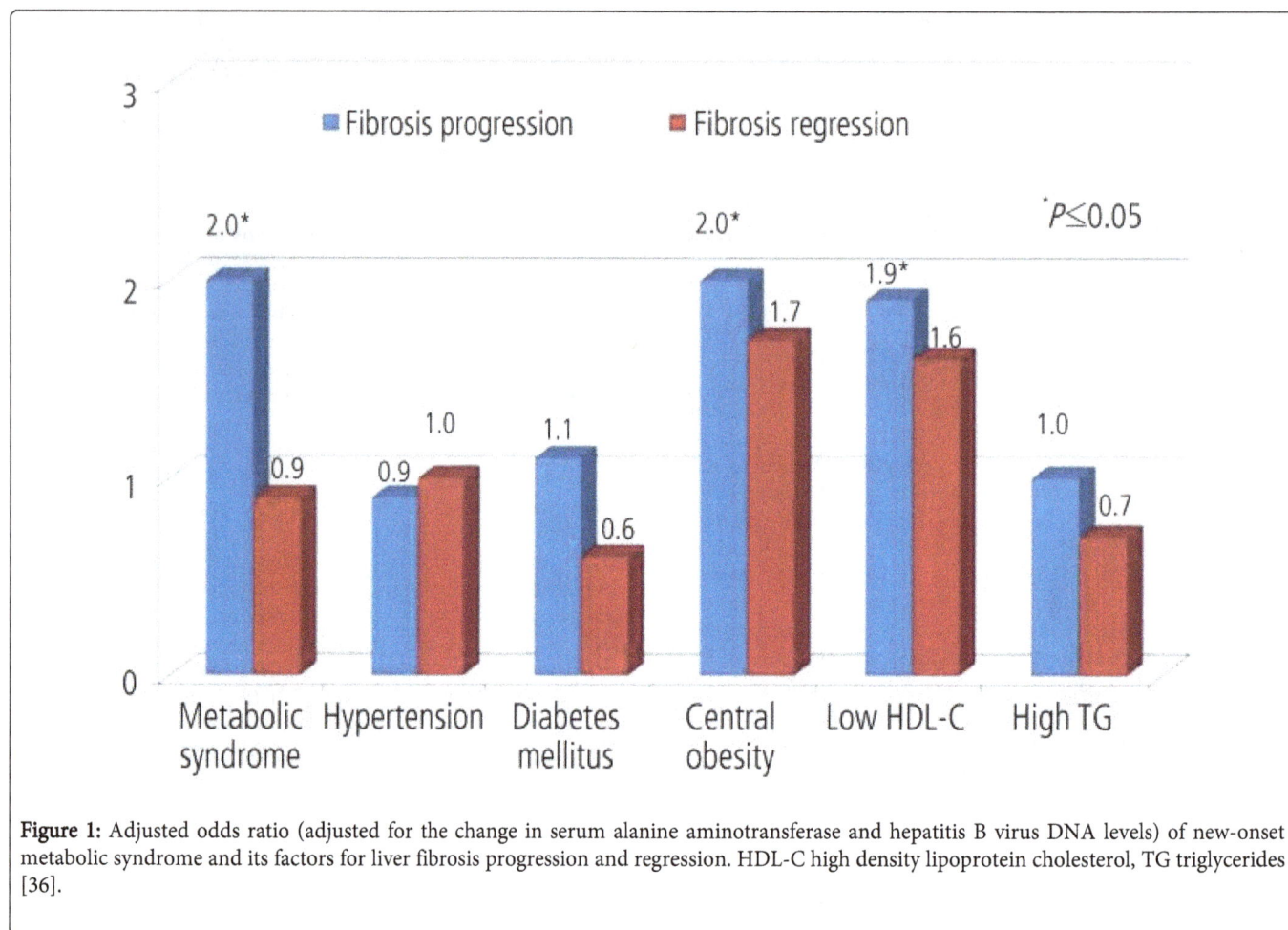

Figure 1: Adjusted odds ratio (adjusted for the change in serum alanine aminotransferase and hepatitis B virus DNA levels) of new-onset metabolic syndrome and its factors for liver fibrosis progression and regression. HDL-C high density lipoprotein cholesterol, TG triglycerides [36].

Conclusion

Obesity and the metabolic syndrome are growing epidemics worldwide. These diseases are associated with both increased risk for, and worsened outcomes of many types liver diseases as well as chronic HBV. In the liver, inflammatory and fibrogenic and angiogenic changes due to underlying insulin resistance and fatty liver disease will likely lead to increased numbers of HBV patients with cirrhosis and HCC in the near future. Much work needs to be done to define more clearly the risks for development of terminal liver disease in those with underlying metabolic syndrome. Screening those at risk, and ultimately, the suitable treatments targeting the underlying mechanisms of pathogenesis would be beneficial.

References

1. Friedman SL (2010) Evolving challenges in hepatic fibrosis. Nat Rev Gastroenterol Hepatol 7: 425-436.

2. Hernandez-Gea V, Friedman SL (2011) Pathogenesis of liver fibrosis. Annu Rev Pathol 6: 425-456.

3. Chan HL, Sung JJ (2006) Hepatocellular carcinoma and hepatitis B virus. Semin Liver Dis 26: 153-161.

4. Wong GL, Chan HL, Chan HY, Tse PC, Tse YK, et al. (2013) Accuracy of risk scores for patients with chronic hepatitis B receiving entecavir treatment. Gastroenterology 144: 933-944.

5. Gristina V, Cupri MG, Torchio M, Mezzogori C, Cacciabue L, et al. (2015) Diabetes and cancer: A critical appraisal of the pathogenetic and therapeutic links. Biomed Rep 3: 131-136.

6. Expert Panel on Detection, Evaluation and Treatment of High Blood Cholesterol in Adults.Executive Summary of The Third Report of The National Cholesterol Education Program (NCEP) Expert Panel on Detection, Evaluation, And Treatment of High Blood Cholesterol In Adults (Adult Treatment Panel III) (2001) JAMA.285: 2486-2497.

7. Dandona P, Aljada A, Chaudhuri A, Mohanty P, Garg R (2005) Metabolic syndrome: a comprehensive perspective based on interactions between obesity, diabetes, and inflammation. Circulation 111: 1448-1454.

8. Kassi E, Pervanidou P, Kaltsas G, Chrousos G (2011) Metabolic syndrome: definitions and controversies. BMC Med 9: 48.

9. Hsu CS, Liu CJ, Liu CH, Chen CL, Lai MY, et al. (2008) Metabolic profiles in patients with chronic hepatitis C: a case-control study. Hepatol Int 2: 250-257.

10. Huang JF, Chuang WL, Yu ML, Yu SH, Huang CF, et al. (2009) Hepatitis C virus infection and metabolic syndrome-a community-based study in an endemic area of Taiwan. Kaohsiung J Med Sci 25: 299-305.

11. Su TC, Lee YT, Cheng TJ, Chien HP, Wang JD (2004) Chronic hepatitis B virus infection and dyslipidemia. J Formos Med Assoc 103: 286-291.

12. Chiang CH, Lai JS, Sheu JC, Yen LL, Liu CJ, et al. (2012) The risky body mass index ranges for significant hepatitis B viral load: A campus-based study. Obes Res Clin Pract 6: e1-e90.

13. Wang SH, Yeh SH, Lin WH, Wang HY, Chen DS, et al. (2009) Identification of androgen response elements in the enhancer I of hepatitis B virus: a mechanism for sex disparity in chronic hepatitis B. Hepatology 50: 1392-1402.

14. Huo TI, Wu JC, Lee PC, Tsay SH, Chang FY, et al. (2000) Diabetes mellitus as a risk factor of liver cirrhosis in patients with chronic hepatitis B virus infection. J Clin Gastroenterol 30: 250-254.

15. Sangiorgio L, Attardo T, Gangemi R, Rubino C, Barone M, et al. (2000) Increased frequency of HCV and HBV infection in type 2 diabetic patients. Diabetes Res Clin Pract 48: 147-151.

16. Lao TT, Tse KY, Chan LY, Tam KF, Ho LF (2003) HBsAg carrier status and the association between gestational diabetes with increased serum ferritin concentration in Chinese women. Diabetes Care 26: 3011-3016

17. Janicko M, Senajová G, Drazilová S, Veselíny E, Fedacko J, et al. (2014) Association between metabolic syndrome and hepatitis B virus infection in the Roma population in eastern Slovakia: a population-based study. Cent Eur J Public Health 22 Suppl: S37-42.

18. Zhao J, Zhao Y, Wang H, Gu X, Ji J, et al. (2011) Association between metabolic abnormalities and HBV related hepatocelluar carcinoma in Chinese: a cross-sectional study. Nutr J 10: 49.

19. Enomoto H, Aizawa N, Nakamura H, Sakai Y, Iwata Y et al (2014). An Increased Ratio of Glycated Albumin to HbA1c Is Associated with the Degree of Liver Fibrosis in Hepatitis B Virus-Positive Patients. Gastroenterol Res Pract 2014:351396.

20. Chen CL, Yang HI, Yang WS, Liu CJ, Chen PJ, et al. (2008) Metabolic factors and risk of hepatocellular carcinoma by chronic hepatitis B/C infection: a follow-up study in Taiwan. Gastroenterology 135: 111-121.

21. Spiegelman BM, Puigserver P, Wu Z (2000) Regulation of adipogenesis and energy balance by PPARgamma and PGC-1. Int J Obes Relat Metab Disord 24 Suppl 4: S8-10.

22. Koo SH, Satoh H, Herzig S, Lee CH, Hedrick S, et al. (2004) PGC-1 promotes insulin resistance in liver through PPAR-alpha-dependent induction of TRB-3. Nat Med 10: 530-534.

23. Lin J, Wu PH, Tarr PT, Lindenberg KS, St-Pierre J, et al. (2004) Defects in adaptive energy metabolism with CNS-linked hyperactivity in PGC-1alpha null mice. Cell 119: 121-135.

24. Arany Z, He H, Lin J, Hoyer K, Handschin C, et al. (2005) Transcriptional coactivator PGC-1 alpha controls the energy state and contractile function of cardiac muscle. Cell Metab 1: 259-271.

25. Shlomai A, Shaul Y (2009) The metabolic activator FOXO1 binds hepatitis B virus DNA and activates its transcription. Biochem Biophys Res Commun 381: 544-548.

26. Finck BN, Kelly DP (2006) PGC-1 coactivators: inducible regulators of energy metabolism in health and disease. J Clin Invest 116: 615-622.

27. Bhalla K, Hwang BJ, Dewi RE, Ou L, Twaddel W et al. (2011) PGC1alpha promotes tumor growth by inducing gene expression programs supporting lipogenesis. Cancer research 71:6888–6898.

28. Hajjou M, Norel R, Carver R, Marion P, Cullen J et al. (2005) cDNA microarray analysis of HBV transgenic mouse liver identifies genes in lipid biosynthetic and growth control pathways affected by HBV. Journal of medical virology 77: 57–65.

29. Calvisi DF, Wang C, Ho C, Ladu S, Lee SA (2011) Increased lipogenesis, induced by AKT-mTORC1-RPS6 signaling, promotes development of human hepatocellular carcinoma. Gastroenterology 140:1071–1083

30. Yoon H, Lee JG, Yoo JH, Son MS, Kim DY, et al. (2013) Effects of metabolic syndrome on fibrosis in chronic viral hepatitis. Gut Liver 7: 469-474.

31. Zhao J, Zhao Y, Wang H, Gu X, Ji J, et al. (2011) Association between metabolic abnormalities and HBV related hepatocelluar carcinoma in Chinese: a cross-sectional study. Nutr J 10: 49.

32. Welzel TM, Graubard BI, Zeuzem S, El-Serag HB, Davila JA, et al. (2011) Metabolic syndrome increases the risk of primary liver cancer in the United States: a study in the SEER-Medicare database. Hepatology 54: 463-471.

33. Wong GL, Wong VW, Choi PC, Chan AW, Chim AM, et al. (2009) Metabolic syndrome increases the risk of liver cirrhosis in chronic hepatitis B. Gut 58: 111-117.

34. Yoon H, Lee JG, Yoo JH, Son MS, Kim DY, et al. (2013) Effects of metabolic syndrome on fibrosis in chronic viral hepatitis. Gut Liver 7: 469-474.

35. Wong GL (2014) Prediction of fibrosis progression in chronic viral hepatitis. Clin Mol Hepatol 20: 228-236.

36. Wong GL, Chan HL, Yu Z, Chan AW, Choi PC, Chim AM, et al. (2014) Coincidental metabolic syndrome increases the risk of liver fibrosis progression in patients with chronic hepatitis B--a prospective cohort study with paired transient elastography examinations. Aliment Pharmacol Ther 39:883–893.

37. Wong GL, Chan HL, Yu Z, Chan AW, Choi PC, et al. (2014) Coincidental metabolic syndrome increases the risk of liver fibrosis progression in patients with chronic hepatitis B—a prospective cohort study with paired transient elastography examinations. Aliment Pharmacol Ther 39:883–893.

14

A New Oral Formulation based on D-Chiro-Inositol/Monacolin K/ Bergamot Extract/Methylfolate and Vitamin K2 in Prevention and Treatment of Metabolic Syndrome in Perimenopausal Women with a BMI>25 Kg/m²

Claudia Tosti, Valentina Cappelli and Vincenzo De Leo[*]

Obstetrics and Gynecology, Department of Molecular and Developmental Medicine, University of Siena, Policlinico "Santa Maria alle Scotte", Viale Bracci, 53100 Siena, Italy

[*]**Corresponding author**: Vincenzo De Leo, MD, Obstetrics and Gynecology, Department of Molecular and Developmental Medicine, University of Siena, Policlinico "Santa Maria alle Scotte", Viale Bracci, 53100 Siena, Italy; E-mail: vincenzo.deleo@unisi.it

Abstract

Background: Insulin resistance is characteristic of patients with metabolic syndrome and it's more pronounced in overweight patients. In the long term there may be cardiovascular and pressor consequences. Lifestyle and diet changes may partly improve these aspects. The use of insulin-sensitizing drugs such as metformin gives good results, although side effects limit its use. Recently, new molecules exerting a similar effect without side effects have been put on the market, such as the d-chiro-inositol, a new insulin-sensitizing molecule. Have been proposed various associations between inositol and ingredients able to potentiate its therapeutic effect.

Materials and methods: This was a prospective study. 40 women were recruited aged>40 years in perimenopause with metabolic syndrome with insulin resistance, altered lipid parameters and with a BMI>25. Were evaluated: BMI, insulin levels and fasting plasma glucose, lipid profile (total cholesterol, HDL, triglycerides). The patients were divided into 2 groups: group A treated with a new oral product containing d-chiro-inositol 100 mg, monacolin-K 3 mg, bergamot extract 250 mg, methylfolate 200 mcg and natural vitamin K2 45 mcg (Mesix®) in tablets for 6 months, one tablet per day. Group B not treated and followed for 6 months.

Results: The results demonstrated a significant reduction in the levels of almost all parameters in the group treated with this new supplement, without any side effect.

Conclusions: This innovative natural supplement, thanks to the synergy of action of its components, can be a new effective alternative in prevention and treatment of metabolic syndrome in perimenopausal women.

Keywords: Metabolic syndrome; Inositol; Natural supplement; Perimenopause

Abbreviations

MS: Metabolic Syndrome; HOMA: Homeostatic Model Assessment; BMI: Bone Mineral Index

Introduction

Metabolic Syndrome (MS) is defined as a disease characterized by the presence of different variable clinical manifestations such as hypertension, abnormal glucose metabolism, abdominal fat distribution, dyslipidemia, and alterations of coagulation. The definition of the International Diabetes Federation (IDF) in 2005 attributed to the abdominal circumference a determining value for the diagnosis [1,2]. In Italy, the prevalence of this syndrome in the general population appears to be approximately 34%, with a peak in the age group between 65 and 74 years [1]. In type 2 diabetics, however, we arrive at a prevalence of 80-90% [1,2]. A high percentage of women after the age of 40 tend to develop hormonal changes that are reflected in an altered metabolic trim. The estrogen deficiency that occurs with advancing age may be a risk factor for the development of insulin resistance; in fact, physiologically estrogen increases the sensitivity of adipose tissue and striated muscle tissue at insulin action and can affect insulin secretion by increasing circulating levels of growth hormone and cortisol [3,4]. Can also be realized that an increase in blood pressure due to several factors: increase in body weight, increase in plasma insulin levels, whose action can be mediated by sympathetic activation, by a saline retention and/or by a hypertrophy, and finally increased vasomotor reactivity to the stimulations. Even the haemocoagulative structure undergoes significant changes to coincide with the decline of ovarian activity that results in a tendency to hypercoagulability and increased risk of thrombotic events [5]. It's therefore established the framework best defined as metabolic syndrome, characterized by: fasting plasma glucose > 110 mg/dl; blood pressure ≥ 130/85 mm Hg; triglycerides ≥ 150 mg/dl; HDL cholesterol < 50 mg/dl in women, associated with a waist circumference>88 cm in women or a waist-hip ratio [WHR] ≥ 0.81 with minor differences related to age and race [6-8].

Insulin resistance was defined as a state (of a cell, tissue or organism) in which is necessary a quantity of higher than normal insulin to quantitatively produce a normal response [9]. This leads to an increased insulin secretion from β cells and to a compensatory hyperinsulinemia. As long as hyperinsulinemia exceeds insulin resistance, glucose levels remain normal; if the compensatory response of the β cells decreases, a relative or absolute insulin deficiency develops that can lead to glucose intolerance and diabetes type 2.

Insulin resistance diagnosis is based on several tests, the simplest is the determination of blood insulin and sugar levels calculated by the HOMA index (HOMA=glucose (mmol/l) × insulin (mU/ml)/22.5). Values>2.5 indicate insulin resistance [10].

Unfortunately there is not a single treatment to treat MS, the approach is to deal with each symptom separately through the administration of various drugs or nutraceuticals as berberine, resveratrol, urosolic acid [11-13]. With regard to insulin-sensitizing drugs the most often used in women of this age group it's undoubtedly metformin but with side effects. In 30% of cases are reported gastro intestinal side effects such as diarrhea, nausea, bloating, loss of appetite, anorexia, metallic taste in the mouth.

In order to reduce the incidence of these side effects, in recent times it has been used inositol, either in the form of myo-inositol that in that of d-chiro-inositol.

While intracellular inositol is almost all (>99%) myo-inositol, in most of the tissues there are significant differences in the concentrations of myo-inositol and d-chiro-inositol, another important stereoisomer present in fat, in muscles and liver. This distribution reflects the different functions that probably the two isomers play in different tissues, and their proportions are maintained thanks to the action of the NAD, NADH-dependent enzyme epimerase that converts myo-inositol in d-chiro-inositol [14]. Some actions of insulin are performed by inositolphosphoglycan (IPG) mediators that are released by cells after stimulation by insulin [15,16]. It was found that a deficiency in a specific d-chiro-inositol-containing IPG (DCI-IPG) may contribute to IR in individuals with impaired glucose tolerance or type 2 diabetes mellitus [17].

Inositol has been associated to other natural substances in order to potentiate the therapeutic effects [18,19]. The aim is to have a unique formulation in a single daily dosing; thanks to the synergic action of its natural components it may help to stabilize the different altered parameters of MS in order to combine efficacy, safety and compliance.

On this bases we have developed a new formulation based on d-chiro-inositol for insulin-resistance along with monacolin k for hypercolesterolemia, bergamot extract for dyslipidemia, natural vitamin K2 for cardiovascular protection and methylfolate for hyperomocisteinemia.

Monacolin K acts on the regulation of the lipid profile. The monacolins are a group of molecules produced by the fermentation of red yeast rice by *Monascus purpureus*. All monacolins and, in particular, the monacolin K, play an important action in the control of cholesterol levels; in particular, they are involved in hepatic metabolism of cholesterol by competing structurally with the 3-hydroxy-3-methyl-CoA-reductase (HMG-CoA-reductase) active site. In this way the metabolic pathway is interrupted and the endogenous cholesterol production is reduced. Numerous clinical studies conducted on the fermented red yeast rice have highlighted the significant reduction of serum cholesterol, in particular LDL cholesterol, with increase, instead, of HDL [20].

The bergamot juice has been recently studied for its important action on dyslipidemia. Pharmacological studies have confirmed the activities already known in folk medicine, cholesterol lowering action and lipid lowering action. These actions are mainly due to the flavonoids. Clinical studies have shown that the activity of individual flavonoid compounds doesn't have the same power of action of the entire plant complex. The lipid-lowering action carried out by the main bioactive compounds (flavonoids) contained in bergamot juice was further confirmed in a major clinical RCT study conducted on 237 patients with hypercholesterolemia either associated to hyperglycemia or not. The results obtained after 30 days have confirmed that treatment with bergamot extract results in a significant reduction of total and LDL-cholesterol, and a significant increase in HDL-cholesterol values [21]. The plant complex of bergamot has demonstrated in vivo to lower triglyceride levels [22-24].

The addition of methylfolate ensures the control on plasma total homocysteine in women with defects in the methylene tetrahydrofolate reductase (MTHFR) as well [25,26], and natural vitamin K2 helps to improve vascular functionality [27].

The aim of this study was to show as the synergic action of nutritional components and plant extracts of this new supplement may help to control the various altered functional states of MS. We have evaluated changes of lipid profile (total cholesterol, HDL, triglycerides), the reduction of BMI and insulin resistance assessed by HOMA index, after taking this new natural product based on d-chiro-inositol/monacolin K/bergamot extract/natural vitamin K2 and methylfolate.

Materials and Methods

After careful clinical and physical evaluation, 40 women were enrolled aged 40-50 years with metabolic syndrome, BMI>25 kg/m^2 and insulin resistance, with HOMA index>2.5. The women have been introduced to our surgery for menstrual irregularities problems ranging from oligomenorrhea to a real amenorrhea with absences of the menstrual cycle for 60-90 days. Five women had a shortened cycle with a flow rate between 20 and 23 days.

The women were divided into two groups of 2 0 each and treated respectively as follows:
- Group A: treated with a natural supplement based on: bergamot extract 250 mg; d-chiro-inositol 100 mg; vitamin K2 45 mcg, methylfolate 200 mcg; monacolin K 3 mg (Mesix®, PharmaSuisse, Italy) at a dose of 1 tablet per day for 6 months.

- Group B: control, not treated and followed for 6 months.

All the women were subjected to gynecological examination, transvaginal ultrasound and blood sampling at baseline, after 3 months and after 6 months. Patients have been analyzed for those parameters which are typical of MS: insulin, glucose (HOMA index), total cholesterol, HDL cholesterol and triglycerides and has been also rated their BMI. It was also carried out a determination of basal levels of follicle-stimulating hormone (FSH), luteinizing hormone (LH), estradiol, prolactin, thyroid stimulating hormone (TSH) to make a diagnosis of perimenopause resulting FSH levels>20 mIU/ml and, at the same time, to exclude pituitary and thyroid pathologies. Pelvic ultrasonography had excluded the presence of uterine fibromatosis and ovarian cysts, therefore, from the gynecological point of view, enrolled women could be considered dysfunctional patients. The patients were not allowed to assume other treatments (drugs or nutraceuticals), to make changes in diet nor life style in order not to affect the results of the study.

Statistical analysis

Data were reported as mean and standard deviation (SD). The comparison between the parameters before and after treatment for each variable was performed by Wilcoxon Signed Ranks test and between the two different groups through the Mann-Whitney test. The data were considered statistically significant for values of p < 0.05. All analyses were performed using SPSS statistical software version 17 (SPSS Chicago, IL, USA).

Results

All patients completed the study and any particular side effects have not been reported.

The baseline characteristics of the patients are reported in Table 1. There are no statistical significant differences between group A and group B.

	Group A	Group B	p
Age	41 ± 1.8	42 ± 2.0	ns
Insulin (mIU/l)	24.5 ± 2	23 ± 3	ns
Blood glucose (mg/dl)	104 ± 3	106 ± 5	ns
HOMA index	6.3 ± 1.2	6.1 ± 1.4	ns
Triglycerides (mg/dl)	128 ± 15	133 ± 14	ns
Total cholesterol (mg/dl)	255 ± 16	248 ± 15	ns
HDL cholesterol (mg/dl)	47 ± 3	45 ± 2	ns
BMI (kg/m^2)	30 ± 2	29.2 ± 1.8	ns
FSH (mIU/ml)	25 ± 4	23 ± 4.5	ns
LH (mIU/ml)	19.2 ± 3.1	18 ± 2.7	ns
E2 (pg/ml)	35 ± 12	39 ± 8	ns
TSH (mIU/ml)	1.3 ± 0.7	1.5 ± 0.9	ns
PRL (ng/ml)	12.1 ± 4	10.3 ± 3.5	ns

Table 1: Patients baseline characteristics (Mean ± SD). Group A: 20 women treated with d-chiro-inositol/monacolin K/bergamot extract/natural vitamin K2 and methylfolate. Group B: 20 women untreated.

Analysis of the results showed a significant reduction in the levels of all individual parameters in the group treated with the supplement. A result to be emphasized is the body weight reduction measured by the BMI (Kg/m^2), which reduced from 30 ± 2 to 24 ± 1 (p<0.05) after 6 months of treatment with the supplement (Group A) with a 20% BMI reduction; in the control group BMI was instead mostly unchanged (Figure 1).

Even insulin levels were significantly reduced in Group A passing from baseline values of 24.5 ± 2 mIU/l to 18.2 ± 4 mIU/l after 3 months up to 15 ± 1.8 mIU/l after 6 months (p<0.05), while in group B the insulin levels were not significantly altered, rather they are slightly increased (Figure 2). Insulin values were reduced by 37.5% in the group treated with the supplement.

Blood glucose levels in Group A decreased (no statistically significant) from 104 ± 3 mg/dl to 93 ± 4 mg/dl after 3 months to achieve the concentration of 90 ± 2 mg/dl after 6 months of treatment compared to group B where levels remained virtually unchanged (106 ± 5 mg/dl; 108 ± 4 mg/dl; 104 ± 5 mg/dl at baseline time, after 3 months and 6 months, respectively). Blood sugar values in group A

have, therefore, been decreased of 14% compared to a reduction of 2% in the group B.

A similar trend was observed for lipid pro ile; total cholesterol in group A decreased from 255 ± 16 mg/dl to 220 ± 8 mg/dl after 3 months up to 212 ± 9 mg/dl after 6 months of treatment (p<0.05) compared to group B, whose concentrations were not significantly changed (Figure 3).

The total cholesterol is therefore decreased by 16% in the group A. The baseline blood levels of HDL cholesterol increased significantly from 47 ± 3 mg/dl to 66 ± 5 mg/dl after 6 months of treatment (p<0.05) in the group A, with an increase of 40%. In this case also the group B showed no significantly changes (Figure 4). Another interesting parameter is triglycerides value reduced in the group A from 128 ± 15 mg/dl to 112 ± 6 mg/dl (no statistically significant). In the group B this parameter has, instead, increased changing from 133± 14 mg/dl to 138 ± 12 mg/dl after 6 months. Group A showed a decrease in triglycerides values of 12.5%, while in the group B there was a slight increase of 3%.

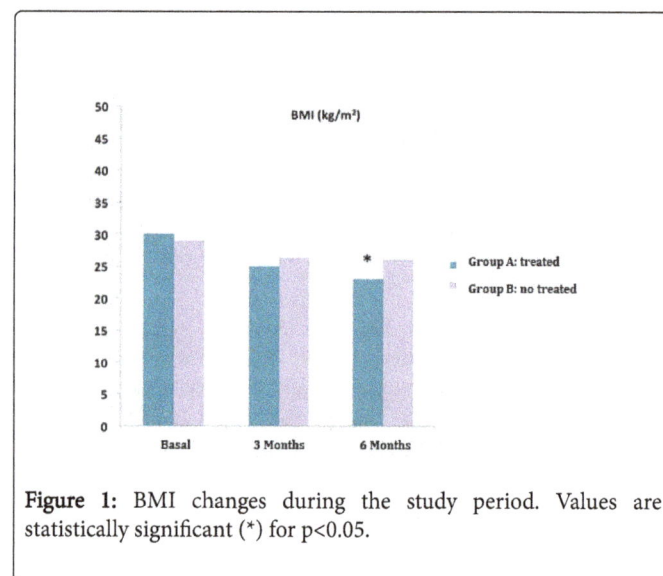

Figure 1: BMI changes during the study period. Values are statistically significant (*) for p<0.05.

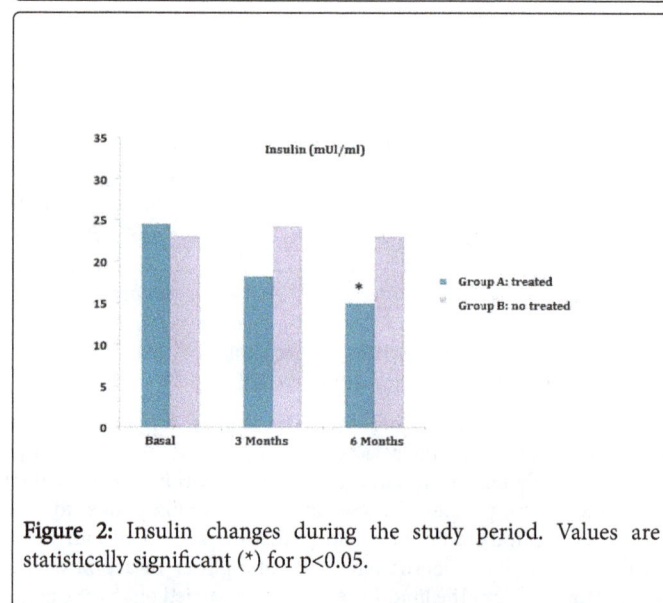

Figure 2: Insulin changes during the study period. Values are statistically significant (*) for p<0.05.

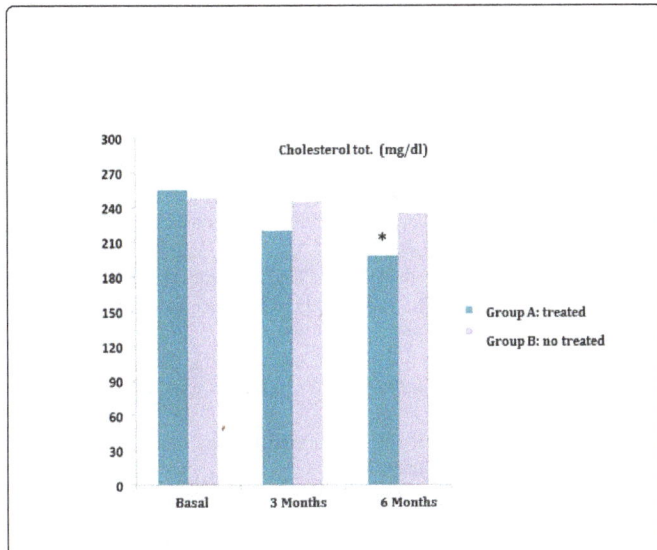

Figure 3: Total cholesterol changes during the study period. Values are statistically significant (*) for p<0.05.

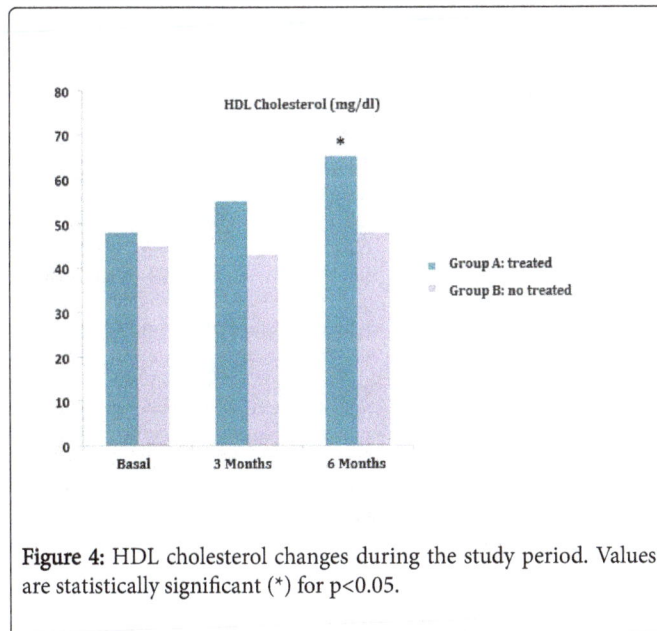

Figure 4: HDL cholesterol changes during the study period. Values are statistically significant (*) for p<0.05.

The HOMA index evaluation has changed significantly in the group of women treated with the supplement (group A) with values that decreased from 6.3 ± 1.2 to 4.1 ± 1.1 after 3 months (p<0.05) and to 3.3 ± 0.6 after 6 months with a variation at the end of the study of 48% from baseline; in the untreated group (Group B), instead, the values increased after 3 months (6.1 ± 1.4 at baseline and 6.48 ± 1.3 at 3 months) and reduced, however not significantly, at the end of study with values that are passed from 6.1 ± 1.4 to 5.9 ± 0.5 with a change of 4% (Figure 5).

Discussion

These data demonstrate that treatment with d-chiro-inositol, monacolin k, bergamot extract, methylfolate and vitamin K2 in perimenopausal overweight women, suffering from metabolic syndrome, improves lipid parameters, insulin resistance, HOMA index and reduces the BMI after 6 months of therapy.

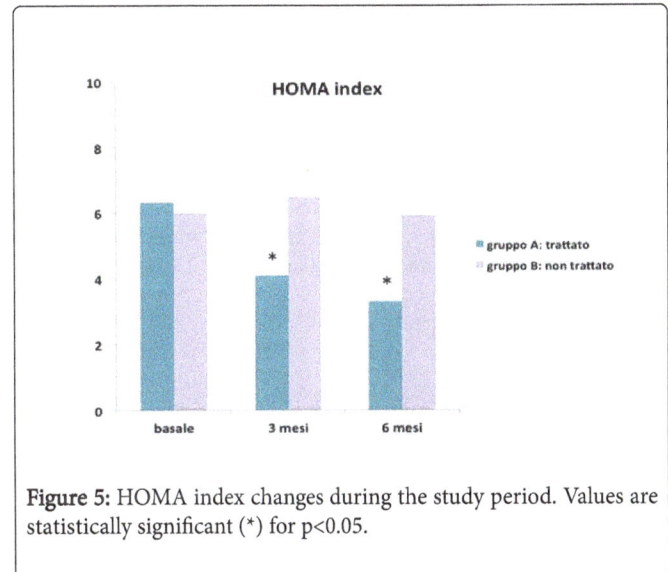

Figure 5: HOMA index changes during the study period. Values are statistically significant (*) for p<0.05.

The BMI was significantly reduced after 6 months in women treated with the supplement and this result has certainly affected the improvement of glucose and lipid metabolism parameters. Regarding the lipid profile, total cholesterol and triglycerides showed a significant decrease while HDL levels have increased. This study demonstrated that the association between d-chiro-inositol, monacolin-K, bergamot extract, methylfolate and vitamin K2 is not limited only to the reduction of total cholesterol, but may increase HDL production that is universally recognized as the most powerful protection factor of cardiovascular risk.

This study confirms the results of previous studies conducted with some of the individual components and, at the same time, gives the evaluated product specific therapeutic characteristics related to the synergistic action of all substances.

A lot of study demonstrated that oral nutritional supplementation with inositol enhances insulin sensitivity and improves the clinical and hormonal characteristics of PCOS patients [28-30].

Recently an International Consensus on Myo-Inositol and d-Chiro-Inositol studied the link between inositol and metabolic syndrome [31].

De Leo et al. demonstrated that the association between monacolin k and inositol improves hormonal and metabolic profiles of women with altered blood value of TG, HDL, LDL and total cholesterol [32].

The endocrine changes that occur in women after age 40, with the reduction in estrogen levels, may contribute to the development of some clinical features of the metabolic syndrome as the different distribution of body fat. In the period of transition from the fertile period to menopause, women are subject to a weight gain with a redistribution of body fat that causes an accumulation of it on the abdomen. In addition to the changes characteristic of the metabolic syndrome such as increased LDL, triglycerides and very low density lipoproteins (VLDL), we observed reduced HDL levels and increased glucose and insulin levels as well. These risk factors may be the result of menopause hormonal deficiency or, alternatively, of the metabolic status due to the redistribution of fat at the central level.

Metabolic syndrome is a condition in which coexist different risk factors and predisposing to the development of diabetes and cardiovascular problems. Risk factors consist of: abdominal obesity, increased triglycerides levels, low HDL cholesterol levels, glucose intolerance, hypertension. In women, a weight gain is achieved with a fat distribution, central or android type, which correlates with a major alteration in blood lipid levels and an increased risk of insulin resistance with compensatory hyperinsulinemia. The latter determines a worsening of atherogenic mechanisms, increasing the risk of cerebrovascular and cardiovascular diseases. Hormonal changes cause, in fact, an increase in total cholesterol, LDL cholesterol, apolipoprotein AI, apolipoprotein B and triglycerides and a decrease in HDL cholesterol plasma concentrations. Lipid alterations, most often associated with the metabolic syndrome, are characterized by elevated levels of triglycerides (>150 mg/dl), low HDL (<50 mg/dl), and LDL levels borderline or high (130/159 mg/dl). This syndrome shows as well significant amounts of small, dense LDL particles with an increased residence time in the circulation for a lower affinity with their receptor and exercising histolesive and inflammatory action on the endothelial tissue.

The synergic action of nutritional components and plant extracts of this new supplement demonstrated to effectively rebalance the altered functional states of the gluco-lipid metabolism and vascular system. The d-chiro-inositol is the most active isomer of inositol. It is an insulin-sensitizing agent, involved in the successful activation of second messenger systems and the insulin receptor. The d-chiro-inositol has contributed, in patients enrolled in this study, to normalize insulin resistance and has been crucial in bringing back the body weight within normal limits. The monacolin K is a phytostatin, for chemical structure and properties very similar to the synthetic statins. It acts as an inhibitor of the HMG-CoA reductase enzyme, involved in the endogenous cholesterol synthesis, exerting cholesterol lowering action with a high degree of clinical evidence, safety and efficacy. The bergamot extract showed multilevel action on the lipid profile (cholesterol, HDL, LDL and triglycerides) and glucose with a mixed mechanism of action, due to the action statin-like and complementary mechanisms of action of the plant complex flavanones. Vitamin K2 (MK-7) biological role is to remove calcium from arteries and soft tissues and help to deposit it on bone tissue, contributing to reduce the risk of cardiovascular diseases. The methylfolate is the active form of folic acid and it doesn't require metabolic transformation by the body. It has shown greater efficacy than folic acid in reducing homocysteine values. Hyperhomocysteinemia is an important cardiovascular factor risk. Based on these results, it can be said that the administration of this innovative natural supplement, Mesix®, thanks to the synergy of action of its components, can be a new and effective alternative in prevention and treatment of metabolic syndrome in perimenopausal women.

Acknowledgment

His study has been supported by PharmaSuisse Laboratories with a not binding contribution

References

1. Kahn R, Buse J, Ferrannini E, Stern M (2005) The metabolic syndrome: time for a critical appraisal: joint statement from the American Diabetes Association and the European Association for the Study of Diabetes. Diabetes Care 28: 2289-2304.

2. Ray JG, Lonn E, Yi Q, Rathe A, Sheridan P, et al. (2007) Venous thromboembolism in association with features of the metabolic syndrome. QJM 100: 679-684.

3. Davis SR, Castelo-Branco C, Chedraui P, Lumsden MA, Nappi RE, et al. (2012) Understanding weight gain at menopause. Climacteric 15: 419-429.

4. Cervellati C, Pansini FS, Bonaccorsi G, Bergamini CM, Patella A, et al. (2011) 17β-estradiol levels and oxidative balance in a population of pre-, peri-, and post-menopausal women. Gynecol Endocrinol 27: 1028-1032.

5. Chae CU, Derby CA (2011) The menopausal transition and cardiovascular risk. Obstet Gynecol Clin North Am 38: 477-488.

6. Alberti KG, Zimmet P, Shaw J (2005) The metabolic syndrome--a new worldwide definition. Lancet 366: 1059-1062.

7. WHO (2000) Obesity: preventing and managing the global epidemic. Report of a WHO consultation. World Health Organ Tech Rep Ser 894: 1-253.

8. Albers JJ, Slee A, O'Brien KD, Robinson JG, Kashyap ML, et al. (2013) Relationship of apolipoproteins A-1 and B, and lipoprotein(a) to cardiovascular outcomes: the AIM-HIGH trial (Atherothrombosis Intervention in Metabolic Syndrome with Low HDL/High Triglyceride and Impact on Global Health Outcomes). J Am Coll Cardiol 62: 1575-1579.

9. Mantzoros CS, Flier JS (1995) Insulin resistance: the clinical spectrum. Adv Endocrinol Metab 6: 193-232.

10. Katz A, Nambi SS, Mather K, Baron AD, Follmann DA, et al. (2000) Quantitative insulin sensitivity check index: a simple, accurate method for assessing insulin sensitivity in humans. J Clin Endocrinol Metab 85: 2402-2410.

11. Martínez-Abundis E, Méndez-Del Villar M, Pérez-Rubio KG, Zuñiga LY, Cortez-Navarrete M, et al. (2016) Novel nutraceutic therapies for the treatment of metabolic syndrome. World J Diabetes 7: 142-152.

12. Sharma BR, Kim HJ, Rhyu DY (2015) Caulerpa lentillifera extract ameliorates insulin resistance and regulates glucose metabolism in C57BL/KsJ-db/db mice via PI3K/AKT signaling pathway in myocytes. J Transl Med 13: 62

13. Sharma BR, Oh J, Kim HA, Kim YJ, Jeong KS, et al. (2015) Anti-Obesity Effects of the Mixture of Eriobotrya japonica and Nelumbo nucifera in Adipocytes and High-Fat Diet-Induced Obese Mice. Am J Chin Med 43: 681-694.

14. Heimark D, McAllister J, Larner J (2014) Decreased myo-inositol to chiro-inositol (M/ C) ratios and increased M/C epimerase activity in PCOS theca cells demonstrate increased insulin sensitivity compared to controls. Endocr J 61: 111-117.

15. Romero G, Larner J (1993) Insulin mediators and the mechanism of insulin action. Adv Pharmacol 24: 21-50.

16. Saltiel AR (1990) Second messengers of insulin action. Diabetes Care 13: 244-256.

17. Asplin I, Galasko G, Larner J (1993) chiro-inositol deficiency and insulin resistance: a comparison of the chiro-inositol- and the myo-inositol-containing insulin mediators isolated from urine, hemodialysate, and muscle of control and type II diabetic subjects. Proc Natl Acad Sci U S A 90: 5924-5928.

18. Thomas RM, Nechamen CA, Mazurkiewicz JE, Ulloa-Aguirre A, Dias JA (2011) The adapter protein APPL1 links FSH receptor to inositol 1,4,5-trisphosphate production and is implicated in intracellular Ca(2+) mobilization. Endocrinology 152: 1691-1701.

19. Grasberger H, Van Sande J, Hag-Dahood Mahameed A, Tenenbaum-Rakover Y, Refetoff S (2007) A familial thyrotropin (TSH) receptor mutation provides in vivo evidence that the inositol phosphates/Ca2+ cascade mediates TSH action on thyroid hormone synthesis. J Clin Endocrinol Metab 92: 2816-2820.

20. Li Y, Jiang L, Jia Z, Xin W, Yang S, et al. (2014) A meta-analysis of red yeast rice: an effective and relatively safe alternative approach for dyslipidemia. PLoS One 9: e98611.

21. Mollace V, Sacco I, Janda E, Malara C, Ventrice D, et al. (2011) Hypolipemic and hypoglycaemic activity of bergamot polyphenols: from animal models to human studies. Fitoterapia 82: 309-316.

22. Miceli N, Mondello MR, Monforte MT, Sdrafkakis V, Dugo P, et al. (2007) Hypolipidemic effects of Citrus bergamia Risso et Poiteau juice in rats fed a hypercholesterolemic diet. J Agric Food Chem 55: 10671-10677.

23. Cappello AR, Dolce V, Iacopetta D, Martello M, Fiorillo M, et al. (2016) Bergamot (Citrus bergamia Risso) Flavonoids and Their Potential Benefits in Human Hyperlipidemia and Atherosclerosis: an Overview. Mini Rev Med Chem 16: 619-629.

24. Cha JY, Cho YS, Kim I, Anno T, Rahman SM, et al. (2001) Effect of hesperetin, a citrus flavonoid, on the liver triacylglycerol contentand phosphatidate phosphohydrolase activity in orotic acid-fed rats. Plant Foods Hum Nutr 56: 349-358.

25. Venn BJ, Green TJ, Moser R, Mann JI (2003) Comparison of the effect of low-dose supplementation with L-5-methyltetrahydrofolate or folic acid on plasma homocysteine: a randomized placebo-controlled study. Am J Clin Nutr 77: 658-662.

26. Villa P, Suriano R, Costantini B, Macrì F, Ricciardi L, et al. (2007) Hyperhomocysteinemia and cardiovascular risk in postmenopausal women: the role of folate supplementation. Clin Chem Lab Med 45: 130-135.

27. Geleijnse JM, Vermeer C, Grobbee DE, Schurgers LJ, Knapen MH, et al. (2004) Dietary intake of menaquinone is associated with a reduced risk of coronary heart disease: the Rotterdam Study. J Nutr 134: 3100-3105.

28. Nestler JE, Jakubowicz DJ, Reamer P, Gunn RD, Allan G (1999) Ovulatory and metabolic effects of D-chiro-inositol in the polycystic ovary syndrome. N Engl J Med 340: 1314-1320.

29. Iuorno MJ, Jakubowicz DJ, Baillargeon JP, Dillon P, Gunn RD, et al. (2002) Effects of d-chiro-inositol in lean women with the polycystic ovary syndrome. Endocr Pract 8: 417-423.

30. Gerli S, Mignosa M, Di Renzo GC (2003) Effects of inositol on ovarian function and metabolic factors in women with PCOS: a randomized double blind placebo-controlled trial. Eur Rev Med Pharmacol Sci 7: 151-159.

31. Facchinetti F, Bizzarri M, Benvenga S, D'Anna R, Lanzone A, et al. (2015) Results from the International Consensus Conference on Myo-inositol and d-chiro-inositol in Obstetrics and Gynecology: the link between metabolic syndrome and PCOS. Eur J Obstet Gynecol Reprod Biol 195: 72-76.

32. De Leo, Musacchio MC, Cappelli V, Di Sabatino A, Tosti C, et al. (2013) A Combined Treatment with Myo-Inositol and Monacolin K Improve the Androgen and Lipid Profiles of Insulin-Resistant PCOS Patients. J Metabolic Synd 2: 127.

15

Low Hepatic Mg^{2+} Content promotes Liver dysmetabolism: Implications for the Metabolic Syndrome

Chesinta Voma[1,2], Zienab Etwebi[2], Danial Amir Soltani[2], Colleen Croniger[3] and Andrea Romani[1*]

[1]Department of Physiology and Biophysics, Case Western Reserve University, USA

[2]Department of Clinical Chemistry, Cleveland State University, USA

[3]Department of Nutrition, Case Western Reserve University, USA

*Corresponding author: Dr. Andrea Romani, Department of Physiology and Biophysics School of Medicine, Case Western Reserve University 10900 Euclid Avenue, Cleveland, OH, 44106-4970, USA; E-mail: amr5@po.cwru.edu

Abstract

Metabolic Syndrome, a pathological condition affecting approximately 35% of the USA population, is characterized by obesity, insulin resistance, and hypertension. Metabolic syndrome is considered the single most common condition predisposing to the development of various chronic diseases including diabetes and hypertension. Hypomagnesaemia has been consistently observed in association with metabolic syndrome, but it is unclear whether reduced Mg^{2+} levels are the consequence or a possible cause for the development of the metabolic syndrome and/or its associated pathologies.

Research performed in our laboratory showed that rats exposed for 2 weeks to a Mg^{2+} deficient diet presented decreased glucose accumulation into the hepatocytes together with low Mg^{2+} level in the circulation and within the liver cells. To better investigate the changes in glucose metabolism, HepG2 were used to mimic in vitro Mg^{2+} deficiency conditions. HepG2 cells cultured in low extracellular Mg^{2+} presented a 20% decrease in total cellular Mg^{2+} content, reduced glucose accumulation, and enhanced glucose 6-phosphate (G6P) transport into the endoplasmic reticulum (ER). The increased G6P transport was associated with its enhanced hydrolysis by the glucose 6-phosphatase, but also conversion to 6-phosphogluconolactone by the glucose 6-phosphate dehydrogenase. The latter process resulted in the increased generation of NADPH within the ER and the increased conversion of cortisone to cortisol by the 11-β-hydroxysteroid dehydrogenase type-1 (11-β-OHSD1).

Taken together, our results provide compelling evidence that Mg^{2+} deficiency precedes and actually promotes some of the hepatic dysmetabolisms typical of the metabolic syndrome. The decrease in intrahepatic Mg^{2+} content up-regulates G6P entry into the hepatic endoplasmic reticulum and its routing into the pentose shunt pathway for energetic purposes. The associated increased in NADPH production within the ER then stimulates cortisol production, setting the conditions for hepatic insulin resistance and further altering liver metabolism.

Keywords: Dietary magnesium; Hepatic Mg^{2+} homeostasis; Metabolic syndrome; Glucose 6 phosphate; Glucose 6 phosphate dehydrogenase; 11 Beta-hydroxysteroid-dehydrogenase-1; Cortisol

Introduction

In the last twenty years the incidence of obesity and type-2 diabetes has dramatically increased in both industrialized and developing countries. In the US, it is currently estimated that more than one-third of the US population is overweight or frankly obese [1], with an economic impact on health care costs estimated at ~$147 per year [2]. To this figure it has to be added the cost of severe medical complications associated with obesity, which include myocardial infarction, cardiovascular diseases, stroke, hypertension, and some forms of cancer (colon and breast cancer, preeminently).

Metabolic syndrome, also known as insulin resistance syndrome, or syndrome X, represents a particular form of obesity. First introduced by Dr. Haller in 1977 [3], the term refers to a cluster of disorders that includes dyslipidemia, hyper-lipoproteinemia, hepatic steatosis, hypertension, obesity, and insulin resistance (or glucose intolerance), and ultimately results in the onset of type 2 diabetes [4]. This definition reflects the view that insulin resistance is the underlying cause of the dysmetabolism [5], and leads to other complications including hypertension [4].

Because of the central role of insulin resistance in the pathophysiology of the metabolic syndrome, the liver becomes a vital organ in coordinating carbohydrate, lipid, and protein metabolism at the whole body level under tight control by circulating hormones such as insulin, catecholamine, cortisol, and glucagon [4]. Abnormal increase in intrahepatic lipid metabolites content directly inhibits insulin-stimulated glucose transport activity in the organ, with major implications for the onset of liver dysmetabolism in the metabolic syndrome.

Interestingly, the increase in the incidence of metabolic syndrome and obesity has coincided with the progressive decrease in dietary magnesium intake [6]. The current Western diet contains approximately 30% to 40% less magnesium than the diet in the late seventies [6] as a result of changes in food processing and water purification. Magnesium is the fourth most abundant cation in the human body, and the second within the cells after potassium [6]. Its distribution is such that approximately 99% of the total magnesium content is within bones, muscles, and soft tissues, leaving ~1% in the circulation [6,7]. Because of this distribution, serum magnesium level is not a reliable indicator of whole body magnesium homeostasis [6].

At the cellular level, magnesium ions (Mg^{2+}) are highly compartmentalized within the cytoplasm, mitochondria, nucleus, and endoplasmic (or sarcoplasmic) reticulum [6,7]. Within these compartments Mg^{2+} is associated with phospholipids, chromatin, ATP, and other phosphonucleotides [7], where by total Mg^{2+} concentrations range between 15 and 18 mM within the cellular organelles, and between 4 to 5 mM in the cytoplasm [7].

Although elevated, these Mg^{2+} concentrations are not static but change dynamically following hormonal stimuli and metabolic conditions [7]. Administration of insulin, for example, promotes Mg^{2+} influx into the hepatocytes [7].

About twenty years ago, Resnick observed that Mg^{2+} content was decreased and Ca^{2+} content increased in erythrocytes from individuals affected by metabolic syndrome [8]. This prompted Resnick to propose the 'ionic theory' whereby these changes in Ca^{2+} and Mg^{2+} concentrations were essential components of the metabolic syndrome. Although Resnick's initial observation was confirmed by several other reports [9], it is still unclear whether Mg^{2+} deficiency proceeds or is a consequence of the metabolic syndrome onset.

In the present study, HepG2 cells were maintained in culture in the presence of physiological (1 mM) or reduced (0.6 mM) extracellular Mg^{2+} to mimic Mg^{2+} deficiency conditions. Changes in glucose accumulation and utilization were assessed by a combination of radio-isotopic distribution techniques or fluorescence methods. The results reported here indicate that Mg^{2+} deficient hepatocyte present reduced glucose accumulation and enhanced G6P entry into the ER of the hepatocyte. This increased G6P entry is associated with an enhanced oxidation to 6-phosphogluconolactone via G6PD, and NADPH production. The production of NADPH, in turn, promotes a marked increase in the conversion of cortisone to cortisol via 11-β-hydroxysteroid-dehydrogenase-1. Taken together, these results suggest that a reduction in intrahepatic Mg^{2+} content changes glucose utilization within the hepatocyte and promotes cortisol production perhaps for gluconeogenetic purposes, setting the conditions for reduced insulin responsiveness.

Materials and Methods

Materials

HepG2 cells were a kind gift from Dr.Cederbaum (Mt. Sinai, New York). 3H-2-deoxyglucose was from Amersham (GE, Pittsburgh, PA). Culture medium and bovine calf serum were from Gibco (Life Science, Grand Island, NY). Antibody anti Glut2 and Glut1 glucose transporters were from Santa Cruz (Dallas, TX). All other reagents were of analytical grade (Sigma, St Louis, MO).

Methods

Cell cultures

HepG2 cells were maintained in MEM medium (M2279, Sigma) containing 0.8mM $MgSO_4$ and 5.5 mM glucose in the presence of 5% CO2 until 85% confluent. Cells were then divided into two groups and cultured in the presence of physiological (0.8 mM) extracellular Mg^{2+} or under Mg^{2+} deficient conditions (0.4 mM extracellular Mg^{2+}). The presence of 10% bovine calf serum increased extracellular Mg^{2+} content to 1 mM and 0.6 mM, respectively (measured by atomic absorbance spectrophotometry).

At confluence, cells were harvested and used to determine Mg^{2+} and ATP content, glucose accumulation, or glucose 6 phosphate dehydrogenase activity.

Cellular Mg^{2+} content: To measure total cellular Mg^{2+} content, normal or Mg^{2+} deficient HepG2 cells were harvested at confluence, washed briefly in PBS (500 rpm for 1 min) and sedimented again (500 rpm for 2 min) in microfuge tubes. The supernatants were removed and the cell pellets dissolved in 10% HNO_3. The acid mixture was sonicated for 10 min in a sonicating bath, and acid-digested overnight. The following morning, the acid mixtures were sonicated again, vortexed, and sedimented at 5000 rpm for 3 min in microfuge tubes. The supernatants were removed and assessed for Mg^{2+} content in a Varian 210 atomic absorbance spectrophotometer (AAS) calibrated with Mg^{2+} standards.

To measure the intracellular Mg^{2+} distribution, HepG2 cells were harvested and washed as described above. The cell pellets were then resuspended in a Mg^{2+} free medium containing (mM) 100 KCl, 10 mM Mops, 1mM $KH2PO_4$, pH 7.2 [10], pre-warmed at 37°C, at the final concentration of 0.5 mg protein per ml. Digitonin (50μg/ml), FCCP (2 μg/ml), and A23187 (1μg/ml) were sequentially added to the cell mixture at 5 min intervals to measure cytoplasmic, mitochondrial, and post mitochondrial Mg^{2+} content, respectively [11]. Prior to the addition of any of these agents, aliquots of the cell mixture were withdrawn in duplicate and sedimented in microfuge tubes (5000 rpm for 3 min). The supernatants were removed and assessed for Mg^{2+} content by AAS. The pellets were digested in 10% HNO_3 and assessed for Mg^{2+} content as reported above. Although indirect, this approach has been successfully used in our laboratory, with results equivalent to those reported by other with different techniques [11].

ATP content

Cellular ATP content was measured by luciferin-luciferase as previously reported [12]. Briefly, HepG2 cells were harvested, washed and sedimented as described above. The cell pellets were then extracted in 10% PCA on ice for 10 min. The mixture was neutralized with one volume of 1M $KHCO_3$ on ice and sedimented in a refrigerated Beckman J6B centrifuge (1800 rpm for 5 min). The supernatant was removed and stored at -20°C until tested. The cellular ATP content was determined by luciferin-luciferase assay (detecting sensitivity in the pmol-nmol/ml range (Sigma) in a LUMAT Berthold LB 9,501 luminometer.

Glucose utilization

Glucose content in the culture medium was measured by glucose kit (Fisher) according to the directions of the producer. Alternatively, glucose accumulation into the cells was measured radio-isotopic distribution. Cells at confluence were serum starved for 3 hours prior to measure glucose accumulation. Cells were then harvested and washed as previously reported. The cell pellets were resuspended at the final concentration of 0.5mg protein/ml in a medium having a composition similar to the MEM medium reported above but containing only 100 μM glucose labeled with 0.5 μCi/ml3H-2-deoxyglucose, at 37°C [13]. At selected time points, 0.5 ml aliquots of the incubation mixture were withdrawn in duplicate and diluted 11 fold in 250 mM 'ice-cold' sucrose containing 20 μM phloretin as a glucose transporter inhibitor. The mixture was rapidly filtered onto Whatman glass fiber filters (GF, 250 nm pore size) under vacuum suction. The filter was washed once under vacuum with 5 ml of 'ice-cold' sucrose (plus phloretin), removed from the filtration device and air-dried. The radioactivity retained onto the filter was measured in a Beckman 6500 β-scintillation counter. For comparison purposes, similar experiments were carried out with glucose labeled with 3H-3-methyl-glucose or 14C-glucose.

Glucose transporter expression

The protein expression of Glut2 and Glut1 transporters was assessed by Western blot analysis using commercially available antibodies against these transporters (Santa Cruz). The blots were routinely stained with Ponceau-S before immune-staining to confirm samples loading and the transfer of equivalent amounts of protein. The membranes were extensively washed with PBS, and the primary antibody binding visualized using peroxidase-conjugated secondary antibody and enhanced chemiluminescent Western blotting detection reagents (Amersham). Densitometry was performed using Scion Image Program (NIH). The bands corresponding to Glut2 and Glut1 isoforms were separately 'framed' for densitometry determination. The obtained results were normalized for GAPDH gene product expression.

Glucose 6-Phosphate dehydrogenase activity

Glucose 6-phosphate dehydrogenase activity was measured as reported by Marcolongo et al. [14]. Briefly, HepG2 cells at confluence were harvested and washed as previously reported. The cells were then resuspended in a medium containing (mM): 100 KCl, 10 MOPS, 1 $KH2PO_4$, pH 7.2, and permeabilized by the addition of 50μg/ml digitonin. Permeabilization was assessed by Trypan Blue exclusion test [12]. Aliquots of the cells were diluted 20-fold in a final volume of 2 ml medium, and transferred to a Perkin Elmer 3 fluorimeter (Perkin Elmer, 3) at 340nm excitation wavelength and 490 nm emission wavelengths [14]. The reaction was started by the addition of 1mM (or different concentration) glucose 6 phosphate, and the production of NADPH recorded for 10-15 min at room temperature. In separate sets of experiments, NADPH production was recorded for a similar period of time at 37°C. For comparison purposes, NADPH production was measured in an Agilent 8453 spectrophotometer equipped with data acquisition software according to the procedure of Senesi et al. [15]. Calibration was carried out by adding known amounts of NADPH standards to aliquots of heat-inactivated permeabilized cells under similar experimental conditions.

Cortisol production

The activity of the 11-β-hydroxysteroid-dehydrogenase-1 (11-β-≅HSD1) in reducing cortisone to cortisol was measured as reported elsewhere [14]. Briefly, HepG2 cells in culture were incubated in the presence of 5μM cortisone for 12 hours. The cells were then placed on

ice, washed once with PBS, and extracted with 500 μl ice cold methanol. The methanol mixture was stored at -20°C. After thawing, the methanol mixture was centrifuged at 18,000 rpm (20,000 g for 10 min at $ C in a Beckman J20 centrifuge. The supernatants were collected, and their cortisone and cortisol contents measured by HPLC (BioRad 1740) using a 5 μm mash C18 reverse phase column HPLC (Waters), and an isocratic methanol: water, 58:42 (vol/vol) mobile phase at a flow rate of 0.7 ml/min. Absorbance was detected at 245 nm (Biorad 1740 UV detector). The peaks corresponding to cortisone and cortisol and their retention time were determined via standards injection [14].

Statistical analysis

Data are reported as means ± S.E. of at least four different preparations for each experimental condition, each tested in duplicate. Data were analyzed by Student T- test set at $p<0.05$ for significance.

Results

HepG2cells cultured in the presence of 0.5 mM extracellular Mg^{2+} presented ~20% less total cellular Mg^{2+} than HepG2 cells maintained in the presence of physiological 1 mM $[Mg^{2+}]o$ (34.2 ± 0.9 versus 42.3 ± 1.2 nmol Mg^{2+}/mg protein, n=8, p<0.05) (Figure1). Assessment of the intracellular Mg^{2+} distribution as reported under Materials and Methods confirmed that Mg^{2+} content decreased in the cytoplasm, mitochondria, and post mitochondrial pools (Figure 1). HepG2 cells maintained in 0.6 mM $[Mg^{2+}]o$ also showed a significant 18% decrease in total ATP content (4.35 ± 0.8 vs. 4.18 ± 1.2 nmol/mg protein, n=10, p<0.05).

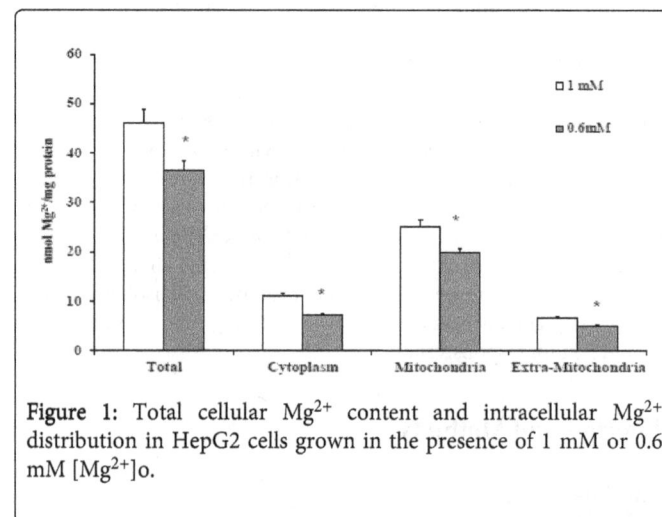

Figure 1: Total cellular Mg^{2+} content and intracellular Mg^{2+} distribution in HepG2 cells grown in the presence of 1 mM or 0.6 mM $[Mg^{2+}]o$.

HepG2 cells maintained in culture in the presence of 1 mM (physiological) or 0.6 mM (Mg^{2+}-deficient) extracellular Mg^{2+} were assessed for total cellular Mg^{2+} content and intracellular Mg^{2+} compartmentalization as described under Materials and Methods. Figure 1 onset reports the time points at which Mg^{2+} content was assessed and the various agents added to the cells. The data are means ± S.E. of 4 different preparations, each assessed in duplicate. *Statistical significant versus the corresponding value in 1 mM HepG2 cells.

Our and others laboratories [13,16] have previously reported that a reduction in extracellular Mg^{2+} concentration impairs glucose accumulation into the cells. To determine whether the reduction in ATP content depended on a reduced transport of glucose into the cells, we measured the changes in medium glucose content at 24 hour intervals by glucose enzymatic kit. Our results indicated that HepG2 cells in 0.6 mM $[Mg^{2+}]o$ accumulated approximated 50% less glucose than HepG2 cells in 1 mM $[Mg^{2+}]$(Figure 2A). Because the reduced glucose utilization could depend on changes in the number of cells and their reduplication rate, we measured glucose transport into the cells by 3H-2-deoxy-glucose radio-isotopic distributions, normalized per number of cells. As Figure 2B shows, 0.6 mM HepG2 cells accumulated less glucose (~85%) than 1 mM HepG2 cells under basal conditions. The glucose accumulation rate in 0.6 mM HepG2 cells did not increase upon administration of 10 nM insulin (Figure 2B), whereas it increased significantly in 1 mM HepG2 cells. Similar results were obtained when glucose was labelled with 3H-3-methyl-glucose or 14C-glucose (data not shown), or when glucose concentrations higher than 100 µM were used (data now shown).

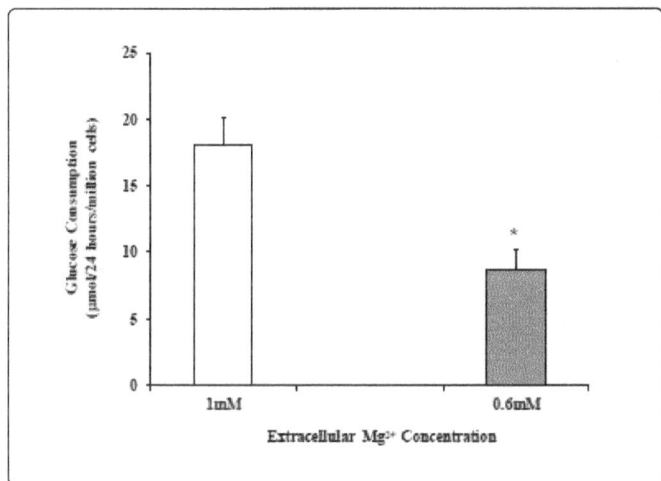

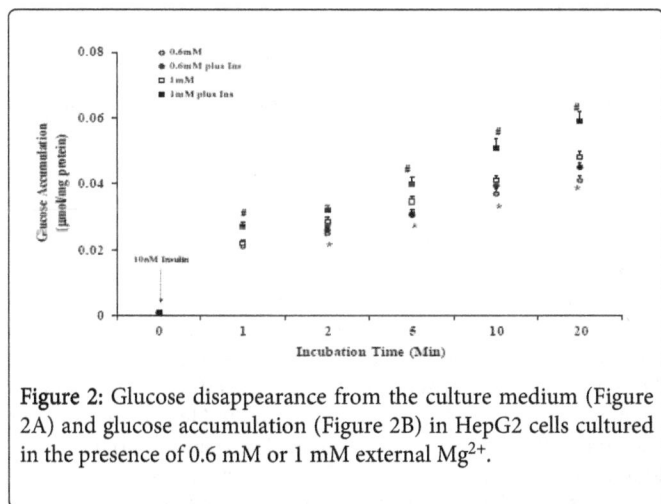

was measured as the amount of radioactivity accumulated within the cells at the indicated time points (Figure 2B). Where indicated, insulin (10 nM) was added to the incubation system, and glucose accumulation carried out for 20 min. Data are means ± S.E. of 4 different experiments, each carried out in duplicate, for all the experimental conditions reported.

*Statistical significant versus the corresponding value in 1 mM HepG2 cells.

#Statistical significant versus the corresponding value in 1 mM HepG2 cells in the absence of insulin stimulation.

To determine whether the defect in glucose accumulation depended on a different expression of glucose transporters Western blot analysis and mRNA expression were carried out for Glut2 and Glut1 under our experimental conditions. As Figure 3 shows, no significant differences in Glut 2 and Glut 1 protein expression were observed.

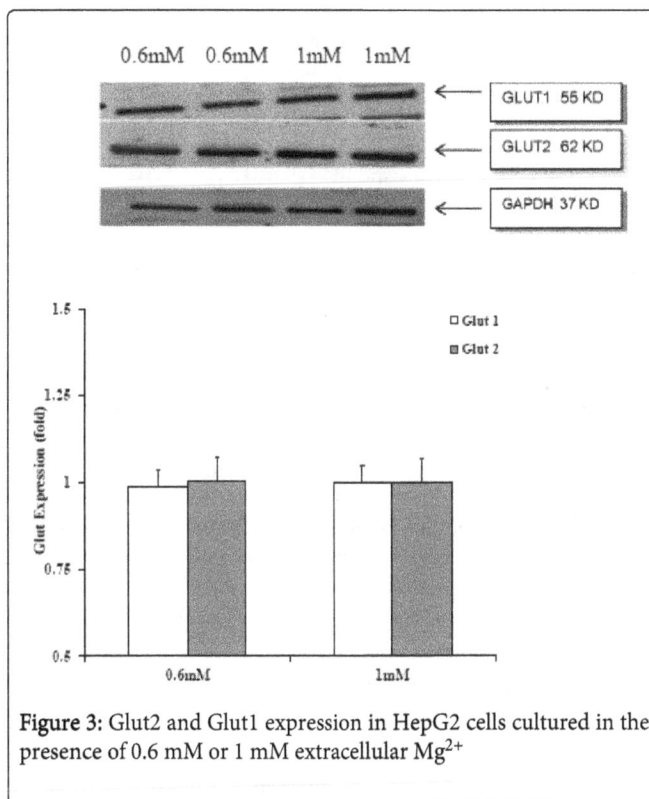

Figure 3: Glut2 and Glut1 expression in HepG2 cells cultured in the presence of 0.6 mM or 1 mM extracellular Mg^{2+}

Figure 2: Glucose disappearance from the culture medium (Figure 2A) and glucose accumulation (Figure 2B) in HepG2 cells cultured in the presence of 0.6 mM or 1 mM external Mg^{2+}.

HepG2 cells were maintained in culture in the presence of 0.6 mM or 1 mM extracellular Mg^{2+}. Glucose disappearance from the medium was measured by glucose assay kit in aliquots of the culture medium withdrawn at 24 hours interval (Figure 2A). Accumulation of glucose (100µM labeled with 0.5mCi/ml 3H-2-deoxy-glucose) into the cells

Assessment of Glut2 and Glut1 protein expression in HepG2 cells was carried by Western blot analysis using commercially available antibodies against the glucose transporters. Densitometry was carried out using Scion program (NIH) as indicated under Materials and Methods. Data are means ± S.E. of three different preparations, each tested in duplicate.

We have previously reported that a decrease in cytoplasmic Mg^{2+} content enhances the transport of glucose 6-phosphate (G6P) into the hepatic endoplasmic reticulum and its hydrolysis by the glucose 6-phosphatase. These results were obtained in both freshly isolated hepatocytes [10] and in microsomal vesicles from livers of Mg^{2+} deficient animals [17]. A similar increase in G6P transport and hydrolysis was observed in permeabilized HepG2 cells (Figure 4), confirming our previous experimental results.

In addition to being hydrolyzed by the G6Pase, G6P is also oxidized within the hepatic ER to 6-phosphogluconolactone by the glucose 6-phosphate dehydrogenase in a process associated with the production of endo-luminal NADPH [14]. The reaction catalyzed by the G6PD represents the limiting step in the pentose shunt, an alternative energetic pathway within the hepatocyte.

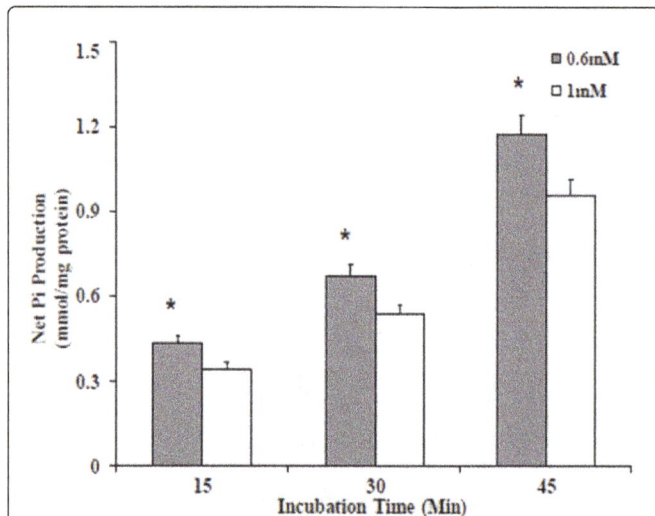

Figure 4: Glucose 6-phosphate hydrolysis in HepG2 cells

HepG2 cells were maintained in culture in the presence of 0.6 mM or 1 mM extracellular Mg^{2+}. At confluence, cells were harvested, and permeabilized by digitonin addition (50 µg/ml). The cells were then washed and incubated in a cytosol-like medium in the presence of 1 mM G6P, at $37°C$. Hydrolysis of G6P by glucose 6-phosphatase was measured as the amount of Pi released into the incubation medium at specific time points. Data are means ± S.E. of 5 different experiments, each carried out in duplicate, for all the experimental conditions reported.

*Statistical significant versus the corresponding value in 1 mM HepG2 cells.

To determine whether also this alternative pathway was enhanced in Mg^{2+} deficient cells, the production of NADPH was measured in HepG2 cells in the presence of various amounts of exogenous G6P. The results reported in Figure 5A indicate 0.6 mM HepG2 cells produced almost twice the amount of NADPH than 1 mM HepG2 cells. The NADPH production rate in 0.6 mM HepG2 cells was reduced by the addition of excess Mg^{2+} excess prior to G6P administration (Figure 5A) but not when a similar (Figure 5B) or a higher (not shown) dose of Mg^{2+} was added after the G6P administration and the NADPH production was already near maximal.

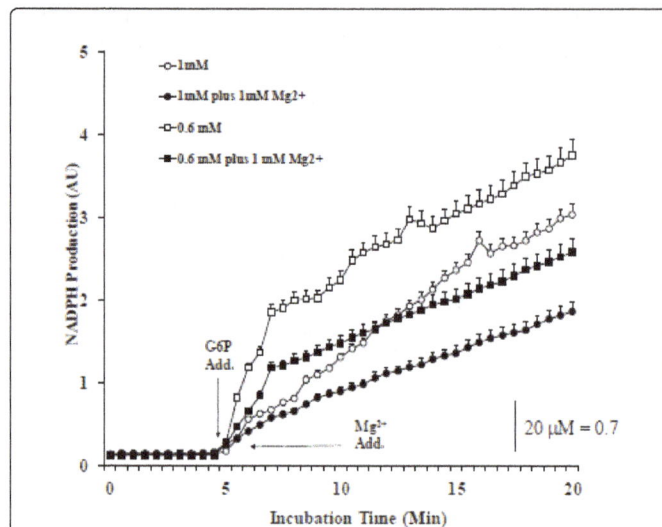

Figure 5A: 0.6 mM HepG2 cells produced twice the amount of NADPH than 1 mM HepG2 cells

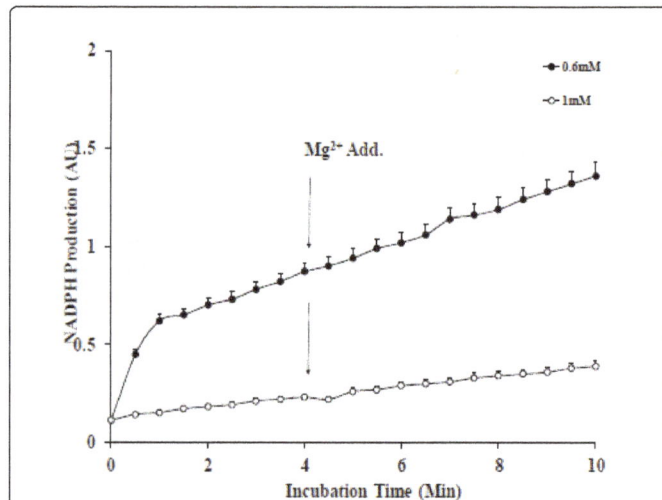

Figure 5: Glucose 6-phosphate dehydrogenase activity in HepG2 cells

HepG2 cells were maintained in culture in the presence of 0.6 mM or 1 mM extracellular Mg^{2+}. At confluence, cells were harvested, and permeabilized by digitonin addition (50µg/ml). The cells were then washed and incubated in a cytosol-like medium in the presence of 1 mM G6P, at $37°C$. NADPH as the by-product of G6P conversion to 6-phosphogluconolactone by the reticular G6PD was measured fluorimetrically as described under Materials and Methods. Calibration was carried out as described in the Methods section. The inhibitory effect of exogenous 1 mM Mg^{2+} added prior to G6P addition is reported in Figure 5A. The lack on an inhibitory effect of exogenous 1 mM Mg^{2+} added following G6P addition is reported in Figure 5B. Data are means ± S.E. of 3 different experiments for all the experimental conditions reported. In both Figure 5A and Figure 5B, all the data points for 0.6 mM following G6P addition and Mg^{2+} addition are statistical significant versus the corresponding values in 1 mM HepG2 cells. Labeling is omitted for simplicity.

Experimental evidence indicates that the production of luminal NADPH through G6PD is coupled to the conversion of cortisone to cortisol by the 11-β-hydroxysteroid-dehydrogenase-1 [14]. Renewed attention has been paid to this enzyme as an increase in its activity and/or expression and the associated production of cortisol have been considered one of the possible causes for increased insulin resistance in certain forms of type-2 diabetes.

To establish whether Mg^{2+}-deficient HepG2 cells could indeed convert cortisone to cortisol at an higher rate than HepG2 cells maintained in the presence of physiological extracellular Mg^{2+}, exogenous cortisone was administered for 12 hours to cells in culture, and the cortisone to cortisol conversion measured by HPLC. The results reported in Figure 6 indicate that Mg^{2+}-deficient HepG2 cells produced approximately 30% more cortisol than cells maintained in physiological Mg^{2+}.

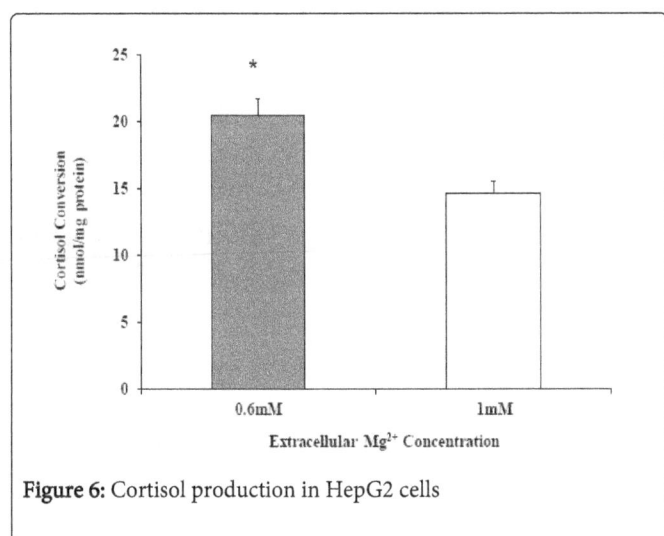

Figure 6: Cortisol production in HepG2 cells

HepG2 cells were maintained in culture in the presence of 0.6 mM or 1 mM extracellular Mg^{2+}. Cortisone (5 μM) was added for 12 hours to cells in culture. The cells were then harvested and processed as described in the Methods section. Cortisone to cortisol conversion by the 11-b-OHSD1 was assessed by HPLC and normalized per mg of protein. Data are means ± S.E. of 3 different experiments for all the experimental conditions reported. *Statistical significant versus the corresponding value in 1 mM HepG2 cells.

Discussion

The incidence of metabolic syndrome in Western countries has markedly increased in the last two decades. Altered ion homeostasis including hypomagnesaemia and reduced cellular Mg^{2+} levels have frequently been observed in patients affected by metabolic syndrome, raising the question as to whether the Mg^{2+} deficiency is consequence or cause of the pathology onset.

Although carried out in liver cells in culture, the results reported here suggest that Mg^{2+} deficiency is a contributing factor. Induction of Mg^{2+} deficiency in liver cells impairs glucose metabolism to a significant extent and in different manners. For one, the decrease in extracellular and cellular Mg^{2+} content reduces the ability of these hepatocytes to accumulate and utilize glucose properly, resulting in a decrease in ATP content. This decrease in glucose accumulation and utilization does not depend on changes in glucose transport expression as both Glut2, the predominant glucose transporter in these cells, and

Glut1 - which is also present to an extent in the cells - are expressed to a comparable extent in cells grown in the presence of low (0.6 mM) or physiological (1 mM) extracellular Mg^{2+}. As we have not measured directly the glucokinase activity, we cannot exclude the possibility that the reduced glucose entry observed in Mg^{2+} deficient cells depends on a reduced activity of this enzyme. However, the reported data on increased G6P transport and hydrolysis by the endo-reticular glucose 6-phosphatase suggest, albeit indirectly, that G6P generated by the glucokinase is routed more rapidly towards the endoplasmic reticulum, resulting in an enhanced glucose-to G6P-to glucose futile cycle [18], with possible implications for the net ATP loss detected in these cells.

Perhaps more pertinent to the metabolic syndrome onset are our results on an increased activity of the glucose 6-phosphate dehydrogenase, the other reticular enzymes involved in metabolizing G6P. This enzyme represents the limiting step in the pentose phosphate shunt pathway, and the conversion of G6P to 6-phosphogluconolactone catalyzed by the enzyme is coupled to the reduction of NADP to NADPH. This endo-reticular pool of reduced pyridine nucleotide can then be used for fatty acids and cholesterol synthesis within the hepatocyte. More importantly, the NADPH reticular pool can be used by the 11-β-hydrosteroid dehydrogenase-1 to reduce cortisone to cortisol within the hepatocyte as attested by the 30% increase in cortisol production under our experimental conditions. Recently, experimental and clinical evidence has associated the increased expression and/or activity of this enzyme with insulin resistance and obesity [14], two stigmata of the metabolic syndrome [3,4]. Preliminary experiments in our laboratory support the idea that Mg^{2+} deficiency results in reduced insulin receptor responsiveness (Romani, personal observation). It remains to be elucidated as to whether the decrease in insulin response depends directly on the Mg^{2+} deficiency, which impairs the autophosphorylation of the insulin receptor and the subsequent activation of the insulin receptor substrate, as observed in skeletal muscles of Mg^{2+} deficient animals [19], or indirectly through the G6PDNADPHcortisol up-regulation observed under our experimental conditions. In this respect, studies are being carried out in our laboratory to determine whether Mg^{2+} deficiency also promotes G6PD gene expression in addition to increasing G6PD enzymatic activity.

Because the hepatocytes are able to interchangeably utilize glucose or fatty acids for energetic purposes, it could be argued that the increased G6PD activity should results in more NADPH being routed towards the synthesis of fatty acids, which the hepatocytes should be able to utilize as energetic substrates for metabolic purposes without experiencing a decrease in ATP content. Yet, this does not appear to be the case. In addition, both fetal and bovine calf serum, which are commonly utilized in cell culture to support cell growth, have significant levels of short chain fatty acids that the HepG2 cells could use for energy purposes. Thus, the possibility that the reduced ATP content measured in HepG2 Mg^{2+}-deficient cells might depend on energetic substrate restriction (i.e. only glucose in the culture medium) is also not supported. Although more detailed experiments need to be carried out to elucidate the reasons behind the inability of Mg^{2+} deficient HepG2 cells to sustain their ATP level, it is possible that less than optimal Mg^{2+} content within the mitochondria, another major cellular pool for this cation [6] affects the organelle β-oxidation.

Irrespective of the mechanism behind the reduced ATP production (or increased ATP consumption), an increase in G6PD activity has been related to increased lipid dysfunction and insulin resistance [20], thus landing support to our observation and its experimental and clinical relevance.

To our knowledge, this is the first study that has provided a cause-effect link between Mg^{2+} deficiency and some of the metabolic alterations present in the metabolic syndrome, namely altered glucose metabolism, insulin resistance, and possibly obesity. Because of the novelty of our observation, several questions are still in need of a more thoroughly investigation including the validation of our data in human subjects.

Acknowledgement

This Study was supported by NIAAA-11593 to Dr. Andrea Romani.

References

1. http://www.cdc.gov/obesity/data/adult.html

2. Finkelstein EA, Khavjou OA, Thompson H, Trogdon JG, Pan L, et al. (2012) Obesity and severe obesity forecasts through 2030. Am J Prev Med 42: 563-570.

3. Haller H (1977) [Epidermiology and associated risk factors of hyperlipoproteinemia]. Z Gesamte Inn Med 32: 124-128.

4. Meshkani R, Adeli K (2009) Hepatic insulin resistance, metabolic syndrome and cardiovascular disease. Clin Biochem 42: 1331-1346.

5. Reaven GM (2005) The insulin resistance syndrome: definition and dietary approaches to treatment. Annu Rev Nutr 25: 391-406.

6. Romani AM (2013) Magnesium in Health and Disease, in Metal Ions in Life Science: Metallomics and the Cell. Basel, Switzerland 49-79.

7. Romani A (2012) Cellular Magnesium Homeostasis in mammalian cells, in Metal Ions in Life Science: Metallomics and the Cell, Sigel A, Sigel H, and Sigel RKO series Eds. Basel, Switzerland 69-118.

8. Resnick LM, Barbagallo M, Gupta RK, Laragh JH (1993) Ionic basis of hypertension in diabetes mellitus. Role of hyperglycemia. Am J Hypertens 6: 413-417.

9. Barbagallo M, Dominguez LJ (2007) Magnesium metabolism in type 2 diabetes mellitus, metabolic syndrome and insulin resistance. Arch Biochem Biophys 458: 40-47.

10. Doleh L, Romani A (2007) Biphasic effect of extra-reticular Mg^{2+} on hepatic G6P transport and hydrolysis. Arch Biochem Biophys 467: 283-290.

11. Fagan TE, Cefaratti C, Romani A (2004) Streptozotocin-induced diabetes impairs Mg^{2+} homeostasis and uptake in rat liver cells. Am J Physiol Endocrinol Metab 286: E184-193.

12. Tessman PA, Romani A (1998) Acute effect of EtOH on Mg^{2+} homeostasis in liver cells: evidence for the activation of an Na+/Mg2+ exchanger. Am J Physiol 275: G1106-1116.

13. Romani AM, Matthews VD, Scarpa A (2000) Parallel stimulation of glucose and $Mg(^{2+})$ accumulation by insulin in rat hearts and cardiac ventricular myocytes. Circ Res 86: 326-333.

14. Marcolongo P, Piccirella S, Senesi S, Wunderlich L, Gerin I, et al. (2007) The glucose-6-phosphate transporter-hexose-6-phosphate dehydrogenase-11beta-hydroxysteroid dehydrogenase type 1 system of the adipose tissue. Endocrinology 148: 2487-2495.

15. Senesi S, Legeza B, Balázs Z, Csala M, Marcolongo P, et al. (2010) Contribution of fructose-6-phosphate to glucocorticoid activation in the endoplasmic reticulum: possible implication in the metabolic syndrome. Endocrinology 151: 4830-4839.

16. Henquin JC, Tamagawa T, Nenquin M, Cogneau M (1983) Glucose modulates Mg^{2+} fluxes in pancreatic islet cells. Nature 301: 73-74.

17. Barfell A, Crumbly A, Romani A (2011) Enhanced glucose 6-phosphatase activity in liver of rats exposed to $Mg(^{2+})$-deficient diet. Arch Biochem Biophys 509: 157-163.

18. Jungermann K, Heilbronn R, Katz N, Sasse D (1982) The glucose/glucose-6-phosphate cycle in the periportal and perivenous zone of rat liver. Eur J Biochem 123: 429-436.

19. Suárez A, Pulido N, Casla A, Casanova B, Arrieta FJ, et al. (1995) Impaired tyrosine-kinase activity of muscle insulin receptors from hypomagnesaemic rats. Diabetologia 38: 1262-1270.

20. Park J, Rho HK, Kim KH, Choe SS, Lee YS, et al. (2005) Overexpression of glucose-6-phosphate dehydrogenase is associated with lipid dysregulation and insulin resistance in obesity. Mol Cell Biol 25: 5146-5157.

16

Bergamot Polyphenols: Pleiotropic Players in the Treatment of Metabolic Syndrome

Micaela Gliozzi, Ross Walker and Vincenzo Mollace[*]

Institute of Research for Food Safety & Health (IRC-FSH), University of Catanzaro "Magna Graecia", Catanzaro, Italy

[*]**Corresponding author:** Vincenzo Mollace, Campus Universitario di Germaneto, Viale Europa, 88100 Catanzaro, Italy; E-mail: mollace@libero.it

Abstract

Metabolic syndrome (MS) represents a clustering of risk factors related to an elevated incidence of cardiovascular disease (CVD) and type 2 diabetes. Despite the possibility of multiple pharmacological interventions to treat metabolic changes related to MS, these therapeutic strategies often exhibit several side effects and inadequately prevents CVD. Among nutraceutical compounds presenting potential efficacy in this regard, bergamot polyphenols, via their multi-action properties, have been shown to positively modulate several mechanisms involved in MS suggesting their benefits as therapy. The purpose of this review is to discuss the beneficial effects of bergamot polyphenols providing a new therapeutic approach in the treatment of MS.

Keywords: Metabolic syndrome; Bergamot polyphenols; Hyperlipidemia; Cardiovascular disease

Introduction

Metabolic syndrome (MS) is a clustering of numerous age-related metabolic abnormalities that together increase the risk for cardiovascular disease (CVD) and type 2 diabetes. They include obesity which is thought to be a cause rather than a consequence of metabolic disturbance, high blood pressure, high blood glucose and dyslipidaemia [1]. In particular, increased concentrations of low-density lipoprotein cholesterol (LDL-C), total blood cholesterol (TC) and triglycerides (TG) comprise the main pathogenic risk profile. Moreover, conditions of insulin resistance such as impaired glucose tolerance or "prediabetes" are often accompanied by low levels of high-density lipoprotein cholesterol (HDL-C) which amplify the risk of CVD [2].

Recent studies highlight a relationship between dietary factors and MS, but the characteristics of an optimal diet to prevent or treat MS have yet to be better clarified [3]. Increasing experimental and epidemiological evidence suggests that dietary polyphenols, in particular flavonoids, may play an important role in ameliorating prediabetes due to their multi-action properties in counteracting pathophysiological mechanisms leading to the development of MS [4].

The health benefits of polyphenols are generally attributed to both non-specific mechanisms, dependent upon a broad anti-oxidant activity, and more specific mechanisms [5]. Indeed, the in vitro activity of polyphenols strongly suggests that their role extends much beyond their ability to limit oxidative processes as they have been also shown to modulate metabolic enzymes, nuclear receptors, gene expression and multiple signaling pathways [6].

Bergamot (Citrus bergamia) is an endemic plant of the Calabrian region in Southern Italy with a unique profile of flavonoid and flavonoid glycosides present in its juice and albedo, such as neoeriocitrin, neohesperidin, naringin, rutin, neodesmin, rhoifolin and poncirin. Bergamot differs from other Citrus fruits not only because of the composition of its flavonoids, but also because of their

particularly high content [7,8]. Among them naringin, present also in grapefruit, has already been reported to be active in animal models of atherosclerosis [9], while neoeriocitrin and rutin have been shown to inhibit LDL oxidation [10]. Importantly, bergamot juice is rich in neohesperidosides of hesperetin and naringenin, such as melitidine and brutieridine. These flavonoids possess a 3-hydroxy-3-methylglutaryl moiety with a structural similarity to the natural substrate of HMG-CoA reductase and exhibit statin-like proprieties [11].

Recently, the therapeutic potential of bergamot derivatives has also been investigated in human studies [12-14]. Here, we provide a brief overview of these findings underlying the mechanism of action hypothesised for bergamot-derived polyphenols which suggests new and important insights in MS therapy.

Bergamot polyphenolic fraction (BPF) and MS

The National Cholesterol Education Program Adult Treatment Panel III (NCEPATP III) clinical definition of MS requires the presence of at least three out of five risk factors which include abdominal obesity, high plasma triglycerides, low plasma HDL, high blood pressure and high fasting plasma glucose [15].

Experimental and epidemiological studies have demonstrated that bergamot polyphenolic fraction (BPF) ameliorates serum lipemic profile and normalizes blood pressure in patients suffering from MS. Previous scientific evidence obtained with Citrus flavonoids and other non-nutritive constituents of Citrus fruits, explain their beneficial effects and to further clarify some mechanisms involved in MS [12,13,16].

Indeed, it has been demonstrated that Citrus peel extracts, rich in pectins and flavonoids, cause lowering of cholesterol levels by modulating hepatic HMG-CoA levels [9,17,18] and bergamot juice has been shown to enhance the excretion of fecal sterols in rats [19] thereby contributing to its hypolipemic and hypoglycemic effect subsequently found in patients on BPF treatment.

A special contribution to the hypolipemic response of BPF seems to be related to the modulatory properties of naringin and neohesperidin. Indeed, evidence exists that dietary hesperetin reduces hepatic TG accumulation and this is associated with the reduced activity of TG synthetic enzymes, such as phosphatidate phosphohydrolase [20]. In addition, in vitro studies suggest that naringenin and hesperein decrease the availability of lipids for assembly of apoB-containing lipoproteins, an effect mediated by reduced activities of acyl CoA: cholesterol acyltransferases (ACAT) [21].

Importantly, BPF is rich in brutieridine and melitidine, which are 3-hydroxy-3-methylglutaryl derivatives of hesperetin and naringenin, respectively. In addition, the classical glycoside derivative of naringenin, which is naringin, has been shown to inhibit hepatic HMG-CoA reductase [22]. Therefore it is likely that melitidine and brutieridine in concert with naringin and other flavonone glycosides might be responsible for the striking potency of BPF in reducing cholesterol levels.

The recent finding that eNOS knockout mice present a cluster of cardiovascular risk factors comparable to those of MS suggests that defects in eNOS function may cause human MS and that its dysfunction induces an impaired vasodilation mediated by reduction of NO levels [15,23,24].

The unifying hypothesis of eNOS-reduced activity and subsequent endothelial dysfunction caused by oxidative stress and inflammatory processes observed in MS might justify the reduced NO-dependent vasodilation.

Well documented antioxidant and anti-inflammatory mechanisms regulated by Citrus flavonoids, such as increasing superoxide dismutase and catalase activities and protection of plasma vitamin E [25], may attenuate overproduction of oxygen reactive species in the vascular wall thereby restoring the imbalanced endothelial function, as also observed in patients under BPF treatment (Figure 1).

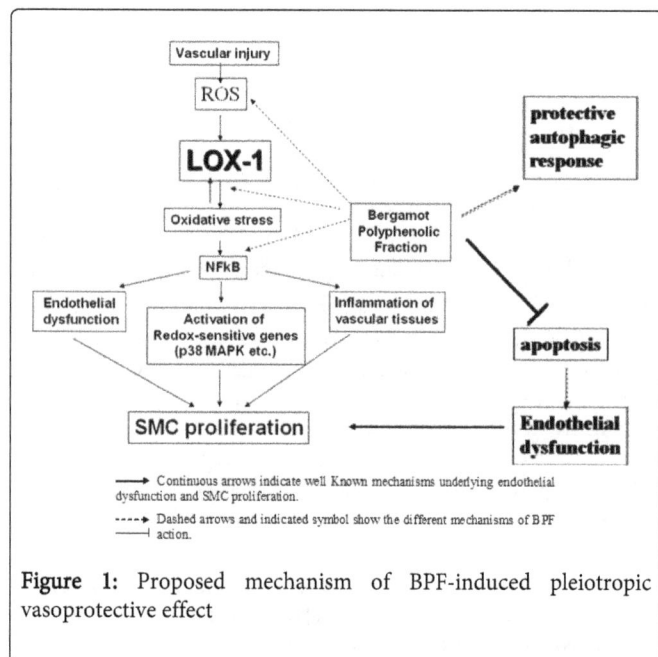

Figure 1: Proposed mechanism of BPF-induced pleiotropic vasoprotective effect

Another potential benefit of BPF is related to its hypoglycemic activity. Among the few mechanistic studies on the hypoglycemic effects of flavonoids, it has been shown that naringenin, similarly to other polyphenols, significantly increased AMP kinase (AMPK) activity and glucose uptake in muscle cells and liver [26,27]. The hypoglycaemic activity of insulin sensitivity and glucose tolerance has been shown in animal models of MS [28].

On the basis of these findings, supplementing an ordinary diet with BPF represents a phytotherapeutic approach for the better management of prediabetic states in patients with MS by lowering plasma cholesterol and lipids, ameliorating NO-dependent vasoreactivity and by reducing blood glucose [12] (Figure 1).

Potential benefits of BPF in reducing statin dosage

A meta-analysis of placebo-controlled "standard dose" statin trials show a reduction in cardiovascular mortality averaging 20% and a decrease in major cardiovascular events by approximately 25% [13]. Treatment with high-dose statins was shown to reduce the morbidity by 36%, and a reduction of cardiovascular events up to 40% [13]. Despite the significant clinical benefits provided by statins, many patients, in particular those with diabetes or metabolic syndrome do not achieve their recommended LDL-C and HDL-C target goals with statins alone [13]. Moreover, statins have been reported to cause dose-related side effects, the more serious including liver disease or severe myopathy, in up to 22% of patients eligible for this therapeutic approach [13]. This limits the use of statins and suggests the need for alternative and/or supplementary therapeutic approaches.

The enriched composition of BPF in naringin, neoeriocitrin and neohesperidin produces antilipidemic effects in patients with pure or mixed hypercholesterolemia. This effect is a prominent reduction of both total cholesterol and LDL-C and a moderate increase of HDL-C, thus suggesting a potential benefit in reducing cardiometabolic risk. Given the structural similarity to HMG-CoA reductase substrate brutieridine and melitidine have been shown to possess statin-like properties, by selective inhibition of HMG-CoA reductase [29]. The direct action of BPF on HMG-CoA reductase activity has been confirmed by a significant reduction of the end product of HMG-CoA reductase activity, mevalonate (MVA), detected in the urine of patients under BPF treatment [12,13,16,30].

This effect of BPF suggests a potential benefit of attenuating statin-induced side effects through the co-administration of bergamot polyphenols and low dose of statins. Indeed, on the basis of this hypothesis, it has been demonstrated that BPF, given orally in patients with mixed hyperlipidemia, allows the reduction of daily dosage for rosuvastatin but maintain target lipid values of hypolipemic treatment. On the other hand, reduction of serum cholesterol in patients taking both BPF and rosuvastatin is accompanied by a significant reduction in triglyceride levels, an effect which has not been found with rosuvastatin alone, and by a further elevation of HDL-C thus suggesting a synergistic role of BPF in statin-induced hypolipidemic response.

The significant synergism of BPF with rosuvastatin is also demonstrated by the further reduction seen in urinary MVA in patients after treatment with both BPF and lower doses of rosuvastatin [13].

The hypolipidemic response found in patients undergoing BPF treatment seems to be related to the modulatory properties of naringin and neo-hesperidin. Indeed, dietary hesperetin not only reduces the hepatic TG accumulation but also reduces apoB levels [31] which together with an enhanced expression of the LDL receptor may explain, at least in part, the hypocholesterolemic properties of BPF. Naringenin shows to act at multiple levels in regulating lipid metabolism in patients [32] probably increasing hepatic fatty acid oxidation through a peroxisome proliferator-activated receptor (PPAR) gamma coactivator alpha/PPARalpha-mediated transcription program, preventing sterol regulatory element-binding protein 1c-mediated lipogenesis in both liver and muscle by reducing fasting hyperinsulinemia and decreasing hepatic cholesterol and cholesterol ester synthesis. Moreover, naringin is able to reduce both VLDL-derived and endogenously synthesized fatty acids, preventing muscle triglyceride accumulation and, finally, improving overall insulin sensitivity and glucose tolerance [33].

In addition to their lipid-lowering properties, BPF synergizes with statins to enhance antioxidant activity. In particular, it has been shown that statins display cholesterol-independent pleiotropic effects including antioxidative actions such as suppression of NADPH oxidase expression and activity [34,35], induction of antioxidant enzymes (SOD1, SOD3, and GPx) [36,37], prevention of eNOS uncoupling [34,35], and enhancement of eNOS expression and activity. All these beneficial properties are limited by well known side effects of statins; however, this restriction may be overcome by the use of a combination therapy with antioxidants [38]. Indeed, in patients with mixed hyperlipidemia, it has been observed that BPF administration enhances antioxidant properties of rosuvastatin inducing a significant reduction of oxidative stress in circulating polymorphonucleates (PMC). In particular, malonyldialdheyde (MDA) levels, a viable marker of lipid peroxidation, in PMC decreases when adding BPF to rosuvastatin [12,13].

Moreover, the measured oxidative stress in the PMC of patients with hyperlipidemia, treatment with rosuvastatin or BPF alone reduced the expression of LOX-1 and Phospho PKB and these effects were enhanced in patients taking both compounds [13].

Since both LOX-1 and phospho PKB expression are relevant biomarkers of vascular cell viability, it is likely that an additional vaso-protective effect when using both statins and BPF may be expected in patients with high or moderate cardiometabolic risk [13].

Effects of BPF on liver steatosis and LDL particles

The effect of BPF in lowering cholesterol, triglycerides and glucose in patients suffering from MS is accompanied by reduction of LDL-C and elevation of HDL-C as described above. This beneficial effect in the lipemic profile of patients suffering MS is also characterized by prominent re-arrangement of lipoprotein particle profile found following 120 day BPF treatment. Indeed, BPF reduced small size, atherogenic LDL particles. This effect, combined with reduction of inflammatory biomarkers, suggests that BPF leads to an attenuation of atherogenic risk in patients with MS [14].

The mechanism of such an effect in lipoprotein particle size is not clear to date. The combined effect of BPF in reducing both cholesterol and triglycerides may well explain lipoprotein re-arrangement due to prolonged BPF treatment. Indeed, an increased clearance of TG-rich lipoprotein particles makes these particles became better substrates for lipoprotein lipase. This would be expected to result in decreased levels of large and medium-sized VLDL and perhaps even intermediate density lipoprotein (IDL), which contains roughly equal amounts of TG and cholesterol [14].

The increased cascade of VLDL to IDL to LDL would result in increased numbers of large LDL particles and provide surface constituents for the formation of large HDL. The formation of small LDL is mainly due to cholesteryl ester transfer protein-mediated exchange of VLDL-TG for LDL cholesterol ester and the subsequent hydrolysis of LDL-TG. The decrease in large and medium VLDL diminishes the cholesteryl ester transfer protein-mediated exchange, decreasing the formation and number of small LDL particles. A similar mechanism may also explain the decrease in the number of medium-sized HDL particles.

Recently, it has been shown that MS is associated with non alcoholic fatty liver disease (NAFLD) [14].

The improvement of hepatocyte function found in patients with MS and associated NAFLD after taking BPF might also contribute in the amelioration in lipoprotein profile thereby attenuating cardiometabolic risk [14].

Some studies have demonstrated that insulin resistance almost universally induces NAFLD [39,40]. It is known that this condition may precede the development of cardiovascular disease [41,42]. To confirm the connection between NAFLD and atherosclerosis, carotid atherosclerosis has recently been detected in patients with NAFLD [43]. Pathogenetic mechanisms responsible for that include an increased lipolysis and increased delivery of free fatty acids to the liver [44]. The improvement of steato test and hepatorenal index in patients with MS and NAFLD following BPF treatment gives a quantitative estimation of steatosis and leads to the conclusion that BPF improves both liver function and signs of chronic liver inflammation, as confirmed by reduction of TNF-α and CRP [14].

Mild to moderate elevations of serum aminotransferases (ALT and AST) found in BPF-treated patients subjects at baseline represents the most common abnormality found in patients with NAFLD. Their serum levels were significantly reduced after BPF, thereby confirming data obtained with steato test and hepatorenal index.

The mechanism of the hepato-protective effect of BPF still remains to be elucidated. However, evidence shows that BPF acts as a cytoprotective agent in liver of rats administered an high cholesterol diet [30,45]. The probable explanation is related to BPF BPF activities in oxidative inflammation and changes in hepatocyte membrane permeability probably via stabilization of the hepatocyte membrane structure, thereby preventing toxins from entering the cells. In addition, other indirect cytoprotective effect may be due to the modulation of hepatic 3-hydroxy-3-methylglutaryl coenzyme A (HMG-CoA) levels, possibly by binding bile acids and increasing the turnover rate of blood and liver cholesterol [46-50], and to the enhancement in the excretion of fecal sterols. As mentioned above, the hypolipidemic response found in patients undergoing BPF treatment may be related to the modulatory properties of naringin and neo-hesperidin, via inhibition of hepatic TG accumulation. Thus, BPF polyphenolic components, through different mechanisms reduce liver accumulation of fat thereby producing an overall improvement of liver function.

Effects of BPF in a balloon injury model

It has been demonstrated that bergamot-derived polyphenols are able to antagonize smooth muscle cell (SMC) proliferation and neointima formation in rat carotid artery subsequent to balloon injury. This effect is clearly related to the antioxidant activity of polyphenols, as shown by the significant reduction of nitrated tyrosine staining into injured blood vessels, an action due to the reduced generation of peroxynitrite, a powerful oxidant free radical. Moreover, BPF prevented balloon injury-related overexpression of LOX-1, the receptor for oxidized-LDL (oxyLDL), underling the imbalance of redox status of arterial blood vessels [51], thereby leading to SMC proliferation. Peroxynitrite generation is a crucial step in activating proliferation of subintimal SMCs which follows vascular injury; also, LOX-1 expression is involved in this process, which leads to the reactive neointima formation [51].

Oxidative stress and LOX-1 expression are early events in the biochemical changes that can be found in vascular tissue after induction of injury, and restoring antioxidant status by treating rats with BPF reduces restenosis of injured arterial vessels by counteracting free radical formation and LOX-1 expression [16].

In summary, our studies suggest that BPF, a natural antioxidant rich fraction of bergamot (citrus bergamia), inhibits oxidative stress which occurs in injured arteries and modulates both LOX-1 expression and neointima formation. This may be relevant as an alternative approach to conventional anti-atherogenic compounds in the treatment of vascular disorders in which proliferation of vascular SMCs and oxyLDL-related endothelial dysfunction occur [16].

Conclusion

The nutraceutical approach for the management of MS may represent a promising strategy in preventing cardiometabolic risk. In particular, polyphenols used in clinical practice have been shown to target the pathogenesis of diabetes mellitus, MS and their complications and to favourably modulate a number of biochemical and clinical endpoints [52].

Bergamot-deriving polyphenolic fraction has been shown to possess beneficial effects in patients suffering MS as demonstrated by a concomitant amelioration of lipemic and glycemic profile and by an improvement of the impaired endothelium-mediated vasodilation. In addition, in patients with MS and NAFLD, BPF substantially reduces liver steatosis.

All these effects are due to multi-action properties of bergamot derivatives which modulate key signalling proteins involved in the pathogenesis of MS and, on the other hand, directly counteract oxidative stress shedding new light on the potential use of BPF for reducing cardiometabolic risk in patients with MS.

Acknowledgements

This paper has been supported by PON a3_00359 and POR Calabria FSE 2007/2013.

References

1. Cameron A (2010) The metabolic syndrome: validity and utility of clinical definitions for cardiovascular disease and diabetes risk prediction. Maturitas 65: 117-121.

2. Lorenzo C, Wagenknecht LE, D'Agostino RB Jr, Rewers MJ, Karter AJ, et al. (2010) Insulin resistance, beta-cell dysfunction, and conversion to type 2 diabetes in a multiethnic population: the Insulin Resistance Atherosclerosis Study. Diabetes Care 33: 67-72.

3. Cannon CP, Steinberg BA, Murphy SA, Mega JL, Braunwald E (2006) Meta-analysis of cardiovascular outcomes trials comparing intensive versus moderate statin therapy. J Am Coll Cardiol 48: 438-445.

4. Cherniack EP (2011) Polyphenols: planting the seeds of treatment for the metabolic syndrome. Nutrition 27: 617-623.

5. Fraga CG, Galleano M, Verstraeten SV, Oteiza PI (2010) Basic biochemical mechanisms behind the health benefits of polyphenols. Mol Aspects Med 31: 435-445.

6. Seeram NP (2008) Berry fruits: compositional elements, biochemical activities, and the impact of their intake on human health, performance, and disease. J Agric Food Chem 56: 627-629.

7. Dugo P, Presti ML, Ohman M, Fazio A, Dugo G, et al. (2005) Determination of flavonoids in citrus juices by micro-HPLC-ESI/MS. J Sep Sci 28: 1149-1156.

8. Nogata Y, Sakamoto K, Shiratsuchi H, Ishii T, Yano M, et al. (2006) Flavonoid composition of fruit tissues of citrus species. Biosci Biotechnol Biochem 70: 178-192.

9. Jeong YJ, Choi YJ, Choi JS, Kwon HM, Kang SW, et al. (2007) Attenuation of monocyte adhesion and oxidised LDL uptake in luteolin-treated human endothelial cells exposed to oxidised LDL. Br J Nutr 97: 447-457.

10. Yu J, Wang L, Walzem RL, Miller EG, Pike LM, et al. (2005) Antioxidant activity of citrus limonoids, flavonoids, and coumarins. J Agric Food Chem 53: 2009-2014.

11. Di Donna L, De Luca G, Mazzotti F, Napoli A, Salerno R, et al. (2009) Statin-like principles of bergamot fruit (Citrus bergamia): isolation of 3-hydroxymethylglutaryl flavonoid glycosides. J Nat Prod 72: 1352-1354.

12. Mollace V, Sacco I, Janda E, Malara C, Ventrice D, et al. (2011) Hypolipemic and hypoglycaemic activity of bergamot polyphenols: from animal models to human studies. Fitoterapia 82: 309-316.

13. Gliozzi M, Walker R, Muscoli S, Vitale C, Gratteri S, et al. (2013) Bergamot polyphenolic fraction enhances rosuvastatin-induced effect on LDL-cholesterol, LOX-1 expression and protein kinase B phosphorylation in patients with hyperlipidemia. Int J Cardiol 170: 140-145.

14. Gliozzi M, Carresi C, Musolino V, Palma E, Muscoli C et al. (2014) The effect of bergamot-derived polyphenolic fraction on LDL small dense particles and non alcoholic fatty liver disease in patients with MS. Advances in Biological Chemistry.

15. Leighton F, Miranda-Rottmann S, Urquiaga I (2006) A central role of eNOS in the protective effect of wine against metabolic syndrome. Cell Biochem Funct 24: 291-298.

16. Mollace V, Ragusa S, Sacco I, Muscoli C, Sculco F, et al. (2008) The protective effect of bergamot oil extract on lecitine-like oxyLDL receptor-1 expression in balloon injury-related neointima formation. J Cardiovasc Pharmacol Ther 13: 120-129.

17. Nogata Y, Sakamoto K, Shiratsuchi H, Ishii T, Yano M, et al. (2006) Flavonoid composition of fruit tissues of citrus species. Biosci Biotechnol Biochem 70: 178-192.

18. Choe SC, Kim HS, Jeong TS, Bok SH, Park YB (2001) Naringin has an antiatherogenic effect with the inhibition of intercellular adhesion molecule-1 in hypercholesterolemic rabbits. J Cardiovasc Pharmacol 38: 947-955.

19. Vinson JA, Liang X, Proch J, Hontz BA, Dancel J, et al. (2002) Polyphenol antioxidants in citrus juices: in vitro and in vivo studies relevant to heart disease. Adv Exp Med Biol 505: 113-122.

20. Cha JY, Cho YS, Kim I, Anno T, Rahman SM, et al. (2001) Effect of hesperetin, a citrus flavonoid, on the liver triacylglycerol content and phosphatidate phosphohydrolase activity in orotic acid-fed rats. Plant Foods Hum Nutr 56: 349-358.

21. Wilcox LJ, Borradaile NM, de Dreu LE, Huff MW (2001) Secretion of hepatocyte apoB is inhibited by the flavonoids, naringenin and hesperetin, via reduced activity and expression of ACAT2 and MTP. J Lipid Res 42: 725-734.

22. Kim HJ, Oh GT, Park YB, Lee MK, Seo HJ, et al. (2004) Naringin alters the cholesterol biosynthesis and antioxidant enzyme activities in LDL receptor-knockout mice under cholesterol fed condition. Life Sci 74: 1621-1634.

23. Mollace V, Muscoli C, Masini E, Cuzzocrea S, Salvemini D (2005) Modulation of prostaglandin biosynthesis by nitric oxide and nitric oxide donors. Pharmacol Rev 57: 217-252.

24. Salvemini D, Kim SF, Mollace V (2013) Reciprocal regulation of the nitric oxide and cyclooxygenase pathway in pathophysiology: relevance and clinical implications. Am J Physiol Regul Integr Comp Physiol 304: R473-487.

25. Jeon SM, Bok SH, Jang MK, Lee MK, Nam KT, et al. (2001) Antioxidative activity of naringin and lovastatin in high cholesterol-fed rabbits. Life Sci 69: 2855-2866.

26. Hwang JT, Kwon DY, Yoon SH (2009) AMP-activated protein kinase: a potential target for the diseases prevention by natural occurring polyphenols. N Biotechnol 26: 17-22.

27. Zygmunt K, Faubert B, MacNeil J, Tsiani E (2010) Naringenin, a citrus flavonoid, increases muscle cell glucose uptake via AMPK. Biochem Biophys Res Commun 398: 178-183.

28. Mulvihill EE, Allister EM, Sutherland BG, Telford DE, Sawyez CG, et al. (2009) Naringenin prevents dyslipidemia, apolipoprotein B overproduction, and hyperinsulinemia in LDL receptor-null mice with diet-induced insulin resistance. Diabetes 58: 2198-2210.

29. Gouédard C, Barouki R, Morel Y (2004) Dietary polyphenols increase paraoxonase 1 gene expression by an aryl hydrocarbon receptor-dependent mechanism. Mol Cell Biol 24: 5209-5222.

30. Miceli N, Mondello MR, Monforte MT, Sdrafkakis V, Dugo P, et al. (2007) Hypolipidemic effects of Citrus bergamia Risso et Poiteau juice in rats fed a hypercholesterolemic diet. J Agric Food Chem 55: 10671-10677.

31. Borradaile NM, Carroll KK, Kurowska EM (1999) Regulation of HepG2 cell apolipoprotein B metabolism by the citrus flavanones hesperetin and naringenin. Lipids 34: 591-598.

32. Huong DT, Takahashi Y, Ide T (2006) Activity and mRNA levels of enzymes involved in hepatic fatty acid oxidation in mice fed citrus flavonoids. Nutrition 22: 546-552.

33. Li JM, Che CT, Lau CB, Leung PS, Cheng CH (2006) Inhibition of intestinal and renal Na+-glucose cotransporter by naringenin. Int J Biochem Cell Biol 38: 985-995.

34. Wenzel P, Daiber A, Oelze M, Brandt M, Closs E, et al. (2008) Mechanisms underlying recoupling of eNOS by HMG-CoA reductase inhibition in a rat model of streptozotocin-induced diabetes mellitus. Atherosclerosis 198: 65-76.

35. Antoniades C, Bakogiannis C, Tousoulis D, Reilly S, Zhang MH, et al. (2010) Preoperative atorvastatin treatment in CABG patients rapidly improves vein graft redox state by inhibition of Rac1 and NADPH-oxidase activity. Circulation 122: S66-73.

36. Carrepeiro MM, Rogero MM, Bertolami MC, Botelho PB, Castro N, et al. (2011) Effect of n-3 fatty acids and statins on oxidative stress in statin-treated hypercholestorelemic and normocholesterolemic women. Atherosclerosis 217: 171-178.

37. Landmesser U, Bahlmann F, Mueller M, Spiekermann S, Kirchhoff N, et al. (2005) Simvastatin versus ezetimibe: pleiotropic and lipid-lowering effects on endothelial function in humans. Circulation 111: 2356-2363.

38. Alsheikh-Ali AA, Karas RH (2009) The relationship of statins to rhabdomyolysis, malignancy, and hepatic toxicity: evidence from clinical trials. Curr Atheroscler Rep 11: 100-104.

39. Sanyal AJ; American Gastroenterological Association (2002) AGA technical review on nonalcoholic fatty liver disease. Gastroenterology 123: 1705-1725.

40. Brea A, Mosquera D, Martín E, Arizti A, Cordero JL, et al. (2005) Nonalcoholic fatty liver disease is associated with carotid atherosclerosis: a case-control study. Arterioscler Thromb Vasc Biol 25: 1045-1050.

41. Marchesini G, Brizi M, Morselli-Labate AM, Bianchi G, Bugianesi E, et al. (1999) Association of nonalcoholic fatty liver disease with insulin resistance. Am J Med 107: 450-455.

42. Hamaguchi M, Kojima T, Takeda N, Nagata C, Takeda J, et al. (2007) Nonalcoholic fatty liver disease is a novel predictor of cardiovascular disease. World J Gastroenterol 13: 1579-1584.

43. Chitturi S, Abeygunasekera S, Farrell GC, Holmes-Walker J, Hui JM, et al. (2002) NASH and insulin resistance: Insulin hypersecretion and specific association with the insulin resistance syndrome. Hepatology 35: 373-379.

44. Choudhury J, Sanyal AJ (2004) Insulin resistance and the pathogenesis of nonalcoholic fatty liver disease. Clin Liver Dis 8: 575-594, ix.

45. Janda E, Parafati M, Aprigliano S, Carresi C, Visalli V, et al. (2013) The antidote effect of quinone oxidoreductase 2 inhibitor against paraquat-induced toxicity in vitro and in vivo. Br J Pharmacol 168: 46-59.

46. Bok SH, Lee SH, Park YB, Bae KH, Son KH, et al. (1999) Plasma and hepatic cholesterol and hepatic activities of 3-hydroxy-3-methyl-glutaryl-CoA reductase and acyl CoA: cholesterol transferase are lower in rats fed citrus peel extract or a mixture of citrus bioflavonoids. J Nutr 129: 1182-1185.

47. Marounek M, Volek Z, Synytsya A, Copíková J (2007) Effect of pectin and amidated pectin on cholesterol homeostasis and cecal metabolism in rats fed a high-cholesterol diet. Physiol Res 56: 433-442.

48. Terpstra AH, Lapre JA, de Vries HT, Beynen AC (1998) Dietary pectin with high viscosity lowers plasma and liver cholesterol concentration and plasma cholesteryl ester transfer protein activity in hamsters. J Nutr 128: 1944-1949.

49. Terpstra AH, Lapré JA, de Vries HT, Beynen AC (2002) The hypocholesterolemic effect of lemon peels, lemon pectin, and the waste stream material of lemon peels in hybrid F1B hamsters. Eur J Nutr 41: 19-26.

50. Garcia-Diez F, Garcia-Mediavilla V, Bayon JE, Gonzalez-Gallego J (1996) Pectin feeding influences fecal bile acid excretion, hepatic bile acid and cholesterol synthesis and serum cholesterol in rats. J Nutr 126: 1766-1771.

51. Muscoli C, Sacco I, Alecce W, Palma E, Nisticò R, et al. (2004) The protective effect of superoxide dismutase mimetic M40401 on balloon injury-related neointima formation: role of the lectin-like oxidized low-density lipoprotein receptor-1. J Pharmacol Exp Ther 311: 44-50.

52. Davì G, Santilli F, Patrono C (2010) Nutraceuticals in diabetes and metabolic syndrome. Cardiovasc Ther 28: 216-226.

17

Metabolic Syndrome after Preeclampsia: A Cohort Study with a Mean Follow Up of 14 Years

Ana Ciléia Pinto Teixeira Henriques[*,1,2], Francisco Herlânio Costa Carvalho[1], Helvécio Neves Feitosa[1], Julio Cesar Garcia de Alencar[1], Lívia Rocha de Miranda Pinto[1] and Francisco Edson de Lucena Feitosa[1]

[1]Federal University of Ceará, Department of Public Health, St Prof. Costa Mendes, 1608 – 5th Floor, Rodolfo Teófilo, Fortaleza, Ceará, Brazil

[2]Metropolitan College of Grande Fortaleza, Assis Chateaubriand Maternity Teaching Hospital, Federal University of Ceará, Brazil

[*]Corresponding author: Ana Ciléia Pinto Teixeira Henriques, Departament of Public Health, St Prof. Costa Mendes, 1608, 5th Floor, Rodolfo Teófilo, Fortaleza, Ceará, Brazil; E-mail: anacileiahenriques@gmail.com

Abstract

Objective: To investigate the occurrence and characterization of metabolic syndrome (MetS) in the long term after pregnancies with preeclampsia. Design: Retrospective cohort study. Setting: Assis Chateaubriand Maternity Teaching Hospital - Federal University of Ceará, Fortaleza, Ceará, Brazil. Sample: 68 patients who gave birth between 1992 and 2002 at the Maternity, 34 patients with a history of preeclampsia and 34 with no history of obstetric complications.

Methods: Blood pressure and body compositional indices were recorded. Fasting blood samples were tested for glucose, total cholesterol, high density lipoprotein-cholesterol, low density lipoprotein-cholesterol and triglycerides. A questionnaire was used to collect demographic data including family history of diseases associated with cardiovascular diseases. Criteria for metabolic syndrome were defined by International Diabetes Federation 2005 (IDF). Main outcome measures: Occurrence and characterization of MetS.

Results: There were 18 (52.9%) diagnoses of MetS in the group of women without a history of obstetric complications and 28 (82.3%) in the group of women with a history of preeclampsia, p=0.01 with a RR of 4.1 (CI 95% 1.4 - 12.2, p=0.009). The number of components to characterize MetS were, respectively, 2.7 (± 1.3) and 3.3 (± 1.3), p=0.05.

Conclusions: Women with a history of preeclampsia have a higher prevalence of MetS 14 years after gestation.

Keywords: Metabolic Syndrome X; Preeclampsia; Cardiovascular Diseases; Retrospective studies

Introduction

Of all the conditions that affect pregnancy and childbirth, preeclampsia is one of the most responsible for high rates of maternal and perinatal mortality in many countries [1,2]. Studies show that women with a history of preeclampsia are at increased risk of cardiovascular disease (CVD) in the long term, as demonstrated by several studies with varied follow-up times and specific outcomes for cardiovascular events [3]. A meta-analysis that evaluated studies with a follow-up period of 10 to 14 years, found a relative risk (RR) of 3.70 for systemic arterial hypertension (SAH), 2.16 for acute myocardial infarction (AMI), 1.84 for strokes and 1.79 for deep venous thrombosis (DVT) in these patients [3]. Preeclampsia and CVD have common underlying mechanisms such as dyslipidemia, inflammation, hypercoagulability and insulin deregulation. These factors are components of the clinical framework of metabolic syndrome (MetS) [4,5].

MetS includes a number of metabolic risk factors including the abnormal distribution of body fat, insulin resistance, atherogenic dyslipidemia and elevated blood pressure [5]. Compared with individuals without MetS, those diagnosed with MetS have a higher incidence of cerebrovascular disease and a higher mortality from these causes [6]. Given the significant association between the two conditions, preeclampsia and metabolic syndrome, with the occurrence of CVD, this study aimed to evaluate the occurrence and characteristics of MetS in the long term in women with history of preeclampsia.

Methods

Study design

This is a retrospective cohort study conducted in the Assis Chateaubriand Maternity Teaching Hospital, Fortaleza, Ceará, Brazil, which cares for patients from the capital and the interior, with medium and high risk pregnancies. The population was composed of women who gave birth in the period from 1992 to 2002 in the aforementioned hospital and who resided in the state capital.

The study included women diagnosed with pure preeclampsia as documented in their medical records when discharged. Preeclampsia was defined as the presence of gestational hypertension and concomitant proteinuria in the second half of pregnancy, have been based on the criteria of the International Society for the Study of Hypertension in Pregnancy [7]. According to the International Society for the Study of Hypertension in Pregnancy criteria, gestational hypertension is defined as diastolic blood pressure more than 90 mm Hg, systolic blood pressure more than 140 mm Hg, or both measured on two or more separate occasions at least 4 hours apart; proteinuria was diagnosed when there was more than 300 mg per 24 hours or when dipstick urinalysis was more than 2+ [7].

The group without a history of preeclampsia was composed of women who gave birth during the same period as the exposed women, selected so that there was one non-exposed patient to each exposed patient. The sample was calculated using STATA ° statistical software,, version 12.0 (Stata Corp, USA), considering a significance level of 5%, 80% power and the averages of the mean systolic arterial blood pressures (SBP) found in the two groups, which was the main outcome found in previous studies, resulting in a sample size equal to 60 with 30 patients in each group. Women with a history of other complications associated with the pregnancy-index (Placental abruption, gestational diabetes and placenta previa) or who were pregnant or postpartum at the time of the invitation for evaluation were excluded from the study. The chart shows how the final number of patients was obtained at the end of the study (Figure 1).

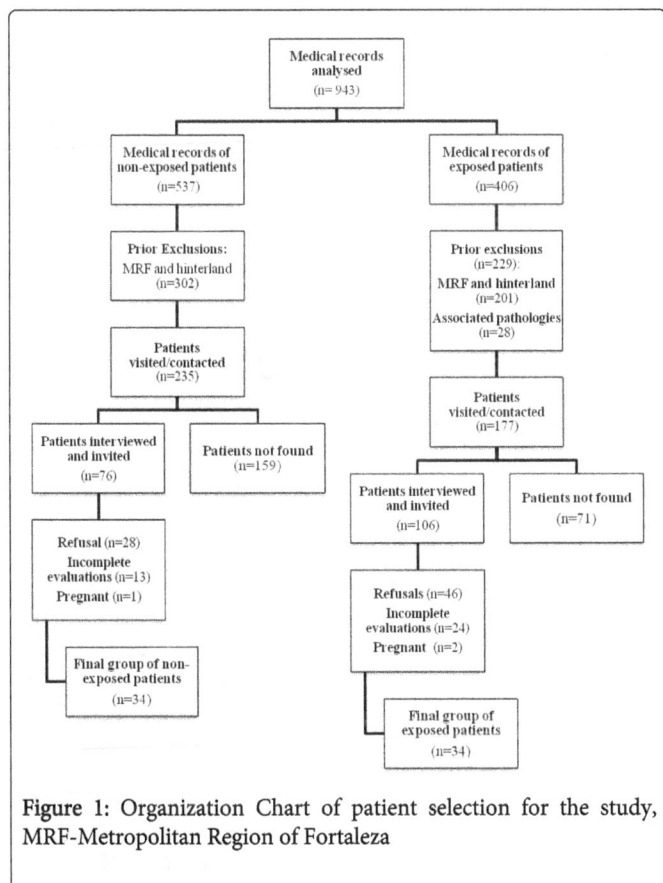

Figure 1: Organization Chart of patient selection for the study, MRF-Metropolitan Region of Fortaleza

Data collection

Interviews were used to collect data on obstetric history (maternal age at the time of delivery, gestational age according to the date of the last menstrual period or by ultrasound before the 20th gestational week in the medical records, type of delivery, number of pregnancies, deliveries and miscarriages and any complications in other pregnancies), socio-demographic data (race, current age, education, income, marital status and occupation), history of current morbidities

and lifestyle (diagnosed conditions and/or receiving treatment, medication use, physical activity, and smoking) and a family history of CVD.

Clinical evaluation was done through the collection of anthropometric and laboratory variables. All analyses were performed by technicians blinded for study group and unaware of the underlying hypothesis. The verification protocol was defined according to international consensus [5,8,9]. Blood pressure was evaluated using the Micro life BP 3BTO-H ° semi-automatic monitor following the recommendations of American Heart Association [9]. The weight and percentage of body fat were measured using the bio impedance technique with the Wiso ° W835 digital analyzer scale with high precision sensors that use infrared and ultrasound technology to analyze body composition to show the percentages of lean body mass, fat, water and bone weight. Height was measured using the Seca ° stadiometer with a scale of 0 to 220 cm and 0.1 cm accuracy. To calculate the Body Mass Index (BMI), the weight in kilograms was divided by the height in meters squared and the evaluation followed the classification of American Heart Association [8].

For the measurement of waist circumference (WC), the patient was requested to remain in a supine position, with their arms relaxed along their sides, wearing light clothing without a belt, taking as reference the last rib and the iliac crest and performing the measurement at the midpoint between them. To measure the abdominal circumference (AC) the same recommendations were followed using the umbilicus as reference. For Caucasian women the International Diabetes Federation sets a waist circumference measurement equal to or above 80 cm as the cut-off point for increased cardiovascular risk [5]. The measurement of the hip circumference (HC) was performed using the greatest curvature of the hip as the reference. For these three measurements non-extendable WCS ° measuring tapes were used with variation in mm and a length of 150 cm.

The waist/hip ratio (WHR), which is the ratio between the circumference of the waist and the hip in cm was calculated using as the cut-off point for women the value of 0.85. The waist-to-height (WHtR), which is the ratio between waist circumference and height in cm, used the cut-off value of 0.53 as presented in the work of Pitanga and Lessa [10]. The Conicity Index (CI) was also calculated, determined by the formula described by Valdez [11], dividing the WC in cm by the constant 0.109, multiplied by the square root of the body weight in kilograms divided by the height in meters using 1.18 as the cutoff point as indicated by Pitanga and Lessa [10].

In addition, the bicipital fold was measured using Innovare 2 Cescorf ° calipers, with the patient in a supine position with her right arm relaxed and extended along the body. The fold was ascertained in the direction of the longitudinal axis of the inside of the arm, precisely at the point of the greatest apparent circumference of the venter of the biceps or located at the midpoint between the acromion and the olecranon. The laboratory evaluation included measurements of total cholesterol and HDL, LDL and VLDL, triglycerides and fasting glucose levels. The patients were instructed to fast for 12 hours and abstain from alcohol the day before venipuncture. The Tinder enzymatic method was used to analyze the samples, fractions of total cholesterol and triglyceride levels and the enzymatic method was employed for the analysis of blood glucose.

To determine MetS, the criteria set by the International Diabetes Federation (IDF) [5], were used, namely: a AC equal to or greater than 80 cm for women, characterized by central obesity and the presence of two or more components, specifically: triglyceride values equal to or greater than 150 mg/dL, HDL less than 50 mg/dL for women; SBP equal to or greater than 130 mmHg and/or a diastolic blood pressure (DBP) equal to or greater than 85 mmHg, or treatment for SAH; fasting glucose equal to or greater than 100 mg/dL, or treatment for diabetes mellitus (DM). Besides the characterization of MetS, the number of components to characterize the MetS was calculated and the frequency of alteration of each component.

Statistical analysis

The collected data were tabulated and analyzed using the STATA ® Program, version 12.0 (StataCorp, USA) and the mean and standard deviation (SD) of clinical and metabolic variables were calculated. The Kolmogorov-Smirnov test was used to test the normality of the variables and the analysis of the differences between exposed and non-exposed women used the T-test for variables with normal distribution and the Mann-Whitney test for non-normal distribution. Pearson's X2 test or the Fisher exact test were used for categorical data. The significance level of $p<0.05$ with a confidence interval (CI) of 95 % was considered. The calculation of Relative Risk (RR) was carried out for variables that showed $p<0.10$ in the first analysis.

The study was approved by the MEAC Ethics Committee under Opinion No. 83/2011.

Results

The study included 68 patients, 34 with a history of preeclampsia and 34 with no history of obstetric complications. The mean age at the time of delivery was 25.7 ± 7.3 years. The average years of follow-up of the unexposed group was 14.8 ± 3.7 years and among the exposed group it was 13.4 ± 2.9, no difference was found between the groups for this variable (p=0.31).

Table 1 presents the characteristics of the current socio-demographic variables. The groups did not differ in age, race, marital status, occupation, education level and family income. The patients were mostly non-white, living with a partner, in paid work either as self-employed or employed formally, with an average of 7.6 ± 3.4 years of schooling and an income of 1.6 ± 6.8 minimum wages.

	Exposure		
	Non-exposed	Exposed	p †
Current age (years) (mean ± DP)	39.1 ± 8.4	40.6 ± 8.1	0.45*
Race (n,%)			
White	7 — 20.6	9 — 26.5	0.56‡
Non-white	27 — 79.4	25 — 73.5	
Civil Status (n,%)			
With a partner	22 — 64.7	25 — 73.5	0.43‡
Without a partner	12 — 35.3	9 — 26.5	
Occupation (n,%)			
Works outside home/Self-employed	17 — 50	20 — 58.8	0.46‡
Unemployed/ Housewife	17 — 50	14 — 41.2	
Schooling (years) (mean ± DP)	7,0 ± 3.2	8.3 ± 3.6	0.13*
Family income (mw) ¥ (mean ± DP)	1,5 ± 0.8	1.7 ± 0.8	0.24*

Table 1: Socio-demographic characteristics of patients with and without a history of preeclampsia - mean follow up of 14 years, MEAC-UFC, Fortaleza, 2012

† Different statistical tests were used in the analysis: * T-Student; ‡ X 2 Test.

¥ mw= minimum wage. Reference value in 2012: R$ 622.00

Table 2 presents data from the current clinical and obstetric history.

	Exposure				
	Non-exposed		Exposed		
	n	%	n	%	p†
Current diseases diagnosed / under treatment	11	32.4	18	52.9	0.08‡
Family history of CVD/CVE ¥	28	82.3	32	94.1	0.3‡‡
Smoking	-	-	4	11.8	0.11‡‡
Doing physical activity	8	23.5	11	32.3	0.41‡
Use of medications					
Antihypertensive	6	17.6	13	38.2	0.05‡
Hypoglycemic	1	2.9	5	14.7	0.19‡‡
Anticoagulants	5	14.7	2	5.9	0.42‡‡
Fibrates / statins	1	2.9	4	11.8	0.35‡‡
Hormonal Contraception	3	8.8	4	11.8	1,00‡‡
Menopausal	5	14.7	6	17.6	0.74‡
Family history of GHS	12	35.3	11	32.3	0.84‡
Family obstetric history (mean ± DP)					
Number of pregnancies	2.7 ± 2.0		3.3 ± 3.6		0.40*
Number of deliveries	2.3 ± 1.7		2.3 ± 2.2		0.85*
Number of miscarriages	0.4 ± 0.7		0.9 ± 1.7		0.11*
Complications in other pregnancies	11	32.3	21	61.8	0.02‡

Table 2: Current clinical and obstetric history for women with and without preeclampsia – Average follow-up of 14 years, MEAC-UFC, Fortaleza, 2012

† Different statistical tests were used in the analysis * T-Student; ‡ X 2 Test; ⌗ Fisher Test.

¥ The patients cited one or more morbid conditions: Systemic arterial hypertension, diabetes mellitus, acute myocardial attack, stroke, congestive heart failure.

CVE= Cardiovascular Event; CVD= Cardiovascular Disease.

GHS= Gestational Hypertensive Syndrome

Hypertension was the most common condition, with a prevalence of 47.1% among the exposed group and 17.6% in the non-exposed group, with a RR of 4.1 (CI 95% 1.4 to 12. 5, p=0.012). The family history of CVD was similar between the groups, which can thus be excluded as a factor for confusion in the analysis of the outcomes. Although all the patients who were currently smokers were in the group with a history of preeclampsia, difference was not found between groups on this variable.

The groups were also similar regarding doing regular physical activity, with the majority of patients (72.1%) reporting that they did not do any physical activity. As for obstetric history, it was found that the women with a history of preeclampsia reported more complications in other pregnancies than non-exposed patients, with a RR of 3.4 (95% CI 1.2 to 9.1, p=0.01).

Table 3 presents the clinical and metabolic findings.

Clinical and metabolic characteristics	Exposure		
	Non-exposed	Exposed	p†
Anthropometric Variables			
Weight (kg)	68.2 ± 9.7	71.4 ± 14.6	0.29*
Height (m)	1.53 ± 0.1	1.52 ± 0.1	0.66*
BMI (kg / m²)	28.2 ± 6.1	28.9 ± 9.2	0.66*
SBP (mmHg)	120.4 ± 14.3	131.0 ± 23.8	0.03*
DBP (mmHg)	79.5 ± 10.7	85.1 ± 14.9	0.08*
AC (cm)	92.9 ± 8.9	95.6 ± 10.4	0.27*
WC (cm)	86.5 ± 8.7	87.7 ± 11.2	0.63*
HC (cm)	102.5 ± 7.7	106.1 ± 10.7	0.11*
WHR	0.8 ± 0.1	0.7 ± 0.2	0.35*
Index C	1.2 ± 0.2	1.1 ± 0.3	0.47*
WHtR	0.54 ± 0.1	0.54 ± 0.2	0.86*
Bicipital fold (mm)	14.2 ± 5.1	15.4 ± 6.9	0.41*
Body fat (%)	42.9 ± 6.3	41.9 ± 7.7	0.58*
Metabolic variables			
Total cholesterol	182.6 ± 41.8	190.5 ± 33.3	0.38*
Triglycerides	143.7 ± 98.6	157.8 ± 62.4	0.05**
LDL cholesterol	109.7 ± 36.1	122.4 ± 31.3	0.05**
HDL cholesterol	43.5 ± 12.3	41.1 ± 8.4	0.34*
Fasting glucose	95.0 ± 11.1	104.1 ± 38.7	0.20*

Table 3: Clinical and metabolic characterization of women with and without preeclampsia– Average follow-up of 14 years, MEAC-UFC, Fortaleza, 2012

†Different statistical tests were used in the analysis: * T-test; **Mann-Whitney.

BMI: Body Mass Index; SBP: Systolic Blood Pressure, DBP: Diastolic Blood Pressure, AC: Abdominal Circumference, WC: Waist Circumference, HC: Hip Circumference, WHR: Waist to Hip Ratio, Index C: Conicity Index, WHtR: Waist-to-Height Ratio, LDL: Low-Density Lipoprotein, HDL: High-Density Lipoprotein.

The patients' average weight was 69.8 ± 12.4 kg, but there was no difference between the two groups with respect to this variable. The mean BMI of 28.6 ± 7.8 kg / m 2 indicates a profile of patients classified as overweight or obese, but without a statistical difference between groups.

The anthropometric measurements of AC and WC had averages above the recommended classification for low cardiometabolic risk, presenting 94.3 ± 9.7 cm and 87.1 ± 9.9 cm, respectively. A difference was detected between the groups in terms of mean SBP, with the group of women with a history of preeclampsia having the highest average. There was a trend towards higher values of DBP, triglycerides and LDL cholesterol in the exposed group. The clinical and metabolic variables were also categorized according to their cut-off points for altered values, there was a higher frequency of change in the group with a history of preeclampsia for the measurements of total cholesterol (values greater than 160 mg/dL) with a RR of 4.9 (95% CI 1.3 to 18.3, p=0.01).

Table 4 shows the data for the characterization of MetS according to the diagnosis, the number of altered components identified in each group and frequency of abnormal factors.

	Exposure				
	Non-exposed		Exposed		
	n	%	n	%	p†
Diagnosis of MetS	18	52.9	28	82.3	0.01‡
Number of MetS components (mean ± SD)	2.7 ± 1.3		3.3 ± 1.3		0.05**
Factors of altered MetS					
AC ≥80 cm	31	91.2	33	97.1	0.61‡‡
Triglycerides ≥ 150 mg / dL	13	38.2	17	50	0.32‡
HDL-c< 50 mg/dL	26	76.5	28	84.8	0.38‡
SBP ≥ 130 mmHg	9	26.5	16	47.1	0.07‡
DBP ≥ 85 mmHg	12	35.3	17	50	0.22‡
Fasting glucose ≥ 100 mg/dL	10	29.4	14	41.2	0.31‡

Table 4: Components and characteristics of Metabolic Syndrome in women with and without a history of preeclampsia – Average follow-up of 14 years MEAC-UFC, Fortaleza, 2012

†† Different statistical tests were used in the analysis: ** Mann-Whitney; ‡ Test X2; ‡‡ Fisher test.

MetS=Metabolic Syndrome; AC=Abdominal Circumference; SBP=Systolic Blood Pressure; DBP= Diastolic Blood Pressure; HDL-High-Density Lipoprotein.

The majority (67.7%) of patients were classified according to the IDF [5] as having metabolic syndrome, and there was a higher prevalence in patients with a history of preeclampsia, with a RR of 4.1 (CI 95% 1.4 to 12.2, p=0.009). There was higher frequency of alteration of the variables for AC (94.1%) and HDL cholesterol (80.1%) in the total population.

Discussion

Main findings

An unfavourable metabolic profile was found among the patients evaluated, with changes in the anthropometric characteristics of central obesity, a major cardiovascular risk factor, and the biochemical measurements that contribute to aggravating this risk, with the majority characterized as having MetS. There was a higher frequency in the group of patients with a history of preeclampsia.

Both groups were alike in their baseline characteristics at the start of the follow up in terms of age, the number of pregnancies, parity, occurrence of miscarriages and smoking status, factors that may influence the outcomes being assessed and demonstrate a recognized association with CVD [4,12,13].

Physical exercise was one important variable analyzed as a possible contributing factor to the composition of MetS, without a difference between groups. There was a low frequency of physical activity in the sample studied, comparable to the results of Ekelund et al. [14] in which the majority of women (59.1%) did not do physical activity or were moderately inactive. The high SBP averages found this study are consistent with the results of other studies that show higher rates of this measurement in women with a history of GHS [15-17].

The AC and WC measurements had averages above the amount considered appropriate; however, this difference was not significant between groups. When analyzing the biochemical blood findings, there was an unfavourable lipid profile, in which all the measurements were altered more frequently in the exposed group. The mean HDL-C values were lower than the amounts recommended as ideal parameters for the female population; this was the second most altered measurement among the exposed patients (84.8%). The presence of factors that characterize metabolic syndrome according to the IDF [5] was evaluated and there were an excessive number of altered values in both groups. In this study, most patients (67.7%) were characterized as having MetS. An analysis of components of MetS showed that AC, an obligatory factor for a classification of MetS, and HDL-C, was one of the most frequent alterations.

Strengths and limitations

It must be emphasized that in the present study, patients with other diagnoses of GHS, such chronic hypertension and preeclampsia superimposed on chronic hypertension were excluded, thereby seeking to evaluate the influence of preeclampsia as a specific disorder of pregnancy predisposing long term metabolic changes.

It is still uncertain whether preeclampsia predisposes women to future CVD mediated by MetS or if it is a manifestation of a subclinical susceptibility to future MetS that predisposes women to preeclampsia [18], which methodologically, cannot be evaluated through retrospective cohort studies, since many factors such as BMI, lipid and glycemic profile analysis and pre-pregnancy anthropometric values are required, which was not possible in this study.

Although some authors discuss the validity of the characterization of MetS, several studies have demonstrated the value of this classification and its association with the occurrence of future cardiovascular events, thus it is important to consider this syndrome

when assessing patients who may have differentiated future cardiometabolic risk factors, such as women with an adverse obstetric history [19].

It may also be considered that the average age of the patients analyzed in this study (39.8 ± 8.2 years) is considered relatively young and may explain why greater changes have not manifested themselves yet, as postulated by Rich-Edwards [20]. Even with the small sample size, significant differences could be found in the profile of morbidities among the group of patients analyzed, showing the need for further evaluation of patients with preeclampsia that also involves the subclinical conditions that may characterize a future adverse cardiovascular profile, so that preventive measures can be taken early, reducing the complications associated with these changes.

Interpretation

Previous studies, with shorter follow-up periods, had already demonstrated this association but no study had ever addressed this assessment in a period over 10 years. Several studies have had longer follow ups for other outcomes, but not for metabolic syndrome [16,18]. A study by Pouta et al. (2004) presented the results of this evaluation with a pregnancy-index range interval up to an evaluation of five months to 11 years [21]. Studies show that women with a history of gestational hypertension syndrome (GHS) tend to have higher frequencies of hypertension, diabetes and use of antihypertensive and hypoglycemic medications, however, the differences between the groups for these variables has not been identified [22-24].

A study by Callaway et al. [25], found that among 191 women with a history of GHS, 32.5% were hypertensive 21 years after delivery, less than in the present study, which showed a frequency of SAH of 47.1% in exposed patients. Studies point to different relative risks for the occurrence of future hypertension in women with a history of GHS, depending on the severity of the condition. For women with a history of gestational hypertension (GH), the RR found by Wilson et al. [24] was 2.47, whereas for preeclampsia/eclampsia, the RR was 3.89.

The profile of the high frequency of changes in anthropometric and metabolic variables are in line with results of other studies, such as Canti et al. [15] that, when analyzing 40 women with a history of preeclampsia and 14 with a history of normotensive pregnancies after a follow-up period of 14.6 years for the exposed group and 15.9 years for the unexposed group, found increased BMI, WC and DBP values in women with a history of PE, with measurements consistent with the characterization of high cardiometabolic risk [8].

Studies show that overweight and obesity represent a serious health threat and are strongly associated with an increased risk of cardiovascular disease, type 2 diabetes mellitus and metabolic disorders [26]. A study conducted by Forest et al. [16] evaluated 168 pairs of women recruited between 1989 and 1997, 7.8 years after labour, 105 with a history of GH and 63 with a history of PE who were compared with 168 controls. They found higher BP averages in patients with a history of GHS and the SBP was equal to 115 mmHg, lower than that shown by the patients in the present study (131.0 ± 23.8 mmHg).

Jie et al. [18] analyzed the prevalence of MetS in 62 women one to three years after a preeclamptic pregnancy. They found that 39% of these women met the IDF criteria for this condition, lower than the findings in the present study. The authors found that abdominal obesity, high blood pressure and decreased HDL-c were the most altered factors in women with history of preeclampsia, whereas fasting glucose was less altered.

Conclusion

An unfavorable clinical and metabolic profile was found, with the patients with a history of preeclampsia having a higher prevalence of MetS diagnoses and a tendency for a higher number of altered components for a characterization of MetS.

Practical recommendations

Reproductive factors are rarely taken into consideration when evaluating an individual's risk for metabolic diseases. However, with an increasing body of evidence indicating that may exist a strong relationship between this conditions, further clinical consideration is required through increased monitoring, risk stratification, and follow-up of individuals with such adverse reproductive histories such as preeclampsia.

Researches recommendations

More research is needed to understand the biological etiology underlying these relationships, including genetic and epigenetic mechanisms, and analyzing larger samples.

Acknowledgements

The authors would like to thank the Conselho Nacional de Desenvolvimento Científico e Tecnológico-CNPq by studentship funding for the principal researcher.

Contribution to Authorship

ACPTH: conception and design of the protocol, acquisition of data, drafting the article approval of the final version; FHCC: conception and design of the protocol, drafting the article, acquisition of data, and approval of the final version; HNF: drafting the article and approval of the final version; JCGA: acquisition of data, drafting the article and approval of the final version; LRMP: acquisition of data, drafting the article and approval of the final version; FELF: drafting the article and approval of the final version.

References

1. Ghulmiyyah L, Sibai B (2012) Maternal mortality from preeclampsia/eclampsia. Semin Perinatol 36: 56-59.

2. Kullima AA, Kawuwa MB, Audu BM, Usman H, Geidam AD (2009) A 5-year review of maternal mortality associated with eclampsia in a tertiary institution in northern Nigeria. Ann Afr Med 8: 81-84.

3. Bellamy L, Casas JP, Hingorani AD, Williams DJ (2007). Preeclampsia and risk of cardiovascular disease and cancer in later life: systematic review and meta-analysis. BMJ 335: 974-977.

4. Sattar N, Greer IA (2002) Pregnancy complications and maternal cardiovascular risk: opportunities for intervention and screening? BMJ 325: 157-160.

5. Alberti KG, Zimmet P, Shaw J (2006) Metabolic syndrome--a new worldwide definition. A Consensus Statement from the International Diabetes Federation. Diabet Med 23: 469-480.

6. Mottillo S, Filion KB, Genest J, Joseph L, Pilote L, et al. (2010) The metabolic syndrome and cardiovascular risk a systematic review and meta-analysis. J Am Coll Cardiol 56: 1113-1132.

7. Brown MA, Lindheimer MD, de Swiet M, Van Assche A, Moutquin JM (2001) The classification and diagnosis of the hypertensive disorders of pregnancy: statement from the International Society for the Study of Hypertension in Pregnancy (ISSHP). Hypertens Pregnancy 20: IX-XIV.

8. Cornier MA, Després JP, Davis N, Grossniklaus DA, Klein S, et al. (2011) Assessing adiposity: a scientific statement from the American Heart Association. Circulation 124: 1996-2019.

9. Pickering TG, Hall JE, Appel LJ, Falkner BE, Graves J, et al. (2005) Recommendations for blood pressure measurement in humans and experimental animals: Part 1: blood pressure measurement in humans: a statement for professionals from the Subcommittee of Professional and Public Education of the American Heart Association Council on High Blood Pressure Research. Hypertension 45: 142-161.

10. Pitanga FJ, Lessa I (2005) [Anthropometric indexes of obesity as an instrument of screening for high coronary risk in adults in the city of Salvador--Bahia]. Arq Bras Cardiol 85: 26-31.

11. Valdez R (1991) A simple model-based index of abdominal adiposity. J Clin Epidemiol 44: 955-956.

12. Sesso HD, Lee IM, Gaziano JM, Rexrode KM, Glynn RJ, et al. (2001) Maternal and paternal history of myocardial infarction and risk of cardiovascular disease in men and women. Circulation 104: 393-398.

13. D'Agostino RB Sr, Vasan RS, Pencina MJ, Wolf PA, Cobain M, et al. (2008) General cardiovascular risk profile for use in primary care: the Framingham Heart Study. Circulation 117: 743-753.

14. Ekelund U, Besson H, Luan J, May AM, Sharp SJ, et al. (2011) Physical activity and gain in abdominal adiposity and body weight: prospective cohort study in 288,498 men and women. Am J Clin Nutr 93: 826-835.

15. Canti IC, Komlós M, Martins-Costa SH, Ramos JG, Capp E, et al. (2010) Risk factors for cardiovascular disease ten years after preeclampsia. Sao Paulo Med J 128: 10-13.

16. Forest JC, Girouard J, Massé J, Moutquin JM, Kharfi A, et al. (2005) Early occurrence of metabolic syndrome after hypertension in pregnancy. Obstet Gynecol 105: 1373-1380.

17. Wolf M, Hubel CA, Lam C, Sampson M, Ecker JL, et al. (2004) Preeclampsia and future cardiovascular disease: potential role of altered angiogenesis and insulin resistance. J Clin Endocrinol Metab 89: 6239-6243.

18. Lu J, Zhao YY, Qiao J, Zhang HJ, Ge L, et al. (2011) A follow-up study of women with a history of severe preeclampsia: relationship between metabolic syndrome and preeclampsia. Chin Med J (Engl) 124: 775-779.

19. Després JP, Arsenault BJ, Côté M, Cartier A, Lemieux I (2008) Abdominal obesity: the cholesterol of the 21st century? Can J Cardiol 24 Suppl D: 7D-12D.

20. Rich-Edwards JW (2012) The predictive pregnancy: what complicated pregnancies tell us about mother's future cardiovascular risk. Circulation 125: 1336-1338.

21. Pouta A, Hartikainen AL, Sovio U, Gissler M, Laitinen J, et al. (2004) Manifestations of metabolic syndrome after hypertensive pregnancy. Hypertension 43: 825-831.

22. Garovic VD, Bailey KR, Boerwinkle E, Hunt SC, Weder AB, et al. (2010) Hypertension in pregnancy as a risk factor for cardiovascular disease later in life. J Hypertens 28: 826-833.

23. Lykke JA, Langhoff-Roos J, Sibai BM, Funai EF, Triche EW, et al. (2009) Hypertensive pregnancy disorders and subsequent cardiovascular morbidity and type 2 diabetes mellitus in the mother. Hypertension 53: 944-951.

24. Wilson BJ, Watson MS, Prescott GJ, Sunderland S, Campbell DM, et al. (2003) Hypertensive diseases of pregnancy and risk of hypertension and stroke in later life: results from cohort study. BMJ 326: 845.

18

Pre-pregnancy Body Mass Index and the Risk of Adverse Pregnancy Outcome in Two Thousand Type 2 Diabetes Mellitus Bangladeshi Women

Samsad Jahan[*1], Chaudhury Meshkat Ahmed[2], Samira Humaira Habib[3], Akter Jahan[4], Farzana Sharmin[5], Md Sakandar Hyet Khan[6] and Manisha Banarjee[7]

[1]Department of Gynaecology & Obstetrics, BIRDEM, Dhaka, Bangladesh

[2]Department of Cardiology, BSMMU, Dhaka, Bangladesh

[3]Health Economics Unit, BADAS, Dhaka, Bangladesh

[4]Govt Homeopathic College, Dhaka, Bangladesh

[5]Department of Obstetrics and Gynecology, BIHS, Dhaka, Bangladesh

[6]Red Crescent Hospital, Cox's Bazar, Bangladesh

[7]Department of Gynecology & Obstetrics, Dhaka Medical College Hospital, Dhaka, Bangladesh

[*]Corresponding author: Samsad Jahan, Department of Gynecology & Obstetrics, Consultant and Associate Professor, BIRDEM, 122 Kazi Nazrul Islam Avenue, Dhaka -1000, Bangladesh; E-mail: shelly_birdem@yahoo.com; dhcdp@dab-bd.org; samirahumaira@yahoo.com

Abstract

Background: The aim of the present study were to evaluate the frequency of maternal complications and adverse fetal outcomes in a group of singleton pregnant women with type 2 diabetes mellitus to compare the outcome in three groups (lean, normal and overweight).

Materials and Methods: The women were categorized into three groups: lean <18.5, normal from 18.5 to 24.9 and overweight >25.0-29.9 kg/m^2. The effect of pre-pregnancy BMI was analyzed by comparing the frequencies of various outcomes in three BMI groups. The results were expressed as odds ratio (ORs) and the corresponding 95% confidence intervals (CIs) & p values.

Results: The risk of late fetal death was consistently increasing with BMI (ORs were 1.2 (0.9-1.7), 1.6 (1.1-2.3) & 2.6 (1.7-3.8) for lean, normal & overweight respectively). The risk of early neonatal death was also higher among women with higher BMI (ORs was 1.6 (1.1-2.3) for overweight). The rate of preeclampsia is higher among women with lean and overweight BMI in compares to normal BMI (the values were 2.5%, 1.8%, & 7.0% for lean, normal & overweight respectively). Hypertensive disorders was also more common among lean (3.8%) and overweight (3.6%) compared to normal (1.6%). The risk of preterm delivery was significantly increased for overweight group (4.2%) and lean (2.4%), as compare to normal. The risk of SGA was significantly more in lean (2.7%) compared to normal weight (1.5%) & overweight group (1.9%).

Conclusion: Pre-pregnancy overweight increases the risk of late fetal death and perinatal mortality.

Keywords: Type 2 diabetes; Body mass index; Pre-pregnancy; Obesity

Introduction

Over the last few decades several studies have shown that women with type1 diabetes mellitus still have a high incidence of adverse maternal, fetal and neonatal morbidity and mortality. [1-9] There is a strongly elevated risk of congenital malformations [1,3,6,7], macrosomia [3,7] and pre-eclampsia [1,7] as well as pre term delivery and increased caesarean section rates[1,6,7]. Neonatal hypoglycemia occurs frequently during the first day after delivery [1]. Elevated plasma glucose levels in first trimester are the major contributor to the development of congenital abnormalities [1,5], in midtrimester pre-eclampsia [10,11] and macrosomia [1,12]. This has suggested to be aimed at reaching normoglycemia or near normoglycemia.

The prevalence of type 2 diabetes is increasing rapidly in all age groups. It is a general clinical observation that the number of pregnant women with pregestational type 2 diabetes has become more frequent in the recent years, however, little knowledge exits concerning the prevalence and outcome of these pregnancies. [13,14]. During the last decade, five surveys have been published which showed maternal, fetal and neonatal outcome in pregestational type 2 diabetes are similar to those in pregnancy with pregestational type1 diabetes [6,15-19]. Pregestational type 2 diabetes is an emerging problem especially since type 2 diabetes has become a global epidemic [20].

This means that type 2 diabetes occurs with increasing frequency in younger age group since at the same time the maternal age of first and subsequent pregnancies has risen in modern society, more and more women are confronted with the problems and burden of type 2 diabetes during pregnancies.

Obesity before pregnancy is associated with an increased risk of fetal macrosomia & perinatal mortality. [21-23]. The mothers being leaner (underweight) than average, on the other hand, is associated with an increased risk of delivering an infant who is small for gestational age and perhaps also the risk of preterm delivery [23-26].

Pregnancies among underweight or overweight women are therefore often regarded as high-risk pregnancies and thin women are frequently advised to gain weight before becoming pregnant. [27-29] and overweight women are advised for weight reduction.

The aim of the study was to examine the association of the maternal Body Mass Index (BMI) and the obstetric and the perinatal outcomes in singleton pregnancies of type 2 DM mother.

Methods and Materials

Two thousand women were categorized into 3 groups on the basis of their maternal Body Mass Index (BMI). The maternal and the neonatal outcome were noted in all groups. The obstetrical outcomes included gestational hypertension or pregnancy induced hypertension, preeclampsia, preterm delivery, shoulder dystocia. The neonatal outcomes included late fetal death, early neonatal deaths, small for gestational age (SGA) and macrosomic baby.

Pregnancy with type 2 diabetes was managed according to our routine procedures. Current treatment with oral hypoglycemic agents was stopped at admission & the women were treated with diet and exercise alone or diet, exercise and insulin. Women treated with diet alone performed home blood glucose measurements before breakfast (fasting) and 2 hours after breakfast, after lunch and after dinner respectively, 2 days per week. Goals were pre-prandial capillary blood glucose levels <6 mmol/L, postprandial levels <7 mmol/L, and a mean <6 mmol/L. If these goals were not obtained treatment with daily dose of insulin (soluble short acting and intermediate acting) was advised.

The women were categorized according to their BMI (kg/m^2): lean <18.5, normal from >18.5 to 24.9 and overweight >25.0-29.9kg/m^2. Information regarding maternal age, parity, complications during pregnancy or delivery and perinatal outcomes were obtained from hospital records. Late fetal death was defined as still birth occurring at 28 or more completed weeks of gestation and early neonatal death as death occurring during the first week after birth, preterm delivery was less than 37 completed weeks of gestation. SGA infants were defined as the birth weight more than 2SD below the mean birth weight for gestational age. Gestational age was calculated based on last menstrual period (LMP) and ultrasound examination performed routinely at less than 12 weeks of gestation. The estimates were adjusted for maternal age, parity, smoking, education, regular menstrual cycle and weight gain during pregnancy. The effect of pre-pregnancy BMI was analyzed by comparing the frequencies of various outcomes in three BMI groups by both univariate and multivariate logistic regression analysis. The results were expressed as odds ratio (ORs) and the corresponding 95% confidence intervals (CIs) & p values.

Statistical Analysis

We used multiple-logistic regression analysis to evaluate the association between pre-pregnancy body-mass index & late fetal death, early neonatal death, preterm delivery & delivery of a small for gestational age infant.

Results

On the basis of the BMI, out of the 2000 women, 348 (17.4%) were underweight or lean group, 1200 (60%) belonged to the normal weight category, while 452 (22.6%) women were from the overweight category.

Factor	Lean	Normal	Overweight
Age	24 ± 5	23 ± 4.5	25 ± 3
Parity	3	2	2
Duration of DM (yrs)	5 ± 1.	6 ± 1.	4 ± 1

Table 1: Maternal Characteristics of 2000 type 2 DM

The maternal complications according to the BMI have been displayed in Table II and III. The mean ± SD age of the study subjects were 25 ± 5 years, the median (range) duration of diabetes was 5 (4-6) years.

Body Mass Index	Early Neonatal Death	Late Fetal Death	Pre-eclampsia	Hypertensive disorders
<18.5	1.1 (0.8-1.6)	1.2 (0.9-1.7)	0.025	3.8 (2.5-5.6)
18.5-24.9	1.3 (0.9-1.9)	1.6 (1.1-2.3)	0.018	1.6 (1.1-2.2)
>25.0-29.9	1.6 (1.1-2.3)	2.6 (1.7-3.8)	0.07	3.6 (2.4-4.5)

Table 2: Adjusted Odd's Ratio for the early and late neonatal death, preeclampsia and Hypertensive disorders associated with pre-pregnancy BMI among type 2 DM mothers

The risk of late fetal death was consistently increasing with BMI (ORs were 1.2 (0.9-1.7), 1.6 (1.1-2.3) & 2.6 (1.7-3.8) for lean, normal & overweight respectively). The risk of early neonatal death was also higher among women with higher BMI (ORs was 1.6 (1.1-2.3) for overweight).

The rate of preeclampsia is higher among women with lean and obese BMI in compare to normal BMI (the values were 2.5%, 1.8%, & 7.0% for lean, normal & overweight respectively). Hypertensive disorders was also more common among lean (3.8%) and overweight (3.6%) compared to normal (1.6%) (ORs 3.8 (2.5-5.6), 1.6 (1.1-2.2) & 3.6 (2.5-4.5) lean, normal and overweight respectively).

Body Mass Index	Pre-term delivery	Small for gestational age (SGA)
<18.5	1.6 (1.3-2.1)	2.7 (1.7-2.8)
18.5-24.9	1.0 (0.8-1.4)	1.2 (0.9-1.5)
>25.0-29.9	2.2 (1.9-2.6)	1.0 (0.6-1.4)

Table 3: Adjusted ODD's Ratios for the preterm delivery & small for gestational age (SGA) associated with pre-pregnancy Body Mass Index among type 2 DM mothers

The risk of preterm delivery was significantly increased for overweight group (2.2%) and lean (1.6%), as compare to normal weight (1.0%) (ORs 1.6 (1.3-2.1), 1.0 (0.8-1.4) & 2.2 (1.9-2.6) lean, normal, overweight respectively). The risk of SGA was significantly more in lean (2.7%) compared to normal weight (1.2%) & overweight group (1.0%) (ORs 2.7 (1.7-2.8), 1.2 (0.9-1.5) & 1.0 (0.6-1.4) respectively).

BMI (kg/m^2)	% of affected	OR Vs Baseline	95% CI
<18.5	1.4	0.9	0.4-2.2
18.5-24.9	1.6	1	0.6-2.3
>25.0-29.9	1.8	1.1	0.5-2.5

Table 4: Shoulder Dystocia associated with pre-pregnancy BMI among type 2 DM mothers

The risk of shoulder dystocia & macrosomic baby was higher in overweight group.

Discussion

Lean BMI has been shown in study to be associated with an increased risk of preterm deliveries, small for gestational age babies [4]. With regards to small for gestational age group (SGA), in our study we found an association of preterm delivery & SGA with the lean BMI group. Apart from an increased risk of SGA, the mothers with a BMI of <18.5 kg/m^2 appeared to be at a lower risk for other labor complications (shoulder dystosia) as compared to the women with higher BMI group, which was consistent with other studies [30,31]. The results of this study showed that lean (underweight) as well as overweight were associated with adverse maternal and perinatal outcomes. The women who were overweight had significantly increased risks for preeclampsia, gestational or pregnancy induced hypertension and large for gestational age babies (macrosomic baby), which was consistent with the findings of other studies [12,13,5]. The neonatal ICU admission rate was more in the overweight group which was attributed to the Macrosomic babies and the diabetic mothers. In another study done by Clansen TD et al. in Netherland while comparing pregnancy outcome of women with type 2 DM during 1996-2001 and women of type2 DM during 1980-92, found higher rate of perinatal mortality in 1996-2001 group. Major congenital malformation and preterm delivery were more in their newer group. Women in this study with newer group were more overweight and more from non nordic Caucasian group. Despite the fact that the newer group in this study had better glycemic control, they showed worse outcome. One of the speculations of the worse outcome in the newer group was probable association of insulin resistant syndrome in this group [15]. As there is different rates of insulin resistance in ethnic group and as the newer group in the study included more patients with overweight and non nordic Caucasian group, it was suggested by the author that further studies to be done to see if rising prevalence of the metabolic syndrome which is higher in proportion in women with non nordic Caucasian and adverse fetal outcome of pregnancy in those populations is related to rising prevalence of the metabolic syndrome [15]. The Asian trait of DM is consisting with higher prevalence of Insulin resistance syndrome. The patients with increased BMI in our study probably reflect the component of insulin resistance. Our study of pregnancy outcome is the diabetic population and in this part of world by showing increase fetal and maternal outcome in overweight group, supports the hypothesis that probably insulin resistance syndrome itself is the cause for increased adverse fetal outcome in this population.

A study which was done by handler et al. [6] evaluated the relationship between the pre pregnancy BMI and the spontaneous preterm birth & they found a significant occurrence of the preterm birth among the lean and obese pregnant women [32-38]. In the present study, correlation of the preterm deliveries was seen in lean BMI group.

Conclusions

Both the extremes of the maternal BMI showed a strong association with pregnancy complications and perinatal morbidity and mortality. Overweight was associated with an increased incidence of preeclampsia, pregnancy induced hypertension, macrosomia and the lean DM women's group is associated with SGA, preterm delivery, PIH, preeclampsia. Women with higher BMI needs medical treatment before and during pregnancy and should reduce the body weight before pregnancy and women with low BMI are advised to take adequate diet to meet the basic requirements of pregnancy.

References

1. Evers IM, de Valk HW, Visser GH (2004) Type 1 diabetic pregnancies are still at high risk for complications: outcome of a nationwide study. BMJ 328: 908-915.

2. Hawthorne G, Robson S, Ryall EA, Sen D, Roberts SH, et al. (1997) Prospective population based survey of outcome of pregnancy in diabetic women: results of the Northern Diabetic Pregnancy Audit, 1994. BMJ 315: 279-281.

3. Casson IF, Clarke CA, Howard CV, McKendrick O, Pennycook S, et al. (1997) Outcomes of pregnancy in insulin dependent diabetic women: results of a five year population cohort study. BMJ 315: 275-278.

4. Temple R, Aldridge V, Greenwood R, Heyburn P, Sampson M, et al. (2002) Association between outcome of pregnancy and glycaemic control in early pregnancy in type 1 diabetes: population based study. BMJ 325: 1275-1276.

5. Suhonen L, Hiilesmaa V, Teramo K (2000) Glycaemic control during early pregnancy and fetal malformations in women with type I diabetes mellitus. Diabetologia 43: 79-82.

6. Boulot P, Chabbert-Buffet N, d'Ercole C, Floriot M, Fontaine P, et al. (2003) French multicentric survey of outcome of pregnancy in women with pregestational diabetes. Diabetes Care 26: 2990-2993.

7. Jensen DM, Damm P, Moelsted-Pedersen L, Ovesen P, Westergaard JG, et al. (2004) Outcomes in type 1 diabetic pregnancies: a nationwide, population-based study. Diabetes Care 27: 2819-2823.

8. Penney GC, Mair G, Pearson DW; Scottish Diabetes in Pregnancy Group (2003) Outcomes of pregnancies in women with type 1 diabetes in Scotland: a national population-based study. BJOG 110: 315-318.

9. Macintosh MC, Fleming KM, Bailey JA, Doyle P, Modder J, et al. (2006) Perinatal mortality and congenital anomalies in babies of women with type 1 or type 2 diabetes in England, Wales, and Northern Ireland: population based study. BMJ 333: 177.

10. Hsu CD, Tan HY, Hong SF, Nickless NA, Copel JA (1996) Strategies for reducing the frequency of preeclampsia in pregnancies with insulin-dependent diabetes mellitus. Am J Perinatol 13: 265-268.

11. Hiilesmaa V, Suhonen L, Teramo K (2000) Glycaemic control is associated with pre-eclampsia but not with pregnancy-induced hypertension in women with type I diabetes mellitus. Diabetologia 43: 1534-1539.

12. Combs CA, Gunderson E, Kitzmiller JL, Gavin LA, Main EK (1992) Relationship of fetal macrosomia to maternal postprandial glucose control during pregnancy. Diabetes Care 15: 1251-1257.

13. Mokdad AH1, Ford ES, Bowman BA, Nelson DE, Engelgau MM, et al. (2000) Diabetes trends in the U.S.: 1990-1998. Diabetes Care 23: 1278-1283.

14. Feig DS, Palda VA (2002) Type 2 diabetes in pregnancy: a growing concern. Lancet 359: 1690-1692.

15. Clausen TD, Mathiesen E, Ekbom P, Hellmuth E, Mandrup-Poulsen T, et al. (2005) Poor pregnancy outcome in women with type 2 diabetes. Diabetes Care 28: 323-328.

16. Dunne F, Brydon P, Smith K, Gee H (2003) Pregnancy in women with Type 2 diabetes: 12 years outcome data 1990-2002. Diabet Med 20: 734-738.

17. Farrell T, Neale L, Cundy T (2002) Congenital anomalies in the offspring of women with type 1, type 2 and gestational diabetes. Diabet Med 19: 322-326.

18. Towner D, Kjos SL, Leung B, Montoro MM, Xiang A, et al. (1995) Congenital malformations in pregnancies complicated by NIDDM. Diabetes Care 18: 1446-1451.

19. Cundy T, Gamble G, Townend K, Henley PG, MacPherson P, et al. (2000) Perinatal mortality in Type 2 diabetes mellitus. Diabet Med 17: 33-39.

20. Feig DS, Palda VA (2002) Type 2 diabetes in pregnancy: a growing concern. Lancet 359: 1690-1692.

21. Kramer MS (1987) Determinants of low birth weight: methodological assessment and meta-analysis. Bull World Health Organ 65: 663-737.

22. Naeye RL (1990) Maternal body weight and pregnancy outcome. Am J Clin Nutr 52: 273-279.

23. Wolfe HM, Zador IE, Gross TL, Martier SS, Sokol RJ (1991) The clinical utility of maternal body mass index in pregnancy. Am J Obstet Gynecol 164: 1306-1310.

24. Kaminski M, Goujard J, Rumeau-Rouquette C (1973) Prediction of low birthweight and prematurity by a multiple regression analysis with maternal characteristics known since the beginning of the pregnancy. Int J Epidemiol 2: 195-204.

25. Meyer MB, Jonas BS, Tonascia JA (1976) Perinatal events associated with maternal smoking during pregnancy. Am J Epidemiol 103: 464-476.

26. Stein ZA, Susser M (1984) Intrauterine growth retardation: epidemiological issues and public health significance. Semin Perinatol 8: 5-14.

27. [No authors listed] (1991) Maternal anthropometry for prediction of pregnancy outcomes: memorandum from a USAID/WHO/PAHO/MotherCare meeting. Bull World Health Organ 69: 523-532.

28. Institute of Medicine (1992) Nutrition during pregnancy and lactation: an implementation guide. Washington, DC. National Academy Press.

29. Wynn AH, Crawford MA, Doyle W, Wynn SW (1991) Nutrition of women in anticipation of pregnancy. Nutr Health 7: 69-88.

30. Weijers RN, Bekedam DJ, Oosting H (1998) The prevalence of type 2 diabetes and gestational diabetes mellitus in an inner city multi-ethnic population. Eur J Epidemiol 14: 693-699.

31. Piacquadio K, Hollingsworth DR, Murphy H (1991) Effects of in-utero exposure to oral hypoglycaemic drugs. Lancet 338: 866-869.

32. HAPO Study Cooperative Research Group1, Metzger BE, Lowe LP, Dyer AR, Trimble ER, et al. (2008) Hyperglycemia and adverse pregnancy outcomes. N Engl J Med 358: 1991-2002.

33. García-Patterson A, Erdozain L, Ginovart G, Adelantado JM, Cubero JM, et al. (2004) In human gestational diabetes mellitus congenital malformations are related to pre-pregnancy body mass index and to severity of diabetes. Diabetologia 47: 509-514.

34. Murphy HR, Steel SA, Roland JM, Morris D, Ball V, et al. (2011) Obstetric and perinatal outcomes in pregnancies complicated by Type 1 and Type 2 diabetes: influences of glycaemic control, obesity and social disadvantage. Diabet Med 28: 1060-1067.

35. Feghali MN, Khoury JC, Timofeev J, Shveiky D, Driggers RW, et al. (2012) Asymmetric large for gestational age newborns in pregnancies complicated by diabetes mellitus: is maternal obesity a culprit? J Matern Fetal Neonatal Med 25: 32-35.

36. Ehrenberg HM, Brian MM, Catalano P (2004) The influence of obesity and diabetes on the prevalence of macrosomia. Am J Obstet Gynecol 191: 964–968

37. Sewell MF, Huston-Presley L, Amini SB, Catalano PM (2007) Body mass index: a true indicator of body fat in obese gravidas. J Reprod Med 52: 907-911.

38. Jarvie E, Hauguel-de-Mouzon S, Nelson SM, Sattar N, Catalano PM, et al. (2010) Lipotoxicity in obese pregnancy and its potential role in adverse pregnancy outcome and obesity in the offspring. Clin Sci (Lond) 119: 123-129.

19

Metformin Combinatorial Therapy for Type 2 Diabetes Mellitus

Keerthi Kupsal[1], Saraswati Mudigonda[1], Nyayapathi VBK Sai[2], Krishnaveni Neelala[2] and Surekha Rani Hanumanth[1*]

[1]Department of Genetics, University College of Science, Osmania University, Telangana, Hyderabad-500007, India

[2]Department of Cardiology, South Central Railway Hospital, Lallaguda-500013, Secunderabad, India

*Corresponding author: Dr. Surekha Rani Hanumanth, M.Sc, PhD, Assistant Professor, Department of Genetics, Osmania University, Hyderabad-500007, Telangana State, India; E-mail: surekharanih@gmail.com

Abstract

Type 2 Diabetes mellitus (T2D) is a worldwide chronic epidemic with increasing incidence. The current algorithm for medical management of type 2 diabetes includes the pharmacological treatment with nine classes of anti-diabetic drugs. Among the nine classes of drugs approved, metformin, an oral hypoglycemic agent from the biguanide family is widely prescribed as the first-line anti-diabetic monotherapy for the treatment of initially diagnosed T2D individuals. The failure of monotherapy to achieve sustain glycemic control prompted the early use of aggressive combination therapies with other anti-diabetic drugs. The primary aim of T2D treatment is to achieve target glycemic control and reducing further complications of diabetes. Hence, fixed dose combination drugs are preferable in order to reduce pill burden and capital investment. Single pill combinations containing drugs for two different diseases can also be prescribed for avoiding extra medication and to reduce further diabetic complications. Our review addresses the mode of action of anti-diabetic drugs and their combinatorial therapy with metformin.

Keywords: Type 2 Diabetes mellitus; Metformin; Anti-diabetic drugs; Combinatorial therapy; Fixed dose combination drugs

Introduction

Type 2 diabetes mellitus (T2D) is a global public health crisis worldwide, facing escalating epidemic particularly in developing countries. It is one of the most challenging health problems and insidious disease in the 21st century. India is a repository to nearly 62 million diabetics making the world's highest diabetes burden country being termed as the 'diabetes capital of the world'. The number of diabetic patients is set to increase to 69.9 million by the year 2025. India's diabetes numbers are expected to cross the 100 million mark by 2030 [1].

T2D is a disastrous disorder characterised by hyperglycemia as a result of insulin resistance, impaired insulin secretion or both. The pharmacological treatment of T2D include eight classes of approved oral anti-diabetic drugs (biguanides, sulfonylureas, thiazolidinediones, glinides, alpha-glucosidase inhibitors, amylin mimetics, glucagon-like peptide 1 mimetics and dipeptidyl peptidase 4 inhibitors). Insulin therapy is recommended for patients with initial HbA1c level greater than 9%.

Over 120 million people worldwide are prescribed metformin, a sole member of biguanide family drug as the first line oral anti-diabetic therapy owing to its safety profile and reduced risk of side effects. It has an exceptional therapeutic index for diabetes to treat hyperglycemia. It is considered as the gold standard anti-diabetic drug due to the insignificant risk of hypoglycemia and prescribed as first-line monotherapy. When metformin monotherapy fails to achieve the recommended standards of care like uncontrolled hyperglycemia, combinatorial therapy with one or two other anti-diabetic drugs along with ongoing metformin therapy is prescribed for effective glycemic control.

Use of metformin is effective in lowering glycosylated haemoglobin (HbA1c) by 1 to 2 percentage points when used as monotherapy or in combination with other anti-diabetic drugs [2]. Substantial evidence indicates that combinatorial therapy can establish superior glycemic control in most of the patients and targets key pathophysiological defects and help to achieve recommended targets in diabetes management. Nine classes of anti-diabetic drugs, their mechanism of action, rationale of combinatorial therapy and the list of combination drugs available in the market are discussed in Tables 1-3.

Metformin - Mode of action

Metformin from the biguanides family is an antihyperglycemic agent and is the drug of first choice to treat initially affected type 2 diabetic cases. It is a safer drug with multiple physiological and molecular effects associated with minimal toxicity. Metformin lowers hyperglycemia by reducing glucose absorption in intestine, increases glucose uptake in peripheral tissues and stimulates insulin secretion from pancreatic beta-cells.

Metformin acutely decreases hepatic glucose output by increasing insulin suppression of gluconeogenesis and reducing the energy supply through activation of AMP-activated protein kinase (AMPK) by inhibition of mitochondrial respiratory-chain complex 1 and consequent increase in NADH oxidation and ultimate reduction in synthesis of ATP (Figure 1).

This mechanism induces glucose uptake into muscle cells, thus lowers the fasting blood glucose in T2D patients [3], (Figure 2). Metformin also regulates its effect in the indirect inhibition of insulin receptor expression and tyrosine kinase activity, thereby enhancing insulin sensitivity and reducing insulin resistance in diabetic patients [4,5].

Sulfonylureas [SU] – Mode of action

SU are the oldest and most widely used medications for the treatment of T2D. These are the insulin secretagogues that enhance pancreatic islet cell function by stimulating insulin secretion from beta-cells, thereby decreasing hepatic glucose production and effectively lowering blood glucose concentrations accompanied by reduction in HbA1c. They also act on the liver, inhibits the production of glucose by stimulating the glycolytic pathway [6].

Drug class	Drug name	Mechanism of action
Biguanides	Metformin	Suppresses gluconeogenesis Reduces glucose absorption in intestine Increases glucose uptake in peripheral tissues Stimulates insulin secretion
Sulfonylureas	Glibencamide, Glimepiride, Glipizide, Glicazide	Stimulates insulin secretion
Thiazolidinediones	Pioglitazone, Rosiglitazone	Increases glucose uptake by skeletal muscle Enhances insulin sensitivity in liver and adipose tissue Rejuvenate Beta cell function
DPP4-Inhibitors	Vidagliptin, Sitagliptin, Saxagliptin	Improves insulin secretion Suppress glucagon secretion
Meglitinides	Repaglinide, Nateglinide	Early insulin secretion
Alpha-glucosidase inhibitors	Acarbose, Miglitol	Inhibits carbohydrate absorption in the small intestine Blocks oligosaccharide catabolism
GLP1-mimetics	Exenatide, Liraglutide	Suppresses glucagon secretion
Amylin mimetics	Pramlinitide	Delays glucose absorption from intestine
Insulin	Insulin	Physiological insulin release

Table 1: Antidiabetic drugs and their mechanism of action.

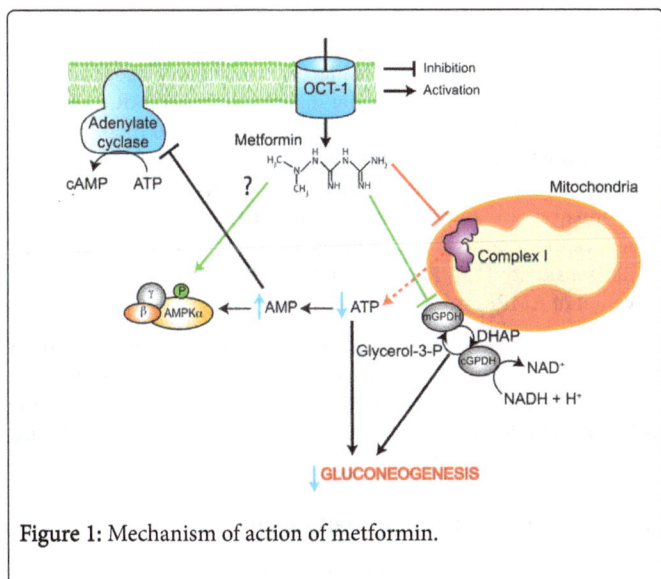

Figure 1: Mechanism of action of metformin.

SU bind to ATP-dependent K$^+$(K-ATP) channel, which is an octameric complex of the inward-rectifier potassium ion channel Kir6.2 and sulfonylurea receptor SUR1 which associate with a stoichiometry of Kir6.24/SUR14 on the cell membrane of pancreatic beta-cells and inhibits potassium efflux, thereby causing the electrical potential to become positive, thus the voltage-gated Ca^{2+} channels are opened leading to intracellular rise in calcium which further leads to increased fusion of insulin granules with cell membrane and finally secretion of insulin from beta-cells [7].

Treatment with SU is associated with a progressive linear decline in beta-cell function [8,9]. Eventual inability to maintain glycemic control reflects an advanced stage of beta-cell failure, thereby leading to hypoglycemia, the most common and most serious adverse event associated with SU therapy. The hypoglycemia episodes can be significant leading to coma or seizures and are seen more often in the elderly.

SU combinatorial therapy with metformin

Due to the adverse effects associated with the use of SU, combinatorial therapy has been focused mainly on adding metformin drug. Metformin and sulfonyl combinatorial therapy is associated with reduced mortality [10,11]. Metformin lowers blood glucose by decreasing hepatic glucose production and by increasing peripheral glucose utilization. SU induces insulin secretion from pancreatic beta-cells [12]. Combining both these drugs at an early stage that act by different individual mechanisms has an advantage of improving glycemic control effectively. This has the potential advantage of increasing the therapeutic effectiveness of both these agents and decreasing the side effects if lower doses could be used.

In an UKPDS experimental study, it has been demonstrated that addition of metformin to SU therapy has increased the proportion of patients who could attain FPG criterion of diabetes (i.e., <40 mg/dl). This study has shown that early progression to metformin and SU combinatorial therapy benefits in maintaining better blood glucose

control that is not possible with single agents. The combination of both these drugs can attain a greater reduction in HbA1c (0.8-1.5%) than either of the monotherapies.

In a study by Reaven GM, et al. administration of 2.5 g/day metformin to sulfonylureas significantly lowered the fasting plasma glucose concentration (12.4 ± 0.8 vs. 8.8 ± 0.7 mmol/l), mean hourly postprandial plasma glucose concentration from 0800-1600 h (14.0 ± 1 vs. 9.4 ± 0.9 mmol/l), and HbA1c (12.3 ± 0.6% vs. 9.0 ± 0.6%) [13].

Drug class combinations	Drug combinations	Mechanism of action	Rationale
Biguanide + Sulfonylureas	Metformin + Glibencamide	Metformin suppresses hepatic gluconeogenesis thus reducing fasting glycemia. Sulfonylureas stimulates insulin secretion from pancreatic beta cells	Provides synergistic effect, reduced mortality, decreases side effects
Biguanide + Thiazolidinediones	Metformin + Pioglitazone	Pioglitazone increases insulin sensitivity in liver and adipose tissue and pancreatic inhibits beta cell loss	Provides synergistic effect, prescribed as late add-on therapy, reduces weight gain
Biguanide + DPP- IV Inhibitors	Metformin + Vidagliptin	Improves insulin secretion from beta cells, decreases output of glucose from pancreatic alpha cells and decreases hepatic gluconeogenesis	Safety and tolerability (used for early combinatorial therapy), Synergistic effect
Biguanide + Meglitinides	Metformin + Repaglinde	Controls postprandial hyperglycemia	Provides synergistic effect
Biguanide + Alpha glucosidase inhibitors	Metformin + Acarbose	Blocks oligosaccharide catabolism, reduces intestinal glucose absorption thus controls postprandial blood glucose	Synergistic effect
Biguanide + GLP1-mimetics	Metformin + Exenatide	Suppresses glucagon secretion thus lowers postprandial blood glucose	Synergistic effect
Biguanide + Amylin mimetics	Metformin + Pramlinitide	Suppresses release of glucagon from pancreatic alpha cells, delays absorption of glucose from intestine	Synergistic effect
Biguanide + Insulin	Metformin + Insulin	Physiological insulin release	Reduces weight gain

Table 2: Combinatorial therapy with metformin and other antidiabetic drugs.

Combination of drugs
Glimepiride + Metformin
Glipizide + Metformin
Glicazide + Metformin
Saxagliptin + Metformin
Sitagliptin + Metformin
Vidagliptin + Metformin
Voglibose + Metformin
Metformin + Rosiglitazone
Pioglitazone + Metformin
Metformin [SR] + Glimepiride + Pioglitazone
Metformin + Glimepiride + Pioglitazone

Table 3: List of antidiabetic combination drugs available in the market.

Thiazolidinediones (TZDs) – Mode of action

TZDs bind to peroxisome proliferator–activated receptors (PPARs), a ligand co-activated transcription factor involved in glucose and lipid metabolism. PPARs exist in several different forms: PPAR-a, PPAR-d, and PPAR-g. PPAR-g is the major target of TZDs, and these receptors are expressed throughout the body in many different tissues, macrophages, and endothelial cells, beta- cells of the pancreas and predominantly in adipose tissue [14]. The drug-PPAR-g complex stimulates the production of proteins like adiponection that enhances insulin sensitivity [15]. Partial insulin sensitivity can be enhanced by activation of AMPK.

TZDs rejuvenate beta cell function thereby delaying progression of the disease and reduce insulin resistance and exhibit no effect on insulin secretion. TZDs lower fasting and postprandial hyperglycemia, fasting insulin levels, free fatty acids suggesting that these drugs improve insulin sensitivity [16].

TZDs combinatorial therapy with metformin

TZDs are prescribed as second line therapy or late add-on therapy as they show no effects on beta-cell function. TZDs should be used in combination with other drugs [17]. Metformin improves insulin sensitivity through the activation of AMPK in liver; TZDs improve insulin sensitivity through activation of PPAR-g in adipocytes. Due to their different sites of action and different cellular mechanisms, this combination results decrease in HbA1c and attains a potential additive and synergistic effect on insulin resistance. The major side effects associated with TZDs include weight gain and fluid retention which typically manifests as peripheral edema. Hence, weight gain can be minimized by using TZDs combined with metformin [18]. Metformin and TZDs combination exhibits cardiovascular benefits also.

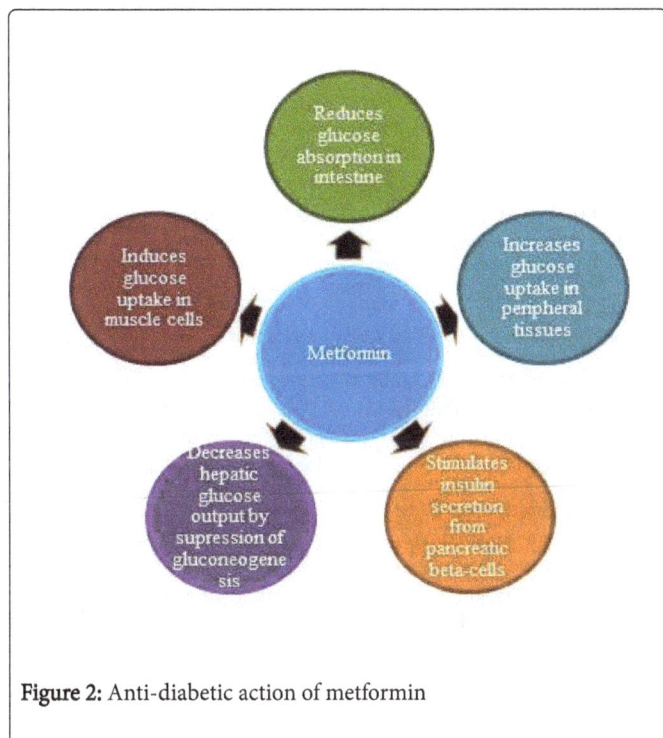

Figure 2: Anti-diabetic action of metformin

Apart from enhancing glycemic control, these drugs lower triglycerides levels, increases high-density lipoprotein cholesterol (HDL) levels, and increases the low-density lipoprotein cholesterol (LDL) particle size. The most commonly approved TZDs in combination with metformin are pioglitazone and rosiglitazone [19]. These drugs have been shown to produce similar reductions in HbA1c of approximately -1.6%, with reductions ranging from -1.2% to -2.3% over 3-12 months of therapy [20-25].

Fixed dose levels of pioglitazone-metformin are approved (15 mg/500 mg and 15 mg/850 mg) for treatment of patients who failed to achieve monotherapy with metformin [26]. In Europe and US, single pill combinations of both pioglitazone-metformin and rosiglitazone-metformin are available in the market [27]. This kind of combination in the same pill often leads to improvement in patient compliance and a decrease in cost.

Dipeptidyl peptidase-IV [DPP-IV] inhibitors – Mode of action

Ingestion of food leads to higher levels of active incretins, the naturally occurring two intestinal glucoregulatory hormones, glucagon-like peptide-1 (GLP-1) and glucose-dependent insulinotropic peptide (GIP) released from small intestine throughout the day. The physiological actions of glucagon-like peptide-1 (GLP-1) includes sensitization of beta-cells, augmentation of glucose stimulated insulin secretion, inhibition of glucagon secretion, thereby reducing the circulating glucose levels and stimulation of insulin biosynthesis

[28,29]. These two incretin hormones play a major role in the postprandial hyperglycemia, for up to 70% of the total insulin is secreted in response to a meal.

In T2D patients, incretin function may be impaired, which leads to reduced postprandial insulin secretion and inadequate glucagon suppression that contribute to postprandial hyperglycemia [28]. DPP-IV inhibitors improve insulin secretion and suppress glucagon secretion by glucose-dependent mechanisms by promoting glucose homeostasis through inhibition of DPP-IV, the key enzyme, responsible for degradation of GLP-1 and GIP. Sitagliptin, vildagliptin and saxagliptin and linagliptin (gliptins) are the licensed agents currently in use for DPP-IV inhibitors.

DPP-IV inhibitors combinatorial therapy with metformin

Progressive decline in beta-cell function is associated in T2D. Vildagliptin improves glycemic control through physiological mechanisms that result in an attenuation of beta-cell decline [30-33]. Vidagliptin prolongs the action of incretins, works in a unique way and improves insulin secretion from the beta-cells of the pancreas and decrease the output of glucagon from the alpha-cells which results in the decrease of hepatic gluconeogenesis.

In an experimental study of 36 patients who were under medication of vidagliptin 50 mg and metformin 500 mg twice daily , the FPG and PPG values were found to be reduced by -76.93 ± 66.55 and reduction in HbA1c levels by - 0.58 ± 0.67 [34,35]. So in patients with T2D the add on of vidagliptin 100 mg to metformin 1000 mg caused a greater reduction in HbA1c [36,37]. The addition of low dose combination of vidagliptin to metformin shows synergistic effect in reducing FPG, PPG and HbA1c.

In a VISION study in Chinese patients, the early use of combinatorial therapy of vidagliptin with ongoing metformin therapy achieved target glycemic goals and improves islet-cell function during fasting stage [37,38]. Saxagliptin at 2.5 mg, 5 mg dosage in combination with 10 mg metformin decreased HbA1c by 0.59%, 0.69%, and 0.58%, respectively [38]. Sitagliptin enhances the postprandial GLP-1 response in a glucose-dependent manner and increases post-meal insulin secretion.

Meglitinides – Mode of action

Glinides are the short acting non-sulfonylureas insulin secretagogues that stimulate the pancreas to produce insulin in response to ingested glucose. Due to their shorter duration of action, they are used as 'prandial drugs' taken just before meals and must be administered more frequently. Two glinides repaglinide and nateglinide are currently in use; of these two glinides, repaglinide is less effective in lowering HbA1c than nateglinide [39]. They act via the ATP dependent potassium channels in pancreatic beta-cell receptors similar to SUs and increases insulin release.

Repaglinide

Repaglinide is the first meglitinide; it stimulates early insulin secretion during postprandial period and causes reduction of postprandial hyperglycemia and reduced HbA1c. It stimulates insulin secretion by blocking ATP-dependent potassium channels (K-ATP) of the pancreatic beta-cell, which is a hetero-octameric complex composed of two different protein subunits, an inwardly rectifying K+ channel (KIR) subunit 6.x and a sulfonylurea receptor (SUR). More than one isoform exists for both Kir6.x (Kir6.1, Kir6.2) and SUR (SUR1, SUR2A, and SUR2B). These subunits Kir6.2 and SUR1 are predominantly expressed in pancreatic beta-cells.

The blocking of K-ATP channels results in depolarization of membrane and influx of calcium through voltage-gated calcium channels leading to an increase in intracellular calcium and subsequent exocytosis of insulin-containing granules [40].

Nateglinide

Nateglinide is a derivative of phenylalanine. Molecular studies have revealed that the binding site of nateglinide is different from that of repaglinide [41]. Nateglinide binds competitively to SURs, inhibits K-ATP channels more rapidly enhancing at a 16-fold when the glucose concentration is raised from 3 mmol/l to 16 mmol/l and shows a higher degree of specificity for SUR1 over SUR2 in a shorter duration of action and stimulates insulin secretion compared to repaglinide where the potency of repaglinide is enhanced 4-fold only. The pharmacodynamic properties of nateglinide are very much unique in several aspects.

The half-life of nateglinide on the receptor is approximately 2 s, very much shorter than that of repaglinide, which is ~3 min. The dissociation from the receptor is 90 times faster when compared to that of repaglinide. It indicates a very short on-off effect of nateglinide on insulin release. Pharmacodynamic studies in T2D patients have revealed that the nateglinide when administered before meals induces early phase insulin secretion and reduces post-prandial hyperglycemia in a dose-dependent manner [42]. Insulin secretion was significantly greater when repaglinide was taken prior to a meal than nateglinide administered in the fasted state [43].

Meglitinides combinatorial therapy with metformin

Metformin regulates basal glucose levels and repaglinide targets postprandial glucose levels, hence the combinatorial therapy of repaglinide with metformin having complementary mechanisms of action are recommended by AACE/ACE for the management of hyperglycemia in patients with HbA1c levels, 9.0%.

Clinical data have shown there is an excellent improvement in glycemic control with combination of repaglinide and metformin over a 4 to 5 months. In a study conducted by Moses et al. [45] metformin and repaglinide combination groups has shown a significant reduction in HbA1c from 8.3% (67 mmol/l) to 6.9% (52 mmol/l) whereas alone metformin and repaglinide groups has shown a remission from 8.6% (70 mmol/l) to 8.3% (67 mmol/l) and from 8.6% (67 mmol/l) to 8.2% (66 mmol/l) respectively [44,45]. Due to their effective combination in maintaining blood glucose, USA has approved this combinatorial therapy in 1997 and in Europe in 1998. In a phase III study in Japanese patients for 16 weeks, HbA1c was reduced by approximately 1% from baseline in patients with metformin and repaglinide combinatorial therapy and achieved significant control in PPG, FPG and postprandial serum insulin [46].

The combination of nateglinide to basal insulin combined with metformin might help in controlling postprandial hyperglycemia. In a study of initial combinatorial therapy of nateglinide with metformin by Horton et al. the patients has shown a significant reduction in HbA1c from a mean baseline of 8.2 ± 0.1% than 0.8% reduction with both monotherapies. Seventy percent of the patients achieved a target HbA1c of <7.0% in nateglinide and metformin combination patients and also FPG and PPG values also reduced [47].

Alpha-glucosidase inhibitors (AGI) - Mode of action

AGI are competitive inhibitors that inhibit alpha-glucosidase enzymes found in the brush border cells lining the small intestine and blocks the oligosaccharide catabolism thus lowering postprandial hyper glycemia and enabling the beta-cells of pancreas to compensate for the first phase insulin secretory defect.

Acarbose and miglitol were the first alpha-glucosidase inhibitors approved in mid-1999 in the U.S. Miglitol, derived from 1-deoxynojirimycin are the first pseudomonosaccharide AGI. Voglibose is weaker at inhibiting sucrase and inhibits most alpha glucosidase enzyme and has minor effect on pancreatic amylase whereas acarbose is an inhibitor of intestinal sucrase and pancreatic amylase [48]. These drugs are administered at the beginning of each meal, and are contraindicated in patients with diseases such as inflammatory bowel disease, partial bowel obstruction, and in severe renal or hepatic disease.

AGI combinatorial therapy with metformin

Hypoglycemia is not typically associated with monotherapy with the alpha-glucosidase inhibitors; hence it is approved as combinatorial therapy with metformin. Acarbose delays glucose absorption and thus attenuates postprandial rises in and blood glucose and insulin.

Metformin suppresses hepatic glucose production. Acarbose in combination with metformin has been shown to improve HbA1c measurement by 0.8% [49], 0.65%, and 0.9% [50]. It has been reported that the combination of acarbose to metformin in sub-optimally controlled patients reduced HbA1c by about 0.8-1.0% [47].

In an observational GLOBE study by Saboo et al., the combination treatment with acarbose/metformin has shown a significant reduction in HbA1c, FBG and PPG by -1.0%, -42.4 mg/dl, and -80.2 mg/dl, respectively [51]. In an another study, acarbose/metformin fixed dose combination (FDC) therapy significantly reduced HbA1c by -1.35%; FPG by -29.5mg/dl, PPG by -41.6mg/dl from baseline. More patients treated with acarbose/metformin FDC achieved HbA1c<7.0% [47.8% vs. 10.7%] [52]. In a study by Rosenstock et al. mean HbA1c achieved a significant reduction by 0.65% in acarbose add-on therapy to metformin [22].

Glucagon like peptide mimetics (GLP-1 mimetics) -Mode of action

GLP-1 mimetics are also known as GLP-1 receptor agonists. GLP-1 is rapidly degraded by DPP-IV enzyme which reduces half-life, thereby limiting its effects, hence may not be given therapeutically. To provide resistance to rapid degradation of GLP-1, GLP-1 mimetics and GLP-1 analogues are given as an injection for therapeutic use which provides longer half-lives than native hormone. On pancreatic beta-cells GLP-1 mimetics bind to GLP-1 receptors, this binding leads to have a longer half-life as the DPP-IV enzyme cannot degrade the homologue or analogue peptides as rapidly as native GLP-1.

GLP-1 mimetics combinatorial therapy with metformin

Exendin and Liraglutide are the first generation GLP-1 analogues. Exendin-4 (exenatide) is the first developed GLP-1-agonist, improves glycemic control similar to the endogenous GLP-1 hormone. Exenatide suppresses glucagon secretion. It is administered subcutaneously twice daily. HbA1c levels are lowered by 0.5-1%, mainly by lowering postprandial blood glucose levels [53].

The add-on therapy of exenatide or rosiglitazone or both with a stable metformin dose in an open-label study in 73 T2D patients has shown controlled mean HbA1c level, 7.8%. [54]. Randomized clinical trials of exenatide in combinatorial therapy with metformin in different dosages have shown a significant reduction in HbA1c [55].

Liraglutide is a GLP-1 analogue with 97% sequence similiar to the human hormone. Due to its structural modifications, it results in reversible albumin binding leading to prolonged duration of action with reduced susceptibility to DPP-IV. It is injected once daily, it reduces fasting blood glucose and glycemic excursions associated with all meals. Liraglutide combined with metformin shows reduced mean HbA1c levels by more than 1% over 26 weeks [56-58].

Amylin mimetics - Mode of action and combinatorial therapy with metformin

Amylin is an amino acid polypeptide hormone produced by the pancreas that is co-localized and co-secreted with insulin in small amounts which slows down the movement of food through the intestine. This suppresses the release of glucagon from pancreatic alpha-cells and delays the absorption of glucose from the intestine which reduces sudden increase in blood glucose. Amylin mimetics are synthetic drugs that are administered before meals; they act like amylin hormone and benefits in weight loss, reducing HbA1c, blood glucose levels and delays gastric emptying [59].

Pramlinitide is a synthetic human amylin analogue, a beta-cell peptide co-secreted with insulin. This has the same actions of native amylin. Pramlintide therapy is not clear as it requires three self-injections daily. At the beginning of the pramlintide therapy, nausea, diarrhoea and headache are the severe side effects. Combination of pramlinitide with metformin shows a significant reduction in HbA1c [60].

Combination of metformin with insulin

Due to progressive deterioration of pancreatic beta-cell function, oral hypoglycaemic agents often fail to maintain adequate glycemic control after few years of treatment. Insulin and metformin combination was more effective than the other combinations shown by a greater reduction in HbA1c after 12 months of treatment and also put on less weight than the other groups [61,62]. Combinatorial therapy with insulin usually refers to the use of daytime oral anti-diabetic agents together with a single injection of intermediate or long-acting insulin at bedtime.

Metformin is usually continued even though the patient is on insulin therapy because it reduces cardiovascular risk in patients with T2D who are overweight. Metformin combined with insulin is associated with decreased weight gain, a lower insulin dosage, and less hypoglycemia when compared with insulin therapy alone. Hence, the efficacy of combinatorial therapy of metformin with other anti-diabetic drugs might have significant achievement in glycemic control.

The landscape combination treatment for management of hyperglycemia in T2D may not achieve desired glycemic goals due to adherence, poor compliance, and persistence to suggested anti-diabetic therapy, flexibility of time of administration and frequent dosages. In order to achieve target glycemic index, improved adherence, decreased incidence of adverse drug reactions, strategies are required for the optimal management of the disease. This problem can be managed by prescribing fixed dose combination drugs (FDCs). The early shift into fixed dose combinatorial therapy is efficient in maintaining glycemic goals and has a chance of preventing diabetic complications.

Fixed dose combination drugs [FDCs]

FDCs are oral pharmaceutical combination formulations with fixed amounts of two or more than two active drugs in a single pill. Use of FDCs reduces prescriber flexibility, simplifies dosage titration along with advantages like ease of administration, convenience, and reduces the pill burden and capital investment. The relative benefits of FDCs compared to monotherapy and combination therapy are discussed in Table 4.

The main aim of T2D treatment is to achieve good glycemic control and to minimize the risk of diabetic complications, macro and micro vascular disorders. The diabetic subjects worldwide rises to double in the next 20 years, as a result of increasing obesity and hypertension [58].

Hence, the development of FDCs of anti-diabetic agents, anti-obesity agents, anti-hypertensive agents and statins [in a single pill-Polypills] can be established to reduce the economic burden which provides an expedience for extra medication without extra tablets.

Several FDC drugs have been developed and available in the market (Table 5). FDCs or polypills when administered in the early onset of the disease might help in improving therapeutic outcomes in diabetes and prevent complications.

Relative benefits	Monotherapy	Combinatorial therapy (free drug combinations)	Fixed dose combinatorial therapy
Response rate	Low	High	High
Dosage simplicity	Simple	Complex	Simple
Compliance	Medium	Medium	High
Tolerability	Medium	High	High
Titration flexibility	High	High	Medium
Ease of administration	Simple	Complex	Simple
Convenience	Simple	Complex	Simple
Cost	Medium	High	Medium

Table 4: Relative benefits of Monotherapy, Combinatorial therapy and FDC therapy

Fixed dose combination of anti-diabetic drugs
Metformin, 500 mg+Glyburide, 5 mg
Metformin, 500 mg+Glipizide, 5 mg
Rosiglitazone, 500 mg+Metformin, 2 mg

Table 5: Fixed dose combination of antidiabetic drugs

Conclusion

T2D is a high profile public health burden reaching pandemic proportions worldwide. Prevention and management of this disease has become a major issue these days and is a special subject in chronic medicine. The main aim is to optimize treatment, personalized management and prevent complications of diabetes. A determined fixed dosage combination drugs for an individual promotes personalized management of T2D reducing pill burden on patients and improving adherence to treatment. In future, extensive research is necessary to understand the potential role of pharmacogenetics in tailoring the safer personalized fixed dose combinatorial therapy and polypill administration for diabetics in reducing further complications.

Acknowledgements

The authors gratefully acknowledge UGC- RFSMS, New Delhi, India.

References

1. Mohan V, Sandeep S, Deepa R, Shah B, Varghese C (2007) Epidemiology of type 2 diabetes: Indian scenario. Indian J Med Res 125: 217-230.

2. Setter SM, Iltz JL, Thams J, Campbell RK (2003) Metformin hydrochloride in the treatment of type 2 diabetes mellitus: a clinical review with a focus on dual therapy. Clin Ther 25: 2991-3026.

3. Viollet B, Guigas B, Garcia NS, Leclerc J, Foretz M, et al. (2012) Cellular and molecular mechanisms of metformin: an overview. Clin Sci 122: 253-270.

4. Pryor R, Cabreiro F (2015) Repurposing metformin: an old drug with new tricks in its binding pockets. Biochem J 471: 307-322.

5. Riedmaier AE, Fisel P, Nies AT, Schaeffeler E, Schwab M (2013) Metformin and Cancer: From The Old Medicine Cabinet To Pharmacological Pitfalls And Prospects. Trends Pharmacol Sci 34: 126-135.

6. Kaku K, Inoue Y, Kaneko T (1995) Extrapancreatic effects of sulfonylurea drugs. Diabetes Res Clin Pract pp: 105-108.

7. Aguilar-Bryan L, Nichols CG, Wechsler SW, Clement JP, Boyd AE, et al. (1995) Cloning of the beta cell high-affinity sulfonylurea receptor: a regulator of insulin secretion. Science 268: 423-426.

8. Turner RC, Cull CA, Frighi V, Holman RR (1999) Glycemic control with diet, sulfonylurea, metformin, or insulin in patients with Type 2 diabetes mellitus: progressive requirement for multiple therapies. JAMA 281: 2005-2012.

9. Del Prato S, Bianchi C, Marchetti P (2007) β-cell function and anti-diabetic pharmacotherapy. Diabetes Metab Res Rev 23: 518-527.

10. Beatriz ARL, Marilia BG (2013) Metformin: an old but still the best treatment for type 2 diabetes. Diabetol Metab Syndr 5: 6.

11. Johnson JA, Majumdar SR, Simpson SH, Toth EL (2002) Decreased Mortality Associated With the Use of Metformin Compared With Sulfonylurea Monotherapy in Type 2 Diabetes. Diabetes Care 25: 2244-2248.

12. Campbell RK, White JR Jr, Saulie BA (1996) Metformin: a new oral biguanide. Clin Ther 18: 360-371.

13. Reaven GM, Johnston P, Hollenbeck CB, Skowronski R, Zhang JC, et al. (1992) Combined metformin-sulfonylurea treatment of patients with noninsulin-dependent diabetes in fair to poor glycemic control. J Clin Endocrinol Metab 74: 1020-1026.

14. Stolar M (2009) Safety and Efficacy of Pioglitazone/Metformin Combination Therapy in Treatment of Type 2 Diabetes: A Rationale for Earlier Use. Clinical Medicine Insights: Therapeutics 1: 289-303.

15. Leonardini A, Laviola L, Perrini S, Natalicchio A, Giorgino F (2009) Cross-Talk between PPARγ and Insulin Signaling and Modulation of Insulin Sensitivity. PPAR Res 2009: 818945.

16. Quinn CE, Hamilton PK, Lockhart CJ, McVeigh GE (2008) Thiazolidinediones: effects on insulin resistance and the cardiovascular system. Br J Pharmacol 153: 636-645.

17. Noble J, Baerlocher MO, Silverberg J (2005) Management of type 2 diabetes mellitus; Role of thiazolidinediones. Can Fam Physician 51: 683-687.

18. Fonseca V (2003) Effect of thiazolidinediones on body weight in patients with diabetes mellitus 115: 42-48.

19. Nesto RW, Bell D, Bonow RO, Fonseca V, Grundy SM, et al. (2003) Thiazolidinedione Use, Fluid Retention, and Congestive Heart Failure A Consensus Statement From the American Heart Association and American Diabetes Association. Circulation 108: 2941-2948.

20. American Association of Clinical Endocrinologists (2007) Medical guidelines for clinical practice for the management of diabetes mellitus. Endocr Pract 13: 3-68.

21. Nathan DM, Buse JB, Davidson MB, Ferrannini E, Holman RR (2009) Diabetes Care 32: 193-203.

22. Rosenstock J, Brown A, Fischer J, Jain A, Littlejohn T, et al. (1998) Efficacy and safety of acarbose in metformin-treated patients with type 2 diabetes. Diabetes Care 21: 2050-2055.

23. Miyazaki Y, DeFronzo RA (2008) Rosiglitazone and pioglitazone similarly improve insulin sensitivity and secretion, glucose tolerance and adipocytokines in type 2 diabetic patients. Diabetes Obes Metab 10: 1204-1211.

24. Norris SL, Carson S, Roberts C (2007) Comparative effectiveness of pioglitazone and rosiglitazone in type 2 diabetes, prediabetes, and the metabolic syndrome: a meta-analysis. Curr Diabetes Rev 3: 127-140.

25. Yamanouchi T, Sakai T, Igarashi K, Ichiyanagi K, Watanabe H (2005) Comparison of metabolic effects of pioglitazone, metformin, and glimepiride over 1 year in Japanese patients with newly diagnosed type 2 diabetes. Diabet Med 22: 980-985.

26. Derosa G, Salvadeo SAT (2009) Glimepiride-pioglitazone Hydrochloride in the Treatment of Type 2 Diabetes. Clinical Medicine: Therapeutics 1: 835-845.

27. Stafford J, Elasy T (2007) Treatment update: Thiazolidinediones in combination with metformin for the treatment of type 2 diabetes. Vascular Health and Risk Management 3: 503-510.

28. Freeman JS (2009) Role of the incretin pathway in the pathogenesis of type 2 diabetes mellitus. Cleve Clin J Med 76: 12-9.

29. Kalra S (2011) Emerging Role of Dipeptidyl Peptidase-IV (DPP-4) Inhibitor Vildagliptin in the Management of Type 2 Diabetes. JAPI 59: 237-245.

30. Nauck MA, Meier JJ (2005) Glucagon-like peptide 1 (GLP-1) and its derivatives in the treatment of diabetes. Regul Pept 128: 135-148.

31. Drucker DJ (2003) Enhancing Incretin Action for the Treatment of Type 2 Diabetes. Diabetes Care 26: 2929-2940.

32. Ahren B (2005) Exenatide: a novel treatment of type 2 diabetes. Therapy 2: 207-222.

33. Ahren B (2006) Vildagliptin: an inhibitor of dipeptidase- 4 with antidiabetic properties. Expert Opin Investig Drugs 4: 431-442.

34. Bhandare B, Satyanarayana V, Jyotirmoy A (2013) A Comparative Study to Evaluate the Efficacy and Safety of Vildagliptin as an Add-on Therapy to a Low-Dose Metformin vs an Uptitration of Metformin in Type 2 DM Patients. Int J Pharm Sci Rev Res 22: 116-120.

35. Scheen AJ (2010) Efficacy and safety of saxagliptin in combination with metformin compared with sitagliptin in combination with metformin in adult patients with type 2 diabetes mellitus. Diabetes Metab Res Rev 26: 540-549.

36. Ji LN, Pan CY, Lu JM, Li H, Li Q, et al. (2013) VISION Study Group. Efficacy and safety of combination therapy with vildagliptin and metformin versus metformin up-titration in Chinese patients with type 2 diabetes mellitus: study design and rationale of the vision study. Cardiovasc Diabetol 12: 118.

37. D'Alessio DA, Denney AM, Hermiller LM, Prigeon RL, Martin JM, et al. (2009) Treatment with the Dipeptidyl Peptidase-4 Inhibitor Vildagliptin Improves Fasting Islet-Cell Function in Subjects with Type 2 Diabetes. J Clin Endocrinol Metab 94: 81-88.

38. DeFronzo RA, Hissa MN, Garber AJ, Gross JL, Duan RY, et al. (2009) The efficacy and safety of saxagliptin when added to metformin therapy in patients with inadequately controlled type 2 diabetes with metformin alone. Diabetes Care 32: 1649-1665.

39. Scheen AJ (2007) Drug-Drug and Food-Drug Pharmacokinetic Interactions with New Insulinotropic Agents Repaglinide and Nateglinide. Clin Pharmacokinet 46: 93-108.

40. Guardado-Mendoza R, Prioletta A, Jiménez-Ceja LM, Sosale A, Folli F (2013) The role of nateglinide and repaglinide, derivatives of meglitinide, in the treatment of type 2 diabetes mellitus. Arch Med Sci 9: 936-943.

41. Gromada J, Dissing S, Kofod H, Frokjaer-Jensen J (1995) Effects of the hypoglycaemic drugs repaglinide and glibenclamide on ATP-sensitive potassium-channels and cytosolic calcium levels in beta TC3 cells and rat pancreatic beta cells. Diabetologia 38: 1025-1032.

42. Gerich J (2013) Pathogenesis and management of postprandial hyperglycemia: role of incretin-based therapies. Int J Gen Med 6: 877-895.

43. Kawamori R, Kaku K, Hanafusa T, Kashiwabara D, Kageyama S, et al. (2012) Efficacy and safety of repaglinide vs nateglinide for treatment of Japanese patients with type 2 diabetes mellitus. J Diabetes Investig 3: 302-308.

44. Moses R, Slobodniuk R, Boyages S, Colagiuri S, Kidson W, et al. (1999) Effect of repaglinide addition to metformin monotherapy on glycemic control in patients with type 2 diabetes. Diabetes Care 22: 119-124.

45. Moses R (1999) Repaglinide in combination therapy with metformin in Type 2 diabetes. Exp Clin Endocrinol Diabetes 107: 136-139.

46. Kawamori R, Kaku K, Hanafusa T, Oikawa T, Kageyama S, et al. (2014) Effect of combination therapy with repaglinide and metformin hydrochloride on glycemic control in Japanese patients with type 2 diabetes mellitus. J Diabetes Invest 5: 72-79.

47. Horton ES, Foley JE, Shen SG, Baron MA (2004) Efficacy and Tolerability of Initial Combination Therapy With Nateglinide and Metformin in Treatment-Naive Patients With Type 2 Diabetes. Curr Med Res Opin 20: 883-889.

48. Revathi P, Jeyaseelan ST, Prakash SK (2011) A Comparative Study of Acarbose and Voglibose on Postprandial Hyperglycemia and serum lipids in Type 2 Diabetic patients. Int J Med Res 2: 121-129.

49. Coniff RF, Shapiro JA, Robbins D, Kleinfield R, Seaton TB, et al. (1995) Reduction of glycosylated hemoglobin and postprandial hyperglycemia by acarbose in patients with NIDDM. Diabetes Care 18: 817-824.

50. Halimi S, Le Berre MA, Grange V (2000) Efficacy and safety of acarbose add-on therapy in the treatment of overweight patients with type 2 diabetes inadequately controlled with metformin: a double-blind, placebo-controlled study. Diabetes Res Clin Pract 50: 49-56.

51. Saboo B, Reddy GC, Juneja S, Kedia AK, Manjrekar P, et al. (2015) Effectiveness and safety of fixed dose combination of acarbose/metformin in Indian Type 2 diabetes patients: Results from observational GLOBE Study. Indian J Endocrinol Metab 19: 129-135.

52. Wang JS, Huang CN, Hung YJ, Kwok CF, Sun JH, et al. (2013) Acarbose plus metformin fixed-dose combination outperforms acarbose monotherapy for type 2 diabetes. Diabetes Res Clin Pract 102: 16-24.

53. IDF Diabetes Atlas (4th edn) Challenges in the Management of Hyperglycaemia in Type 2 Diabetes.

54. Stolar MW (2010) Defining and Achieving Treatment Success in Patients with Type 2 Diabetes Mellitus. Mayo Clin Proc 85: S50-S59.

55. Bond A (2006) Exenatide (Byetta) as a novel treatment option for type 2 diabetes mellitus. Proc (Bayl Univ Med Cent) 19: 281-284.

56. Marre M, Shaw J, Brändle M, Bebakar WM, Kamaruddin NA, et al. (2009) Liraglutide, a once-daily human GLP-1 analogue, added to a sulphonylurea over 26 weeks produces greater improvements in glycaemic and weight control compared with adding rosiglitazone or placebo in subjects with type 2 diabetes (LEAD-1 SU). Diabet Med 26: 268-278.

57. Nauck M, Frid A, Hermansen K, Shah NS, Tankova T, et al. (2009) Efficacy and safety comparison of liraglutide, glimepiride, and placebo, all in combination with metformin, in type 2 diabetes: the LEAD (Liraglutide Effect and Action in Diabetes)-2 Study. Diabetes Care 32: 84-90.

58. Zinman B, Gerich J, Buse JB, Lewin A, Schwartz S, et al. (2009) Efficacy and safety of the human GLP-1 analogliraglutide in combination with metformin and TZD in patients with type 2 diabetes mellitus (LEAD-4 Met+TZD). Diabetes Care 32: 1224-1230.

59. Jonas D, Van Scoyoc E, Gerrald K, Wines R, Amick H, et al. (2011) Drug Class Review: Newer Diabetes Medications, TZDs, and Combinations: Final Original Report. Drug Class Reviews.

60. Verspohl EJ (2012) Novel Pharmacological Approaches to the Treatment of Type 2 Diabetes. Pharmacol Rev 64: 188-237.

61. Burke J (2004) Combination treatment with insulin and oral agents in type 2 diabetes mellitus. Br J Diabetes Vasc 4: 71–76.

62. Ekoe JM, Zimmet P, Williams R (2001) The Epidemology of Diabetes Mellitus: An international perspective, Wiley Online Library.

20

Multiplicity of Dysmetabolic Components in Males is Associated with Elevated Cardiac Troponin T Concentrations

Assi Milwidsky[1*], **Arie Steinvil**[2], **Itzhak Shapira**[1], **Sivan Letourneau-Shesaf**[1], **Rona Limor**[3], **Sharon Greenberg**[1], **Shlomo Berliner**[1] and **OriRogowski**[1]

[1]*Department of Medicine "C" and "E", of the Tel Aviv Sourasky Medical Center, Affiliated to the Sackler Faculty of Medicine, Tel Aviv University, Tel Aviv, Israel*

[2]*Department of Cardiology, of the Tel Aviv Sourasky Medical Center, Affiliated to the Sackler Faculty of Medicine, Tel Aviv University, Tel Aviv, Israel*

[3]*Department of Laboratory, of the Tel Aviv Sourasky Medical Center, Affiliated to the Sackler Faculty of Medicine, Tel Aviv University, Tel Aviv, Israel*

*Corresponding author: Dr. Assi Milwidsky, Department of Internal Medicine "E", The Tel-Aviv Sourasky Medical Center, 6 Weizman St, Tel Aviv, 64239, Israel; E-mail: assi_mil@hotmail.com

Abstract

Background: There are multiple lines of evidence to suggest that chronic myocardial stress and increased cardiovascular risk is associated with the enhanced release of cardiac troponin in patients with ischemic heart disease. However, there is a paucity of data regarding the relation of cardiac troponin to the metabolic syndrome (MetS), a leading risk factor for cardiovascular morbidity.

Methods: We determined the prevalence of measurable high sensitivity cardiac Troponin T (hs-cTnT) with a fifth generation assay and evaluated its association to the presence of the male metabolic syndrome (MetS) components in a cohort of patients undergoing a health survey in the Tel Aviv Medical Center Inflammation Survey (TAMCIS).

Results: A total of 1,641 men with no known cardiovascular disease were recruited and MetS was diagnosed in 330 (20.1%) of them. Hs-cTnT concentrations were higher in patients with MetS (p<0.001). The number of MetS components was associated with the concentration ofhs-cTnT (p<0.001 for trend). The 99th percentile concentration was 27.6 ng/l and 16.03 ng/l for those with and without the MetS, respectively. Five percent of patients with MetS had hs-cTnT concentrations higher than the 99th percentile predetermined by the manufacturer.

Conclusions: The MetS in males is associated with higher levels of hs-cTnT than the general population, with each component increasing hs-cTnT value.

Keywords: Metabolic syndrome; Troponin T; Cardiovascular risk

Introduction

There are multiple lines of evidence to suggest that chronic myocardial stress and increased cardiovascular risk is associated with the enhanced release of cardiac troponin in patients with coronary artery disease and in apparently healthy individuals [1-4]. Increased Hs-cTnT levels had been described in some of the metabolic syndrome (MetS) components [5-7] and particularly in patients with diabetes and obesity. However, there is paucity of data regarding the relation of hs-cTnT to the MetS as a complex, and whether increasing number of MetS components is associated with increased troponin concentration and elevated cardiovascular risk.

We determined the prevalence of measurable hs-cTnT with a fifth generation assay, recently introduced into the Tel-Aviv Medical Centre Inflammation Survey (TAMCIS), [8-10] a relatively large health screening program of the Tel-Aviv Medical Center in Tel-Aviv, Israel. We then evaluated associations of cTnT with the MetS and its distinctive components.

Methods

Study population

We have analyzed data that has been collected during the period of September 2010 to June 2012 in the TAMCIS, a registered data bank of the Israeli ministry of justice [8-10]. This is a relatively large cohort of individuals who attended our medical center for a routine annual check-up and who gave their written informed consent for participation according to the instructions of the local ethics committee. Included were1,891 male subjects for whom hs-cTnT were obtained. Based on the medical history found in the medical charts of TAMCIS, We later excluded 250 subjects due to any previous vascular event (myocardial infarction, pulmonary emboli, venous thromboembolism or a cerebrovascular accident), a previous diagnosis of ischemic heart disease or immunosuppressive therapy, steroidal or antibiotic treatment or recent acute infection or previous malignancy. Following these exclusions the study group was comprised of 1,641 apparently healthy males with no known cardiovascular disease.

Definition of the metabolic syndrome

The diagnosis of the metabolic syndrome was based on the joint interim statement of the International Diabetes Federation Task Force on Epidemiology and Prevention, National Heart, Lung, and Blood

Institute, American Heart Association, World Heart Federation, International Atherosclerosis Society, and International Association for the Study of Obesity [11]. In short, elevated waist circumference was defined as ≥94 cm (37 inches) in men as recommended for Europe and the Middle East. Elevated triglycerides (TG) were defined as ≥150 mg/dl (1.7 mmol/l) or on drug treatment for elevated triglycerides; reduced HDL-C was defined as <40 mg/dL (1.0 mmol/l, all participants were men) or on drug treatment for reduced HDL-C; elevated blood pressure was defined as ≥130 mm Hg systolic blood pressure or ≥85 mm Hg diastolic blood pressure or on antihypertensive drug treatment in a patient with a history of hypertension; elevated fasting glucose was defined as ≥100 mg/dl (5.55 mmol/l), drug treatment of elevated glucose was an alternate indicator. Smokers were defined as individuals who smoked at least 5 cigarettes per day while past smokers had quit smoking for at least 30 days prior to examination.

Laboratory methods

All blood samples were drawn following a 12 hour fasting period. Cardiac troponin T levels were measured with a novel pre-commercial highly sensitive assay (Elecsys Troponin T; Roche Diagnostics, Indianapolis, IN), as described previously [4]. The lower limit of detection of the novel assay is 3ng/L. The coefficient of variation of <10% is 13 ng/L and the 99th percentile value for cTnT published by the manufacturer is14 ng/L.

The complete blood count parameters were measured using a coulter STKS electronic counter. Quantitative fibrinogen was measured by the Claus [12] method, and the high sensitivity C-Reactive Protein (hs-CRP) was performed by using the Behring BN II Nephelometer (DADE Behring, Marburg, Germany) analyzer and a method described by Rifai et al. [13]. Triglycerides were measured by an adaptation of the fossati 3 step enzymatic reactions with the Bayer Advia 1650 chemistry analyzer. Serum triglycerides were determined calorimetrically with an enzyme that produces hydrogen peroxide [14]. HDL-C was determined by a method developed by Izawa et al as described before [15] using the Bayer Advia 1650 chemistry analyzer. LDL-C was derived from the measured concentrations of total cholesterol, HDL-C and triglycerides using the Fried wald equation: LDL-C=Total Cholesterol – HDL-C – TG/5.

Statistical Analysis

All continuous variables were displayed as mean (standard deviation [SD]), while categorical variables were displayed as number (percent) of patients within each group. Since the hs-cTnT displayed non-normal distribution, all analyses were non-parametric. Comparison of all continuous variables was done using the Mann-Whitney U analysis while for categorical variables the Fischer exact test was used.

The level of significance used for all analyses was two-tailed (p<0.05). The SPSS 19.0 statistical package was used to perform all statistical analyses (SSPS Inc., Chicago, IL, USA).

Results

We have presently included a total of 1,641 men, at a mean age ± SD [range] of 47.4 ± 10.1 [24-78] years. Demographic, medical history

and laboratory values of subjects with and without the MetS are presented in Table 1. A diagnosis of the Metabolic Syndrome, according to the harmonized criteria was present in 330 (20.1%) subjects.

		Metabolic Syndrome		P Value
		No	Yes	
Medical history	Age	46.5	50.9	0.59
	Hypertension, %	21.7	61.2	<0.001
	Current smoking, %	11	9.4	<0.001
	Diabetes mellitus, %	1.5	15.5	<0.001
	Systolic blood pressure, mm hg	124	134	0.22
	Diastolic blood pressure, mm hg	78	84	0.49
Laboratory data	Total cholesterol, mg/dL	184	186	0.2
	HDL-C, mg/dL	51	40	<0.001
	Triglycerides, mg/dL	101	179	<0.001
	eGFR, mL/min	80.5	77.8	<0.001
	hs-CRP, mg/L	1.9	2.8	0.008
	Hemoglobin A1C, %	5.4	5.8	<0.001
Medications	Aspirin, %	4.3	14.8	<0.001
	Antihypertensive, %	10	30	<0.001
	Statins, %	14.4	28.5	<0.001

Table 1: Baseline characteristics according to the metabolic syndrome

HDL-C – high density lipoprotein cholesterol, eGFR – estimated glomerular filtration rate, hs-CRP – high sensitive C-Reactive Protein.

The percentage of subjects with one, two, three, four and five components of the MetS was 20%, 31%, 28.8%, 14% and 5.1%, respectively. Mean and percentile values of hs-cTnT were calculated for each group. The 75th percentile for hs-cTnT was3.88 ng/l and 5.4 ng/l for patients without and with MetS, respectively. The 25th and 50th percentiles were 3.0 for both. The 99th percentile was 16.03 ng/l and 27.6 ng/l for those without and with MetS, respectively. Data is presented in Table 2. Waist ≥ 94 cm (37 inches). HTN (hypertension) - ≥ 130 mm Hg systolic blood pressure or ≥ 85 mm Hg diastolic blood pressure or on antihypertensive drug treatment. IFG (Impaired Fasting Glucose) - ≥ 100 mg/dl (5.55 mmol/l) or †on glucose lowering treatment. TG (elevated triglycerides) - ≥ 150 mg/dl (1.7 mmol/l) or on drug treatment for elevated triglycerides. HDL (reduced HDL-c) was defined as <40 mg/dL (1.0 mmol/l) or on drug treatment for reduced HDL-C.

		Number of patients	Hs-cTnT concentrations ng/L					
			Min	Max	25th percentile	Median	75th percentile	99th percentile
Positive MetS comp. *	Waist	959	3.0	35.8	3.0	3.0	4.7	19.1
	HTN	783	3.0	35.8	3.0	3.0	5.0	18.9
	IFG†	120	3.0	26.6	3.0	3.2	6.9	25.0
	TG	343	3.0	35.8	3.0	3.0	4.5	27.4
	HDL	355	3.0	35.8	3.0	3.0	4.1	18.5
Number of positive MetS comp.*	0	329	3.0	43.8	3.0	3.0	3.0	10.6
	1	509	3.0	35.8	3.0	3.0	3.8	16.6
	2	473	3.0	24.6	3.0	3.0	4.7	16.3
	3	229	3.0	28.7	3.0	3.0	5.4	25.6
	4 or 5	101	3.0	35.8	3.0	3.0	6.0	35.6
MetS	No	1,311	3.0	43.8	3.0	3.0	3.9	16.0
	Yes	330	3.0	35.8	3.0	3.0	5.4	27.6

Table 2: hs-cTnT concentrations relation to Metabolic Syndrome components

Hs-cTnT: High sensitive cardiac troponin T, MetS: Metabolic syndrome, Min: Minimum, Max- maximum, Comp: components.

* Positivity of MetS components was based upon the harmonized criteria.

A graphical presentation of hs-cTnT concentrations in individuals with and without the MetS is presented in figure 1. As can be seen, subjects with the MetS had higher measurements of hs-cTnT (p<0.001).

(the median). The ends of the whiskers represent the lowest datum still within 1.5 the inter quartile range (IQR) of the lower quartile, and the highest datum still within 1.5 IQR of the upper quartile. The circles represent outliers in the range of 1.5 to 3 IQR and the stars represent extreme outliers, of more than 3 IQR.

The number of MetS components was associated with the level of hs-cTnT (p<0.001 for trend), with each additional component (e.g. increased waist circumference) increasing the hs-cTnT level (Figure 2).

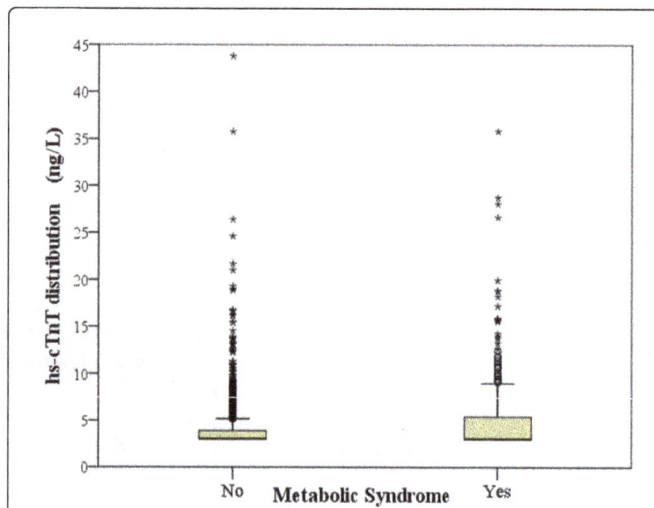

Figure 1: Increased hs-cTnT concentration for subjects with the metabolic syndrome

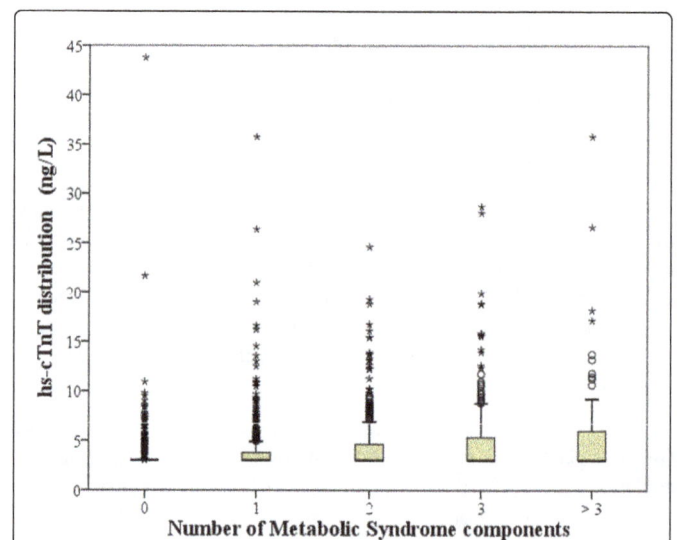

Figure 2: A trend for higher mean hs-cTnT concentration with increasing number of Metabolic syndrome components

Box and whisker plots of the distribution of hs-cTnT: the bottom and top of the box represent the first and third quartiles (25th and 75th percentile), and the bold band inside the box is the second quartile

Hs-cTnT concentrations for each of the metabolic syndrome components and according to the number of positive Mets components are presented in Table 2.

Box and whisker plots of the distribution of hs-cTnT: the bottom and top of the box represent the first and third quartiles (25th and 75th percentile), and the bold band inside the box is the second quartile (the median). The ends of the whiskers represent the lowest datum still within 1.5 the inter quartile range (IQR) of the lower quartile, and the highest datum still within 1.5 IQR of the upper quartile. The circles represent outliers in the range of 1.5 to 3 IQR and the stars represent extreme outliers, of more than 3 IQR.

Discussion

The main finding of the current study is the association of dysmetabolism with the eventual presence of chronic myocardial stress, expressed by elevated hs-cTnT concentrations in males with no known cardiovascular disease.

This is the first large report suggesting that the MetS is associated with elevated hs-cTnT concentrations in adult men. The findings are consistent with a previous work studying the relation of hs-cTnT and the MetS in children and adolescents [6], showing that circulating concentrations of hs-cTnT in obese children with MetS are higher than those without the MetS and the non-obese children. A previous work in adults [16] found that hs-cTnT was directly associated with metabolic risk (P<0.001). However the study did not compare levels of cardiac troponin between those with and without the MetS, nor did it use the harmonized criteria of the metabolic syndrome, currently the most widespread definition used.

We have presently shown that the baseline concentrations of hs-cTnT are influenced by the components of the MetS, a factor not currently included in the depiction of troponin elevation.

Hs-cTnT concentration was above the 99th percentile for almost 5% of patients with the MetS and for

Concentrations increase in relation to increasing number of MetS components, which was statistically significant (p<0.001 for trend). In accordance with the finding of Wallace et al. of four predictors of elevated cTnT levels, one of which was diabetes mellitus [17] The above association might raise a multiple-hit theory for the presence of increased cTnT concentrations in apparently healthy individuals, meaning that MetS components may have an additive value in increasing hs-cTnT levels, a marker of myocardial stress. Despite of being too limited to find out what is the main determinant for the presence of enhanced cTnT concentrations in the peripheral blood, the results do point toward a multiple-hit possibility. Looking at the potential contributors for the metabolic health, one might accept that similar factors are those patients the 99th percentile was 27.6 ng/l, substantially higher than that determined by the manufacturer, at 14 ng/l. This finding is consistent with a previous work by Saunders et.al. [4] who found that actual 99th percentile concentrations were substantially higher than those determined by the manufacturer, a fact that further stresses that need to calibrate threshold values based on local empiric observations.

An additional significant finding of the present study is the association between multiplicities of dysmetabolic risk factors with absolute hs-cTnT concentrations. Although troponin levels were mildly lower in the group with 5 MetS components compared to those with 4 components, this group comprised of only 84 (5.1%)

participants, thus the statistical significance of such minor variability could not be reliably analyzed. Therefore we determined the trend for hs-cTnT involved in the process of cardiomyocytes damage.

Limitations

Only male patients were included in the current analysis because most of the TAMCIS survey population consists of males, unfortunately we were under powered to include females in the study. In the statistical analysis we were unable to exclude factors closely related to the metabolic syndrome (e.g. hypertension, dyslipidemia and diabetes) or use a control group that would isolate their influence on troponin concentration without omitting major influences of the MetS itself. However, we examined patients with MetS as a group with multiple comorbidities by definition, thus an attempt to isolate one of its' critical components seems not necessary.

Conclusion

Elevated concentrations of cTnT might be present in the peripheral blood of men with the metabolic syndrome. The association with multiplicity of dysmetabolic risk factors point toward the possibility of a multiple-hit mechanism that is involved in cardiomyocytes damage. No one dysmetabolic component could be singled out as the most dominant in this report, suggesting the need to improve most, if not all, of the dysmetabolic components in order to protect against cardiomyocytes damage.

References

1. Wang TJ, Wollert KC, Larson MG, Coglianese E, McCabe EL, et al. (2012) Prognostic utility of novel biomarkers of cardiovascular stress: the Framingham Heart Study. Circulation 126: 1596-1604.

2. Omland T, de Lemos JA, Sabatine MS, Christophi CA, Rice MM, et al. (2009) A sensitive cardiac troponin T assay in stable coronary artery disease. N Engl J Med 361: 2538-2547.

3. Leistner DM, Klotsche J, Pieper L, Stalla GK, Lehnert H, et al. (2012) Circulating troponin as measured by a sensitive assay for cardiovascular risk assessment in primary prevention. Clin Chem 58: 200-208.

4. Saunders JT, Nambi V, de Lemos JA, Chambless LE, Virani SS, et al. (2011) Cardiac troponin T measured by a highly sensitive assay predicts coronary heart disease, heart failure, and mortality in the Atherosclerosis Risk in Communities Study. Circulation 123: 1367-1376.

5. de Lemos JA, Drazner MH, Omland T, Ayers CR, Khera A, et al. (2010) Association of troponin T detected with a highly sensitive assay and cardiac structure and mortality risk in the general population. JAMA 304: 2503-2512.

6. Pervanidou P, Akalestos A, Bastaki D, Apostolakou F, Papassotiriou I, et al. (2013) Increased circulating High-Sensitivity Troponin T concentrations in children and adolescents with obesity and the metabolic syndrome: a marker for early cardiac damage? Metabolism 62: 527-531.

7. Zheng J, Ye P, Luo L, Xiao W, Xu R, et al. (2012) Association between blood glucose levels and high-sensitivity cardiac troponin T in an overt cardiovascular disease-free community-based study. Diabetes Res Clin Pract 97: 139-45.

8. Rogowski O, Shapira I, Peretz H, Berliner S (2008) Glycohaemoglobin as a determinant of increased fibrinogen concentrations and low-grade inflammation in apparently healthy nondiabetic individuals. Clin Endocrinol (Oxf) 68: 182-189.

9. Rogowski O, Shapira I, Shirom A, Melamed S, Toker S, et al. (2007) Heart rate and microinflammation in men: a relevant atherothrombotic link. Heart 93: 940-944.

10. Steinvil A, Shirom A, Melamed S, Toker S, Justo D, et al. (2008) Relation of educational level to inflammation-sensitive biomarker level. Am J Cardiol 102: 1034-1039.

11. Alberti KG, Eckel RH, Grundy SM, et al. (2009) Harmonizing the metabolic syndrome: a joint interim statement of the International Diabetes Federation Task Force on Epidemiology and Prevention; National Heart, Lung, and Blood Institute; American Heart Association; World Heart Federation; International Atherosclerosis Society; and International Association for the Study of Obesity. Circulation 120: 1640-1645.

12. CLAUSS A (1957) [Rapid physiological coagulation method in determination of fibrinogen]. Acta Haematol 17: 237-246.

13. Rifai N, Tracy RP, Ridker PM (1999) Clinical efficacy of an automated high-sensitivity C-reactive protein assay. Clin Chem 45: 2136-2141.

14. Fossati P, Prencipe L (1982) Serum triglycerides determined colorimetrically with an enzyme that produces hydrogen peroxide. Clin Chem 28: 2077-2080.

15. Steinvil A, Shapira I, Ben-Bassat OK, Cohen M, Vered Y, et al. (2010) The association of higher levels of within-normal-limits liver enzymes and the prevalence of the metabolic syndrome. Cardiovasc Diabetol 9: 30.

16. Siervo M, Ruggiero D, Sorice R, Nutile T, Aversano M, et al. (2010) Angiogenesis and biomarkers of cardiovascular risk in adults with metabolic syndrome. J Intern Med 268: 338-347.

17. Wallace TW1, Abdullah SM, Drazner MH, Das SR, Khera A, et al. (2006) Prevalence and determinants of troponin T elevation in the general population. Circulation 113: 1958-1965.

21

Palmitoleic Acid Infusion Alters Circulating Glucose and Insulin Levels

Long NM, Burns TA, Volpi Lagreca G, Alende M and Duckett SK[*]

Department of Animal and Veterinary Sciences, Clemson University, Clemson, SC 29634, USA

[*]**Corresponding author:** Susan K Duckett, Department of Animal and Veterinary Science, 146 Poole Agricultural Center, Box 340311, Clemson, SC 29634-0311, USA; E-mail: sducket@clemson.edu

Abstract

Objectives: The objectives of these studies are to evaluate: 1) uptake of a pulse dose of $^{13}C16:1$ cis-9 at varying levels into the blood and 2) glucose and insulin changes after pulse dose of 0 or 5 mg C16:1 cis-9/kg body weight (BW) under challenge conditions in obese lambs.

Methods: Two experiments were conducted to evaluate uptake of U-$^{13}C16:1$ cis-9 into the blood and changes in glucose and insulin under challenges. In the first experiment, lambs (67.4 ± 1.4 kg BW, n=3) received jugular catheters and were used in a 3 x 3 Latin square. Treatments were 0, 2 or 5 mg/kg BW of U-$^{13}C16:1$ cis-9 in 40% (wt/v) ethanol and blood samples were collected post infusion for glucose, fatty acid and insulin analyses. In the second experiment, lambs (86.7 ± 1.5 kg BW; n=4) received jugular catheters. Treatments were 0 or 5 mg/kg BW of C16:1 in 40% (wt/v) ethanol immediately followed by a glucose (0.25 g/kg) or insulin (0.02 mIU/kg) challenge.

Results: Both the 2 and 5 mg/kg BW dose of U-$^{13}C16:1$ cis-9increased (P=0.003) C16:1 cis-9in serum compared to 0 mg/kg BW. The 5 mg/kg BW dose had a greater magnitude of increase for serum C16:1 and resulted in increased whole blood glucose levels for first 60 min and altered insulin levels for first 30 min. During the glucose tolerance test, C16:1bolus infusion increased (P=0.02) peak, overall, and area under the curve for plasma glucose levels. During the insulin challenge, C16:1-treated lambs had increased glucose levels (P=0.04) and peak, overall, and area under the curve plasma insulin (P=0.0001).

Conclusion: Palmitoleic acid infusion results in immediate uptake and clearance of serum palmitoleic acid, increases plasma glucose levels, and alters circulating insulin levels.

Keywords: Palmitoleic acid; Glucose; Insulin; Stable isotope; Fatty acid

Introduction

Palmitoleic (C16:1 cis-9) acid is an omega-7 monounsaturated fatty acid that is produced via desaturation of palmitic acid by stearoyl-CoA desaturase (SCD-1). Palmitoleic acid has been proposed to function as a lipokine, a fatty acid that stimulates muscle insulin action [1]. Previous research [2,3] has shown that palmitoleic (C16:1 cis-9) acid addition to bovine primary adipocytes decreases lipogenesis and increases β-oxidation. Cao et al. [1] reported exogenous administration of palmitoleic acid (C16:1 cis-9) decreased lipogenesis in liver and increased insulin sensitivity in skeletal muscle of mice.

Glucose and insulin regulation in animals and humans is interplay between insulin sensitivity, how responsive a cell or tissue is to insulin binding, and responsiveness of the post receptor signing events [4]. Ruminants are less insulin sensitive compared to monogastrics [5]. The insulin resistance in ruminants has been attributed to decreased activity of glucose transporter proteins fusing to the plasma membrane of muscle during insulin stimulation [6]. Dietary lipids like fish oil, high in long-chain n-3 polyunsaturated fatty acids, increased tissues response to insulin (insulin sensitivity) in rats, miniature pigs and lambs [7-10]. Fish oil infused in the abomasum of steers resulted in increased insulin sensitivity [11]. These differences in insulin sensitivity appears to be due to longchain n-3 polyunsaturated fatty

acids since feeding an saturated fatty acids did not result in changes in insulin and glucose responses [12]. Therefore it should be expected that other unsaturated fatty acids could have effects on glucose and insulin regulation in ruminants. The objectives of these studies are to evaluate: 1)uptake of a pulse dose of $^{13}C16:1$ cis-9 at varying levels into the blood and 2) glucose and insulin changes after pulse dose of 0 or 5 mg C16:1 cis-9/kg BW under challenge conditions in finished lambs.

Methods

Animals

All experimental procedures involving animals were reviewed and approved by the Clemson University Institutional Animal Care and Use Committee.

Experiment 1: Three Southdown yearling wethers (14 months of age; 67.4 ± 1.4 kg BW) were used in a 3 3 Latin square design. Animals were fed approximately 2 kg per day of a high energy, corn-based diet (give Southern State Hi-Energy Lamb starter-Grower , Richmond, VA) designed to meet or exceed NRC (2007) requirements for finishing lambs in addition to ad libitum access to Coastal Bermudagrasshay (11.6% CP, 1.36 McalNEm/kg, and 37.1% ADF on a DM basis) and water. Lambs were housed at the Clemson University Brick Barn (Pendleton, SC) and were maintained in individual pens (1.49 m_2 floor space) during each experimental challenge. Treatments were a pulse dose infusion of 0 (CON), 2 or 5 mg/kg BW of U-$^{13}C16:1$

cis-9 (Isotech, Inc., Miamisburg, OH) in 40% ethanol (wt/vol). Blood samples (~6 ml) were collected at -30, 15, and 0 minutes before pulse lipid infusion, every 15 minutes for 2 hours, and then every 30 minutes for an addition hour post infusion. Immediately after blood collection, whole blood glucose was measured via Alpha Trak handheld glucometer (Abbot; North Chicago, IL) in duplicate (2.2% CV between duplicate readings) as part of normal infusion protocols. Lambs were fasted 12 h prior to each treatment with 10 days rest between tests.

Experiment 2: Four Southdown yearling wethers (18 months of age; 86.7 ± 1.7 kg BW) estimated to have at least 0.91 cm backfat, which equates to about 30% body fat, were used in this study to evaluate changes in glucose and insulin under challenge. Animals were housed and fed as previously described above before and during each experimental challenge. Lambs were fasted 18 h prior to each treatment with 44 h rest between tests. Treatments were a pulse dose infusion of 0 (CON) or 5 mg/kg BW of C16:1 (Sigma-Aldrich, >98.5% C16:1 cis-9) in 40% (wt/vol) ethanol in combination with intravenous administration of 0.25 g glucose/kg BW (intravenous glucose tolerance test, IVGTT; 50% dextrose solution; VedcoInc, ST. Jospeh, MO) at 0 min on the first 2 test days consistent with a crossover design. Ethanol served as the control infusate in sheep receiving 0 mg C16:1/kg BW dose. The crossover design was repeated for 2 additional test days with lambs receiving 0 or 5 mg/kg BW C16:1 pulse dose in combination with an insulin challenge (IC; 0.02 mIU/kg BW, Sigma-Aldridge, St. Louis, MO). On each test day, blood samples (6 ml) were collected at -15 min, immediately prior to infusion, and 2, 4, 6, 8, 10, 12, 15, 20, 25, 30, 35, 40, 50, 60, 70, 80, 100, 120, and 150 min after C16:1 infusion.

A 16-ga indwelling jugular catheter (Abbocath, 16 gauge, Abbott Laboratories, North Chicago, IL, USA) was inserted and sutured to the skin 1 d prior to initiation of the first test for substrate administration and blood sampling. Catheters were kept patent with 4% sodium citrate in sterile saline (Jorgensen Laboratories, Inc., Loveland, CO). Immediately after each sample collection, whole blood was placed into serum and heparinized vacuum tubes. Serum tubes were allowed to clot for 2 h at room temperature, held overnight at 4°C, and centrifuged at 2,000 x g for 15 min to obtain serum. Heparinized tubes were immediately centrifuged at 2,000 x g for 15 min. Plasma aliquots were collected and frozen at -20°C for later analysis of glucose, insulin, and fatty acid concentrations. Serum and plasma aliquots were collected and frozen at -20°C for subsequent analyses of long-chain fatty acids (serum) and glucose and insulin (plasma).

Fatty acids

For fatty acid analysis, serum aliquots (1 mL in duplicate) from each lamb and time point were lyophilized (Lab Conco, Kansas City, MO) and transmethylated according to Park and Goins [13]. Fatty acid methyl esters (FAME) were analyzed using an Agilent 6850 gas chromatograph (GC) equipped with an Agilent 7673A automatic sampler (Agilent Technologies, Inc., Santa Clara, CA). Separations were accomplished using a 100-m Supelco SP-2560 (Supelco, Inc., Bellefonte, PA) capillary column (0.25 mm i.d. and 0.20 μm film thicknesses) according to Duckett et al. [14]. Individual fatty acids were identified by comparison of retention times with known standards (Sigma, St. Louis, MO; Matreya, Pleasant Gap, PA). Fatty acids were quantified by incorporating an internal standard, methyl tricosanoic (C23:0) acid, into each sample during methylation and expressed as a weight percentage.

For stable isotope analyses, FAME samples were analyzed with an Agilent 6890N GC equipped with an Agilent 5973 mass spectrometer (MS) using a 100-m Varian CP7489 (Varian Instruments Inc., Walnut Creek, CA) capillary column (0.25 mm i.d. and 0.20 μm film thickness). Samples were run in chemical ionization mode with He as the carrier gas and CH4 as the reagent gas. Ions of mass-to-charge ratio (m/z) 268 (m) and 284 (m + 16) were selectively measured to calculate the isotopic enrichment of C16:1 in serum. Results were calculated according to [15] and presented as molar percent excess.

Glucose and Insulin

For glucose and insulin concentration during the IVGTT and IC in experiment 2 the -15, 0, 4, 8, 10, 15, 20, 25, 30, 40, 50, 60, 70, 80, 100, 120, and 150 minutes samples were analyzed and all serum samples were analyzed for insulin concentrations in experiment 1. Glucose was measured colorimetrically in triplicate using Liquid Glucose Hexokinase Reagent (Pointe Scientific Inc., Canton, MI), as described by Long and Schafer (2013), and a Bio Tek Synergy HT (Winooski, VT) microplate reader. Mean intra- and inter assay CV were 3.3 and 6.3%, respectively. Insulin was measured in duplicate by commercial RIA [16; Siemens Medical Solutions Diagnostics, Los Angeles, CA], with intra-assay CV of 8.05%, and a sensitivity of 1.5 μIU/mL.

Statistics

For experiment 1, serum U-^{13}C16:1cis-9 molar percent excess, insulin concentration, whole blood glucose, and a calculated insulin to glucose ratio were analyzed as a repeated measures using the Proc Mixed procedure of SAS 9.2 (SAS Institute Inc., Cary, NC) with treatment, time and the two-way interaction as fixed effects and period (order of lipid dosing) as a random effect. Post hoc t-tests were performed to determine treatment differences within a time point. For experiment 2, Graph pad Prism (Graph Pad Software Inc, La Jolla, CA) was used to calculate the area under the curve (AUC) for plasma glucose and insulin response curves during the IVGTT and IC. Plasma metabolite and insulin concentrations were analyzed as a repeated measures using Proc MIXED procedure of SAS using the previously mentioned model. Each AUC for the challenges were analyzed using Proc MIXED procedure of SAS with treatment in the model and period as a random effect. In addition, insulin to glucose ratio was calculated from the AUC from both the IVGTT and IC for each animal treatment combination as previously described [17] and this value was analyzed using the Proc MIXED procedure of SAS with treatment in the model and period as a random effect. Data are presented as least square means ± SEM, and differences considered significant at P<0.05, with a tendency at P<0.10.

Results

Palmitoleic Acid Uptake

Serum concentrations of palmitoleic (C16:1 cis-9) acid and enrichment of U-^{13}C16:1cis 9 are shown in Figure 1a. Serum C16:1 cis-9 levels peaked (P<0.01) at 15 min and returned to baseline levels by 30 min post pulse dose. These results show that exogenous palmitoleic acid is quickly removed (<30 min) from the blood after a single pulse dose. Dosage levels, 2 and 5 mg/kg BW C16:1 cis-9, increased the percentage of C16:1 cis-9 in serum; however, the magnitude of the increase was greater for 5 mg/kg BW (3% of total) than for 2 mg/kg BW (1.5% of total). Serum U-^{13}C16:1 cis-9 as a molar % excess increased (P<0.05) above baseline at 15 min post pulse dose (Figure 1b). For the 2 mg/kg BW dose, serum U-^{13}C16:1 cis-9 remained elevated (P<0.05) above baseline for 60 min. For the 5 mg/kg BW dose, serum U-^{13}C16:1 cis-9 remained elevated (P<0.05) above baseline for 180 min post pulse dose.

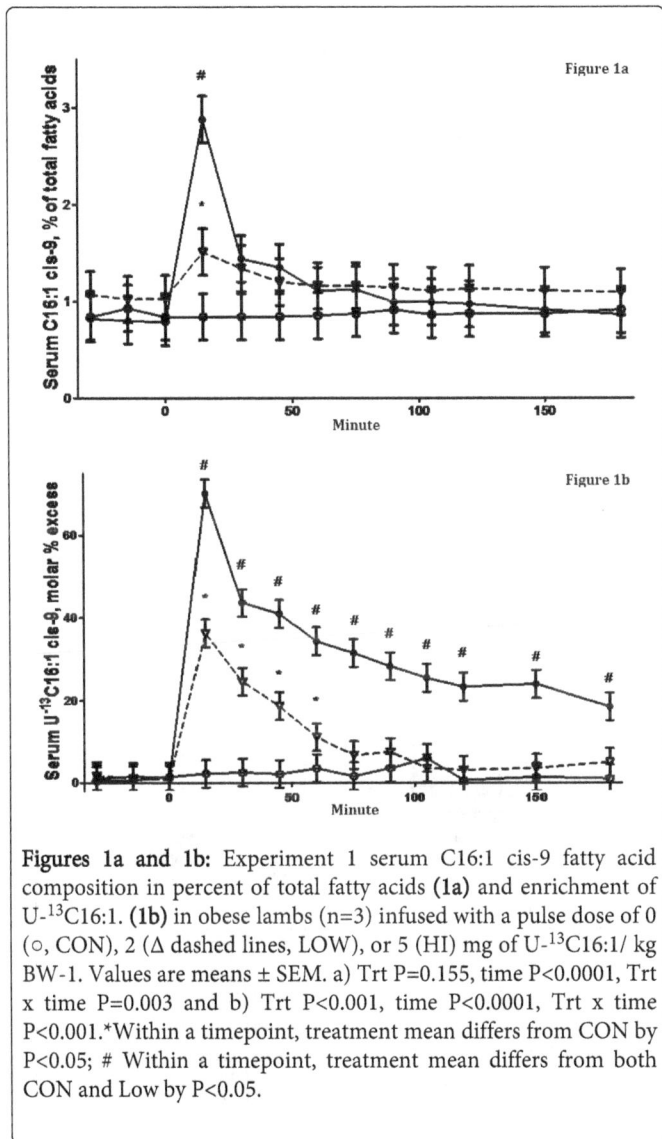

Figures 1a and 1b: Experiment 1 serum C16:1 cis-9 fatty acid composition in percent of total fatty acids (**1a**) and enrichment of U-^{13}C16:1. (**1b**) in obese lambs (n=3) infused with a pulse dose of 0 (○, CON), 2 (Δ dashed lines, LOW), or 5 (HI) mg of U-^{13}C16:1/ kg BW-1. Values are means ± SEM. a) Trt P=0.155, time P<0.0001, Trt x time P=0.003 and b) Trt P<0.001, time P<0.0001, Trt x time P<0.001.*Within a timepoint, treatment mean differs from CON by P<0.05; # Within a timepoint, treatment mean differs from both CON and Low by P<0.05.

Glucose and Insulin

Whole blood glucose concentrations increased (P<0.05) in the 5 mg/kg BW dose of U ^{13}C16:1 cis-9at 15 to 60 minutes post bolus infusion (Figure 2a). For serum insulin, there was a treatment by time interaction (P=0.039; Figure 2b). Serum insulin levels in 5 mg/kg BW U-^{13}C16:1 cis-9 treated animals were elevated over controls at 15 min post doing; however, serum insulin levels decreased below controls at 30 min post dosing. There were no changes in whole blood plasma glucose or serum insulin levels at the 2 mg/kg dose of U-^{13}C16:1 cis-9. These alterations in glucose and insulin reduced (P<0.05) the insulin to glucose ratio from 30 to 75 min post infusion in the 5 mg/kg dose of C16:1 cis-9 group compared to the other two doses (0 and 2 mg/kg BW; Figure 2c).

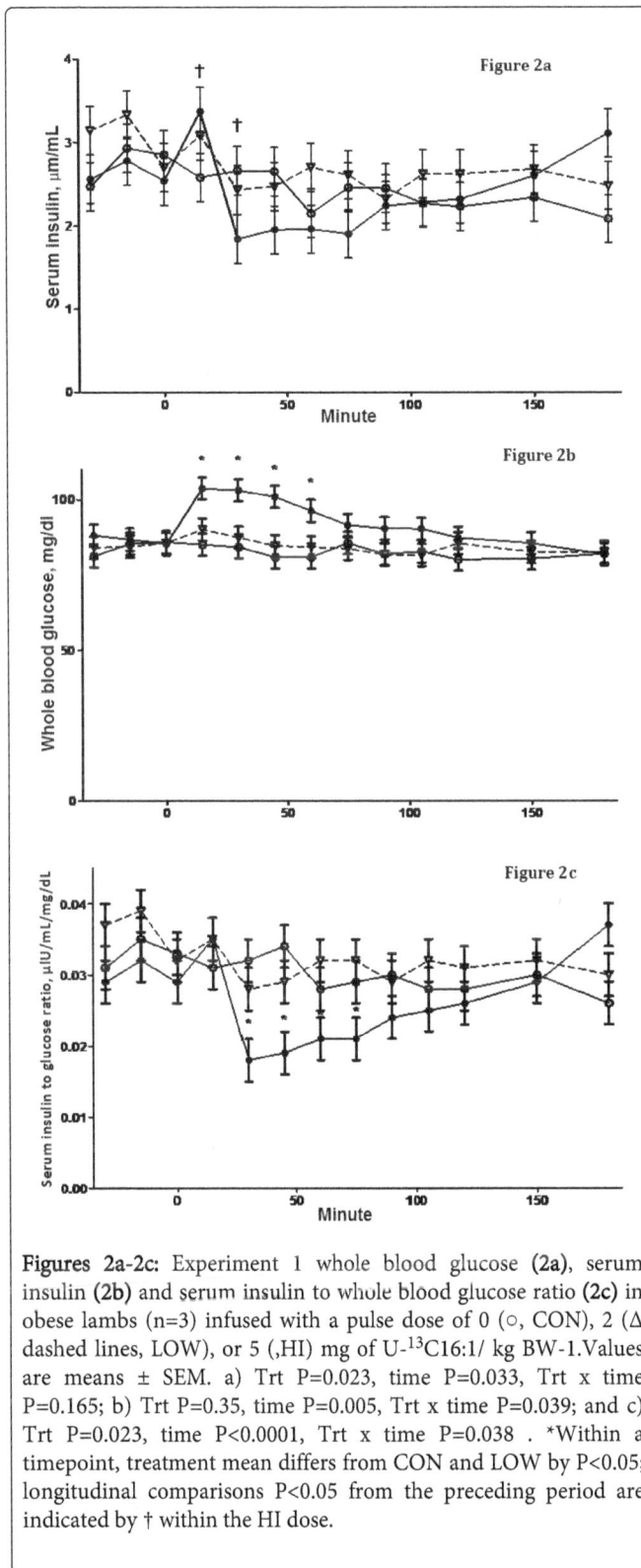

Figures 2a-2c: Experiment 1 whole blood glucose (**2a**), serum insulin (**2b**) and serum insulin to whole blood glucose ratio (**2c**) in obese lambs (n=3) infused with a pulse dose of 0 (○, CON), 2 (Δ dashed lines, LOW), or 5 (,HI) mg of U-^{13}C16:1/ kg BW-1.Values are means ± SEM. a) Trt P=0.023, time P=0.033, Trt x time P=0.165; b) Trt P=0.35, time P=0.005, Trt x time P=0.039; and c) Trt P=0.023, time P<0.0001, Trt x time P=0.038 . *Within a timepoint, treatment mean differs from CON and LOW by P<0.05; longitudinal comparisons P<0.05 from the preceding period are indicated by † within the HI dose.

Glucose Challenge

Serum C16:1 cis-9 as a percent of total serum fatty acids increased (P<0.01) from2 to 15 min post dosing with 5 mg/kg BW bolus infusion of C16:1 cis-9 associated with the glucose administration during

IVGTT (Figure 3a). In response to the 5 mg bolus infusion of C16:1 cis-9, plasma glucose was elevated at 10 min and from 30 to 150 min post infusion compared to the control group (Figure 3b). This difference was confirmed by the 5 mg bolus infusion of C16:1 cis 9 having a greater (P=0.01) AUC for plasma glucose during IVGTT. There was no difference (P=0.95) in plasma insulin between treatments during the IVGTT (Figure 3c). The AUC for plasma insulin was also similar (P=0.89) between treatments. The insulin to glucose ratio during the IVGTT was reduced (P=0.005) in the treated lambs compared to control (0.19 ± 0.03 vs 0.29 ± 0.03, respectively).

Figure 3: Experiment 2 plasma palmitoleic acid. **(a)** glucose **(b)** and insulin **(c)** responses during an intravenous glucose tolerance test in obese lambs pulse infused with 0 (○, n=4) or 5 mg/kg BW of C16:1 (•, n=4). Values are means ± SEM. a) Trt P<0.0001, time P<0.0001, Trt x time P<0.0001; b) Trt P=0.951, time P<0.0001, Trt x time P=0.952; and c) Trt P=0.91, time P<0.0001, Trt x time P=0.95. * Mean differences (P<0.05) and ** mean differences (P<0.01) at a specific time point between treatments.

Insulin Challenge

Serum C16:1 cis-9 as a percent of total serum fatty acids increased (P<0.05) in response to a 5 mg bolus infusion of C16:1 cis 9 from 2 to 30 min post infusion associated with the insulin administration during IC (Figure 4a). During the IC, plasma glucose was increased (P<0.05) at 20, 25 and 100 min post infusion in the 5 mg bolus infusion of C16:1 cis-9 compared to control (Figure 4b). There was an overall increase (P=0.04) in plasma glucose AUC in the 5 mg bolus infusion of C16:1 cis-9 compared to control AUC for plasma glucose during IC. Plasma insulin was increased (P<0.05) initially (2 min. post dosing) and remained elevated through 15 min in the 5 mg bolus infusion of C16:1 cis-9 compared to control (Figure 4c). There was increased plasma insulin AUC during the IC in the 5 mg/kg treated group compared to control (P=0.02). The insulin to glucose ratio during the IC was similar (P=0.62) in the treated lambs compared to control (0.09 ± 0.01 vs. 0.09 ± 0.01, respectively).

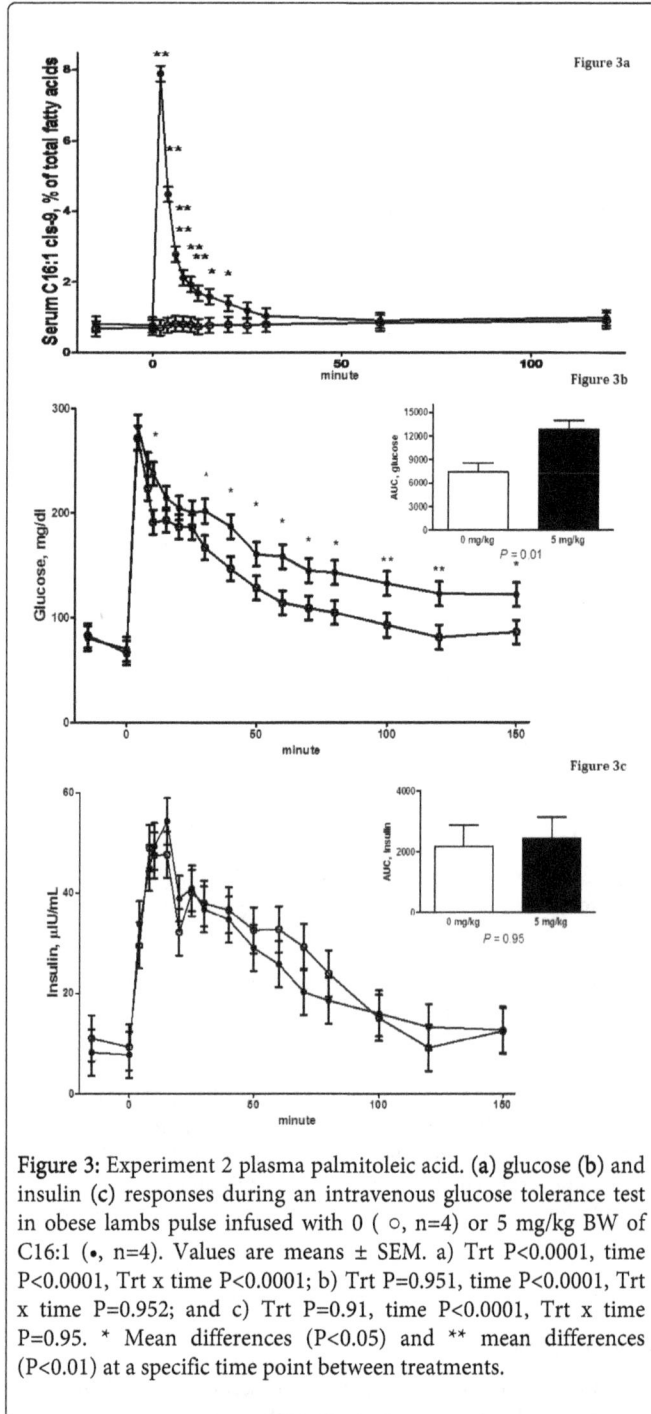

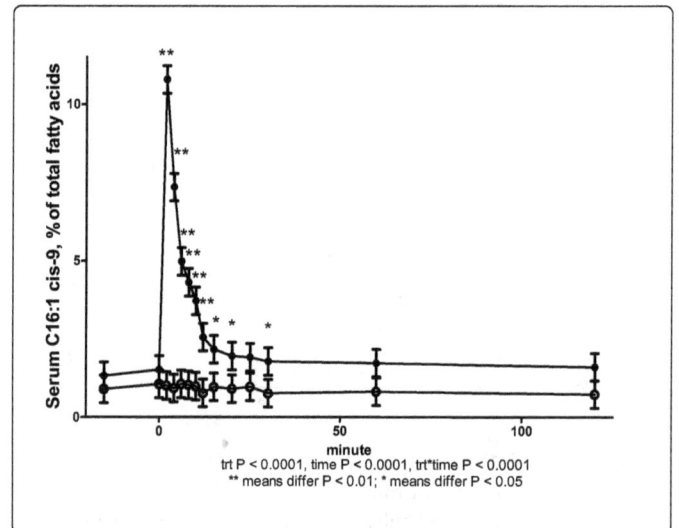

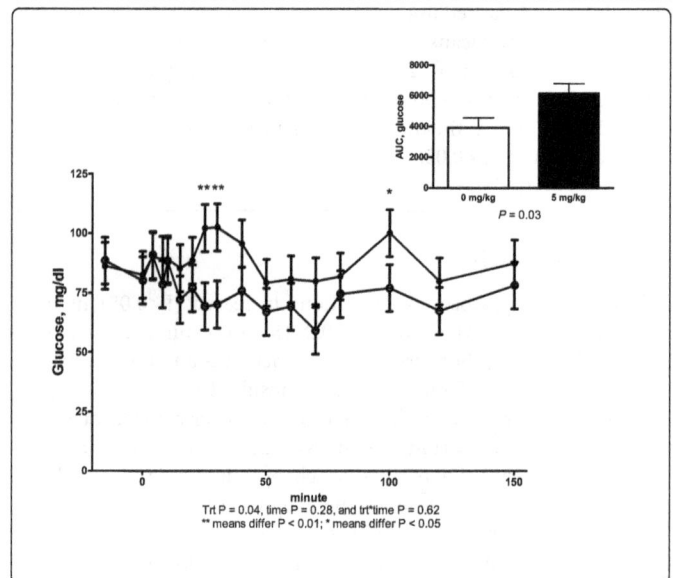

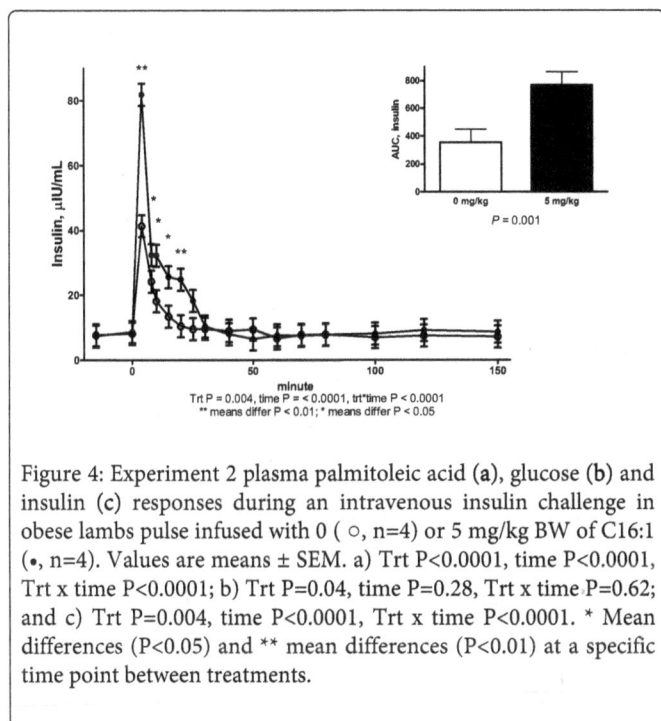

Figure 4: Experiment 2 plasma palmitoleic acid (a), glucose (b) and insulin (c) responses during an intravenous insulin challenge in obese lambs pulse infused with 0 (o, n=4) or 5 mg/kg BW of C16:1 (•, n=4). Values are means ± SEM. a) Trt P<0.0001, time P<0.0001, Trt x time P<0.0001; b) Trt P=0.04, time P=0.28, Trt x time P=0.62; and c) Trt P=0.004, time P<0.0001, Trt x time P<0.0001. * Mean differences (P<0.05) and ** mean differences (P<0.01) at a specific time point between treatments.

Discussion

The objectives of this research were to evaluate uptake of a pulse dose of [13]C16:1 cis-9 at varying levels into the blood and changes in glucose and insulin after pulse dose of 0 or 5 mg C16:1 cis-9/kg BW under challenge conditions in finished lambs. Palmitoleic (C16:1 cis-9) acid is an omega-7 monounsaturated fatty acid that is endogenously produced via de-saturation of palmitic acid by SCD-1. Dietary supply of palmitoleic acid is very low as sources of it in the diet are limited. This research shows that palmitoleic acid, given as a pulse-dose infusion in sheep, is rapidly taken up in the blood stream and returns to baseline levels by 30 minutes post dosing. The magnitude of response was dependent on dose level administered with 5 mg/kg BW dose resulting in a greater peak of C16:1 percentage than 2 mg/kg BW. The level of palmitoleic acid in serum of normal sheep is very low (<1% of total fatty acids). Therefore, we utilized U-[13]C16:1 cis-9 as a tracer so we could specifically measure uptake of this labeled, exogenous fatty acid in the bloodstream. Based on the results, serum palmitoleic acid levels were elevated for a longer time period than could be determined without the use of the stable isotope. Palmitoleic acid concentration was elevated above baseline for 60 and 180 minutes post dosing for 2 and 5 mg/kg BW dose, respectively. Similarly, Persson et al. [15] reported a rapid uptake of free fatty acids into circulation using stable isotope labelled palmitic acid. In bovine adipocytes, palmitoleic acid uptake into the cell responds in a dose responsive manner with maximal inhibition of lipogenesis and de-saturation at 150 μM [3]. This reduction of lipogenesis and desaturation was the result of down regulation of fatty acid synthase (FASN) and stearoyl-CoA desaturase (SCD1), respectively.

There clearly appears to be different effects of the palmitoleic acid pulse dose infusion on plasma glucose and insulin responses depending on whether the animal was in a hyperglycemic or normal glycemic state in the current studies. In all experiments, palmitoleic acid infusion at the 5 mg/kg BW level resulted in increased plasma

glucose above the control (0 mg/kg BW C16:1. During normal glycemic state (Expt. 1) and under IC, serum insulin levels were elevated with palmitoleic acid infusion (5 mg/kg BW). However under a hyperglycemic state (IVGTT), palmitoleic acid infusion did not alter serum insulin levels, thus indicating no difference in insulin release by the β-cells of the pancreas under a stimulated state. These results indicate that palmitoleic acid infusion may alter glucose uptake by peripheral tissues thereby elevating circulating glucose levels. In vitro experiments show that palmitoleate stimulates glucose uptake into C2C12 cells similar to that of insulin [1] and into L6 myotubes in a dose response manner with maximal levels of uptake at 16 h of incubation [18]. Cao et al. [1] found that this increase in glucose uptake was not associated with changes in Glut1 or Glut4 proteins. Dimopoulus et al. [16] found that palmitoleate induced glucose uptake response was enhanced by elevated plasma membrane abundance of both Glut1 and Glut4 indicating that palmitoleate recruits these transporters from sub cellular locations. Rahman et al. [19] found that SCD1-/- mice, which are unable to produce endogenous palmitoleate, had increased glucose uptake and increased Glut4 protein levels compared to SCD1+/+ mice. These authors suggest that loss of SCD1 down regulates protein-tyrosine phosphatase that would regulate phosphorylation of insulin receptor (IR) and insulin receptor substrate (IRS-1) to attenuate the insulin response and increases glucose uptake into cells.

The lack of glucose decline during the IC clearly indicates that these sheep regardless of lipid infusion were experiencing insulin resistance. This is probable due to a number of factors including that ruminants are less insulin sensitive compared to monogastrics [5]. The sheep used in this study were 18 months of age and equal physiologically to early twenties humans [20]. However these sheep used in this study had a large amount of adipose tissue and increased amounts of adipose tissue has been shown to increase insulin resistance in similar aged lambs [20]. In physiologically younger ruminants that did not have increased amounts of adipose tissue a similar insulin challenge resulted in a 50% reduction in plasma glucose compared to baseline values [21]. However, in similar aged lambs insulin resistance was noted in a very lean state (5% Body fat) and this insulin resistance increased as lambs increased in body fat (20% body fat) due to maternal obesity [17].

Palmitoleic acid has been proposed to function as a lipokine, a fatty acid that stimulates muscle insulin action [1]. These authors reported exogenous administration of tripalmitoleate decreased lipogenesis in liver and increased insulin sensitivity in skeletal muscle of mice. Yang et al. [22] orally fed KK-A[y] mice, a model for type 2 diabetes, 300 mg/kg of palmitoleic acid and found that it improved hyperglycemia by increasing insulin sensitivity. It appeared to work in part by down regulating pro-inflammatory gene expression (TNFα and resistin) and by reducing hepatic triglyceride levels. In humans, circulating palmitoleic acid levels are strongly related to insulin sensitivity as measured by oral glucose tolerance test and euglycemic clamp [23] or C-peptide concentrations [24]. Bergman et al. [25] reported that unesterified palmitoleic acid level in plasma was positively related to insulin sensitivity in normal humans but not in subjects with type 1 diabetes. Subjects with type 1 diabetes had lower levels of circulating unesterified palmitoleic acid, which suggests that palmitoleic acid promotes insulin sensitization. Knockout of the SCD-1 gene in mice reduces adipose tissue deposition, increases insulin sensitivity, and makes animals resistant to diet-induced weight gain [26]. SCD1-/- mice had lower fasting insulin and glucose levels on a normal chow diet but glucose tolerance was improved.

The results of this research show that palmitoleic acid infusion increases circulating glucose levels in normal conditions and under glucose challenge; whereas circulating insulin levels were increased with palmitoleic acid infusion during insulin challenge. The changes in plasma glucose levels with palmitoleic acid infusion could result from changes in uptake by peripheral tissues possibly mediated through down regulation of glucose transporters. The increase in insulin by palmitoleic acid infusion under insulin challenge appears related to stimulation of insulin release in islets of Langerhans. Gravena et al. [27] reported increased insulin release from rat and human islets in batch incubations with exposure to palmitoleate and different levels of glucose for 90 minutes. Acute exogenous administration of palmitoleic acid in obese sheep can alter glucose and insulin dynamics. Additional research is needed to examine how long-term exposure to palmitoleic acid regulates glucose and insulin levels *in vivo*. In conclusion, palmitoleic acid infusion results in immediate uptake and clearance of serum palmitoleic acid, increases plasma glucose levels, and alters circulating insulin levels. Additional research is needed to examine how long-term exposure to palmitoleic acid regulates glucose and insulin levels *in vivo*.

Acknowledgements

Technical Contribution No. 6199 of the Clemson University Experiment Station. This material is based upon work supported by the NIFA/USDA, under project number SC-1700439.This project was funded in part by USDA-NIFA grant award 2010-38942-20745.

References

1. Cao H, Gerhold K, Mayers JR, Wiest MM, Watkins SM, et al. (2008) Identification of a lipokine, a lipid hormone linking adipose tissue to systemic metabolism. Cell 134: 933-944.

2. Burns TA, Kadegowda AK, Duckett SK, Pratt SL, Jenkins TC (2012) Palmitoleic (16:1 cis-9) and cis-vaccenic (18:1 cis-11) acid alter lipogenesis in bovine adipocyte cultures. Lipids 47: 1143-1153.

3. Burns TA, Duckett SK, Pratt SL, Jenkins TC (2012) Supplemental palmitoleic (C16:1 cis-9) acid reduces lipogenesis and desaturation in bovine adipocyte cultures. J Anim Sci 90: 3433-3441.

4. Kahn CR (1978) Insulin resistance, insulin insensitivity, and insulin unresponsiveness: a necessary distinction. Metabolism 27: 1893-1902.

5. Kaske M, Elmahdi B, von Engelhardt W, Sallmann HP (2001) Insulin responsiveness of sheep, ponies, miniature pigs and camels: results of hyperinsulinemic clamps using porcine insulin. J Comp Physiol B 171: 549-556.

6. Duhlmeier R, Hacker A, Widdel A, von Engelhardt W, Sallmann HP (2005) Mechanisms of insulin-dependent glucose transport into porcine and bovine skeletal muscle. Am J Physiol Regul Integr Comp Physiol 289: R187-197.

7. Liu S, Baracos VE, Quinney HA, Clandinin MT (1994) Dietary omega-3 and polyunsaturated fatty acids modify fatty acyl composition and insulin binding in skeletal-muscle sarcolemma. Biochem J 299 : 831-837.

8. Behme MT (1996) Dietary fish oil enhances insulin sensitivity in miniature pigs. J Nutr 126: 1549-1553.

9. Ponnampalam EN, Sinclair AJ, Egan AR, Blakeley SJ, Li D, et al. (2001) Effect of dietary modification of muscle long-chain n-3 fatty acid on plasma insulin and lipid metabolites, carcass traits, and fat deposition in lambs. J Anim Sci 79: 895-903.

10. Taouis M, Dagou C, Ster C, Durand G, Pinault M, et al. (2002) N-3 polyunsaturated fatty acids prevent the defect of insulin receptor signaling in muscle. Am J Physiol Endocrinol Metab 282: E664-671.

11. Gingras AA, White PJ, Chouinard PY, Julien P, Davis TA, et al. (2007) Long-chain omega-3 fatty acids regulate bovine whole-body protein metabolism by promoting muscle insulin signalling to the Akt-mTOR-S6K1 pathway and insulin sensitivity. J Physiol 579: 269-284.

12. Cartiff SE, Fellner V, Eisemann JH (2013) Eicosapentaenoic and docosahexaenoic acids increase insulin sensitivity in growing steers. J Anim Sci 91: 2332-2342.

13. Park PW and Goins RE (1994) In situ preparation of FAME for analysis of fatty acid composition in foods. J Food Sci 59: 1262-1266

14. Duckett SK, Neel JP, Lewis RM, Fontenot JP, Clapham WM (2013) Effects of forage species or concentrate finishing on animal performance, carcass and meat quality. J Anim Sci 91: 1454-1467.

15. Persson XM, Blachnio-Zabielska AU, Jensen MD (2010) Rapid measurement of plasma free fatty acid concentration and isotopic enrichment using LC/MS. J Lipid Res 51: 2761-2765.

16. Long NM and Schafer DM (2013) Sex effects on plasma leptin concentrations in newborn and postnatal beef calves. Prof Anim Sci 29:601-605

17. Long NM, Shasa DR, Ford SP, Nathanielsz PW (2012) Growth and insulin dynamics in two generations of female offspring of mothers receiving a single course of synthetic glucocorticoids. Am J Obstet Gynecol 207: 203.

18. Dimopoulos N, Watson M, Sakamoto K, Hundal HS (2006) Differential effects of palmitate and palmitoleate on insulin action and glucose utilization in rat L6 skeletal muscle cells. Biochem J 399: 473-481.

19. Rahman SM, Dobrzyn A, Lee SH, Dobrzyn P, Miyazaki M, et al. (2005) Stearoyl-CoA desaturase 1 deficiency increases insulin signaling and glycogen accumulation in brown adipose tissue. Am J Physiol Endocrinol Metab 288: E381-387.

20. Long NM, George LA, Uthlaut AB, Smith DT, Nijland MJ, et al. (2010) Maternal obesity and increased nutrient intake before and during gestation in the ewe results in altered growth, adiposity, and glucose tolerance in adult offspring. J Anim Sci 88: 3546-3553.

21. Long NM, Prado-Cooper MJ, Krehbiel CR, Wettemann RP (2010) Effects of nutrient restriction of bovine dams during early gestation on postnatal growth and regulation of plasma glucose. J Anim Sci 88: 3262-3268.

22. Yang G, Li L, Fang C, Zhang L, Li Q, et al. (2005) Effects of free fatty acids on plasma resistin and insulin resistance in awake rats. Metabolism 54: 1142-1146.

23. Stefan N, Kantartzis K, Celebi N, Staiger H, Machann J, et al. (2010) Circulating palmitoleate strongly and independently predicts insulin sensitivity in humans. Diabetes Care 33: 405-407.

24. Kurotani K, Sato M, Ejima Y, Nanri A, Yi S, et al. (2012) High levels of stearic acid, palmitoleic acid, and dihomo-γ³-linolenic acid and low levels of linoleic acid in serum cholesterol ester are associated with high insulin resistance. Nutr Res 32: 669-675.

25. Bergman BC, Howard D, Schauer IE, Maahs DM, Snell-Bergeon JK, et al. (2013) The importance of palmitoleic acid to adipocyte insulin resistance and whole-body insulin sensitivity in type 1 diabetes. J Clin Endocrinol Metab 98: E40-50.

26. Ntambi JM, Miyazaki M, Stoehr JP, Lan H, Kendziorski CM, et al. (2002) Loss of stearoyl-CoA desaturase-1 function protects mice against adiposity. Proc Natl Acad Sci U S A 99: 11482-11486.

27. Gravena C, Mathias PC, Ashcroft SJ (2002) Acute effects of fatty acids on insulin secretion from rat and human islets of Langerhans. J Endocrinol 173: 73-80.

22

Metabolic Syndrome Biomarkers in Type II Diabetic Ethiopian Patients

Fitsum Girma Tadesse[1*], Yesehak Worku[2], Yeweyenhareg Feleke[3] and Tarek H. El-Metwally[4]

[1]Department of Medical Microbiology, Radboud Institute for Molecular Life Sciences, Route 268, Geert Grooteplein 26-28, Nijmegen 6525 GA, Netherlands

[2]Department of Biochemistry, College of Medicine, Addis Ababa University, Addis Ababa, Ethiopia

[3]Department of Internal Medicine, Faculty of Medicine, Addis Ababa University, Addis Ababa, Ethiopia

[4]Faculty of Medicine, Assiut University, Assiut, POB: 71526, Egypt

[*]**Corresponding author:** Fitsum Girma Tadesse, Department of Medical Microbiology, Radboud Institute for Molecular Life Sciences, Route 268, Geert Grooteplein 26-28, Nijmegen 6525 GA, Netherlands; E-mail: fitsezemichael@gmail.com, fitsum.girma@aau.edu.et

Abstract

Background: Insulin resistance, which precedes by many years the onset of and accompanies type II diabetes (T2D), is strongly associated with a clustering of cardiovascular risk factors, termed metabolic syndrome (MetS).

Objectives: The aim of this study was to investigate the extent of MetS risk in T2D Ethiopian patients.

Methods: A total of 72 T2D patients and 20 normal healthy controls without MetS were studied. Based on the world health organization criteria, 59.72% (43/72) of the patients had MetS.

Results: Type 2 diabetic patients with MetS (0.953 ± 0.007) were significantly ($P<0.01$) obese than those without (0.913 ± 0.012). Plasma total triglyceride (TG) (206.9 ± 16.91) and blood pressure (138.8 ± 3.247) were strongly significantly high ($P<0.001$) in patients with MetS as compared to those without MetS (104.4 ± 6.766 and 122.8 ± 2.725, respectively). On the other hand, plasma high density lipoprotein-cholesterol (40.91 ± 3.070) and total peroxide (0.055 ± 0.001) were found at a significantly ($P<0.05$) lower amounts in patients with MetS as compared to those without (50.90 ± 2.601 and 0.052 ± 0.001, respectively). In patients with MetS, the IR index showed a significant association ($P<0.05$) with the dyslipidemia markers: TG ($r=0.254$), low density lipoprotein-cholesterol ($r=0.262$), and total cholesterol ($r=0.320$). Waist-hip circumference ratio showed a positive significant correlation with blood pressure ($r=0.330$, $P<0.05$) and C-reactive protein was strongly associated with serum insulin concentration ($r=0.382$, $P<0.01$).

Conclusion: Ethiopian T2D patients with MetS are at a greater risk of hypertensive, dyslipidemia and oxidative stress states, and developing cardiovascular disorders. Interventions should be planned to help those patients avoid/delay onset of cardiovascular complications anticipated upon the accumulation of predisposing factors that are components of MetS.

Keywords: Metabolic syndrome; Type II diabetes; C-reactive protein; Total peroxides; Dyslipidemia; Insulin resistance; Central obesity

Introduction

Type II diabetes (T2D) is a complex and progressive disease that is strongly associated with obesity and Insulin Resistance (IR) as its main characteristic features[1]. Insulin resistance is an early event and precedes the onset of T2D by many years [2]. However, during its early stage IR is compensated by hyperinsulinemia, thus preserving normal glucose tolerance. Deterioration into impaired glucose tolerance occurs when either IR increases or the insulin secretory response of the β-cells decreases, or both [3]. This is partly induced by the apparent hyperglycemia that translates into progressive deterioration and degranulation of β-cells, often accompanied by a decreased β-cell mass [1].

Insulin resistance coexists not only with T2D but also with a constellation of cardiovascular risk factors that world health organization (WHO) designated as metabolic syndrome (MetS) [4].

Insulin resistance is thought to be the mechanism driving the other components of MetS [5]. Furthermore, MetS is accompanied by a proinflammatory and prothrombotic state [6] that enhances the potential for acute thrombosis through hypercoagulability and impaired fibrinolysis [7] to finally precipitate cardiovascular disease (CVD). An emerging body of evidence documents associations of elevated low-grade inflammation markers such as C-reactive protein (CRP) concentrations in individuals with IR [8].

On the other hand, IR can be induced and aggravated by increased oxidative stress (OxS), which is common in T2D [9]. Association of IR with OxS resembles a vicious circle. Oxidative stress increases IR through interference with intracellular insulin signaling [10]. Chronic hyperinsulinemia secondary to IR can, in turn, be responsible for the generation of free radicals and decrease in antioxidant enzyme activity [9,11]. Given the risk of CVD to diabetic patients, there is a need to investigate the underlying alteration in the constellation of components of MetS in T2D patients in order to improve recognition of individuals at risk of future CVD and alleviate the complications patients could face. Studies have evaluated this association among other ethnic groups. However, to our knowledge, there was no report on the Ethiopian T2D patients. We, therefore, sought to evaluate the underlying alterations in Ethiopian T2D patients with MetS.

Materials and Methods

The study proposal was reviewed and approved by the Ethical Review Committee of the Faculty of Medicine of Addis Ababa University. Permission to conduct the study was also obtained from the department of Internal Medicine. Before starting the study, all voluntary participants were given an explanation on the purposes and methods of the study. Informed written consent was obtained from each study participant prior to his/her enrolment in the study.

This project applied a cross-sectional study design and conducted at Tikur Anbessa Specialized Hospital, Faculty of Medicine, Addis Ababa University, Addis Ababa, Ethiopia. A total of 72 T2D patients (36 men and 36 women) regularly attending the diabetic clinic participated in the study. Socio-economically matching 20 (12 males and 8 females) normal healthy subjects were included in the study. They were staff members and post-graduate students of the faculty with normal BMI and without MetS (Table 1).

Parameter	Control(n = 20)	Patient (n = 72)	P values < (Unpaired t-test)
BMI (Kg/m2)	22.55 ± 0.698	25.56 ± 0.470	0.01
WC (cm)	83.05 ± 2.660	96.05 ± 1.214	0.001
HC (cm)	94.65 ± 1.864	102.7 ± 1.197	0.01
WHR	0.87 ± 0.014	0.937 ± 0.007	0.001
SBP (mmHg)	118.50 ± 1.957	132.4 ± 2.404	0.01
DBP (mmHg)	75.00 ± 1.539	81.21 ± 1.138	0.01
FBG (mg/dL)	76.45 ± 2.775	180.8 ± 7.562	0.001
CRP (mg/dL)	1.48 ± 0.208	21.7 ± 4.605	0.05
HDL-C (mg/dL)	61.35 ± 3.721	44.95 ± 2.176	0.01
LDL-C (mg/dL)	50.83 ± 6.599	89.65 ± 5.753	0.05
TG (mg/dL)	147.40 ± 11.410	161 ± 10.190	NS
Insulin (mU/L)	4.75 ± 0.288	5.205 ± 0.212	NS
TP (µM)	0.051 ± 0.001	0.054 ± 0.001	NS
HOMA-IR (mU/L.mM)	0.913 ± 0.079	2.319 ± 0.145	0.01

Table 1: Anthropometric, clinical and biochemical characteristics assessment of the study Ethiopian Type II diabetic patients and healthy controls. **Abbreviations:** BMI = Body Mass Index; DBP = Diastolic Blood Pressure; CRP = C-Reactive Protein; FBG = Fasting Blood Glucose; HC = Hip Circumference; HDL-C = High Density Lipoprotein-Cholesterol; HOMA-IR = Homeostasis Model Assessment-Insulin Resistance; LDL-C = Low Density Lipoprotein-Cholesterol; SBP = Systolic Blood Pressure; TG = Triglycerides; TP = Total Peroxide; WC = Waist Circumference; WHR = Waist-Hip Circumference Ratio; NS = Non-Significant Difference. Data presented are means ± SEM.

After an overnight fasting 5 mL blood was drawn from antecubital vein of the arm of each study participant into anti-coagulant free blood collection vacutainer tubes. The whole blood was left to stand vertically for 30 minutes on ice and the serum from the sample was processed and collected by centrifugation at 3000 rpm for 10 minutes at 4°C. The separated serum was aliquot stored at -70°C until further analysis.

Medical history (age, sex, drugs, smoking, alcohol consumption, and duration of diabetes) and anthropometric measurements (height, weight, waist, and hip circumference) were taken. Waist circumference (WC) was measured with a soft measuring tape on standing subjects midway between the lowest rib and the iliac crest to the nearest 0.1 cm at minimal respiration. Hip circumference (HC) was taken at the greatest gluteal protuberance to the nearest 0.1 cm. The WC-HC ratio was calculated to get the WHR. Weight was measured with a lever balance, to the nearest 100 g, while subjects wore light clothing without shoes. Height was measured, to the nearest 0.5 cm, without shoes, with a measuring tape, with eyes looking straight ahead, with a right-angle triangle resting of the scalp against the wall. Body mass index (BMI) was calculated as weight in kilogram divided by height in meter square expressed in kg/m^2.

Blood Pressure measurements were taken on the right arm twice after the subject had been seated in supine position for at least 5 minutes, with a standard sphygmomanometer, and the mean blood pressure value in mmHg was used. A questionnaire was administered for each participant, both patients and normal controls, to collect other demographic details.

Fasting blood glucose (FBG), high density lipoprotein-cholesterol (HDL-C), total triglyceride (TG) were assayed by enzymatic methods (Biocon® Diagnostik, Vöhl-Marienhagen, Germany). C-reactive protein was assayed with a quantitative turbidimetric immunoassay (Linear Chemicals, S.L., Barcelona, Spain). Insulin was assayed with a solid phase two-site immunoassay (Mercodia AB, Uppsala, Sweden). Total peroxide (TP) concentration was determined using the ferric–xylenol orange "FOX" method [12]. Low density lipoprotein-cholesterol (LDL-C) was determined using Friedewald's equation [13].

The present study used the WHO criteria to identify patients with MetS [5]. Homeostasis model assessment of IR (HOMA-IR) was used for measurement of insulin sensitivity [14].

To avoid confounding by exogenously taken insulin, patients under insulin therapy were excluded. Further, patients with liver disease, thyroid disease, Cushing's syndrome, alcoholics, smokers, those taking lipid lowering drugs, patients suffering from arthritis, and patients with HIV on anti-retroviral drug were excluded.

Information obtained from questionnaire and laboratory analyses was analyzed using Prism 3.0 package (GraphPad Software, Inc, San Diego, CA, USA) and Microsoft Excel 2003. The minimum level of statistical significance was set at p<0.05. The data was expressed as Mean ± SEM. Results were analyzed statistically using column statistics and t-test for comparison of unpaired two-tailed variables. Group differences were determined by analysis of variance (ANOVA) with post hoc testing using the Newman-Keuls method. Correlation among the investigated parameters in each group was tested by the non-parametric Spearman's analysis.

Results

Table 1 shows that means of anthropometric and clinical parameters were significantly different between healthy controls and T2D patients in general. Biochemical investigation of serum FBG, CRP, HDL-C and LDL-C revealed significant mean differences between control groups and T2D patients. Differences in mean serum TG, TP, and insulin concentration remained insignificantly high in T2D patients, however. The mean age of the controls and patients was 35.45 ± 1.019 and 54.85 ± 1.242, respectively.

Table 2 presents ANOVA results on the differences in the mean values of investigated parameters in healthy control subjects as compared to T2D patients sub grouped on the basis of MetS, with and without.

Parameter	Control vs. Without	Control vs. With	Without vs. With
WHR	0.05	0.001	0.01
HDL-C	0.05	0.001	0.05
SBP/DBP	NS	0.001	0.001
TG	NS	0.01	0.001
TP	NS	0.05	0.05
CRP	0.05	0.01	NS
LDL-C	0.01	0.05	NS
HOMA-IR	0.001	0.001	NS

Table 2: Anthropometric, clinical and biochemical characteristics assessment of the study Ethiopian Type II diabetic patients stratified by metabolic syndrome as compared to healthy control groups. **Abbreviations:** DBP = Diastolic Blood Pressure; CRP = C-Reactive Protein; HDL-C = High Density Liporotein-Cholesterol; HOMA-IR = homeostasis model assessment-Insulin Resistance; LDL-C = Low Density Liporpotein-Cholesterol; SBP = Systolic Blood Pressure; TG = Triglycerides; TP = Total Peroxide; WHR = Waist-Hip Circumference Ratio; NS = non-significant difference; Values are means ± SEM.

Comparing between all the three groups (Healthy controls, patients without MetS and patients with MetS), waist-hip circumference ratio (WHR) (0.876 ± 0.014) was significantly lower in controls than that of patients without MetS (0.913 ± 0.012; P<0.05) and with MetS (0.953 ± 0.007; P<0.001). Comparing the two patients' subgroups (with vs. without MetS) revealed a significant difference (P<0.01) too. High density lipoprotein-cholesterol control level (61.35 ± 3.740 mg/dL) was significantly higher than patients without MetS (50.90 ± 2.601 mg/dL, P<0.05) and patients with MetS (40.91 ± 3.070 mg/dL; P<0.001). Comparing patients' subgroups revealed a significant difference (P<0.05).

Systolic blood pressure (SBP), TG and TP resulted in insignificant differences when comparing healthy controls with T2D patients without MetS. However, the controls' level of SBP (118.5 ± 1.957 mmHg) was significantly lower than that of patients with MetS (138.8 ± 3.247 mmHg, P<0.001), with very strong significant difference (P<0.001) between patient subgroups. Total TG in healthy control subjects (147.4 ± 11.41) was significantly lower than patients with MetS (206.9 ± 16.91 mg/dL; P<0.01). Comparison of patients' subgroups revealed a highly significant difference (P<0.001). Serum

TP in healthy control volunteer subjects (0.051 ± 0.001) as compared to that of patients with MetS were significantly lower (0.056 ± 0.001; P<0.05).

On the other hand, HOMA-IR, CRP and LDL-C revealed insignificant differences between patients' subgroups. Healthy controls' IR index (0.913 ± 0.079) was strongly significantly lower (P<0.001) as compared to that of patients without (2.148 ± 0.259) and with MetS (2.434 ± 0.169). Serum CRP in healthy volunteer subjects (1.480 ± 0.208 mg/dL) was significantly lower than patients without MetS (21.31 ± 7.926 mg/dL) and patients with MetS (21.880 ± 5.651 mg/dL), P<0.05 and P<0.01 respectively. The values of LDL-C in healthy subjects (50.83 ± 6.599 mg/dL) was significantly lower than each of patients without MetS (98.52 ± 9.744 mg/dL) and with MetS (81.53 ± 6.733 mg/dL), P<0.01 and P<0.05 respectively.

In a correlation analyses in T2D patients with MetS, IR state significantly positively (P<0.05) associated with each of the dyslipidemia markers; TG (r=0.254), LDL-C (r=0.262) and TC (r=0.320). Waist-hip circumference ratio significantly positively (P<0.05) correlated with each of the SBP (r=0.259) and DBP (r=0.330). C-reactive protein revealed a strongly significant positive (P<0.01) correlation with serum insulin concentration (r=0.382).

Among parameters investigated in T2D patients population as a whole serum insulin concentration revealed a significant negative (r=-0.243, P<0.05) association with HDL-C and a positive significant association with WC (r=0.409, P<0.001) and DBP (r=0.238, P<0.05). WHR showed a significant positive correlation with SBP (r=0.288, P<0.01) and DBP (r=0.329, P<0.01). Total triglyceride showed a significant negative correlation with SBP (r=0.273, P<0.05), DBP (r=0.341, P<0.01), and TP (r=0.271, P<0.05). Insulin resistance revealed a significant positive correlation with DBP (r=0.239, P<0.05), CRP (r=0.221, P<0.05), and TG (r=0.260, P<0.05). C-reactive protein showed a significant negative association with TAC (r=-0.243, P<0.05).

Discussion

Type II diabetes patients with MetS in the present study were significantly obese as compared to those without MetS. In addition to that, dyslipidemia, an increase in circulating TG and a low level in HDL-C, characterized them. In the association study, dyslipidemia was highly correlated with IR index of patients with MetS. The current dominant paradigm is that IR leads to dyslipidemia although it is still possible that dyslipidemia may also cause IR [15]. The vicious "dyslipidemia-IR-hyperinsulinemia" cycle has been forwarded to explain this phenomenon [16].

It is not all the possible list of dyslipidemia, however, that could possibly be causal factors or results of IR. Instead, dyslipidemia consisting of high TGs and low HDL-C is a widely recognized lipid pattern that is frequently associated with IR and subsequent development of chronic heart disease (CHD). Furthermore, in Framingham Heart Study incident CHD risk that is associated with low plasma HDL-C or hypertriglyceridemia was significantly increased only in the presence of IR [17]. Taken together, these results implicate that the study subjects with MetS in this study are at increased risk of developing CVD, as they had hypertriglyceridemia and low HDL-C.

Although there are several causes of CVD, atherosclerosis (leading to CHD) and/or hypertension are the most common ones. The dyslipidemic and obesity state in this study is accompanied by a pronounced increase in blood pressure in patients with MetS. Excess weight gain contributes to increased blood pressure, partly due to activation of the sympathetic nervous system in the kidney that results in increased renal sodium reabsorption and impaired pressure natriuresis, which appears to be mediated in part by increased levels of the adipocyte-derived hormone leptin [18].

There are emerging biochemical explanations for the association of dyslipidemia with CHD, in the presence of IR. In a hyperlipidemic animal model an increased ROS generation and an over expression of the NADPH oxidase gp91phox subunit have been demonstrated [19]. This indicates that the patients in the present study were at increased risk of developing CHD as they had elevated TP in their sera. Currently, OxS is considered as a novel component of the MetS. Assessment of plasma OxS may contribute to identify a subset of MetS patients at increased cardiovascular risk, candidates to more intensive therapies [20]. Previous study reported higher OxS level in subjects with more MetS components [21].

The OxS in diabetics is possibly mediated to a significant extent via increased production of ROS from the high glucose, possibly in concert with fatty acids. Oxidative stress activates a number of cellular stress response pathways [10]. These pathways lead to both IR and impaired insulin secretion. Reports highlighted that central obesity, IR and dyslipidemia significantly correlate with antioxidant enzymes activity [21]. Although all body cells are bathed in the hyperglycemic state in T2D, endothelial cells are extremely vulnerable. Exposure of endothelial cells to high glucose leads to augmented production of superoxide anion, which may quench nitric oxide, a potent endothelium-derived vasodilator that participates in the general homeostasis of the vasculature [22]. With all these effects increases in OxS may contribute to impaired vascular function, inflammation, thrombosis, and atherosclerosis and ultimately give rise to vascular disease [23].

In addition to OxS, subjects with MetS have a higher inflammation status [24]. In clinical studies it is confirmed that inflammation contributes towards the early stages of CHD [25].Correlation analysis, in the present study, revealed that serum insulin concentration is strongly correlating with CRP which is in line with previous reports. In Peruvian adults elevated CRP was significantly associated with increased mean fasting insulin [8]. In addition, the level of CRP was found higher in U.S. youth who had the MetS[26].One of the mechanisms that could explain the inflammation that was observed in the present study could be obesity state of the patients. A study in Portuguese implicated an increase in inflammation (level of CRP) with severity of obesity and high blood pressure [27].The Nod Like Receptor (NLR) family of innate immune cell sensors like the Nlrp3 inflammasome senses obesity-associated 'danger-signals', such as ceramide. Nlrp3 contributes to obesity-induced inflammation and IR [28]. This is worsened by the accumulation of macrophages that secrete proinflammatory mediators [29]. All culminate into a combination of altered functions of insulin target cells; such as in adipose tissue, liver, and skeletal muscle [30].

Above all the OxS and inflammation states are cross-talking with one another and could ultimately exert devastating effects. Inflammation increases the production of ROS resulting in an increased OxS with over-activation of NADPH oxidase [31]. This process reduces the bioavailability of NO. On the other hand, OxS alters the nature, pattern, and magnitude of cytokines produced. With all these effects OxS could play the central role in the alterations observed in patients with MetS increased. This is in agreement with a

Japanese report which indicated that OxS in accumulated fat is an important pathogenic mechanism of obesity-associated MetS [32].

Taken together, in our Ethiopian T2D patients, central obesity, followed by dyslipidemia and low-grade inflammation and OxS, are the main pathogenic mechanism underlying the metabolic changes observed in the study subjects with MetS that predisposes T2D patients to hypertension and risk of CVD. In a proof, patients without MetS had comparable state of blood pressure, lipid profile, and OxS as compared to controls. Since patients with the MetS have greater risk of developing the CVD, this study can help make proper guidelines for prevention and screening, at early time, in T2D Ethiopian patients.

Acknowledgement

The study was financially supported by Addis Ababa University

References

1. Kahn SE, Hull RL, Utzschneider KM (2006) Mechanisms linking obesity to insulin resistance and type 2 diabetes. Nature 444: 840-846.

2. Evans JL, Goldfine ID, Maddux BA, Grodsky GM (2002) Oxidative stress and stress-activated signaling pathways: a unifying hypothesis of type 2 diabetes. Endocr Rev 23: 599-622.

3. Poitout V, Robertson RP (2008) Glucolipotoxicity: fuel excess and beta-cell dysfunction. Endocr Rev 29: 351-366.

4. Metascreen Writing Committee, Bonadonna R, Cucinotta D, Fedele D, Riccardi G, et al. (2006) The metabolic syndrome is a risk indicator of microvascular and macrovascular complications in diabetes: results from Metascreen, a multicenter diabetes clinic-based survey. Diabetes Care 29: 2701-2707.

5. Stolar M (2007) Metabolic syndrome: controversial but useful. Cleve Clin J Med 74: 199-202, 205-8.

6. Deen D (2004) Metabolic syndrome: time for action. Am Fam Physician 69: 2875-2882.

7. Wannamethee SG, Lowe GD, Shaper AG, Rumley A, Lennon L, et al. (2005) The metabolic syndrome and insulin resistance: relationship to haemostatic and inflammatory markers in older non-diabetic men. Atherosclerosis 181: 101-108.

8. Gelaye B, Revilla L, Lopez T, Suarez L, Sanchez SE, et al. (2010) Association between insulin resistance and c-reactive protein among Peruvian adults. DiabetolMetabSyndr 2: 30.

9. Sarafidis PA, Grekas DM (2007) Insulin resistance and oxidant stress: an interrelation with deleterious renal consequences? J CardiometabSyndr 2: 139-142.

10. Evans JL, Goldfine ID, Maddux BA, Grodsky GM (2003) Are oxidative stress-activated signaling pathways mediators of insulin resistance and beta-cell dysfunction? Diabetes 52: 1-8.

11. Bloch-Damti A, Bashan N (2005) Proposed mechanisms for the induction of insulin resistance by oxidative stress. Antioxid Redox Signal 7: 1553-1567.

12. Harma M, Harma M, Erel O (2005) Measurement of the total antioxidant response in preeclampsia with a novel automated method. Eur J ObstetGynecolReprodBiol 118: 47-51.

13. Friedewald WT, Levy RI, Fredrickson DS (1972) Estimation of the concentration of low-density lipoprotein cholesterol in plasma, without use of the preparative ultracentrifuge. ClinChem 18: 499-502.

14. Matthews DR, Hosker JP, Rudenski AS, Naylor BA, Treacher DF, et al. (1985) Homeostasis model assessment: insulin resistance and beta-cell function from fasting plasma glucose and insulin concentrations in man. Diabetologia 28: 412-419.

15. Reaven G (2012) Insulin resistance and coronary heart disease in nondiabetic individuals. ArteriosclerThrombVascBiol 32: 1754-1759.

16. Li N, Fu J, Koonen DP3, Kuivenhoven JA3, Snieder H4, et al. (2014) Are hypertriglyceridemia and low HDL causal factors in the development of insulin resistance? Atherosclerosis 233: 130-138.

17. Robins SJ, Lyass A, Zachariah JP, Massaro JM, Vasan RS (2011) Insulin resistance and the relationship of a dyslipidemia to coronary heart disease: the Framingham Heart Study. ArteriosclerThrombVascBiol 31: 1208-1214.

18. Hall JE, da Silva AA, do Carmo JM, Dubinion J, Hamza S, et al. (2010) Obesity-induced hypertension: role of sympathetic nervous system, leptin, and melanocortins. J BiolChem 285: 17271-17276.

19. Maeda K, Yasunari K, Sato EF, Inoue M (2005) Enhanced oxidative stress in neutrophils from hyperlipidemic guinea pig. Atherosclerosis 181: 87-92.

20. Hopps E, Noto D, Caimi G, Averna MR (2010) A novel component of the metabolic syndrome: the oxidative stress. NutrMetabCardiovasc Dis 20: 72-77.

21. Yubero-Serrano EM, Delgado-Lista J, Peña-Orihuela P, Perez-Martinez P, Fuentes F, et al. (2013) Oxidative stress is associated with the number of components of metabolic syndrome: LIPGENE study. Exp Mol Med 45: e28.

22. Giugliano D, Ceriello A, Paolisso G (1996) Oxidative stress and diabetic vascular complications. Diabetes Care 19: 257-267.

23. Berliner JA, Navab M, Fogelman AM, Frank JS, Demer LL, et al. (1995) Atherosclerosis: basic mechanisms. Oxidation, inflammation, and genetics. Circulation 91: 2488-2496.

24. Chen SJ, Yen CH, Huang YC, Lee BJ, Hsia S, et al. (2012) Relationships between inflammation, adiponectin, and oxidative stress in metabolic syndrome. PLoS One 7: e45693.

25. Luc G, Bard JM, Juhan-Vague I, Ferrieres J, Evans A, et al. (2003) C-reactive protein, interleukin-6, and fibrinogen as predictors of coronary heart disease: the PRIME Study. ArteriosclerThrombVascBiol 23: 1255-1261.

26. Ford ES, Ajani UA, Mokdad AH; National Health and Nutrition Examination (2005) The metabolic syndrome and concentrations of C-reactive protein among U.S. youth. Diabetes Care 28: 878-881.

27. Santos AC, Lopes C, Guimarães JT, Barros H (2005) Central obesity as a major determinant of increased high-sensitivity C-reactive protein in metabolic syndrome. Int J Obes (Lond) 29: 1452-1456.

28. Vandanmagsar B, Youm YH, Ravussin A, Galgani JE, Stadler K, et al. (2011) The NLRP3 inflammasome instigates obesity-induced inflammation and insulin resistance. Nat Med 17: 179-188.

29. Olefsky JM, Glass CK (2010) Macrophages, inflammation, and insulin resistance. Annu Rev Physiol 72: 219-246.

30. Schenk S, Saberi M, Olefsky JM (2008) Insulin sensitivity: modulation by nutrients and inflammation. J Clin Invest 118: 2992-3002.

31. Rivera J, Sobey CG, Walduck AK, Drummond GR (2010) Nox isoforms in vascular pathophysiology: insights from transgenic and knockout mouse models. Redox Rep 15: 50-63.

32. Furukawa S, Fujita T, Shimabukuro M, Iwaki M, Yamada Y, et al. (2004) Increased oxidative stress in obesity and its impact on metabolic syndrome. J Clin Invest 114: 1752-1761.

23

Prophylactic Fixation of Impending Fractures

Bahaa Kornah[1,2*]**, Hesham Safwat**[1,2]**, Tharwat Abdel Ghany**[1,2] **and Mohamed Abdel-AAl**[1,2]

[1]*Al-Azhar University, Cairo, Egypt*

[2]*Manshet El bakey Hospital, Alazhar University, Cairo, Egypt*

*Corresponding author: Bahaa Kornah, MD, Consultant Orthopedic Surgeon, Al-Azhar University, Cairo, Egypt, 90 D Ahmed Orabi St. Mohandessin, Giza, Egypt; E-mail: bkornah@yahoo.co.uk

Abstract

Aim: Pathologic fractures occur as a result of weakening of the mechanical properties of bone. There are many conditions, which lead to bone softening. There are neoplastic and non-neoplastic diseases that cause pathologic fractures. The aim is to evaluate and to highlight on value of prophylactic fixation of impending fractures in abnormal bone situation to prevent occurrence of pathological fracture and its complications.

Patients and methods: Between 2003 and 2009, study on forty-nine patient (35 females and 14 males) between the age of 20 and 65 years with an average age of 49.9 years with expected possibility of fractures of lower extremities. The entire patient with fractures risks prophylactic fixation has done. Different types of fixation either surface plating (dynamic hip screws), medullary (Gamma nails or locking nail) or external fixation in cases unsuitable for surgery was used according to the type and the site of the deformity in combination of management of primary condition.

Results: Most patients had significant relief of pain. 35 (71.5%) of patients with impending fracture were ambulatory after therapy and able to walk outdoor while 10 (20.5%) of patients could walk inside door. Three patients (6%) using wheel chair, and they were on renal dialysis. Only one patient (2%) was not able to walk, and he was not cooperative for unknown reason. The mean duration of hospitalization was 21 days (range from 7 to 35 days). That time included preoperative period of investigation and preparation and post-operative surgery and rehabilitation.

Discussion: Pathological fractures create a serious morbidity in patients with bone disease. Orthopedic surgeons who look after patients with skeletal lesions should focus on proactive treatments designed to prevent pathologic fractures before they occur. Prophylactic fixations have decreased morbidity compared with patient's sustained fractures before fixation.

Conclusion: Surgical fixation of fractures in weight-bearing long bones with impending fractures provides pain relief, and a functionally stable and durable construct. It helps early an ambulation and prevents fracture's complication. It allows independent function and avoids irretrievable catastrophes.

Keywords: Fractures; Prophylactic fixation; Pathological fractures; Impending fractures

Introduction

Changes in the bone are the results from a continuous process of bone resorption and bone formation known as "bone remodeling" which involves bone growth, changes in bone density and calcium level regulation in the body. This process occurs throughout a life span. Once the bone mass has been achieved, bone formation generally equal to bone resorption and bone density remains unchanged. This is called peak bone density [1]. In normal bone, shear stresses are distributed evenly in cross section.

Pathological fractures occur as a result of an underlying process; the so-called bone softening disease; that weakens the mechanical properties of bone. There are neoplastic and non-neoplastic diseases that cause pathological fractures [2]. Bone softening is a condition which occurs almost only in adults, and is due to a loss of the lime-salts

of the bone. The disease, which is comparatively rare, affect's women, principally. Many diseases that affect the metabolism typically result in bone softening because the osteoid, which is the bone matrix, does not calcify how it should, resulting in bones that bend, twist and fracture. Many medical conditions and chemical drug therapy can affect the bone strength, e.g. vitamin D deficiency and Phenytoin for treatment of epilepsy produce osteomalacia. The strength and integrity of bones depend on maintaining a delicate balance between bone resorption by osteoclasts and bone formation by osteoblasts [3].

Factors affect the biomechanics of bone and lead to pathological fractures are Bone defect size, Biological behavior of bone lesion, and the anatomic location of the lesion. Bone in these situations is subjected to what is called impending pathological fractures which definition is controversial. Diagnosis and estimation of fracture at risk with its decision for prophylactic fixation are difficult.

Pain; mostly, in the pelvis, is the first symptom with the bone softening disease. The pain could radiate towards the spinal column or thighs, and at first it is often thought to be rheumatic. Soon, however, an uncertain dragging or peculiarly waddling gait becomes noticeable. Sitting causes pain and the bones bend. The spinal column is no longer able to carry the weight of the body. It curves backward and as a result; the patients grow shorter. When the disease has reached a more advanced stage, walking becomes impossible and the patients must remain in bed. The fractures typically are sustained after a low-energy mechanism with the presence of an existing characteristic stress fracture. However, it is unclear whether these patients are best treated conservatively or operatively.

Many authors recommend prophylactic osteosynthesis for all impending pathological fractures [4-7]. Many options are available to the orthopedic surgeon for reconstruction of long bones; this includes the usage of plates and screws, intramedullary nails, reconstruction nails, endoprosthesis and customized or massive endoprosthesis [2]. In literatures, little is mentioned about prophylactic fixation for non-neoplastic diseases that cause pathologic fractures.

Patients and Methods

Patient's population

Between 2003 and 2009, forty-nine patients (35 females (71.4%) and 14 (28.6%) males) with an average age of 49.9 years (20-65 years) and an expected lower extremities fractures were treated.

Cause of bone softening	No. of patients
Osteomalacia and osteoporosis	25
Renal dialysis	6
Secondary bone metastasis	11
Rheumatoid arthritis	1
Hyperparathyroidism	2
Bone cyst	3
Primary bone Malignant	1
Total	49

Table 1: Clinical Data.

Pain was the most common symptom and was present in 35 patients (71.4%). Other symptoms and signs were difficult to walk and limping. 25 patients (51%) had looser zone and progressive decrease in neck shaft angle. Those patients were diagnosed as having osteomalacia. The remaining 24 patients (49%) had different bone softening conditions (Table 1). The femur was affected in 35 patients (71%), and the tibia was affected in 14 patients (29%) (Table 2).

Patient's evaluation

The diagnosis in all cases was done in a combined work between orthopedic, rheumatology, internal medicine and other necessary specialties. This was done by history, clinical, radiological and laboratory findings, in addition to biopsy.

Estimation of fracture at risk is a very important step to do prophylactic fixation. The fracture at risk is based on radiographic findings. The occurrence of pathological fractures depended upon many factors such as bone defect size, biological behavior of bone lesion, and the anatomic location.

Site affected	Number of patients	Method of fixation	Female	Male
Femur	12	Interlocking femoral nail and gamma nail	5	7
Neck of femur	20	DHS	13	7
Distal femur	2	distal locked femur plate	1	1
Tibia	12	Interlocking nail	6	6
Tibia	2	Locked plate	1	1
Femur	1	External fixators		1
Total	49		26	23

Table 2: Site Affected and Method of Management.

Harington's criteria:

>50% destruction of diaphyseal cortices

>50-75% destruction of metaphysis (>2.5 cm)

Permeative destruction of the subtrochanteric femoral region

Persistent pain following irradiation

The size of pathological defects is classified as two types [8]:

1. Lesions less than the diameter of the involved bone and

2. Lesion that is greater than the diameter of bone on the maximum dimension.

Prophylactic fixation is recommended for lesions finer than 2.5 cm or finer than 50% of the cross-sectional bone destruction [9]. The use of imaging in treatment planning depends on whether the differential diagnosis includes primary benign or malignant lesions. In benign lesions, the diagnosis depends upon the age, radiological characteristics and location of the lesions and the presence or absence of progressive or multiple lesions. The natural history of some tumors may require more advanced imaging [10].

The traditional surgical treatment of benign bone tumors has been curettage and autologous bone graft or marginal resection of expendable bone lesions [10] and prophylactic fixation if doubt of segment stability. Biopsy was done for lesions to type of lesion exclude malignancy and then treats and fix prophylactic ally like the primary lesions.

Scoring system was proposed [11] in an attempt to identify the risk of sustaining a pathological fracture through a metastatic defect in long bone. This system is based on four characteristics: (1) site of lesion; (2) nature of lesion; (3) size of a lesion; and (4) pain. All the features were assigned in progressive scores ranging from 1 to 3. According to Mirels' recommendation, prophylactic fixation is highly indicated for a lesion with an overall score of 9 or greater [11] (Table 3).

Mirels' score clinical recommendation is if ≤7 then radiotherapy and observation, if 8 then use clinical judgment and ≥9 then Prophylactic fixation.

Excluded from this study is any patient who already developed pathological fracture. Different types of fixation either surface plating (dynamic hip screws) (Figures 1 and 2). Medullary (Gamma nails) (Figure 3) or external fixation in cases unsuitable for surgery (Figure 4) were used according to the type and the site of the deformity. In tibial cases, we used the tourniquet without blood evacuation in the limb.

Variable	Score		
	1	2	3
Site	Upper limb	Lower limb	Peritrochanter
Pain	Mild	Moderate	Functional
Lesion	Basic	Mixed	Lytic
Size	<1/3	1/3-2/3	>2/3

Table 3: Mirel's scoring system (Mirels, 1989). It is based on four charecteristics: site of lesion, pain, nature of lesion and size of lesion. All the features were assigned progressive scores ranging from 1 to 3.

All patients with medical conditions were first managed by the specialist to treat the primary causes and all patients were evaluated post operatively regarding to: discharge destination, mortality, morbidity, pain status and daily activity.

Postoperative care

The postoperative physical therapy largely depends on the type of construct used and the intra-operative observations made by the surgeon regarding the quality of bone, screw purchase, and overall stability of the construct. The goal is to achieve mobility and independence in order to improve the quality of life and to decrease cardiopulmonary complications that are associated with immobility in the elderly patient. Adequate pain control is necessary for participation in physical therapy.

DVT prophylaxis is very important in cancer patients that are immobilized. Bisphosphonates, radiation therapy, and chemotherapy should be used as indicated, keeping in mind that radiation and chemotherapy decrease wound healing and may be delayed.

Results

In this study, all patients with impending fracture lesions with an overall score of 9 or greater went for prophylactic fixation [11]. There were 35 female (71.4%) and 14 male (28.6%) between the age of twenty and 65 years with an average age of 49.9 years with bending fractures of lower extremities. The average duration of follow-up was 2.2 years (range, 6- 48 months). The average blood loss was 250 ml, and the average surgery time was 135 minutes (45 minutes to 180 minutes). Most of blood loss was in the femoral cases.

All patients began to stand up within the first week after surgery and ambulated partially from the second week. Two cases of hyperparathyroidism had a combined orthopedic and general surgical treatment. In this series of patients, there were no cases of wound infection, deep venous thrombosis or decubitus ulcer. Wound drainage was seen in two cases; one was hepatic patient with blood Coagulopathy and was fixed by external fixation. The discharge was sterile and was treated by plasma transfusion and control blood bleeding profile.

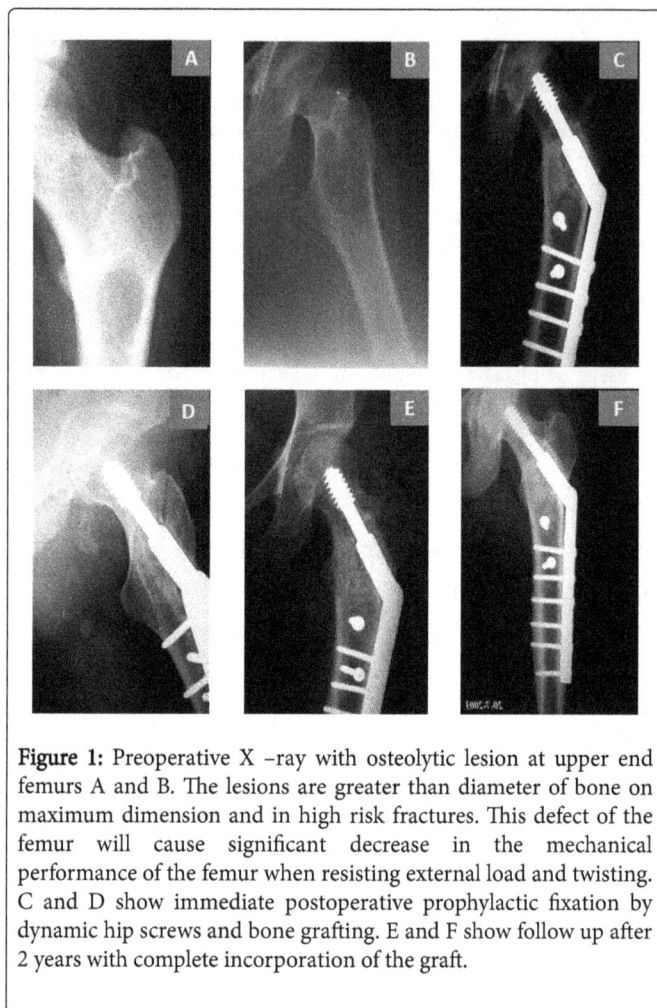

Figure 1: Preoperative X –ray with osteolytic lesion at upper end femurs A and B. The lesions are greater than diameter of bone on maximum dimension and in high risk fractures. This defect of the femur will cause significant decrease in the mechanical performance of the femur when resisting external load and twisting. C and D show immediate postoperative prophylactic fixation by dynamic hip screws and bone grafting. E and F show follow up after 2 years with complete incorporation of the graft.

The second case was treated by antibiotic after debridement, the culture of which was negative and resolved during 2 months. There was no instrumentation failure, loosening or mortality.

Most patients had significant relief of pain. 35 (71.5%) of patients with impending fracture were ambulatory after therapy and able to walk outdoor, while 10 (20.5%) of patients were able to walk inside door. We had 3 (6%) patients using wheel chair and they were on renal dialysis. Only one patient (2%) was not able to walk and he was not cooperative for unknown reason (Figure 5).

Discussion

Pathological fractures create a serious morbidity in patients with bone disease. Orthopedic surgeons who treat patients with skeletal lesions should focus on proactive treatments designed to prevent pathological fractures before they occur. Prophylactic fixations have decreased morbidity compared with patient's sustained fractures before fixation [11]. The difficulty lies in determining patients requiring prophylactic fixation. Many different criteria have been suggested including, pain over the site of lesion, size and location of the lesion, whether the lesion is blastic or lytic or mixed, irradiation of the lesion and the type of primary tumor in metastatic lesions [12].

bone and those that are greater than the diameter of bone on the maximum dimension. Smaller lesions called stress riser while a large defects called open section defect [8].

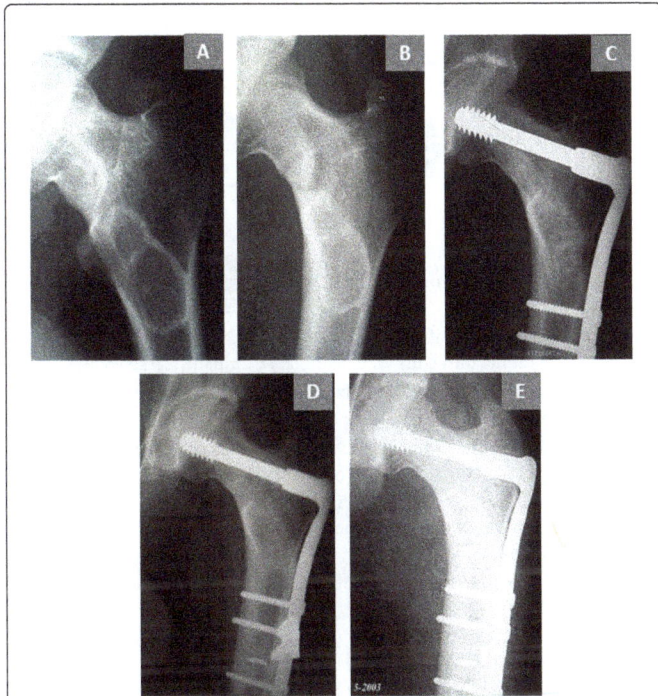

Figure 2: Preoperative X-rays of a lesion at the proximal end and neck of the femur (loser zone), the lesion is more than half of the diameter with an impending fracture at the neck of the femurs (A and B). C and D post-operative prophylactic fractures fixation by dynamic condylar plate. E shows 2 years follow up.

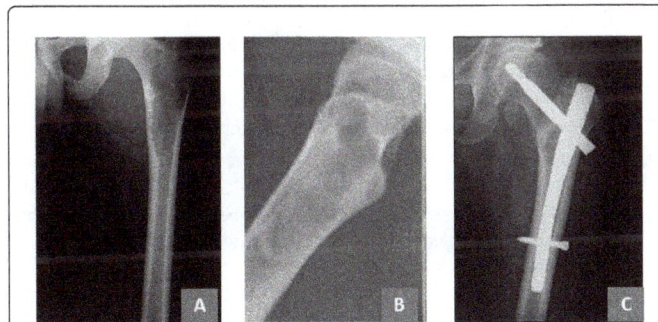

Figure 3: A and B Show an osteolytic lesion of the proximal end femur with high risk factors by increasing pain, the size of the lesion, radiographic appearance, localization, transverse/axial/circumferential involvement of the cortex and the scoring system of Mirels. C Shows post-operative fixation after one year with mild resolution of the cyst and heterotrophic calcification at site of nail insertion and head of femur.

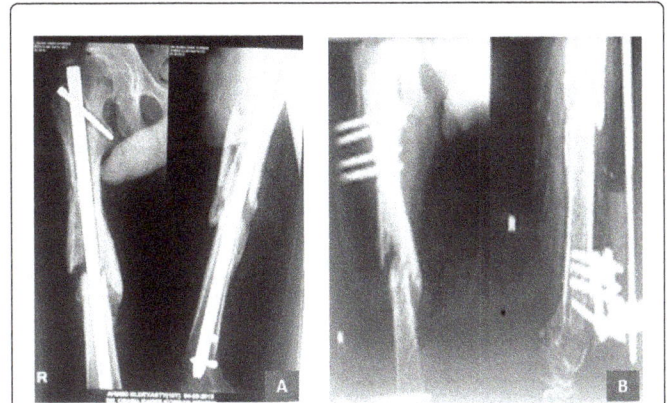

Figure 4: A) Shows an x-ray with post traumatic infected interlocking nail and partial healing of the fracture. B) After debridement of the infection, removal of the nail with the risk of sustaining a pathological fracture through a defect in long bone. A prophylactic external fixator was applied to avoid a pathological fracture.

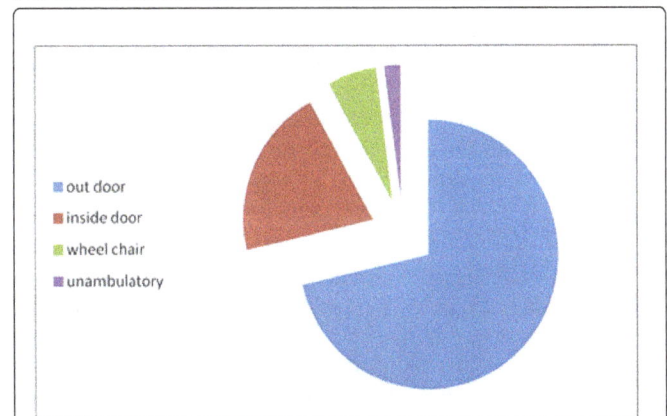

Figure 5: The mean duration of hospitalization was 21 days (range from 7 to 35 days). That time included preoperative period of investigation and preparation and post-operative surgery and rehabilitation.

In order to determine which patient require prophylactic fixation to prevent pathological fracture, it is necessary to perform accurate and reliable risk evaluations. Many factors, including patient himself, non-neoplastic diseases that cause pathologic fractures, tumor nature (malignant or benign), pain and lastly, responsiveness to non-surgical treatment can affect the discussion [11]. The potential for pathological fracture can be assisted by size as the bone defect which could be classified under two types, these less than the diameter of the involved

It is of importance to stress on the anatomic location of the bony lesions for the assessment of potential fractures [13]. As the lower limbs to support body weight for ambulation, so, lesions in these areas are at increased risk for pathological fracture, specifically, those lesions in the proximal femur which are considered to be at the greatest risk for fracture among all long bone lesions [14].

The most important factor to be considered in deciding the treatment option for the management of impending bone fracture due to bone softening disease is the level of the patient's dysfunction and pain. Severe dysfunction or pain demands a treatment that predictably leads to a quick resumption of the painless activities of daily living and to prevent fractures. Prophylactic surgical treatment of impending fractures has been shown to improve outcomes [15]. Early management will help the patient to continue and shorten the treatment period and the need for assistance.

Prophylactic fixation has been recommended for lesions finer than 2.5 cm or finer than 50% of cross sectional bone destruction [9]. The consequences of pathological fracture in this area are significant so that prophylactic fixation prevents pathological complications [12,16].

Biologic behavior of bony lesions is another factor in determining the possibility for pathological fracture. Biologic aggressiveness can be inferred from whether the lesion is lytic or blastic or mixed (lytic and blastic). Zickel and Mouradian [17] reviewed 34 patients and found that lesions could be listed in ascending order of least likely to fracture are blastic lesions, mixed blastic and lytic lesion then purely lytic lesions, which are the most prone to pathological fracture.

The treatment of patients with an expected short life span as those suffering from metastatic disease is considered to be very important to help them. A bone that has lost its structural integrity, even though not grossly fractured, will not support weight bearing for months even if the metastasis is eliminated. Control of the metastatic tumor does not always equate with return to function [18].

It is a reasonable goal to avoid bone softening or bone metastasis to progress to pathological fracture. Function can almost always be returned to these patients with impending fractures. This can be done by surgical stabilization, which may be the best way to return the patient's function while he/she is being treated postoperatively with medical therapy, radiotherapy or chemotherapy.

Comprehensive management of patients with soft bone disease requires the participation of an orthopedic surgeon early in the clinical course. The orthopedic surgeon's role should be more than patching together fractured bones that have not responded to other treatment modalities. Early consultation and mutual follow-up will benefit a patient in maintaining independent function and avoid irretrievable catastrophes.

In this study, many devices were used. Most of the cases with hip affection due to osteomalacia were fixed by dynamic hip screws. These devices allow an open exposure of lesions' sites, which is useful in cases that require open biopsy and diagnostic confirmation. Intramedullary nails can be used for femoral shaft lesion if there is permeate destruction without significant focal size area of cortical loss. For most patients with impending fracture from femoral metastasis, insertion of reconstruction nail is favorable. This technique provides resistance to be torsional stresses as well as angular displacement throughout the full length of the femur, including the intertrochanteric and femoral neck areas [6].

External fixators were used in patients with medical conditions that prevent surgical interference. Active and prompt treatment of pathological fractures is justified. In the present series, all patients were relieved of pain immediately after fixation and as a consequence of the fracture treatment; it became easier to mobilize them. The length of the hospital stay is reduced and for those patients who cannot be mobilized because of their primary disease, the nursing care is made easier.

Conclusion

Surgical fixation of fractures in weight-bearing long bones with impending fractures provides pain relief, and a functionally stable and durable construct. It helps an early ambulation and prevents fracture complications. It allows independent function and avoids irretrievable catastrophes.

References

1. Hadjidakis DJ, Androulakis II (2006) Bone remodeling. Ann N Y Acad Sci 1092: 385-396.

2. Levine AM, Aboulafia AJ (2008) Pathologic Fractures in Browner: Skeletal Trauma (4th edn) W. B. Saunders Company, United States.

3. Rodan GA, Martin TJ (2000) Therapeutic Approaches to Bone Diseases. Science 289: 1508-1514.

4. Altman H (1953) Metallic fixation for pathologic fracture and impending fracture of long bones. J Int Coll Surg 19: 612-617.

5. Bremner RA, Jelliffe AM (1958) The management of pathological fracture of the major long bones from metastatic cancer. J Bone Joint Surg Br 40: 652-659.

6. Johnson EW (1957) Intramedullary fixation of pathological fractures. JAMA 163: 417-419.

7. Katzner M, Petit R, Schvingt E (1974) Surgical treatment of metastases and metastaic fractures of the long bones. Apropos of 53 palliative osteosynthesis. Rev Chir Orthop Reparatrice Appar Mot 60: 387-400.

8. Haentjens P, Casteleyn PP, Opdecam P (1993) Evaluation of impending fractures and indications for prophylactic fixation of metastases in long bones. Review of the literature. Acta Orthop Belg 59: 6-11.

9. Hipp JA, Springfield DS, Hayes WC (1995) Predicting pathologic fracture risk in the management of metastatic bone defects. Clin Orthop Relat Res 312: 120-135.

10. Gibbs CP, Lewis VO, Peabody T (2005) Beyond bone grafting: techniques in the surgical management of benign bone tumors. Instr Course Lect 54: 497-503.

11. Mirels H (1989) Metastatic disease in long bones. A proposed scoring system for diagnosing impending pathologic fractures. Clin Orthop Relat Res 249: 256-264.

12. O'Donnell P (2013) Impending Fracture & Prophylactic Fixation.

13. Harrington KD (1986) Impending pathologic fractures from metastatic malignancy: evaluation and management. Instr Course Lect 35: 357-381.

14. Keene JS, Sellinger DS, McBeath AA, Engber WD (1986) Metastatic breast cancer in the femur. A search for the lesion at risk of fracture. Clin Orthop Relat Res 203: 282-288.

15. Ward WG, Holsenbeck S, Dorey FJ, Spang J, Howe D (2003) Metastatic disease of the femur: surgical treatment. Clin Orthop Relat Res 415: S230-S244.

16. Van Geffen E, Wobbes T, Veth RP, Gelderman WA (1997) Operative management of impending pathological fractures: a critical analysis of therapy. J Surg Oncol 64: 190-194.

17. Zickel RE, Mouradian WH (1976) Intramedullary fixation of pathological fractures and lesions of the Subtrochanteric region of the femur. J Bone Joint Surg 58: 1061-1066.

18. Colyer RA (1986) Surgical stabilization of pathological neoplastic fractures. Curr Probl Cancer 10: 117-168.

24

Oral Aspects of Metabolic Disorders

Ankita Bohra* and Bhateja S

P.G Oral Medicine and Radiology Department, Vyas Dental College and Hospital, Jodhpur, India

*Corresponding author:Ankita Bohra, P.G Oral Medicine and Radiology Department, Vyas Dental College and Hospital, Jodhpur, India;
E-mail: aav1423@hotmail.com

Abstract

Metabolism is a complex process that involves a series of chemical reactions in the human body. Alterations in these metabolic processes constitute the disturbances of metabolism causing metabolic disorders. The breakdown of carbohydrate by the oral microorganisms has been the subject of numerous investigations. This review discusses the oral aspects of metabolic diseases.

Keywords: Metabolism; Oral flora; Metabolic disorder

Introduction

Metabolism

Duncan defined metabolism as "the sum total of tissue activity as considered in terms of physicochemical changes associated with and regulated by the availability, utilization and disposal of protein, fat, carbohydrate, vitamins, minerals, water and the influences which the endocrines exert on these processes". Metabolism is a complex process that involves a series of chemical reactions in the human body. Some reactions produce the energy which is stored in the form of ATP while other reactions consume energy to manufacture complex compounds. The process of metabolism includes 2 types of mechanisms, i.e, catabolism and anabolism [1].

Catabolism is a process which involves release of energy by breaking complex organic compounds into simple molecules. Thus, in this process energy is been produced.

Anabolism is a process that requires energy for synthesis of complex compounds from small molecules. In this process energy is been utilized.

Alterations in these metabolic processes constitute the disturbances of metabolism causing metabolic disorders. The breakdown of carbohydrate by the oral microorganisms has been the subject of numerous investigations [2]. It is believed by many that the intraoral production of acids from carbohydrate, arising from incomplete oxidation, is a factor in the production of dental caries, periodontal diseases, oral malodor, bone loss and other associated metabolic diseases [3].

Types of Metabolic Disorders [4,5]

- Disturbances in Protein metabolism
- Disturbances in Lipid metabolism
- Disturbances in Carbohydrate metabolism
- Disturbances in hormone metabolism
- Lysosomal storage disorders
- Mitochondrial storage disorders

Disturbances of protein metabolism

Amyloidosis: It is a rare disease that results from accumulation of inappropriately folded proteins. These misfolded proteins are called amyloids. When proteins that are normally soluble in water fold to become amyloids, they become insoluble and deposit in organs or tissues, disrupting normal function.

Protein energy malnutrition: PEM includes Kwashiorkor (protein malnutrition predominant), Marasmus (deficiency in calorie intake), Marasmic Kwashiorkor (marked protein deficiency and marked calorie insufficiency signs present, sometimes referred to as the most severe form of malnutrition) PEM is fairly common worldwide in both children and adults and accounts for 6 million deaths annually. PEM may be secondary to other conditions such as chronic renal disease or cancer cachexia in which protein energy wasting may occur.

Porphyria: The porphyrias are a group of rare diseases in which chemical substances called porphyrins accumulate. The body requires porphyrins to produce heme, which carries oxygen in the blood; but, in the porphyrias, there is a deficiency (inherited or acquired) of the enzymes that transform the various porphyrins into others, leading to abnormally high levels of one or more of these substances. This manifests with either neurological complications or skin problems or occasionally both.

Erythropoietic uroporphyria: It is caused by genetic defects which lead to deficiency of the enzyme uroporphyrinogen III cosynthase (UROS). The disease is characterised by extreme photosensitivity (abnormal cutaneous reaction to sunlight) which can leave severe scarring, blister formation and the loss of digits or other features. Damaged skin can become infected, leading to further necrosis and deformities. The face, hands and arms are the most significantly affected as they are frequently exposed; sometimes presenting as severe disfiguration.

Disturbances in carbohydrate metabolism [6]

Mucopolysacchridoses result from abnormal degradation of glycosaminoglycans. Disorders in carbohydrate metabolism include Mucopolysacchridoses (MPS) type I, II, III, IV, VIa, VIb, VII.

MPS Type I includes Hurler and Scheie syndrome: It is a cutaneous condition characterized by mild mental retardation and corneal clouding (Figure 1).

MPS Type II includes Hunter syndrome: (mild to severe form) It is a lysosomal storage disease caused by a deficient or absent enzyme, iduronate-2-sulfatase (I2S). The accumulated substrates in Hunter syndrome are heparan sulfate and dermatan sulfate. The syndrome has X-linked recessive inheritance.

MPS Type III includes Sanfillippo syndrome: It is a metabolism disorder passed down through families. It makes the body unable to properly break down long chains of sugar molecules called glycosaminoglycans (formerly called mucopolysaccharides). The syndrome belongs to a group of diseases called mucopolysaccharidoses (MPS).

MPS Type IV includes Morquio syndrome: It is an autosomal recessive mucopolysaccharide storage disease usually inherited. It is a rare type of birth defect with serious consequences like cardiovascular and ophthalmic defects.

MPS Type VIa includes Maroteaux- Lamy syndrome (classic form) MPS Type VIb includes Maroteaux- Lamy syndrome (mild form): It is a form of mucopolysaccharidosis caused by a deficiency in arylsulfatase B (ARSB). Symptoms include neurological complications like clouded corneas, deafness, thickening of the dura and pain caused by compressed or traumatized nerves and nerve roots.

MPS Type VII includes beta glucuronidase deficiency: It is a very rare genetic disorder with high mortality rate. Congenital defect in multiple organs with gender predilection for males.

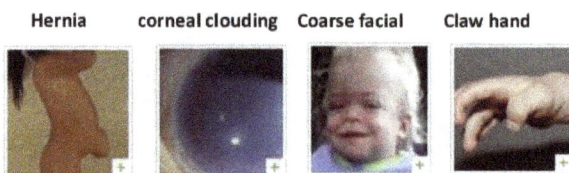

Figure 1: Showing key features of Hurler syndrome.

Disturbances in lipid metabolism [7]

Gaucher's disease: It is a genetic disease in which glucosylceramide accumulate in cells and certain organs. The disorder is characterized by bruising, fatigue, anaemia, low blood platelets, and enlargement of the liver and spleen. It is caused by a hereditary deficiency of the enzyme glucocerebrosidase.

Niemann-Pick disease: It is one of a group of lysosomal storage diseases that affect metabolism and that are caused by genetic mutations. Enlargement of the liver and spleen (hepatosplenomegaly) may cause reduced appetite, abdominal distension, and pain.

Letterer-Siwe disease: It is the acute disseminated multisystem form of Langerhans cell histiocytosis characterised by proliferation of nonlipid histiocytes in the viscera and bones. Clinical features include a variety of skin lesions, osteolytic lesions, lymphadenopathy, hepatosplenomegaly, pulmonary infiltration, spiking fever, anaemia, thrombocytopenia, mandibular hyperplasia, gingival inflammation, loss of teeth, otitis media, hemorrhages, failure to thrive, cachexia.

Disturbances in Hormone metabolism [8]

Pituitary hormone: Hypopituitarism: Symptoms include fatigue, low blood pressure, weight loss, weakness, depression, nausea, or vomiting, constipation, weight gain, sensitivity to cold, decreased energy, and muscle weakness or aching. In women, symptoms include irregular or stopped menstrual periods and infertility. Hyperpituitarism: Symptoms includes headaches, visual disturbance, and growth failure, weight gain. Hirsutism and premature adrenarche may occur in prepubertal children. Pubertal arrest, acne, fatigue, and depression are also common.

Thyroid hormone: Hyperthyroidim includes irritability, muscle weakness, sleeping problems, a fast heartbeat, poor tolerance of heat, diarrhea, enlargement of the thyroid gland, exopthalamus and weight loss. Hypothyroidsm includes poor ability to tolerate cold, a feeling of tiredness, and weight gain. In children, hypothyroidism leads to delays in growth and intellectual development which is called cretinism.

Parathyroid hormone: Hyperparathyroidism includes depression, fatigue, polydypsia and polyuria, feeling sick and losing your appetite, muscle weakness, constipation, tummy pain, loss of concentration. Hypoparathyroidism includes muscle aches or cramps, tingling, burning, or numbness in fingertips, toes, and lips, muscle spasms, especially around the mouth, patchy hair loss, dry skin, brittle nails, fatigue, anxiety or depression.

Lysosomal storage disorders [9,10]

Lysomal storage disorders are a group of approximately 50 rare inherited metabolic disorders results from defects in lysosomal function. Lysosomes are sacs of enzymes within cells that digest large molecules and pass the fragments on to other parts of the cell for recycling. This process requires several critical enzymes. If one of these enzymes is defective, because of a mutation, the large molecules accumulate within the cell, eventually killing it. The symptoms of lysosomal storage disease vary, depending on the particular disorder and other variables like the age of onset, and can be mild to severe. They include developmental delay, movement disorders, seizures dementia, deafness and/or blindness, hepatomegaly splenomegaly and cardiac problems, and bones that grow abnormally. Some examples are listed below.

Schinder disease/Kanzaki disease: Schindler disease results from the deficient activity of the enzyme alpha-N-acetylgalactosaminidase (alpha-galactosidase B), with the accumulation of sialylated-asialo-glycopeptide and oligosaccharide with alpha-N-acetylgalactosamilnyl residues.

Faber disease: (Farber's lipogranulomatosis, ceramidase deficiency) is an extremely rare (80 cases reported worldwide to this day) autosomal recessive lysosomal storage disease marked by a deficiency in the enzyme ceramidase that causes an accumulation of fatty material lipids leading to abnormalities in the joints, liver, throat, tissues and central nervous system.

Krabbe disease: (globoid cell leukodystrophy) is a rare, often fatal degenerative disorder that affects the myelin sheath of the nervous system. It is a form of sphingolipidosis, as it involves dysfunctional metabolism of sphingolipids. This condition is inherited in an autosomal recessive pattern.

Tay-Sachs and Sandhoff diseases: is a rare autosomal recessive genetic disorder. It causes a progressive deterioration of nerve cells and of mental and physical abilities that begins around six months of age and usually results in death by the age of four.

Pyknodysostosis: also known as osteopetrosis acro-osteolytica or Toulouse-Lautrec syndrome is a rare autosomal recessive bone dysplasia, characterised by osteosclerosis and short stature.

Mitochondrial diseases [11]

Mitochondrial disease is a group of disorders caused by dysfunctional mitochondria, the organelles that generate energy for the cell. Mitochondrial disorders may be caused by mutations, acquired or inherited, in mitochondrial DNA (mtDNA) or in nuclear genes that code for mitochondrial components. They may also be the result of acquired mitochondrial dysfunction due to adverse effects of drugs, infections, or other environmental causes. Symptoms include poor growth, loss of muscle coordination, muscle weakness, visual problems, hearing problems, learning disabilities, heart disease, liver disease, kidney disease, gastrointestinal disorders, respiratory disorders, neurological problems, autonomic dysfunction and dementia. Examples of mitochondrial diseases include-

Luft disease: Consist of Hypermetabolism, with fever, heat intolerance, profuse perspiration, polyphagia, polydipsia, ragged-red fibers, and resting tachycardia. Exercise intolerance with mild weakness.

Leigh syndrome: Consist of subacute sclerosing encephalopathy after normal development the disease usually begins late in the first year of life, although onset may occur in adulthood. A rapid decline in function occurs and is marked by seizures, altered states of consciousness, dementia, ventilatory failure (Figure 2).

Alpers disease: Also called as Progressive Infantile Poliodystrophy. Symptoms include seizures, dementia, spasticity, blindness, liver dysfunction, and cerebral degeneration.

Pearson marrow syndrome: It is a mitochondrial disease characterized by sideroblastic anaemia and exocrine pancreas dysfunction. Clinical features includes failure to thrive, pancreatic fibrosis, muscle and neurologic impairment, and, frequently, early death.

Wilson disease: is an autosomal recessive disorder in which copper accumulates in tissues this manifests as neurological or psychiatric symptoms and liver disease. It is treated with medication that reduces copper absorption or removes the excess copper from the body, but occasionally a liver transplant is required.

Batten disease: It is a rare, fatal autosomal recessive neurodegenerative disorder that begins in childhood. Early signs may be subtle personality and behaviour changes, slow learning or regression, repetitive speech or echolalia, clumsiness, or stumbling. There may be slowing head growth in the infantile form, poor

circulation in lower extremities (legs and feet), decreased body fat and muscle mass, curvature of the spine, hyperventilation and/or breath-holding spells, teeth grinding, and constipation.

Menkes disease: It is a disorder that affects copper levels in the body leading to copper deficiency. It is an x linked recessive disorder, and is therefore considerably more common in males: females require two defective alleles to develop the disease. Signs and symptoms of this disorder include weak muscle tone (hypotonia), sagging facial features, seizures, intellectual disability, blue sclera and developmental delay. The patients have brittle hair and metaphyseal widening. In rare cases, symptoms begin later in childhood and are less severe. Affected infants may be born prematurely.

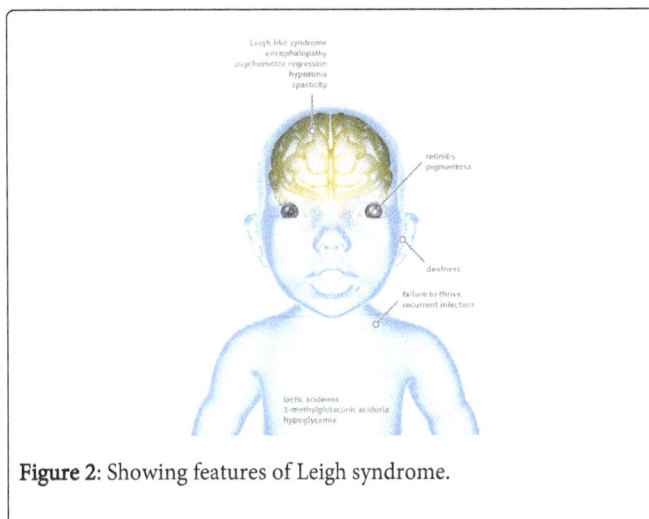

Figure 2: Showing features of Leigh syndrome.

Conclusion

Process of metabolism is very complex and intermingled with multiple factors responsible for homeostasis. Oral microbial flora also plays a vital role in this process. Any kind of change in the pathway from cellular to macroscopic level may give rise to number of metabolic diseases associated with local and systemic changes. This review enlightens various types of metabolic disorders and their associated oral conditions.

References

1. Ebenhöh O, Heinrich R (2001) Evolutionary optimization of metabolic pathways. Theoretical reconstruction of the stoichiometry of ATP and NADH producing systems. Bull Math Biol 63: 21-55.

2. Takahashi N, Sato T (2002) Dipeptide utilization by the periodontal pathogens Porphyromonas gingivalis, Prevotella intermedia, Prevotella nigrescens and Fusobacterium nucleatum. Oral Microbiol Immunol 17: 50-54.

3. Niederman R, Zhang J, Kashket S (1997) Short-chain carboxylic-acid-stimulated, PMN-mediated gingival inflammation. Crit Rev Oral Biol Med 8: 269-290.

4. Takahashi N, Saito K, Schachtele CF, Yamada T (1997) Acid tolerance of growth and neutralizing activity of Porphyromonas gingivalis, Prevotella intermedia and Fusobacterium nucleatum. Oral Microbiol Immunol 12: 323-328.

5. Mayanagi G, SatoT, Shimauchi H, Takahashi N (2004) Detection frequency of periodontitis-associated bacteria by polymerase chain reaction in subgingival and supragingival plaque of subjects with periodontitis and healthy subjects. Oral Microbiol Immunol 19: 379-385.

6. Saito K, Takahashi N, Horiuchi H, Yamada T (2001) Effects of glucose on formation of cytotoxic end-products and proteolytic activity of Prevotella intermedia and Prevotella nigrescens. J Periodontal Res 36: 355-360.

7. Ratcliff PA, Johnson PW (1999) The relationship between oral malodor, gingivitis, and periodontitis. A review. J Periodontol 70: 485-489.

8. Winchester B, Vellodi A, Young E (2000) The molecular basis of lysosomal storage diseases and their treatment. Biochem Soc Trans 28: 150-154.

9. Ponder KP, Haskins ME (2007) Gene therapy for mucopolysaccharidosis. Expert Opin Biol Ther 7: 1333-1345.

10. Finsterer J (2007) Hematological manifestations of primary mitochondrial disorders Acta Haematol 118: 88–98.

11. Marriage B, Clandinin MT, Glerum DM (2003) Nutritional cofactor treatment in mitochondrial disorders. J Am Diet Assoc 103: 1029-1038.

25

Readiness of Primary Health Care Facilities in Jimma Zone to Provide Diabetic Services for Diabetic Clients, Jimma Zone, South West Ethiopia, March, 2013

Fikru Tafese[1], Elias Teferi[2*], Beyene Wondafirash[1], Sintayehu Fekadu[1], Garumma Tolu[1] and Gugsa Nemarra[1]

[1]Department of Health Service Management, School of Public Health, Jimma University, Jimma, Ethiopia

[2]Department of Public health, College of Medicine and Health Sciences, Ambo University, Addis Ambo, Ethiopia

*Corresponding author: Elias Teferi, Ambo University, Ambo, Ethiopia; E-mail: eliasteferi2015@gmail.com

Abstract

Background: Diabetes is one of the commonest non-communicable diseases of the 21st century. Global burden of diabetes in 2010 was estimated at 285 million and projected to increase to 438 million by the year 2030, if no interventions are put in place. The primary health care facilities are the first level of contact for such rising cases of diabetes, despite of this fact there is no study done on the capabilities of primary health care facilities to accommodate diabetic services. Hence, the objective of this study is to assess the readiness of selected primary public hospitals and health centers to accommodate diabetic care in Jimma zone south west Ethiopia.

Methods: Health facility based cross-sectional study design using quantitative and qualitative method of data collection was conducted from Feb 1-March 1, 2013. After checking the completeness, and coding of questionnaires, the quantitative data were entered into computer software and analyzed using SPSS version 20.0.

Results: All of the facilities have at least some of the drugs and medical supplies and other resources required for the diagnosis and management of diabetes never the less there was no specific plan to deal with diabetic management at health facilities. Majority of patients were first diagnosed in other health facilities and referred to the current health institutions for follow up and there is no routine screening for diabetics in adult outpatient department in some health facilities.

Conclusion and recommendation: Required drugs and medical supplies are not regularly fulfilled, health facilities have no plan for diabetic management, and health workers did not get training on management of diabetics. No routine screening at adult patients at outpatient departments. Hence the Woreda and the zone have to work on the capacity of the health workers and health facilities to handle diabetic care at health center level.

Keywords: Diabetics; PHC; Ethiopia; Jimma University

Introduction

Diabetes mellitus is a chronic metabolic disorder that occurs when the pancreas does not produce enough insulin, or when the body cannot effectively use the insulin it produces or both [1]. This results in elevated blood sugar (hyperglycemia) and other metabolic derangements which over time lead to multiple organ damage. The common complications of diabetes include eye complications, damage to heart, blood vessels, kidneys, nervous system and foot complications leading to amputations [1]. Diabetes is one of the commonest non-communicable diseases of the 21st century. In 2007 the global burden of diabetes was estimated to be 246 million people. In its 2009 Diabetes atlas publication, the international Diabetes federation, the global burden of diabetes in 2010 was estimated at 285 million and projected to increase to 438 million by the year 2030, if no interventions are put in place [2].

This rise in diabetes is associated with demographic and social changes such as globalization, urbanization, aging population and adoption of unhealthy lifestyles such as consumption of unhealthy diets and physical inactivity. Despite the higher prevalence of diabetes in high-income countries, the majority of the disease burden from

diabetes, more than 70%, is in the developing regions because of their larger populations. The prevalence of diabetes in traditional rural African communities is less than 1% but escalates up to 30% in cities [2].

The predisposing factors include advancing age, family history, excessive body weight, excessive alcohol consumption, lack of physical inactivity, Stress, Unhealthy diet, Gestational Diabetes mellitus and chronic use of steroids [1,3,4]. Diabetes mellitus often goes undiagnosed because many of its symptoms though serious are often missed or are treated as common ailments [5].

Ethiopia, which is one of the developing nations, is at a risk of increased diabetes incidence. In Ethiopia, the number of deaths attributed to diabetes reached over 21,000 in 2007 [6]. Community based studies are non-existent at the national level and hospitals may give figures of those who come for treatment and follow up. As a result, the national estimate is based on neighboring countries with similar socio-economic situations and accordingly, 2%-3% of the population is estimated to live with diabetes in Ethiopia. No population-based prevalence study exists in Ethiopia but from hospital based studies it can be seen that the prevalence of diabetes admission has increased from 1.9% in 1970 to 9.5% in 1999 of all medical admissions [4-7].

WHO estimated the number of diabetics in Ethiopia to be about 800,000 cases by the year 2000, and the number is expected to increase to 1.8 million by 2030 [8]. In Ethiopia, the average age at death of people with Type 1 diabetes is of just 32 years [9]. In urban areas, Type 2 diabetes accounts for 71% of the people with the condition. When compared with the urban population, the proportion of people in the rural areas who are known to have Type 2 diabetes appears to be relatively very low 23% of the people with the condition [9].

An assessment conducted by FMOH Ethiopia in 2008 has revealed that non communicable diseases such as cardiovascular diseases, diabetes mellitus and cancers are among the major Contributors to the high level of mortality and morbidity. The combined prevalence of impaired fasting glucose and glucose tolerance test was 14.8% in Jimma town [10] and the overall prevalence of chronic non communicable disease in Gilgel Gibe Field Research Center was 8.9% (7.8% men and 9.8% women). The specific observed prevalence was 0.5% for diabetes mellitus in this Fielded research [11]. Slow implementation of programmes to tackle NCDs is one of the challenge forwarded by HSDP III and it is recommended (by HSDP IV) undertaking the necessary preparedness with regard to growing burden of non-communicable diseases and emerging medical conditions.

The overall goal of diabetes management is to help individuals with diabetes and their families gain the necessary knowledge life skills, resources, and support them to achieve optimal health. This is done through team effort and in a stepwise approach. The approaches to diabetes management are nutritional management, physical exercise, psychological support, drug treatment: using insulin and or oral anti-diabetic drugs depending on the type of diabetes and the individual patient, monitoring of blood glucose [1,3,4].

Therefore, despite its multi-system effects, diabetes is a controllable disease, and enormous human and economic toll can be significantly reduced by early and aggressive ongoing therapeutic intervention specifically at primary level of care. Therefore if diabetes care is to achieve the health benefits that modern science has made possible, it must be continuous, proactive, planned, patient centered, and population based at the point of first contact in health system especially in resource limited settings. The purpose of this study is therefore, to determine the level to which the primary level healthcare facilities accommodate services for diabetic clients.

Methods and Materials

Study area and period

The study was conducted in PHC facilities in Jimma zone from Feb1-March 1, 2013. Jimma zone is one of the 18 Zones in Oromia Regional State in which its main city is located at about 357 km away from the capital in the Southwest. According to the Ethiopian 2007 census report, the zone has a total population of 2,692,740 [12]. The majority of the population lives in rural area and engaged in farming activities. Politically the zone is subdivided in to 18 administrative Woredas, which are further subdivided in to 545 administrative Kebeles (515 rural and 30 urban Kebeles).

In the zone eight health centers, namely Serbo , Assan Daboo, Omo Nada, Sheki, Seka, Shebe, Yebu and Agaro were giving chronic non communicable disease services (epilepsy, diabetes and cardiovascular diseases) in collaboration with Jimma University and tropical health and education Trust (THET) and the British council project. Jimma

University and tropical health and education Trust mainly train health officers and nurses in those health centers and provide supplies and drugs for screaming and management of theses chronic diseases [13]. But other PHCs in Jimma zone were providing these services by the government budget.

Study design

Health facility based cross-sectional study design that with quantitative and qualitative method of data collection was conducted.

Sample size, sampling technique and population

All diabetic patients that fulfill the inclusion criteria were interviewed, the average number of diabetic patients on follow up in the month before data collection was 15 per each health facility, therefore based on this 240 patients are expected. All health care providers working in the facilities during data collection period (320, that means 120 for facilities under THET project and 200 for facilities not under THET project) were included.

Five patient provider interactions at each health facility were observed. For qualitative study one key informant from zonal health office, each selected Woredas' chronic disease program coordinator and each selected PHC facility heads were purpose fully selected for in-depth interview.

As source population, all diagnosed diabetic patients who were on follow up in Jimma Zone PHC facilities during the data collection period were considered. All healthcare providers working in the PHC facilities during the data collection period and the focal persons from zonal health office, and each selected Woredas' chronic disease program coordinator were also taken as source population.

Inclusion criteria

Adults who came for diabetic follow at selected facilities during the study period.

Exclusion criteria

Diabetic patients who were unstable due to complications of diabetes like diabetic keto acidosis (DKA) and other co-morbidities were excluded.

Operational definitions

Resource for diabetic care: Includes laboratory equipment and reagents, staffs, registration format and plan documents at PHC facility level.

Provider's knowledge: It is measured based on modules and guide lines to manage Diabetes at PHC level. These include mentioning main sign and symptom of diabetes, laboratory investigation, drug management, and health information and when to refer the diabetic patient).

Healthcare providers' attitude: It was measured on five-point likert scale using four questions. The attitude score was standardized as a percentage of maximum scale score so that the score was between ranges 0 and 100.

PHC facilities: This includes primary hospitals and health centers.

Readiness of facility: It was measured by resources, health workers knowledge and attitude, and plan documents for diabetic services based on WHO guideline [14].

Study variables, data collection instruments and procedures: Measurements Variables that have been theoretically, empirically and conceptually linked to Resource for diabetic care, Provider's knowledge, Healthcare providers' attitude, Readiness of facility were used in this study.

Accordingly, Socio-demographic variables (Age, marital status, educational status, religion, occupation and residence), Availability of logistics and supplies (urine test kits, glucose test kits, glucometer, swabs, lancets, 45% DW), Availability diabetic drugs and diagnostic set ups, Availability of trained staffs, Availability of local plans were taken as independent variables. The dependent variables were Patients perception, Healthcare providers' knowledge and Healthcare providers' attitude.

Quantitative data collection tools were adapted after review of relevant literatures [15] and modified to the local situation. For qualitative data collection, FGD guide in-depth interview guide and checklist were developed based on national guideline. The exit interviews were conducted by five trained diploma nurses who can speak Afan Oromo (local language) fluently. Key informants were interviewed by four BSC holders in public health. FGD was conducted by PI and two masters of public health holders.

Data quality control

To ensure quality of the data, adapted questionnaires were used for data collection. In addition, pre- testing of all the data collection tools on 5% of the study subjects on Jimma University specialized hospital was done prior to the actual conduction of study. Moreover, training was given for three consecutive days in interview technique, and ethical issues, emphasizing the importance of safety of the participants and interviewers, minimization of under reporting and maintaining confidentiality.

Data analysis

After checking the completeness, and coding of questionnaires, the quantitative data were entered into computer software and analyzed using SPSS version 17.0 windows. The findings were presented in mainly tables. The qualitative data was analyzed thematically and presented by narrating and triangulated to the quantitative findings.

Ethical considerations

Before field work, ethical clearance was obtained from the ethical review board of the College of Public Health and Medical Science, Jimma University. Jimma zonal health department and respective Woreda health office were informed to get the official letters to conduct the study.

After a brief explanation on the purpose of the research, clients who gave verbal consent were interviewed at the end of their visit by trained interviewers who were not members of the clinics' staffs. Participants' involvement in the study was on voluntary basis. Farther more, confidentiality was assured by excluding name of the clients from any response obtained.

Results

Socio demographic characteristics

Eight health facilities (one primary hospital and seven health centers were assessed and 207 patients on chronic follow up were interviewed. The mean age of the patients was 42 years, majority of them are from rural area 128(61.8). More than half of them were farmers 115(55.6) (Table 1).

Variables	N=207	No	%
Residence	Urban	79	38.2
	Rural	128	61.8
Ethnicity	Oromo	167	80.7
	Amhara	25	12.1
	Others	15	7.2
Religion	Musilim	139	67.1
	Christan	67	32.1
	Others	1	0.5
Marital status	Married	141	68.1
	Single	42	20.3
	Others	24	11.6
Occupation	Farmer	115	55.6
	Merchant	30	14.5
	Civil servant	27	13
	House wife	14	6.8
Educational status	Illiterates	82	39.6
	Read and write only	53	25.6
	Primary school (1-8)	32	15.5
	Secondary school	16	7.7
	Grade 12 and above	24	11.6

Table 1: Major socio- demographic characteristics of the study subjects in Jimma Zone, south west Majority of the patients were diagnosed in year 2002 and more than half of them were first diagnosed in other health facilities and came to the health facilities where they have been interviewed for follow up.

Availability of resources

All of the health facilities have had some of the resources to treat chronic non communicable diseases at the time of data collection. The distribution of available resources at each health facility is presented in Table 2.

Even though the above drugs and medical supplies are there during the visit, most of the key informants have said that these resources are not regularly there and not planned according to the expected number of patients.

Knowledge and attitude of health workers

Thirty two health workers who were working at different department were assessed on their knowledge about diabetes management, twenty three (71%) of them were male, majority of them were nurse 22(87%), the minimum, maximum and mean service year of the health workers respectively was 1,21 and 6.7 with 6.34 Standard deviation. The minimum, maximum, mean age and Standard deviation of the health workers was 2,46,28.6 and 6.1 respectively. Majority of the respondents 25(78.1%) mentioned RBS/FBS as the major diagnostic approach to diabetes. Twenty nine (90.6%) of the respondents mentioned polyphagia as major symptom of diabetes. More than 80% of the respondent mentioned polydepsia as major symptom of diabetes. Polyuria was mentioned by 28(87.5%) of the health works as major symptom of diabetes.

Resources	Health facilities							
	Agaro HC	Limmu Hospital	Setema HC	Toba HC	Sheik HC	Shebe HC	Asandabo HC	Sokoru HC
Hb, WBC, ESR	yes	Yes	Yes	Yes	Yes	Yes	Yes	Yes
Fasting Blood Sugar	Yes	Yes	Yes	Yes	Yes	Yes	Yes	Yes
Cllini test	Yes	Yes	Yes	Yes	Yes	Yes	Yes	Yes
BUN and Creatinine	No	Yes	no	no	no	yes	yes	Yes
Lipid	no	Yes	no	no	no	no	no	no
HbA1c	no	Yes	no	no	no	no	no	no
Specific drugs for diabetes management	Yes	Yes	Yes	Yes	Yes	Yes	Yes	Yes
Insulin	Yes	Yes	Yes	Yes	Yes	Yes	Yes	Yes
Insulin syringes								
OHA	no	no	no	no	no	no	no	no
Drugs for management of complications of diabetes	no	Yes	no	no	no	no	no	no
Aldomet	Yes	Yes	Yes	Yes	Yes	Yes	Yes	Yes
Propranolol	Yes	Yes	Yes	Yes	Yes	Yes	Yes	Yes
Hydrochlorothiazide	Yes	Yes	Yes	Yes	Yes	Yes	Yes	Yes
Lasix	Yes	Yes	Yes	Yes	Yes	Yes	Yes	Yes
Digoxin								
Human power	Yes	Yes	Yes	Yes	Yes	Yes	Yes	Yes
Average number of Doctors	0	4	0	0	0	0	0	0
Average number of Nurses	5	12	4	6	4	6	6	8
Average number of laboratory technicians	3	4	2	2	2	2	3	3

Table 2: Availability of drugs, medical supplies and other resources in the health facilities, Jimma zone, south west Ethiopia, March 2013.

Majority of the health workers had no in-service training on diabetes management. The key informants have also supported this finding because most of them said that in-service trainings are mostly given on common infectious diseases like Tb, HIV and malaria.

Patients' perception on the services

Majority of patients 190 (91.8%) agreed that they regularly get the health care provider on their each follow-up. However thirty two 15.5% of them reported that they usually do not get the drug at their visit to health facilities for follow up. Almost all of the patients 200 (96.6%) reported that they come for the services regularly according to their appointment and majority of them have good perception that the health workers give them enough time to present their problems. 10% of the patients disagree that the health care providers did not tell about their current health problems. 17% of the patients disagree that the dose and frequency of their drug were well explained to them by health care providers. Almost 20% of the patients disagree that the health care provider did explain healthy life style to them (Table 3).

Discussion

In this study it is attempted to assess the readiness of primary health facilities to provide diabetes care. As there are few studies done on this area literatures are few to compare especially in Ethiopia. This study may also be limited. Since we have interviewed patients at health facility they might give the positive information only. But we have interviewed the facilities head and checked resources and plan availability to support quantitative findings. The availability of resources like drugs and laboratory facilities are there even though they are in comprehensive way not established well during data collection which is also supported by study done in Addis Abeba heath care facilities [16]. All key informants have also addressed that there is no specific plan to address this health problem at health facilities which made it difficult to address the resource issue comprehensively.

Heath care provider gave you enough time to explain complaints	Number	Percent
Strongly disagree	32	15.5
Disagree	20	9.7
Undecided	19	9.2
Agree	91	44.0
Strongly agree	45	21.7
Health care provider told you what could worsen health condition and what should the patient take care of		
Strongly disagree	24	11.6
Disagree	18	8.7
Undecided	36	17.4
Agree	76	36.7
Strongly agree	53	25.6
Health care provider has well explained to you the type, dose and frequency of the drug I should take		
Strongly disagree	12	5.8
Disagree	22	10.6
Undecided	31	15.0
Agree	85	41.1
Strongly agree	57	27.5

Table 3: Patients' perception to health care providers practice in giving them enough time for patients compliant (N=207), Jimma zone, south west Ethiopia, March 2013.

Majority of the patients were also diagnosed in other health facilities like Jimma university specialized hospital that also shows the current facilities are mostly receiving referred cases. It was also pointed out by key informants that there is no regular follow-up of the service since it is not in their priority plans. Even though majority of patients reported that they can get the health care providers during their follow-up visits, considerable number of them didn't get the drugs that they have to get. This is similar with the finding from study conducted in Egypt in which 87% of the patients said they were visiting their physician regularly [17]. Majority of the health care providers had good attitude

to the services as reported by majorities of the patients. However, this is not supported by patient's perception to what health care provider told them about what worsens their current problem and this could be due to lack of comprehensive knowledge about the disease. There is also no guideline for health care providers to help manage this problem which may also justify this patient's perception. concerning the drug and dose frequency, 17% of the patients disagree that the health care provider explained this issue for them, this may also be due to knowledge gap and facilities readiness in availing information that help these issues.

Health life style advice to patients was also not agreed by considerable number of patients and this has been very critical information equal to drug information, again this gap may be justified by health care providers' knowledge.

Conclusion and Recommendation

In conclusion, Required drugs and medical supplies are not regularly fulfilled, health facilities have no plan for diabetic management, health workers particularly working at the outpatient departments had not given training on the management of this problem and there is no guideline that support what they are doing. Majority of the outpatient departments were run by nurses. There was no routine screening of adult patients at outpatient departments. Generally the facilities are not ready to accommodate this service. The Woreda and the zone have to work on the capacity of the health workers and health facilities to handle diabetic care at health center level.

Acknowledgements

We are very much grateful to Jimma University for its financial support for undertaking this study. We thank primary health care in Jimma zone, for providing us important information though out the study. Our thanks also go to the study participants for their willingness to participate in the research.

References

1. National Institute of Diabetes and Digestive and Kidney Diseases (2008) National Diabetes Statistics.

2. International Diabetes federation (2012) Diabetes Atlas (5th edn) Brussels: IDF.

3. University of Michigan Health System (2009) History of Diabetes.

4. Wexler D (2015) Type 1 diabetes.

5. Wexler D, Zieve D (2015) Type 2 diabetes.

6. Diabetes (2008) NIH Senior Health.

7. http://familydoctor.org/online/famdocen/home/women/pregnancy/complications/075.html

8. Diseases and Conditions diabetes (2014) Mayo Clinic.

9. Alemu S, Watkins P (2004) Access to diabetic care in northern Ethiopia. Diabetes Voice 49.

10. Diabetes Complications. Medline Plus. National institute of Health.

11. Muluneh AT, Haileamlak A, Tessema F, Alemseged F, Woldemichael K, et al. (2012) Population based survey of chronic non-communicable diseases at gilgel gibe field research center, southwest ethiopia. Ethiop J Health Sci 22: 7-18.

12. Ethiopia Demographic and Health Survey (2011) Final Report: Addis Ababa, Ethiopia, and Calverton, Maryland, USA, CSA and ORC Macro.

13. Jimma zonal health department second quarter activity achievement report of 2003 EC.

14. World health organization guideline for prevention and control of non-communicable diseases a guideline for primary health care in low-resource settings.

15. Rangasami JJ, Greenwood DC, McSporran B, Smail PJ, Patterson CC, et al. (1997) Rising incidence of type 1 diabetes in Scottish children, 1984-93. The Scottish Study Group for the Care of Young Diabetics. Arch Dis Child 77: 210-213.

16. Diabetes treatment: Medications for type 2 diabetes (2014) Mayo Clinic.

17. El-Shazly M, Abdel-Fattah M, Zaki A, Bedwani R, Assad S, et al. (2000) Health care for diabetic patients in developing countries: a case from Egypt 114: 276-281.

26

MicroRNAs Regulation by Nutrients, the New Ray of Hope in Obesity Related Glucose and Lipid Metabolic Disorders

Seyed Rafie Arefhosseini[1], Mehrangiz Ebrahimi-Mamaeghani[2] and Somayeh Mohammadi[3*]

1Department of food technology, Faculty of Nutrition sciences, Tabriz University of Medical sciences, Tabriz, Iran

2Nutrition Research center, Faculty of Nutrition sciences, Tabriz University of Medical sciences, Tabriz, Iran

3Department of Nutrition, Faculty of Nutrition sciences, Tabriz University of Medical Sciences, Tabriz, Iran

*Corresponding author: Somayeh Mohammadi, Department of Nutrition, Faculty of Nutrition sciences, Tabriz University of Medical Sciences, Tabriz, Iran; E-mail: Mohammadis.phd@gmail.com

Abstract

Glucose and lipid metabolic disorders are two most prevalent complications of obesity. Regarding increasing rates of obesity and its metabolic disorders, more effective approaches are needed for prevention or treatment of related metabolic disorders. Therefore, understanding molecular mechanisms involved in metabolic syndrome would be open new way in maintaining homeostasis in these circumstances. miRNAs are non-coding small RNAs with transcriptional and posttranscriptional regulatory effects on gene expression, however, any disturbance of them could be involved in the pathogenesis of obesity and its related lipid and glucose metabolic disorders. miRNAs are proposed as an ideal non-invasive biological markers for rapid prediction of some obesity related metabolic diseases because of their stability and measurable concentrations in body fluids. Recent evidences reported changes of some important miRNAs profile with regulatory effects on glucose and lipid metabolic pathways even years before the onset and/or diagnosis of these obesity related metabolic disorders. Nutrition and dietary components as significant epigenetic factors have an important role in posttranscriptional regulations of lipid and glucose metabolism genes by modulating of related key miRNAs. Epigenetic suggests the importance of personalized nutrition according to miRNAs profile in prevention, control and treatment of obesity and related metabolic disorders. In this review we summarize evidences regarding the influence of nutrients and food components on some important related circulating miRNAs and their signature as new diagnosis, prognosis and therapeutic agents in obesity related lipid metabolism and diabetes as dietary-derived disorders.

Keywords: MicroRNAs; Nutrition; Obesity; Metabolism

Introduction

Obesity is one of the most important risk factors for chronic diseases, such as diabetes and cardiovascular diseases. In the early twentieth century, obesity has been considered prevalent and WHO announced its epidemic prevalence in the worldwide [1-3]. Obesity is known as one of the main causes of insulin resistance, impaired insulin secretion from pancreatic beta cells and diabetes. Diabetes mellitus is a common metabolic disorder in the world and as a result of its increasing trend that accompanied with aging of the populations, the number of diabetic subjects would be doubled over two decades [4-6]. Complications of this disease, including diabetic nephropathy are also rising [7]. Despite of these increasing rates, more effective approaches to prevention and treatment of glucose and lipid disorders should be selected. Until now, only a small part of the molecular mechanisms of diabetes and the occurrence of diabetes complications have been identified in obese and overweight patients. Its molecular mechanism should be studied more. The relationship between obesity and diabetes with non-coding RNAs has recently been proposed. Some current studies have been reported specific signature of some types of non-coding RNAs in obesity related metabolic diseases such as cardiovascular disease, lipid metabolism disturbances and type 2 diabetes mellitus [8].

microRNAs (miRNAs) are non-coding small RNAs that function as post-transcriptional regulators of gene expression and modulators of the diverse biological processes and pathologies [9,10]. miRNAs are key modulator factors in response to different environmental conditions and stresses that could assist the maintenance of homeostasis in these conditions. Besides, in conditions of sever or long stress they provide a mechanism for the expression of genes to create a new scheme for adapting themselves. Any disturbance in this area would be involved in the pathogenesis of some chronic diseases such as cancer, cardiovascular diseases, type 2 diabetes and obesity [11]. In obesity and its related metabolic diseases, miRNAs are involved in several important biological processes, including adipocytes differentiation, lipid metabolism and insulin sensitivity [12]. These RNAs are stable and measurable in the body fluids such as blood and urine. Therefore, they are proposed as ideal non-invasive biological markers for rapid prediction of some diseases such as obesity and diabetes complications. It is now clear that the miRNA profile in tissues with insulin resistance, changes years before the onset and/or diagnosis of type 2 diabetes. Studies have found that its circulating level reflects an expression pattern of miRNA [13,14]. So, early detection of disease with the help of miRNAs profile can significantly increase the quality of clinical management of chronic disease and improve their outcomes. Impaired expression of some types of miRNAs in obesity and diabetes opens a new window on our way to treat the problem.

It is well known that metabolic syndrome and related chronic diseases are caused by the modulating effect of the imbalanced dietary energy intake and expenditure, unhealthy nutrients and dietary components on genetic factors. Current results have shown the critical impact of nutrients as the significant epigenetic factors have an important role in the regulation of many genes. Impact of nutrition on non-coding RNAs that involved in adipogenesis, adipocytes differentiation, adipokines synthesis and secretion [15,16], insulin resistance, glucose and lipid metabolism [17,18], is the base for the Nutrigenomics science.

In this review we assessed existing valid scientific proofs and summarized evidences regarding the influence of nutrients and food components on some related circulating miRNAs and their signature as a new diagnosis tool, prognosis and therapeutic agents in obesity related lipid metabolism and diabetes as dietary-derived disorders.

History of miRNAs

Diagnosis and biogenesis

miRNAss are a class of short non-coding RNAs with about 22 nucleotides that discovered in 1993 and recognized as a class of biological regulators in the early 2000s [19]. These molecules found in prokaryotic and eukaryotic organisms such as plants, animals, and some viruses, that regulate gene expression by an effect on translation and / or stability of mRNAs through base-pairing with complementary target sequences within mRNA molecules, or in other cases, post transcriptional regulation by changing the protein's function [8,20]. miRNA is made from stem loop regions of long primary transcriptional precursors [21,22] which are usually transcribed by RNA polymerase II (Pol II) [23,24]. The resulting transcript of polymerase is capped with a specially modified nucleotide at the 5` end. It polyadenylated with multiple adenosines (a poly A tail), [24,25] and becomes more elongated molecules of miRNA (the primary miRNA or pri-miRNA). Under nuclear processing with the enzyme Drosha, hairpins liberated from pri-miRNA by cleaving about eleven nucleotides from hair pin base. This structure with two-nucleotide overhang at its 3` end, with 3` hydroxyl and 5` phosphate groups, called as pre-miRNA (precursor-miRNA). Each hair pin loop is composed of about 70 nucleotides. Pre-miRNA hairpins exported of the nucleus to the cytoplasm where the pre-miRNA hairpin is cleaved by the RNase III enzyme Dicer, yielding an imperfect miRNA (double-stranded miRNA) with about 22 nucleotides [26]. Although each strand of the duplex may potentially act as a functional miRNA, only one strand as a mature miRNA is usually incorporated into the RNA-induced silencing complex (RISC) where the miRNA molecules bind to the 3' UTR of free mRNA and affect the post translation gene expression (mostly inhibit). Some reports on translation silencing nuclear genes, show that the mature cytoplasmic miRNAs could return to nucleolus and affect the translation by targeting mRNAs and connecting to a promoter region [27]. Recently miRNA researches have revealed multiple roles for these regulatory molecules in negative regulation (transcript degradation and sequestering, translational suppression) and possible involvement in positive regulation (activation of transcription and translation) [28-30]. Up to now the 19th Edition database miRBase (http://www.mirbase.org), identified about 25521 miRNAs in more than 193 different varieties which may target about 60% of mammalian genes and are abundant in many human cell types [31,32]. Besides, miRNAs are involved in most of biological processes.

miRNAs as Regulators of Lipid and glucose metabolism pathways

Current evidences have determined important roles for particular miRNAs in regulation of lipid and glucose metabolism pathways. Determining the miRNAs profile of abdominal fat cells and subcutaneous adipose tissue in humans has been shown the increased expression of miR-29a, miR-935, miR-100, miR-125b, miR-221 and miR-34a in obesity and decreased expression of these miRNAs in the differentiation and maturation stages of fat cells [33]. A significant positive correlation was observed between miR-143 expression, which involves in regulating of adipocytes differentiation, with body weight and visceral fat in mice under high-fat diet [33]. Respect to the recent scientific results, dyslipidemia, impaired lipolysis and impaired blood triglyceride levels are some consequences of disrupting miRNAs and involved in cholesterol metabolism, trigger of some metabolic disorders and could cause insulin resistance (IR). Some miRNAs such as miR-33 [34] and miR-122 [35] that we will discuss in the following sections are shown as the post-translational regulators of cholesterol homeostasis, fatty acid metabolism and lypogenesis (Table 1).

miR-33

In humans, the miR-33 family consists of two members named mir-33a and mir-33b, these two human intronic miRNAs are located in intron-16 within two protein-coding genes for Sterol regulatory element-binding proteins (SREBF), SREBP-2 and SREBP-1 respectively. SREBP is a key regulator of genes involved in cholesterol absorption and synthesis. Under the condition of cholesterol reduction, miR-33a and SREBF-2 are transcribed simultaneously and regulate the expression of several genes involved in cholesterol transport, fatty acid oxidation and blood lipid profile including HDL-C [36].

ATP-binding cassette transporters A1 and G1 (ABCA1, ABCG1) are the cholesterol membrane transporters and important target genes of both miR-33 [34]. The entry of miR-33 to mouse macrophages down regulates ABCA1 and ABCG1 and reduces the cholesterol efflux to protein APOA1, a protein which involved in the transport of cholesterol from tissues to the liver for excretion. In contrast, the inhibition of endogenous miR-33 simultaneously increases ABCA1 and ABCG1 protein expression (first step in the production of nascent HDL-c) and cholesterol transfer to Apoa1. ABCA1 leads to a modest but significant rise in plasma HDL-c levels. The endolysosomal transport protein, Niemann-Pick type C1 protein (NPC1), is another target gene of miR-33 [30,37]. NPC1 along with ABCA1 participates in cholesterol efflux to APOA1 [38].

Injection of anti-miR-33 to LDL-c receptor knock-out causes increased hepatic expression of ABCA1, higher levels and size of circulating HDL-c and enhanced reverse cholesterol transport. Reverse cholesterol transport results increased transport of cholesterol from extra-hepatic tissues to HDL-c and supports the impact of miR-33 target genes (ABCA1 and ABCG1) on the liver as well as other tissues [37,39]. These results are accompanied by a reduction in size and lipid content of atherosclerotic plaques, increased markers of plaque stability and decreased inflammatory gene expression. In general, it is suggested that antagonism of miR-33 could protect the cardiovascular system [40]. Injection of anti-miR-33 oligonucleotide increased the hepatic expression of ABCA1 in African green monkeys. It was also induced a sustained increase in plasma HDL-c and reduced plasma levels of very-low-density lipoprotein (VLDL), it's also accompanied by the reduction in triglycerides levels [34].

The decreased expression of miR-33 a/b target various genes in fatty acid oxidation pathways, including Peroxisomal carnitine O-octanoyltransferase (CROT), Mitochondrial carnitine palmitoyltransferase 1a (CPT1A), hydroxyacyl-CoA dehydrogenase/3-ketoacyl-CoA thiolase/enoyl-CoA hydratase β-subunit (HADHB) and Protein kinase AMP-activated alpha 1 catalytic subunit (PRKAA1). The decreased expression of miR-33 a/b also, regulate certain genes that involved in the synthesis of fatty acids such as Fatty acid synthase (FASN), ATP citrate lyase (ACLY), Acetyl-CoA carboxylase α (ACACA), hepatocellular Sirtuin-6 (SIRT6) and the expression of insulin receptor substrates 2 (IRS2), one critical component of the insulin signal transduction pathway in the liver [34,41].

miR-33b in cooperation with SREBF1 inversely affects on glucose metabolism in hepatocytes, through pyruvate carboxy kinase (PCK1) and glucose-6 - phosphate (G6PC) pathways. It is a key regulatory enzyme of hepatic gluconeogenesis pathways. miR-33b also contributes to the regulation of cholesterol and fatty acid homeostasis by targeting key transcriptional regulators of lipid metabolism, including steroid receptor co-activator 1 (SRC1), steroid receptor co-activator 3 (SRC3), nuclear transcription factor Y, gamma, (NFYC), and nuclear receptor-interacting protein 1 (RIP140) [42,43]. These results show regulation of various lipid and glucose metabolic pathways by miR-33, including cholesterol efflux, fatty acid metabolism and insulin signaling. Also, the key transcriptional regulators of glucose and lipid metabolism also targeted, indicating to the clinical significance and manipulation of miR-33a/b as a new therapeutic target in metabolic diseases.

miR-122

Besides of miR-33, miR-122 is another important miRNA that conserved between vertebrate specie. Approximately 70% of total liver miRNA expression belongs to MiR-122 that is most abundant miRNAs in the liver, and is prominently involved in the regulation of lipid and glucose metabolism [44,45]. miR-122 has a key role in hepatitis C infection and its down-regulation has been found in hepatocellular carcinoma (HCC) [45,46]. In patients with non-alcoholic fatty liver disease (NAFLD) the hepatic and serum miR-122 levels associates with hepatic steatosis and fibrosis, suggesting serum miR-122 level as a useful predictive marker of liver fibrosis in patients with NAFLD [47].

In vivo experiments suggest the miR-122 importance in maintenance of liver function through down-regulation of several genes involved in liver lipid and glucose metabolism and increasing the expression of some other related genes that are normally repressed in hepatocytes [45,46]. Hepatic miR-122 inhibition down-regulates hepatic expression of several genes involved in regulation of lipid biosynthesis and oxidation such as acetyl-CoA carboxylase α and β (ACC1, ACC2), stearoyl-CoA desaturase (SCD1), ATP citrate lyase (ACLY) and Fatty acid synthase (FAS) and therefore, caused sustain reduction of total plasma cholesterol levels by 30% (in dose dependent manner), decreased HDL-c, apolipoprotein AI, LDL-c and apolipoprotein B, increased hepatic fatty acid oxidation, decreased hepatic fatty acid and cholesterol synthesis rates. Although the mechanisms are not clearly known, probably some large part of them is related to the impact of miR-122 on AMP- activated protein kinase (AMPK). miR-122 directly suppresses AMPK, the important regulator of metabolism that promotes ATP-generating pathways like fatty acid

oxidation and inhibits energy storage through fatty acid synthesis. Hepatic miR-122 inhibition increases AMPK activation that inhibits ACC2 and induce energy usage from fatty acids [45,46]. Also, recent evidences show connections of miR-122 to the PPAR family, a family of nuclear receptors with regulating effect on metabolism. Up-regulation of PPARβ/δ has been reported upon hepatic miR-122 inactivation [48]. Although hepatic functions of PPARβ/δ have not yet been clearly studied, an interaction between the PPARβ/δ and AMPK pathways was shown recently in muscle. Therefore, it is hypothesized that liver miR-122 depletion increased hepatic fatty acid oxidation probably indirectly activating by AMPK through higher PPARβ/δ protein levels [44,49].

Besides, miR-122 reduces lactate production and increases oxygen consumption, by targeting many of glycolytic genes, especially by the reduced pyruvate kinase (PK) gene expression (Isoform M2 (PKM2) in human hepatocellular carcinoma. PK level is significantly associated with poor clinical outcomes of HCC patients [50]. These evidences demonstrated the regulatory role of miR-122 in lipid and glucose metabolism, having an implication of therapeutic intervention targeting in metabolic syndrome.

miR-375

miRNAs have an important role in the development and secretory function of pancreas [36,37], but their accurate functional pathways except for miR-375 is not completely clear [38]. miR-375 is one most abundant pancreatic miRNA and involved in the development of the endocrine pancreas. miR-375 targets two key transcriptional factors, Pdx-1 (Pancreatic and duodenal homeobox 1) and Neuro D1, 2 (Neuronal differentiation 1,2) [39]. key target genes of Pdx1 are involved in glucose-stimulated insulin transcription and secretion including Glut2 (Glucose transporter2), glucokinase, MafA, insulin and GLP1 (glucagon-like peptide 1) [51]. Previous studies have shown that Pdx1, MafA and NeuroD1 synergistically activate the insulin promoter [52]. Pdx-1 and Neuro D1, 2 mediate pancreas development , differentiation of β-cell and non-β-cells into insulin-producing cells, insulin gene transcription in β-cells and this cells maintenance [52,53]. Therefore, miR-375 inhibition results in pancreas developmental disorders, impaired β-cell function, glucose-induced insulin secretion and increased blood glucose levels [30,37,38]. In diabetic mice, inhibition of miR- 375 leads to increased blood glucose levels through increased glucagon and reduced the number of pancreatic β and α cell [54]. Genetic deletion of miR-375 in obese mice (375/ob) significantly reduced adaptive β-cell expansion in response to increasing insulin demand in insulin resistance tissues and resulted in a severely diabetic state [55].

Recently, Ling et al. showed increased expression of miR-375 and some evidences of 3T3-L1 adipocyte differentiation such as increased PPARγ (Peroxisome proliferator-activated receptor γ) and aP2 (Adipocyte Protein 2) mRNA levels and suppressed phosphorylation of ERK1/2 (Extracellular-signal-regulated kinases). In contrast, anti-miR-375 increased ERK1/2 phosphorylation levels in pre-adipocytes after stimulation of adipogenic differentiation [56]. Also, in some previous evidences have been reported the effects of ERK-PPARγ pathway on adipocyte differentiation and adipogenesis, by activating mitogen-activated protein kinases (MAPKs), an essential kinase in adipocyte differentiation pathway [57-59]. Therefore this study reported the effect of miR-375 in the differentiation of pre-adipocytes and adipocytes with targeting ERK, PPARγ and aP2 pathways [56] and suggesting the probable importance of miR-375 in obesity induced peripheral insulin resistance by targeting ERK 1/2 phosphorylation .

In general, miR-375 targets β-cells from multiple pathways such as insulin gene expression and secretion, beta cell proliferation and dealing with insulin resistance; so that the blood levels of this miRNA could be used as a biomarker of beta cell death and diabetes [60].

miR-29

The important mammalian target organs for miR-29 family (a, b and c) are muscle, adipose and liver tissues that strongly deregulated by hyperglycemia and hyperinsulinemia [61]. Plasma signatures of some miRNAs including miR-29b, can accurately differentiate patients with a high risk of developing diabetes from healthy controls [62]. In diabetic mice and humans [13,63,64] elevated circulating and cellular levels of miR-29a have been reported in β -cells that exposed to high levels of glucose. The effects of increased levels of glucose in human INS-1E β-cells on miR-29a gene expression, β- cells proliferation and glucose induced insulin secretion, introduced miR-29a as a causing factors of the β-cell dysfunction in glucose-induced insulin secretion [65]. In β- cells treated with high glucose levels, the over-expression of miR-29a reduced Syntaxin1A (Stx-1a) expression ,one of two t-SNAREs involved in insulin exocytose from the β cell, suggests mediatory role of miR-29a in glucose-induced down-regulation of Stx-1a in β-cells [66]. In contrast in obese diabetic rat, miR-29 family (a-c) gene expression increases in hepatocytes exposed with reduced blood glucose through inhibition of hepatic gluconeogenesis pathways including Glucose 6-phosphatase (G6Pase) and Peroxisome proliferator-activated receptor gamma co-activator 1-alpha (PGC-1α) [66].

Obesity-induced molecular changes and environmental signals strongly deregulate miRNAs in adipose tissue. miR-29a and miR-29b gene expression increases in the in vitro incubation of 3T3-L1 adipocytes with high glucose and insulin. Their increased expression with reduced insulin-dependent glucose uptake in these cells, indicate the role of miR-29 in the development of adipocytes insulin resistance and inhibition of insulin signal transduction through AKT (Protein Kinase B (phosphorylation pathway [67,68].

Adiponectin is an insulin sensitizing cytokines. Recent findings demonstrate a significant inverse association of adiponectin with insulin resistance and inflammation status in diabetic patients [69-71]. Activating transcription factor 3 (ATF3), a member of the ATF/cAMP-responsive element-binding protein family of transcription factors and a stress-inducible transcriptional repressor, suppress adiponectin gene expression. In genetically predisposed mice to type 2 diabetes, high fat diet significantly increased AFT3, serum IL-6, TNF-α and miR-29a levels and decrease serum adiponectin levels. This study shows a significant relation between miR-29a over-expression and decreased serum adiponectin [72]. Also, a restricted information exist about the effect of miR-29 on the expression of adiponectin, this study suggests that in obesity induced insulin resistance, miR-29a could be believed to be a selective repressor of adiponectin gene.

Down-regulation of miR-29b in diabetic mice in response to advanced glycation end (AGE) product is associated with progressive diabetic kidney injury, micro-albuminuria, renal fibrosis, and inflammation [73]. High glucose-induced cell apoptosis was prevented in db/db mice with knockdown of miR-29c. In a recent study, over-expression of miR-29c targeted Spry1 protein, activated Rho kinase and induction of podocyte apoptosis. Anti-miR-29c significantly reduced albuminuria and kidney mesangial matrix accumulation [74]. These findings identify miR-29 b/c not only as novel targets in glucose and lipid metabolic disorder, but also as key mediators in diabetic complications specially nephropathy.

miR-103 & miR-107

miR-103 and miR-107 are another important miRNAs target multiple mRNA involve in human cellular acetyl-CoA pathways and lipid metabolism. miR-103 and miR-107 exist within introns of the pantothenate kinase (PANK) genes in vertebrate genomes. PANK enzymes also affect cellular acetyl-CoA and lipid metabolic pathways. Therefore, the miR-103 and miR-107 act synergistically with 'host' gene [75]. Genome-wide miRNA profiling studies, identify that in pre-adipocytes ectopic expression of the miR-103 increases speed of adipogenesis by up-regulation of many adipogenesis involved markers specially Peroxisome proliferators-activated receptor gamma (PPARγ) and Fatty Acid Binding Protein 4 (FABP4). It also, increases triglyceride accumulation at an early stage of adipogenesis [76]. Several anti-adipogenic factors such as Aryl hydrocarbon receptor nuclear translocator (ARNT), Frizzled homolog 1 (FZD1), and Runt-related transcription factor 1 (RUNX1T1/ETO/MTG8) may be involved in adipogenesis as targets of miR-103 and miR-107 [76]. These results showed the importance of miR-103 and miR-107 in adipose biology. Hepatic miR-103 up-regulation in hyperglycemic rats suggests its role in the pathophysiology of type 2 diabetes [68]. Silencing the up-regulation of miR-103 and miR-107 in obese mice improve glucose homeostasis and their up-regulation act on the contrary in adipose and liver tissues. So, subsequently they have a key role in insulin sensitivity and glucose homeostasis.

Another target gene of miR-103/107 is Caveolin-1, a critical regulator of insulin receptor. Up-regulated Caveolin in adipocytes upon inhibition of miR-103/107 is simultaneous with insulin receptor stabilization, enhanced insulin signaling, decreased adipocyte size and enhanced insulin-stimulated glucose uptake [77]. Recently miRNAs microarray in ob/ob streptozotocin (STZ)-induced type 1 diabetic mice with NAFLD, showed the up-regulation of eight miRNAs including miR-103 and miR-107 and down-regulation of four miRNAs such as miR-29c, and miR-122 in comparison to normal C57BL/6 mice [78].

In general, these evidences lead to a suggestion that miR-103 and miR-107 represent potential targets for the regulation of lipid and glucose metabolism, hepatic energy, adipogenesis, insulin sensitivity and associate with the pathophysiological processes of Type 2 diabetes and NAFLD. Table 1 has been summarized discussed key metabolic miRNAs together with their targets in lipid and glucose metabolism.

Effect of nutrition on miRNA expression

Differences of tissue and circulating miRNAs profile in subjects with metabolic syndrome from healthy subjects and various gene expression between diet induced obese and non-obese mice [54,79,80] and humans [33,81] have proposed involvement of diet-dependent epigenetic mechanisms in regulation of gene expression. Dietary components including macro nutrients (proteins and amino acids, carbohydrates and fatty acids) and micro nutrients (vitamins and minerals) can exert some of their epigenetic effects through affecting miRNAs expression and functions. The scientific evidences that have demonstrated these relations would be discussed in the following parts.

miRANs	Target genes	Target pathway	References
miR-33	ABCA1, ABCG1	Cholesterol membrane transporters	35
	NPC1	Cholesterol efflux	31, 38
	CROT, CPT1A, HADHB, PRKAA1	Fatty acids oxidation	35
	FASN, ACLY, ACACA, SIRT6	Fatty acids synthesis	35, 42
	IRS2	Insulin signal transduction	35, 42
	PCK1, G6PC	Hepatic gluconeogenesis	43, 44
	SRC1, SRC3, NFYC, RIP140	Lipid metabolism (Transcriptional regulation)	43, 44
miR-122	ACC1, ACC2, SCD1, ACLY,	Lipid biosynthesis	46
	FAS	Lipid oxidation	46, 47
	AMPK	ATP-generating pathways	46, 47
	PK	Glycolitic pathways	49
miR-375	Pdx-1, Neuro D1, 2	Transcriptional pathway in pancreas	40
	ERK, PPARγ, aP2	Pre-adipocytes and adipocytes differentiation	52
	Pancreatic β-cells and α cell	Insulin and glucagon production, Cells development and proliferation	50-53
miR-29	Stx-1a	Insulin exocytose	59
	AKT	Insulin signal transduction	60,61
	Adiponectin	Insulin resistance	65
	Spry1 protein and Rho kinase	Podocyte apoptosis	67
	G6Pase, PGC-1α	G,ucose metabolism	59
miR-103	PPARγ, FABP4	Adipogenesis	69
miR-103/ 107	ARNT, FZD1, RUNX1T1/ETO/MTG8	Adipogenesis	69
	Caveolin-1	Regulation of insulin receptor	70

Table 1: miRNAs with regulatory effects on glucose and lipid metabolic pathways

The impact of macronutrients on microRNA

Phytochemicals

Dietary polyphenols are found to improve dyslipidemia [82,83] and insulin resistance [84-86] in rodents with metabolic syndrome. Each polyphenol targets specific hepatic miRNAs [87-89]. Proanthocyanidins are most abundant polyphenol class in the human diets. In hepatocytes of obese rat treated with grape seed proanthocyanidins (GSP), hepatic cholesterol efflux increased by repressing miR-33 and its target gene (ABCA1) to produce new HDL-c particles and lipogenesis is reduced by silencing miR-122 [90]. In T2DM hypertensive patients long-term supplementation with grape extract containing Resveratrol (RES) decreases the expression of some key pro-inflammatory cytokines through modulation of related miRNAs in circulating immune cells. This evidence indicates a beneficial immunomodulatory effect of grape extract containing Resveratrol in these patients [91]. Because of richer phenolic compounds of GPE (grape proanthocyandin extract) in comparing with Grape seed proanthocyandin extract (GSPE), various compositions of grape extracts and different molecular structure of each polyphenols, diverse influences of polyphenols have been demonstrated on miR-33a and miR-122 expression in hepatic cells.

In hepatic cells of rats and humans, GSPE reduces both miR-122 and miR-33a levels, but GPE reduces miR-122 and increases miR-33a expression. Also, in this study RES and epigallocatechin gallate

(EGCG) repressed miR-33a and miR-122 [92]. Chronic treatment of GSPE in healthy rats, in a dose-dependent manner can improve tolerance to lipid overload and postprandial lipemia through repressing liver miR-33a and miR-122 and decreasing their target genes even in population with normal-dose intake [93]. In diet-induced hyperlipidemic mice plant-derived polyphenols prevented fatty liver disease by regulating expression of miR-103/107 and miR-122 and changes in lipid and glucose metabolism [94]. The nature of binding polyphenols such as green tea catechins to miRNAs and proteins have shown in some recent studies [95,96]. In general, considering these significant effects of polyphenolic compound on the expression of some essential miRNAs involved in metabolic pathways, introduce polyphenols as new posttranscriptional modulators of metabolic pathways including lipid and glucose metabolism.

Fatty acids

Fatty acids are other dietary components with impact on miRNA expression levels that have been demonstrated in various cell lines. Increased butyrate, a short-chain fatty acid produced in the mammalian colon by colonizing bacteria with effect on cell differentiation, in human colonic cells and stem cells enhances the expression of miR-375 [97]. This finding suggests that at least some parts of butyrate impact on cell differentiation can be related to its modulator effect on miRNA expression.

Over-expressions of miR-375 and miR-107 have been reported with increased PUFA n-3 in the early stages of mice colon cancer [98]. High fat diet is supposed as an important agent in pathogenesis of obesity and obesity related metabolic diseases that could change the expression of miRNAs. Down-regulation of hepatic miR-122 has been reported in murine [99] and rat [100] fed with high fat diet, but there are conflicting results for miR-103 and miR-107. In murine models high fat diet resulted in miR-103 and miR -107 up-regulation [101] while, some other evidences showed down-regulation of these miRNAs [77].

The expression of miR-33 increased in response to reduced sterols in human macrophages, whereas in rats with both normal and high-fat diet, dietary cholesterol intake caused miR-33 over-expression in peritoneal and peripheral macrophages [34].

Maternal consumption of a high-fat diet during pregnancy and lactation lead to hepatic lipid metabolism disturbances in offspring and their adulthood, by modulating various related genes in offspring including increased hepatic IκB kinase and β-oxidation-related gene and down-regulation of miR-122 [102]. Moreover, maternal high-fat diet consumption before conception down-expressed some miRNAs including miR-122 during pregnancy and lactation. Early miRNAs disturbances can result metabolic disorders in adult life. These evidences suggest an epigenetic mechanism of diet that can explain how dietary induced early changes in gene expression is maintained until adulthood [103].

Dietary supplementation with Conjugated linoleic acid (CLA) in many mammalian species is considered for reducing body fat stores particularly abdominal white adipose tissue and increasing lean body mass. CLA works with the mechanism of enhancing lipolysis in adipose tissue, increasing fat oxidation in muscle cells, reducing the uptake and storage of fatty acids in adipose tissue, fat cell apoptosis, reducing the size of fat cells, inhibition of enzymes involved in lipid metabolism, increasing energy metabolism and changing gene expression of proteins involved in lipid metabolism [104,105]. Therefore, it reduces insulin resistance and increase insulin sensitivity in adipose tissue and muscle cells. An animal study was performed to investigate the impacts of CLA supplementation on mice adipose tissue gene expressions. Results showed the effects of CLA on miR-103 and mi-R-107 down-regulation in mice fed standard fat-diet [99]. In general dietary fatty acids are considered as important modulator factor in regulations of miRNAs involved in lipid and glucose metabolism pathways.

Amino acids

miRNAs expression is significantly responsive to nitrogen (N) and amino acids starvations. Recently, miRNAs were shown to act in plant nutrient metabolism. Sequencing technology in plants showed that in response to N deficiency, members of same miRNA families have different expressions. Upon these conditions the expression of some miRNAs was repressed and that of some others was induced [106]. Consumption of methionine-choline-deficient diet in mice as experimental animal, lead to diet-induced NAFLD, liver steatosis and over-expression of some miRNAs in liver metabolic pathways [107]. Also, amino acid deficient diets stimulate the expression of proteins that compete with miRNAs for binding to their target mRNAs. miR-122 represses the expression of cationic amino acid transporter 1 (CAT-1) mRNA in human hepatocytes, but evidences demonstrated that in various stressful conditions for cells, such as amino acid deprivation, oxidative stresses and reticulum stress, miR-122 is

inhibited and this repression is relieved. Binding of HuR, an AU-rich-element binding protein, to the 3'UTR of CAT-1 mRNA results down-regulation of CAT-1 and suggesting that proteins interacting with the 3'UTR act as modulators of miRNAs potential to repress gene expression [108].

Rapidly up- or down-regulation of specific genes in human skeletal muscle during insulin infusion [109], fasting [110] or a high-glycemic meal [110,111] lead to this concept that essential amino acids (EAA) ingestion alters the expression of miRNAs and genes associated with muscle growth. It is suggested that some miRNAs levels increased after administration of essential amino acids including histidine, isoleucine, leucine, methionine, phenylalanine, threonine and valine [112]. Therefore both quality and quantity of dietary amino acids can alter miRNAs expression in various metabolic pathways, also further studies needed for identifying dietary protein effects on the expression of key regulatory miRNAs involved in lipid and glucose metabolism.

Carbohydrates

Circulating levels or availability of glucose has been recognized as the modulating factor of miRNA expression [113]. As mentioned before, hyperglycemia reported as a factor that increase some miRNAs involved in glucose metabolism and insulin resistances such as miR-375 and miR-33 [55,63]. However, different miR-122 and miR-375 profile between healthy and glucose intolerant subject's islets indicate the effect of hyperglycemia and insulin sensitivity on the expression of miRNA involved in glucose metabolisms [114].

A maternal low protein-high carbohydrate diet during pregnancy causes over-expression of hepatic G6PC and alters some related miRNAs expression in male piglets, which suggests epigenetic effects of high carbohydrate diet on early onset of hyperglycemia in adulthood [115].

High carbohydrate diet consumption for just 6 days in healthy subjects significantly reduced circulating levels of some miRNAs including miR-29 [116]. miR-29b down-regulation have previously been demonstrated as a predictor of type 2 diabetes development and its complications such as nephropathy [73]. In conflict with miR-29 b, hyperglycemic conditions enhance the expression of miR29c and reduce the expression of its target Sprouty Homolog 1 (Spry1). This condition induces cell apoptosis and fibronectin synthesis, which are characteristics of diabetic nephropathy [74]. It was concluded that the dietary macronutrients composition and serum glucose levels involve in the regulation of the level of serum miRNAs, and consequently may lead to regulate insulin signaling, glucose uptake and cause the development and complications of type 2 diabetes.

Micronutrients which found their impact on miRNA expression

Only a few studies have investigated the effects of vitamins, mineral and their derivatives on the expression of miRNAs that involved in glucose and lipid metabolisms in different experimental models.

Vitamin A is one of these micro nutrients. Vitamin A is a lipophilic micronutrient (VA, Retinol) that has long been implicated as an essential nutritional factor in human health for its roles in the development and maturation of various cells (growth), anti-infective and immunity booster activities. Retinoid acid (RA) is active metabolite of vitamin A and is in attention due to its numerous effects on immunity, cell differentiations and regulation of gene expressions.

Adipose tissue is a place for vitamin A storage and retinol conversion to its active metabolite RA. The importance of vitamin A in adipose tissue biology, obesity and type II diabetes has been shown in recent years [117,118].

Dietary components	Target miRNAs	Change	Subjects or type of cells	References
Polyphenols				
GSP	miR-33a, miR-122	Down-regulation	Rats hepatocyte	83
GPE	miR-33a, miR-122	Up-regulation-Down-regulation	Rats and humans hepatocyte	85
GSPE	miR.33a, miR-122	Down-regulation	Rats and humans hepatocyte	85
GSPE	miR.33a, miR-122	Down-regulation	Healthy rats	86
RES	miR.33a, miR-122	Down-regulation	Rats and humans hepatocyte	85
EGCG	miR.33a, miR-122	Down-regulation	Rats and humans hepatocyte	85
Polypenoics	miR-103/107, miR-122	Up-regulation-Down-regulation	Hyperlipidemic mice	87
Fatty acids				
Butyrate	miR-375	Up- regulation	Human colon and stem cells	90
PUFA n-3	miR-375, miR-107	Up- regulation	Mice colon cancer cells	91
High fat diet	miR-122	Down-regulation	Murine and rats, Humans	92, 96
	miR-103/107	Up or down- regulation	Murine and rats	92, 70
Cholesterol	miR-33	Up- regulation	Rats	35
CLA	miR-103/107	Down-regulation	Mice	92
Protein				
Protein deficiency	miR-122	Up- regulation	Human hepatoma cells	101
Carbohydrates				
Hyperglycemia	miR-375, miR-33 ,miR-122	Up- regulation	Mice, human islets of Langerhans	51, 56, 107
High carbohydrate diet	miR-29 ,miR-29b, miR29c	Down-regulation-Up- regulation	Humans	109
Vitamins				
RA	miR-103	Up- regulation	Human neuroblastoma cells	121, 122
1, 25- dihydroxyvitamin D3	miR-29a, miR-29b	Up- regulation	human prostate cancer cells	126
Vitamin E deficiency	miR-122a		Rats and humans hepatocytes	133

Table 2: Dietary polyphenols and nutrients effects on miRNAs involved in glucose and lipid metabolic pathways

There are multiple isomeric forms of RA, such as all-trans RA and 9-cis RA [119] that modulates gene expression through the activation of two families of nuclear receptors and RA receptors by all-trans RA and RXRs through 9-cis RA [120,121].

Srebp-1c expression, transcription and maturation are induced by synergistic effect of Retinal and vitamin A with insulin in primary hepatocytes that is followed by regulation of the Srebp-1c target gene, FASN. This up-regulation is done via binding of the general transcription factors and the diet-associated transcription factors like SREBP-1c to proximal promoter of FASN .Also, Retinoids and retinal can regulate hepatic Srebp-1c expression through activation of RXR [122,123]. These evidences show the importance of vitamin A in regulation of genes targets in glucose metabolic pathway and lipogenesis.

Trans-RA acts as a potent anti- tumor retinoid derivative by inhibiting of cell proliferation, cell differentiation and apoptosis [124,125]. Inadequate supply of all trans-RA (atRA) leads to the repressed transcriptional expression of retinoic acid-responsive genes and in reverse manner adequate pharmacological atRA can reverse this effect with targeting miRNAs involvement pathways [126,127]. miR-103 is one of these genes that is up-regulated by retinoic acid (RA) in human neuroblastoma cells [128]. Besides some other evidences demonstrated the impact of atRA on neuronal cells differentiation by up-regulation of miR-9 and miR-103 [129] suggests that some of RA effects on cell differentiation could be mediated by their impact on miRNAs profile expressions.

Altered vitamin D metabolism in type 2 diabetic mice, suggests the protective effects of vitamin D metabolites against diabetic complications specially diabetic nephropathy [130]. It is appeared that vitamin D enhances the intracellular mechanisms of insulin action. It is mediated by vitamin D receptor (VDR) and Insulin receptor substrate (IRS-1). In vitamin D treated mice under high fat diet significant weight loss, muscle VDR down-regulation, liver VDR up-regulation, increased muscle IRS-1 transcriptional levels and down-regulation of hepatic IRS-1 have been reported in compared to control group [131]. The physiologically active form of vitamin D3, 1,25-Dihydroxyvitamin D3, plays a key role in cell differentiation and inhibits porcine pre-adipocyte differentiation in a dose-dependent manner through down-regulating the expression of adipogenesis-related genes [132]. Therefore, vitamin D could regulate post translational expression of genes involved in metabolic syndrome, lipid and glucose metabolism. Co-administration of 1,25-dihydroxy vitamin D3 with testosterone modulate lipid metabolism in human prostate cancer cells through up-regulation of the miRNAs that target peroxisome proliferators-activated receptor alpha (PPAR-α) such as miR-29a, miR-29b and increased lipogenesis [133] . Plasma levels of 25 (OH) vitamin D in early pregnancy are significantly associated with some maternal peripheral blood gene expression and post-transcription regulation of miRNAs [134].

Vitamin E, its main congener is α-tocopherol (αT), consists of two classes of compounds: tocopherols and tocotrienols. Synthetic ligands of PPAR-α and PPAR-γ are currently used for treating hyperlipidemia and diabetes. Tocotrienol-enriched palm oil as PPAR modulator increases insulin sensitivity reduces blood glucose levels and improves whole body glucose utilization in patients and preclinical animal diabetic db/db mice [135,136]. Vitamin E regulates gene expression by modulating mRNA concentrations in various tissues of mammals [137-139]. Vitamin E deficiency caused a reduced concentration of hepatic miRNA-122a, suggesting vitamin E as an important regulator of lipid metabolism with up-regulation of miR-122 as the most abundant miRNA in rat and human liver [140]. Other evidences confirmed that the increased dietary Vitamin E decreases the activity of superoxide dismutase (SOD) and increases the expression of hepatic miRNAs such as miR-122 in Nile tilapia [141]. There aren't any reported evidences about other micro nutrients including minerals and gene expression of miRNAs involved in glucose and lipid metabolism pathways.

In general, despite recent evidences reported in this review, so far little studies have been conducted about the effects of nutrients and nutritional factors on the miRNA involved in glucose and lipid metabolism. So, further studies are necessary recommended for identifying more miRNAs' probable influence by nutrients.

Conclusion

Emerging evidences suggest that miRNAs play important roles in the development or treatment of obesity related glucose and lipid metabolism. Expression profiling studies have revealed that some miRNAs are deregulated in obesity and metabolic syndrome possibly involved in the pathogenesis of various these metabolic disorders. miRNAs are stable in body biological fluids and measurable as ideal biomarkers for non-invasive and rapid diseases prediction and diagnosis. Early detection significantly increases the quality of clinical nutrition management and improves complications of chronic diseases. Investigation of miRNAs in obesity and related metabolic disorders, genetic targets of miRNAs and their influence by dietary modulators can potentially identify novel pathways involved in metabolic disorders and influence future therapeutic approaches. In

recent years, nutrition, dietary modulators and phytochemicals have been interested as important epigenetic factors involved in post-transcriptional regulations of adipogenesis, lipid and glucose metabolism genes. We can use of miRNA profiling as a useful aid for designing therapeutic approaches, assessment of the nutritional status and planning the suitable diet in obesity related metabolic diseases.

In a contest of epigenetic effects of nutritional factors on miRNAs and their host gene expression, the personalized nutrition is in its infancy. Up to now, only few nutritional factors and phytocemicals have been demonstrated in this field, but can discuss them in the field of personalized nutrition, as a good way to predict and treat metabolic complications of obesity. Also multi-faceted mechanism of action is likely for effects of nutrition and nutritional components on involved miRNAs in metabolic disorders.

With further researches on principal that involved miRNAs expression and nutritional factors, in complement with the absorption of food derived exogenous miRNAs [142] and breast milk miRNAs with immune-modulator activities [143] in humans, we can reach the famous phrase that "you are what you eat".

References

1. Caballero B (2007) The global epidemic of obesity: an overview. Epidemiol Rev 29: 1-5.

2. Organization WH (2011) Obesity and overweight. 2011.

3. Rashidy-Pour A, Malek M, Eskandarian R, Ghorbani R (2009) Obesity in the Iranian population. Obes Rev 10: 2-6.

4. Maori L, Ezekiel D and Bilal J Prevalence of Diabetes in Zambuk General Hospital.

5. Wild S, Roglic G, Green A, Sicree R, King H (2004) Global prevalence of diabetes: estimates for the year 2000 and projections for 2030. Diabetes Care 27: 1047-1053.

6. Shaw JE, Sicree RA, Zimmet PZ (2010) Global estimates of the prevalence of diabetes for 2010 and 2030. Diabetes Res Clin Pract 87: 4-14.

7. Hayden PS, Iyengar SK, Schelling JR, Sedor JR (2003) Kidney disease, genotype and the pathogenesis of vasculopathy. Curr Opin Nephrol Hypertens 12: 71-78.

8. Kusenda B, Mraz M, Mayer J, Pospisilova S (2006) MicroRNA biogenesis, functionality and cancer relevance. Biomed Pap Med Fac Univ Palacky Olomouc Czech Repub 150: 205-215.

9. Chen K, Rajewsky N (2007) The evolution of gene regulation by transcription factors and microRNAs. Nat Rev Genet 8: 93-103.

10. Bentwich I, Avniel A, Karov Y, Aharonov R, Gilad S, et al. (2005) Identification of hundreds of conserved and nonconserved human microRNAs. Nat Genet 37: 766-770.

11. Ali AS, Ali S, Ahmad A, Bao B, Philip PA, et al. (2011) Expression of microRNAs: potential molecular link between obesity, diabetes and cancer. Obes Rev 12: 1050-1062.

12. McGregor RA, Choi MS (2011) microRNAs in the regulation of adipogenesis and obesity. Curr Mol Med 11: 304-316.

13. Kong L, Zhu J, Han W, Jiang X, Xu M, et al. (2011) Significance of serum microRNAs in pre-diabetes and newly diagnosed type 2 diabetes: a clinical study. Acta Diabetol 48: 61-69.

14. Turchinovich A, Weiz L, Langheinz A, Burwinkel B (2011) Characterization of extracellular circulating microRNA. Nucleic Acids Res 39: 7223-7233.

15. Fenech M, El-Sohemy A, Cahill L, Ferguson LR, French TA, et al. (2011) Nutrigenetics and nutrigenomics: viewpoints on the current status and applications in nutrition research and practice. J Nutrigenet Nutrigenomics 4: 69-89.

16. Jousse C, Parry L, Lambert-Langlais S, Maurin AC, Averous J, et al. (2011) Perinatal undernutrition affects the methylation and expression of

the leptin gene in adults: implication for the understanding of metabolic syndrome. FASEB J 25: 3271-3278.

17. Ng SF, Lin RC, Laybutt DR, Barres R, Owens JA, et al. (2010) Chronic high-fat diet in fathers programs β-cell dysfunction in female rat offspring. Nature 467: 963-966.

18. Raychaudhuri N, Raychaudhuri S, Thamotharan M, Devaskar SU (2008) Histone code modifications repress glucose transporter 4 expression in the intrauterine growth-restricted offspring. J Biol Chem 283: 13611-13626.

19. Lee RC, Feinbaum RL, Ambros V (1993) The C. elegans heterochronic gene lin-4 encodes small RNAs with antisense complementarity to lin-14. Cell 75: 843-854.

20. Bartel DP (2009) MicroRNAs: target recognition and regulatory functions. Cell 136: 215-233.

21. Thomason MK, Storz G (2010) Bacterial antisense RNAs: how many are there, and what are they doing? Annu Rev Genet 44: 167-188.

22. Carthew RW, Sontheimer EJ (2009) Origins and Mechanisms of miRNAs and siRNAs. Cell 136: 642-655.

23. Zhou X, Ruan J, Wang G, Zhang W (2007) Characterization and identification of microRNA core promoters in four model species. PLoS Comput Biol 3: e37.

24. Lee Y, Kim M, Han J, Yeom KH, Lee S, et al. (2004) MicroRNA genes are transcribed by RNA polymerase II. EMBO J 23: 4051-4060.

25. Cai X, Hagedorn CH, Cullen BR (2004) Human microRNAs are processed from capped, polyadenylated transcripts that can also function as mRNAs. RNA 10: 1957-1966.

26. Lund E, Dahlberg JE (2006) Substrate selectivity of exportin 5 and Dicer in the biogenesis of microRNAs. Cold Spring Harb Symp Quant Biol 71: 59-66.

27. Zhang X, Rossi JJ (2011) Phylogenetic comparison of small RNA-triggered transcriptional gene silencing. J Biol Chem 286: 29443-29448.

28. Brennecke J, Hipfner DR, Stark A, Russell RB, Cohen SM (2003) bantam encodes a developmentally regulated microRNA that controls cell proliferation and regulates the proapoptotic gene hid in Drosophila. Cell 113: 25-36.

29. Cuellar TL, McManus MT (2005) MicroRNAs and endocrine biology. J Endocrinol 187: 327-332.

30. Poy MN, Eliasson L, Krutzfeldt J, Kuwajima S, Ma X, et al. (2004) A pancreatic islet-specific microRNA regulates insulin secretion. Nature 432: 226-230.

31. Lewis BP, Burge CB, Bartel DP (2005) Conserved seed pairing, often flanked by adenosines, indicates that thousands of human genes are microRNA targets. Cell 120: 15-20.

32. Friedman RC, Farh KK, Burge CB, Bartel DP (2009) Most mammalian mRNAs are conserved targets of microRNAs. Genome Res 19: 92-105.

33. Ortega FJ, Moreno-Navarrete JM, Pardo G, Sabater M, Hummel M, et al. (2010) MiRNA expression profile of human subcutaneous adipose and during adipocyte differentiation. PLoS One 5: e9022.

34. Rayner KJ, Suárez Y, Dávalos A, Parathath S, Fitzgerald ML, et al. (2010) MiR-33 contributes to the regulation of cholesterol homeostasis. Science 328: 1570-1573.

35. Iliopoulos D, Drosatos K, Hiyama Y, Goldberg IJ, Zannis VI (2010) MicroRNA-370 controls the expression of microRNA-122 and Cpt1alpha and affects lipid metabolism. J Lipid Res 51: 1513-1523.

36. Correa-Medina M, Bravo-Egana V, Rosero S, Ricordi C, Edlund H, et al. (2009) MicroRNA miR-7 is preferentially expressed in endocrine cells of the developing and adult human pancreas. Gene Expr Patterns 9: 193-199.

37. Joglekar MV, Joglekar VM, Hardikar AA (2009) Expression of islet-specific microRNAs during human pancreatic development. Gene Expr Patterns 9: 109-113.

38. Kloosterman WP, Lagendijk AK, Ketting RF, Moulton JD, Plasterk RH (2007) Targeted inhibition of miRNA maturation with morpholinos reveals a role for miR-375 in pancreatic islet development. PLoS Biol 5: e203.

39. Keller DM, McWeeney S, Arsenlis A, Drouin J, Wright CV, et al. (2007) Characterization of pancreatic transcription factor Pdx-1 binding sites using promoter microarray and serial analysis of chromatin occupancy. J Biol Chem 282: 32084-32092.

40. Rayner KJ, Sheedy FJ, Esau CC, Hussain FN, Temel RE, et al. (2011) Antagonism of miR-33 in mice promotes reverse cholesterol transport and regression of atherosclerosis. J Clin Invest 121: 2921-2931.

41. Dávalos A, Goedeke L, Smibert P, Ramírez CM, Warrier NP, et al. (2011) miR-33a/b contribute to the regulation of fatty acid metabolism and insulin signaling. Proc Natl Acad Sci U S A 108: 9232-9237.

42. Lagos-Quintana M, Rauhut R, Yalcin A, Meyer J, Lendeckel W, et al. (2002) Identification of tissue-specific microRNAs from mouse. Curr Biol 12: 735-739.

43. Goedeke L, Vales-Lara FM, Fenstermaker M, Cirera-Salinas D, Chamorro-Jorganes A, et al. (2013) A regulatory role for microRNA 33* in controlling lipid metabolism gene expression. Mol Cell Biol 33: 2339-2352.

44. Esau C, Davis S, Murray SF, Yu XX, Pandey SK, et al. (2006) miR-122 regulation of lipid metabolism revealed by in vivo antisense targeting. Cell Metab 3: 87-98.

45. Elmén J, Lindow M, Silahtaroglu A, Bak M, Christensen M, et al. (2008) Antagonism of microRNA-122 in mice by systemically administered LNA-antimiR leads to up-regulation of a large set of predicted target mRNAs in the liver. Nucleic Acids Res 36: 1153-1162.

46. Lanford RE, Hildebrandt-Eriksen ES, Petri A, Persson R, Lindow M, et al. (2010) Therapeutic silencing of microRNA-122 in primates with chronic hepatitis C virus infection. Science 327: 198-201.

47. Miyaaki H, Ichikawa T, Kamo Y, Taura N, Honda T, et al. (2014) Significance of serum and hepatic microRNA-122 levels in patients with non-alcoholic fatty liver disease. Liver Int 34: e302-307.

48. Yang X, Downes M, Yu RT, Bookout AL, He W, et al. (2006) Nuclear receptor expression links the circadian clock to metabolism. Cell 126: 801-810.

49. Narkar VA, Downes M, Yu RT, Embler E, Wang YX, et al. (2008) AMPK and PPARdelta agonists are exercise mimetics. Cell 134: 405-415.

50. Liu AM, Xu Z2, Shek FH3, Wong KF4, Lee NP3, et al. (2014) miR-122 targets pyruvate kinase M2 and affects metabolism of hepatocellular carcinoma. PLoS One 9: e86872.

51. Babu DA, Deering TG, Mirmira RG (2007) A feat of metabolic proportions: Pdx1 orchestrates islet development and function in the maintenance of glucose homeostasis. Mol Genet Metab 92: 43-55.

52. Yang Y, Chang BH, Samson SL, Li MV, Chan L (2009) The Krüppel-like zinc finger protein Glis3 directly and indirectly activates insulin gene transcription. Nucleic Acids Res 37: 2529-2538.

53. Miyatsuka T, Matsuoka T-a and Kaneto H (2008) Transcription factors as therapeutic targets for diabetes.

54. Zhao E, Keller MP, Rabaglia ME, Oler AT, Stapleton DS, et al. (2009) Obesity and genetics regulate microRNAs in islets, liver, and adipose of diabetic mice. Mamm Genome 20: 476-485.

55. Poy MN, Hausser J, Trajkovski M, Braun M, Collins S, et al. (2009) miR-375 maintains normal pancreatic alpha- and beta-cell mass. Proc Natl Acad Sci U S A 106: 5813-5818.

56. Ling HY, Wen GB, Feng SD, Tuo QH, Ou HS, et al. (2011) MicroRNA-375 promotes 3T3-L1 adipocyte differentiation through modulation of extracellular signal-regulated kinase signalling. Clin Exp Pharmacol Physiol 38: 239-246.

57. Bost F, Aouadi M, Caron L, Binétruy B (2005) The role of MAPKs in adipocyte differentiation and obesity. Biochimie 87: 51-56.

58. Kim KA, Kim JH, Wang Y, Sul HS (2007) Pref-1 (preadipocyte factor 1) activates the MEK/extracellular signal-regulated kinase pathway to inhibit adipocyte differentiation. Mol Cell Biol 27: 2294-2308.

59. Tanabe Y, Koga M, Saito M, Matsunaga Y, Nakayama K (2004) Inhibition of adipocyte differentiation by mechanical stretching through ERK-mediated downregulation of PPARgamma2. J Cell Sci 117: 3605-3614.

60. Erener S, Mojibian M, Fox JK, Denroche HC, Kieffer TJ (2013) Circulating miR-375 as a biomarker of Î²-cell death and diabetes in mice. Endocrinology 154: 603-608.

61. Rottiers V, Näär AM (2012) MicroRNAs in metabolism and metabolic disorders. Nat Rev Mol Cell Biol 13: 239-250.

62. Zampetaki A, Kiechl S, Drozdov I, Willeit P, Mayr U, et al. (2010) Plasma microRNA profiling reveals loss of endothelial miR-126 and other microRNAs in type 2 diabetes. Circ Res 107: 810-817.

63. Bagge A, Clausen TR, Larsen S, Ladefoged M, Rosenstierne MW, et al. (2012) MicroRNA-29a is up-regulated in beta-cells by glucose and decreases glucose-stimulated insulin secretion. Biochem Biophys Res Commun 426: 266-272.

64. Karolina DS, Armugam A, Tavintharan S, Wong MT, Lim SC, et al. (2011) MicroRNA 144 impairs insulin signaling by inhibiting the expression of insulin receptor substrate 1 in type 2 diabetes mellitus. PLoS One 6: e22839.

65. Bagge A, Dahmcke CM, Dalgaard LT (2013) Syntaxin-1a is a direct target of miR-29a in insulin-producing Î²-cells. Horm Metab Res 45: 463-466.

66. Liang J, Liu C, Qiao A, Cui Y, Zhang H, et al. (2013) MicroRNA-29a-c decrease fasting blood glucose levels by negatively regulating hepatic gluconeogenesis. J Hepatol 58: 535-542.

67. Herrera BM, Lockstone HE, Taylor JM, Wills QF, Kaisaki PJ, et al. (2009) MicroRNA-125a is over-expressed in insulin target tissues in a spontaneous rat model of Type 2 Diabetes. BMC Med Genomics 2: 54.

68. Herrera BM, Lockstone HE, Taylor JM, Ria M, Barrett A, et al. (2010) Global microRNA expression profiles in insulin target tissues in a spontaneous rat model of type 2 diabetes. Diabetologia 53: 1099-1109.

69. Mirza S, Hossain M, Mathews C, Martinez P, Pino P, et al. (2012) Type 2-diabetes is associated with elevated levels of TNF-alpha, IL-6 and adiponectin and low levels of leptin in a population of Mexican Americans: a cross-sectional study. Cytokine 57: 136-142.

70. Mohammadi S, Hosseinzadeh-Attar MJ, Hosseinnezhad A, Hosseini SH, Eshraghian MR, et al. (2011) Compare the effects of different visfatin concentration on cardiovascular risk factors, adiponectin and insulin resistance in patients with T2DM. Diabetes & Metabolic Syndrome: Clinical Research & Reviews 5:71-75.

71. Attar MJH, Mohammadi S, Karimi M, Hosseinnezhad A, Hosseini SH, et al. (2013) Association of adiponectin with dietary factors and cardiovascular risk factors in type 2 diabetes mellitus patients. Diabetes & Metabolic Syndrome: Clinical Research & Reviews 7:3-7.

72. Adi N, Adi J, Cesar L, Hollar D, Kurlansky P, et al. (2008) Decreased Adiponectin Levels in Obese Mice with Polygenetic Susceptibility to Type 2 Diabetes Is Linked to Altered miRNA Levels of the ATF3 Gene In Visceral Adipose Tissue. CIRCULATION, LIPPINCOTT WILLIAMS & WILKINS 530 WALNUT ST, PHILADELPHIA, PA 19106-3621 USA, pp. S278-S278

73. Chen HY, Zhong X, Huang XR, Meng XM, You Y, et al. (2014) MicroRNA-29b inhibits diabetic nephropathy in db/db mice. Mol Ther 22: 842-853.

74. Long J, Wang Y, Wang W, Chang BH, Danesh FR (2011) MicroRNA-29c is a signature microRNA under high glucose conditions that targets Sprouty homolog , and its in vivo knockdown prevents progression of diabetic nephropathy. J Biol Chem 286: 11837-11848.

75. Wilfred BR, Wang WX, Nelson PT (2007) Energizing miRNA research: a review of the role of miRNAs in lipid metabolism, with a prediction that miR-103/107 regulates human metabolic pathways. Mol Genet Metab 91: 209-217.

76. Xie H, Lim B, Lodish HF (2009) MicroRNAs induced during adipogenesis that accelerate fat cell development are downregulated in obesity. Diabetes 58: 1050-1057.

77. Trajkovski M, Hausser J, Soutschek J, Bhat B, Akin A, et al. (2011) MicroRNAs 103 and 107 regulate insulin sensitivity. Nature 474: 649-653.

78. Li S, Chen X, Zhang H, Liang X, Xiang Y, et al. (2009) Differential expression of microRNAs in mouse liver under aberrant energy metabolic status. J Lipid Res 50: 1756-1765.

79. Nakanishi N, Nakagawa Y, Tokushige N, Aoki N, Matsuzaka T, et al. (2009) The up-regulation of microRNA-335 is associated with lipid metabolism in liver and white adipose tissue of genetically obese mice. Biochem Biophys Res Commun 385: 492-496.

80. Park JH, Ahn J, Kim S, Kwon DY, Ha TY (2011) Murine hepatic miRNAs expression and regulation of gene expression in diet-induced obese mice. Mol Cells 31: 33-38.

81. Heneghan H, Miller N, McAnena O, O'Brien T and Kerin M (2011) Differential miRNA expression in omental adipose tissue and in the circulation of obese patients identifies novel metabolic biomarkers. The Journal of Clinical Endocrinology & Metabolism 96:E846-E850.

82. Quesada H, Del Bas J, Pajuelo D, Diaz S, Fernandez-Larrea J, et al. (2009) Grape seed proanthocyanidins correct dyslipidemia associated with a high-fat diet in rats and repress genes controlling lipogenesis and VLDL assembling in liver. International journal of obesity 33:1007-1012.

83. Chen YK, Cheung C, Reuhl KR, Liu AB, Lee MJ, et al. (2011) Effects of green tea polyphenol (-)-epigallocatechin-3-gallate on newly developed high-fat/Western-style diet-induced obesity and metabolic syndrome in mice. J Agric Food Chem 59: 11862-11871.

84. Hininger-Favier I, Benaraba R, Coves S, Anderson RA, Roussel AM (2009) Green tea extract decreases oxidative stress and improves insulin sensitivity in an animal model of insulin resistance, the fructose-fed rat. J Am Coll Nutr 28: 355-361.

85. Wolfram S, Raederstorff D, Preller M, Wang Y, Teixeira SR, et al. (2006) Epigallocatechin gallate supplementation alleviates diabetes in rodents. J Nutr 136: 2512-2518.

86. Rivera L, Morón R, Sánchez M, Zarzuelo A, Galisteo M (2008) Quercetin ameliorates metabolic syndrome and improves the inflammatory status in obese Zucker rats. Obesity (Silver Spring) 16: 2081-2087.

87. Baselga-Escudero L, Arola-Arnal A, Pascual-Serrano A, Ribas-Latre A, Casanova E, et al. (2013) Chronic administration of proanthocyanidins or docosahexaenoic acid reverses the increase of miR-33a and miR-122 in dyslipidemic obese rats. PLoS One 8: e69817.

88. Arola-Arnal A, Bladé C (2011) Proanthocyanidins modulate microRNA expression in human HepG2 cells. PLoS One 6: e25982.

89. Milenkovic D, Deval C, Gouranton E, Landrier JF, Scalbert A, et al. (2012) Modulation of miRNA expression by dietary polyphenols in apoE deficient mice: a new mechanism of the action of polyphenols. PLoS One 7: e29837.

90. Baselga-Escudero L, Bladé C, Ribas-Latre A, Casanova E, Salvadó MJ, et al. (2012) Grape seed proanthocyanidins repress the hepatic lipid regulators miR-33 and miR-122 in rats. Mol Nutr Food Res 56: 1636-1646.

91. Tomé-Carneiro J, Larrosa M, Yáñez-Gascón MJ, Dávalos A, Gil-Zamorano J, et al. (2013) One-year supplementation with a grape extract containing resveratrol modulates inflammatory-related microRNAs and cytokines expression in peripheral blood mononuclear cells of type 2 diabetes and hypertensive patients with coronary artery disease. Pharmacol Res 72: 69-82.

92. Baselga-Escudero L, Blade C, Ribas-Latre A, Casanova E, Suárez M, et al. (2014) Resveratrol and EGCG bind directly and distinctively to miR-33a and miR-122 and modulate divergently their levels in hepatic cells. Nucleic Acids Res 42: 882-892.

93. Baselga-Escudero L, Bladé C, Ribas-Latre A, Casanova E, Salvadó MJ, et al. (2012) Grape seed proanthocyanidins repress the hepatic lipid regulators miR-33 and miR-122 in rats. Mol Nutr Food Res 56: 1636-1646.

94. Joven J, Espinel E, Rull A, Aragonès G, Rodríguez-Gallego E, et al. (2012) Plant-derived polyphenols regulate expression of miRNA paralogs miR-103/107 and miR-122 and prevent diet-induced fatty liver disease in hyperlipidemic mice. Biochimica et Biophysica Acta (BBA)-General Subjects 1820:894-899.

95. Kuzuhara T, Sei Y, Yamaguchi K, Suganuma M, Fujiki H (2006) DNA and RNA as new binding targets of green tea catechins. J Biol Chem 281: 17446-17456.

96. Xiao J, Kai G (2012) A review of dietary polyphenol-plasma protein interactions: characterization, influence on the bioactivity, and structure-affinity relationship. Crit Rev Food Sci Nutr 52: 85-101.

97. Tzur G, Levy A, Meiri E, Barad O, Spector Y, et al. (2008) MicroRNA expression patterns and function in endodermal differentiation of human embryonic stem cells. PLoS One 3: e3726.

98. Davidson LA, Wang N, Shah MS, Lupton JR, Ivanov I, et al. (2009) n-3 Polyunsaturated fatty acids modulate carcinogen-directed non-coding microRNA signatures in rat colon. Carcinogenesis 30: 2077-2084.

99. Parra P, Serra F, Palou A (2010) Expression of adipose microRNAs is sensitive to dietary conjugated linoleic acid treatment in mice. PLoS One 5: e13005.

100. Brueckner B, Stresemann C, Kuner R, Mund C, Musch T, et al. (2007) The human let-7a-3 locus contains an epigenetically regulated microRNA gene with oncogenic function. Cancer Res 67: 1419-1423.

101. Alisi A, Da Sacco L, Bruscalupi G, Piemonte F, Panera N, et al. (2011) Mirnome analysis reveals novel molecular determinants in the pathogenesis of diet-induced nonalcoholic fatty liver disease. Lab Invest 91: 283-293.

102. Benatti RO, Melo AM2, Borges FO2, Ignacio-Souza LM3, Simino LA2, et al. (2014) Maternal high-fat diet consumption modulates hepatic lipid metabolism and microRNA-122 (miR-122) and microRNA-370 (miR-370) expression in offspring. Br J Nutr 111: 2112-2122.

103. Zhang J, Zhang F, Didelot X, Bruce KD, Cagampang FR, et al. (2009) Maternal high fat diet during pregnancy and lactation alters hepatic expression of insulin like growth factor-2 and key microRNAs in the adult offspring. BMC Genomics 10: 478.

104. Fischer-Posovszky P, Kukulus V, Zulet MA, Debatin KM, Wabitsch M (2007) Conjugated linoleic acids promote human fat cell apoptosis. Horm Metab Res 39: 186-191.

105. Domeneghini C, Di Giancamillo A, Corino C (2006) Conjugated linoleic acids (CLAs) and white adipose tissue: how both in vitro and in vivo studies tell the story of a relationship. Histol Histopathol 21: 663-672.

106. Liang G, He H, Yu D (2012) Identification of nitrogen starvation-responsive microRNAs in Arabidopsis thaliana. PLoS One 7: e48951.

107. Dolganiuc A, Petrasek J, Kodys K, Catalano D, Mandrekar P, et al. (2009) MicroRNA Expression Profile in Lieber-DeCarli Diet-Induced Alcoholic and Methionine Choline Deficient Diet-Induced Nonalcoholic Steatohepatitis Models in Mice. Alcoholism: Clinical and Experimental Research 33:1704-1710.

108. Bhattacharyya SN, Habermacher R, Martine U, Closs EI, Filipowicz W (2006) Relief of microRNA-mediated translational repression in human cells subjected to stress. Cell 125: 1111-1124.

109. Coletta DK, Balas B, Chavez AO, Baig M, Abdul-Ghani M, et al. (2008) Effect of acute physiological hyperinsulinemia on gene expression in human skeletal muscle in vivo. Am J Physiol Endocrinol Metab 294: E910-917.

110. Pilegaard H, Saltin B, Neufer PD (2003) Effect of short-term fasting and refeeding on transcriptional regulation of metabolic genes in human skeletal muscle. Diabetes 52: 657-662.

111. Vissing K, Andersen JL, Schjerling P (2005) Are exercise-induced genes induced by exercise? FASEB J 19: 94-96.

112. Drummond MJ, Glynn EL, Fry CS, Dhanani S, Volpi E, et al. (2009) Essential amino acids increase microRNA-499, -208b, and -23a and downregulate myostatin and myocyte enhancer factor 2C mRNA expression in human skeletal muscle. J Nutr 139: 2279-2284.

113. Druz A, Betenbaugh M, Shiloach J (2012) Glucose depletion activates mmu-miR-466h-5p expression through oxidative stress and inhibition of histone deacetylation. Nucleic Acids Res 40: 7291-7302.

114. Bolmeson C, Esguerra JL, Salehi A, Speidel D, Eliasson L, et al. (2011) Differences in islet-enriched miRNAs in healthy and glucose intolerant human subjects. Biochem Biophys Res Commun 404: 16-22.

115. Jia Y, Cong R, Li R, Yang X, Sun Q, et al. (2012) Maternal low-protein diet induces gender-dependent changes in epigenetic regulation of the glucose-6-phosphatase gene in newborn piglet liver. J Nutr 142: 1659-1665.

116. Rundblad SA (2012) A Diet Rich in Carbohydrates Induces Changes in Serum microRNA Levels Associated with Type 2 Diabetes Development.

117. Hessel S, Eichinger A, Isken A, Amengual J, Hunzelmann S, et al. (2007) CMO1 deficiency abolishes vitamin A production from beta-carotene and alters lipid metabolism in mice. J Biol Chem 282: 33553-33561.

118. Lobo GP, Amengual J, Li HNM, Golczak M, Bonet ML, et al. (2010) ß, ß-carotene decreases peroxisome proliferator receptor ? activity and reduces lipid storage capacity of adipocytes in a ß, ß-carotene oxygenase 1-dependent manner. Journal of biological chemistry 285:27891-27899.

119. Ross AC (2003) Retinoid production and catabolism: role of diet in regulating retinol esterification and retinoic Acid oxidation. J Nutr 133: 291S-296S.

120. Napoli JL (1999) Interactions of retinoid binding proteins and enzymes in retinoid metabolism. Biochim Biophys Acta 1440: 139-162.

121. Zhang Y, Li R, Li Y, Chen W, Zhao S, et al. (2012) Vitamin A status affects obesity development and hepatic expression of key genes for fuel metabolism in Zucker fatty rats. Biochem Cell Biol 90: 548-557.

122. Li R, Chen W, Li Y, Zhang Y, Chen G (2011) Retinoids synergized with insulin to induce Srebp-1c expression and activated its promoter via the two liver X receptor binding sites that mediate insulin action. Biochem Biophys Res Commun 406: 268-272.

123. Roder K, Schweizer M (2007) Retinoic acid-mediated transcription and maturation of SREBP-1c regulates fatty acid synthase via cis-elements responsible for nutritional regulation. Biochem Soc Trans 35: 1211-1214.

124. Toma S, Isnardi L, Raffo P, Dastoli G, De Francisci E, et al. (1997) Effects of all-trans-retinoic acid and 13-cis-retinoic acid on breast-cancer cell lines: growth inhibition and apoptosis induction. Int J Cancer 70: 619-627.

125. Warrell RP Jr, Frankel SR, Miller WH Jr, Scheinberg DA, Itri LM, et al. (1991) Differentiation therapy of acute promyelocytic leukemia with tretinoin (all-trans-retinoic acid). N Engl J Med 324: 1385-1393.

126. Melnick A, Licht JD (1999) Deconstructing a disease: RARalpha, its fusion partners, and their roles in the pathogenesis of acute promyelocytic leukemia. Blood 93: 3167-3215.

127. Garzon R, Pichiorri F, Palumbo T, Visentini M, Aqeilan R, et al. (2007) MicroRNA gene expression during retinoic acid-induced differentiation of human acute promyelocytic leukemia. Oncogene 26: 4148-4157.

128. Laneve P, Di Marcotullio L, Gioia U, Fiori ME, Ferretti E, et al.(2007) The interplay between microRNAs and the neurotrophin receptor tropomyosin-related kinase C controls proliferation of human neuroblastoma cells. Proceedings of the National Academy of Sciences 104:7957-7962.

129. Annibali D, Gioia U, Savino M, Laneve P, Caffarelli E, et al. (2012) A new module in neural differentiation control: two microRNAs upregulated by retinoic acid, miR-9 and -103, target the differentiation inhibitor ID2. PLoS One 7: e40269.

130. Wang Y, Zhou J, Minto AW, Hack BK, Alexander JJ, et al. (2006) Altered vitamin D metabolism in type II diabetic mouse glomeruli may provide protection from diabetic nephropathy. Kidney Int 70: 882-891.

131. Alkharfy KM, Al-Daghri NM, Yakout SM, Hussain T, Mohammed AK, et al. (2013) Influence of vitamin D treatment on transcriptional regulation of insulin-sensitive genes. Metab Syndr Relat Disord 11: 283-288.

132. Zhuang H, Lin Y, Yang G (2007) Effects of ,25-dihydroxyvitamin D3 on proliferation and differentiation of porcine preadipocyte in vitro. Chem Biol Interact 170: 114-123.

133. Wang WL, Chatterjee N, Chittur SV, Welsh J, Tenniswood MP (2011) Effects of 1İ±,25 dihydroxyvitamin D3 and testosterone on miRNA and mRNA expression in LNCaP cells. Mol Cancer 10: 58.

134. Enquobahrie DA, Williams MA, Qiu C, Siscovick DS, Sorensen TK (2011) Global maternal early pregnancy peripheral blood mRNA and miRNA expression profiles according to plasma 25-hydroxyvitamin D concentrations. J Matern Fetal Neonatal Med 24: 1002-1012.

135. Fang F, Kang Z and Wong C (2010) Vitamin E tocotrienols improve insulin sensitivity through activating peroxisome proliferator-activated receptors. Molecular nutrition & food research 54:345-352.

136. Kasimanickam RK, Kasimanickam VR (2011) Effect of tocopherol supplementation on serum 8-epi-prostaglandin F2 alpha and adiponectin concentrations, and mRNA expression of PPARĨ³ and related genes in ovine placenta and uterus. Theriogenology 76: 482-491.

137. Ricciarelli R, Zingg JM, Azzi A (2000) Vitamin E reduces the uptake of oxidized LDL by inhibiting CD36 scavenger receptor expression in cultured aortic smooth muscle cells. Circulation 102: 82-87.

138. Vasu VT, Hobson B, Gohil K, Cross CE (2007) Genome-wide screening of alpha-tocopherol sensitive genes in heart tissue from alpha-tocopherol transfer protein null mice (ATTP(-/-)). FEBS Lett 581: 1572-1578.

139. Hundhausen C, Frank JR, Rimbach G, Stoecklin E, Muller PY, et al. (2006) Effect of vitamin E on cytochrome P450 mRNA levels in cultured hepatocytes (HepG2) and in rat liver. Cancer Genomics-Proteomics 3:183-190.

140. Gaedicke S, Zhang X, Schmelzer C, Lou Y, Doering F, et al. (2008) Vitamin E dependent microRNA regulation in rat liver. FEBS Lett 582: 3542-3546.

141. Tang XL, Xu MJ, Li ZH, Pan Q, Fu JH (2013) Effects of vitamin E on expressions of eight microRNAs in the liver of Nile tilapia (Oreochromis niloticus). Fish Shellfish Immunol 34: 1470-1475.

142. Zhang L, Hou D, Chen X, Li D, Zhu L, et al. (2012) Exogenous plant MIR168a specifically targets mammalian LDLRAP1: evidence of cross-kingdom regulation by microRNA. Cell Res 22: 107-126.

143. Zhou Q, Li M, Wang X, Li Q, Wang T, et al. (2012) Immune-related microRNAs are abundant in breast milk exosomes. Int J Biol Sci 8: 118-123.

27

Metabolic Syndrome and its Impact on Cardiovascular Diseases

Nilesh Kumar J Patel[1*], Sushruth Edla[2], Sohil Golwala[3], Deepak Asti[1], Nilay Patel[4], Achint Patel[5], Nikhil Nalluri[1], Shantanu Solanki[5], Shilp Kumar Arora[5], Hafiz Khan[1], Ritesh Kanotra[1], Pandya Bhavi[1], Abhishek Deshmukh[6], Apurva O Badheka[4], James Lafferty[1] and Jeffrey Rothman[1]

[1]Staten Island University Hospital, Staten Island, New York, USA

[2]St Vincent Charity Medical Center, Cleveland, Ohio, USA

[3]American University of The Caribbean, Sint Maarten, Corel Gables, Florida, USA

[5]Icahn School of Medicine at Mount Sinai, New York, USA

[6]University of Arkansas, Little Rock, UALR, USA

*Corresponding author: Nilesh Kumar J Patel, Staten Island University Hospital, 212, North Rail Road Ave, Apt 1C, Staten Island, New York-10304, USA; E-mail: dr.nilesh.j.patel@gmail.com

Abstract

Over the past decade, metabolic syndrome has gained recognition as a significant contributor to cardiovascular mortality. Isolated metabolic syndrome, without diabetes mellitus, plays an increasingly essential role in the pathogenesis of Coronary Artery Disease (CAD). The risk factors for metabolic syndrome act synergistically to promote the development of Cardiovascular Disease (CVD); the more the risk factors, the higher the likelihood of developing CVD. Among these risk factors, obesity is the biggest culprit as it leads to an increase in the levels of free fatty acids (FFAs), thereby resulting in insulin resistance. This, in turn, causes impaired intracellular glucose metabolism and consequent production of free radicals that reduce nitrous oxide levels and cause endothelial dysfunction, leading to atherosclerosis. Also, visceral fat, being a source of C-reactive protein, indirectly promotes inflammation and atherosclerosis. However, in certain races, insulin resistance is fairly common, even in non-obese individuals. This implies the possibilities of multiple complex mechanisms at the microcellular level, causing insulin resistance over and above the aforementioned mechanisms occurring due to obesity. In spite of this fact, control of obesity still remains the first line of defense against metabolic syndrome and resulting cardiovascular mortality. Measures like proper diet and physical exercise, and medications such as statins, fibrates, niacin, and ACE inhibitors are the cornerstones of management of metabolic syndrome. Additionally, clinical trials using medications affecting peroxisome proliferator-activated receptors (PPARs) and intestinal enteropeptidases have shown promising results for treatment of metabolic syndrome. Moreover, current research is also focused on the role of adipokines, semicarbazide-sensitive amine oxidase/vascular adhesion protein-1 (SSAO/VAP-1), 5-HT2c receptors, and the LKB1/AMPK pathway in influencing the mechanisms of insulin resistance. In the near future, newly discovered mechanisms and highly potent novel drugs may reduce the prevalence of metabolic syndrome and subsequent cardiovascular mortality.

Keywords: Metabolic syndrome; Cardiovascular diseases; Cardiovascular mortality

Introduction

Metabolic syndrome is defined by a group of risk factors that have been known to independently and synergistically increase the risk of developing cardiovascular disease, including, but not limited to coronary artery disease (CAD) and heart failure. According to the National Cholesterol Education Program (NCEP)/Adult Treatment Panel (ATP III), metabolic syndrome is defined as the presence of any three of the following five traits [1]:

1. Abdominal obesity, defined as a waist circumference in men ≥102 cm (40 in) and in women ≥88 cm (35 in).

2. Serum triglycerides ≥150 mg/dL (1.7mmol/L) or drug treatment for elevated triglycerides.

3. Serum HDL cholesterol <40 mg/dL (1mmol/L) in men and <50 mg/dL (1.3 mmol/L) in women or drug treatment for low HDL-C.

4. Blood pressure ≥130/85 mmHg or drug treatment for elevated blood pressure.

5. Fasting plasma glucose (FPG) ≥100 mg/dL (5.6 mmol/L) or drug treatment for elevated blood glucose.

Epidemiology

The prevalence of metabolic syndrome among US adults is close to 22% [2], which equates to about 47 million people. About 44% of those are above 50 years of age [3]. It is important to note that almost 64% of men and 42% of women with impaired glucose tolerance, and 84% of men and 78% of women with type 2 diabetes mellitus have metabolic syndrome [4]. In addition, increased body weight appears to be an important risk factor for metabolic syndrome. In NHANES III, metabolic syndrome was present in 5% of individuals with normal weight, 22% of those who were overweight and in 60% of those who were obese [5]. Obesity proves to be a major risk factor for metabolic syndrome in diabetics as well as non-diabetics.

Isolated metabolic syndrome, without diabetes mellitus, significantly increases the risk of developing cardiovascular disease. Multiple sub analyses, such as the Scandinavian Simvastatin Survival Study (4S) and the Air Force/Texas Coronary Atherosclerosis Prevention Study (AFCAPS/TexCAPS) showed that placebo controls with isolated metabolic syndrome (without type 2 diabetes) were at ~1.5 time's higher risk of coronary events than those without metabolic syndrome [6]. According to the NHANES-III trial, among the participants with age 50 years or more, the prevalence of CAD was found to be the highest among patients with both metabolic syndrome and type 2 diabetes at 19.2%. Similarly, patients with isolated metabolic syndrome (without type 2 diabetes) had a prevalence of 13.2%.

Lastly, the risk of developing cardiovascular disease in metabolic syndrome increases synergistically with each risk factor, proving that the more the risk factors of metabolic syndrome, the higher the likelihood of developing CVD. As shown in the Prospective Cardiovascular Munster (PROCAM) study, the 4 year risk of having a myocardial infarction among men between ages 40 and 65 increased 2.5 times in the presence of either diabetes or hypertension, 8 times in the presence of both diabetes and hypertension, and 19 times in the presence of all 3 risk factors including hypertension, diabetes, and dyslipidemia. Hence, the risk factors associated with metabolic syndrome significantly contribute to the development of cardiovascular disease.

Pathogenesis

ATP III recognized six major components that account for the pathogenesis of metabolic syndrome.

1. Abdominal obesity

2. Insulin resistance [7]

3. Dyslipidemia [8]

4. Hypertension

5. Prothrombotic state, with elevated fibrinogen and plasminogen activator inhibitor (PAI-1)

6. Pro-inflammatory state, with an increase in acute phase reactants.

Abdominal obesity

ATP III considers abdominal obesity to be one of the prime culprits for the rising prevalence of metabolic syndrome. Contrary to the former concept of adipose tissue being inert, there is growing evidence that fat is implicit in the secretion of cytokines and other inflammatory markers like PAI-1 and adiponectin. The excess release of free fatty acids (FFA) by visceral fat or intra-abdominal fat leads to an adverse effect on insulin action and glucose metabolism in several tissues [9], in part by increasing the triglyceride reserves in the liver and muscle tissue, thereby depressing insulin action and increasing the output of VLDLs by the liver [10]. Weight loss in obese individuals has been associated with a marked reduction in visceral fat and in turn a reduction in FFA levels leading to improved insulin sensitivity [11,12].

The differences in distribution of fat in men and women may explain, in part, the higher prevalence of CAD in men than in women [13]. The abdominal distribution of fat seen in men, as opposed to the gluteofemoral distribution of fat in women, has a stronger predisposition for development of CAD [14]. Despite the above observation, it is important to note that patients of normal weight can also be insulin resistant. These have been labeled as metabolically obese, normal-weight individuals.

The impact of obesity on cardiovascular disease is well documented. In the Framingham Heart Study cohort, Wilson et al. showed that an increase in weight of 2.25 kg or more over 16 years was associated with a 21 to 45 percent increase in the risk for developing the syndrome [15]. A large waist circumference alone identifies up to 46% of individuals who could develop metabolic syndrome in the next five years [16]. The International Day of Evaluation of Abdominal Obesity [17], the largest study to assess the frequency of obesity in primary care patients, showed that abdominal obesity, measured by the waist circumference, showed a graded relationship with both CVD and diabetes at all levels of BMI. The Heart Outcomes Prevention Evaluation (HOPE) study concluded that abdominal adiposity worsens the prognosis of patients with CVD and that a weight reduction program should be integrated into the management of these patients [18]. There are a variety of alterations in the intrinsic structure and function of the heart which take place secondary to excess accumulation of adipose tissue. Cardiomyopathy of Obesity, also known as Adipositas Cordis is a phenomenon in which cardiac myocytes accumulate fat between them. This leads to pressure-induced atrophy from the intervening fat, resulting in myocyte degeneration and cardiac dysfunction. Those pathological processes related to obesity predispose the individual to an array of cardiovascular abnormalities such as Coronary Artery Disease (CAD), heart failure and sudden cardiac death. Hence, obesity plays a crucial role in the development of cardiovascular disease in metabolic syndrome, primarily via release of excessive FFAs.

Insulin resistance

It is the defect in insulin action that results in hyperinsulinemia, necessary to maintain euglycemia. A major culprit in the development of insulin resistance is the excessive FFAs released by the visceral fat. FFAs work by inhibiting insulin-mediated glucose uptake, thereby leading to reduced insulin sensitivity. Many investigators continue to argue that this is by far the most important component of metabolic syndrome, so much so that it was named Insulin Resistance Syndrome until recently [19]. It is difficult to assess the specific nature of insulin resistance individually given that it is linked to obesity. It is simplistic to note that increasing levels of body fat are associated with decreasing levels of insulin sensitivity [20] but what dilutes this concept is that there is a broad variation in sensitivities even within the obese population [21]. In certain racial populations like south Asians, insulin resistance is common even in individuals with BMI <25 kg/m^2. But even in these populations with a higher predisposition, the incidence of insulin resistance increases with increased visceral fat. Furthermore, insulin resistance, as identified by increased C-peptide levels, is significantly related to hazards of cardiovascular death in non-diabetic adults [22]. Multiple studies have demonstrated a strong association between metabolic syndrome and the risk of developing type 2 diabetes mellitus [23]. Meta-analysis of 16 multi-ethnic cohort studies by Ford et al. showed that the relative risk of developing diabetes in an individual with metabolic syndrome ranged from 3.53 to 5.17 based on the patient population [24]. Another interesting finding in this study was that the relative risk for incidence of diabetes was increased 2.1-fold if ATP III definition was used and a 3.6-fold if the WHO definition for metabolic syndrome was considered. This difference highlights the importance of insulin resistance, which is a required characteristic of the WHO definition, in the pathogenesis of type 2 diabetes.

Another growing school of thought with regards to the association of insulin resistance and cardiovascular disease is a theory that links endothelial dysfunction with insulin resistance. Endothelial dysfunction is a strong contributor in the pathophysiology of coronary artery disease. Deficiency of endothelial derived Nitric Oxide (NO) is the primary defect that leads to inadequate vasodilation and paradoxical vasoconstriction in coronary vasculature. Nitric Oxide production and release is markedly reduced in the presence of high levels of free radicals like Reactive Oxygen Species (ROS) and Reactive Nitrogen Species (RNS), which are produced as a result of impaired intracellular glucose and lipid metabolism. Endothelial dysfunction, in turn, leads to impaired insulin action due to inadequate transcapillary passage of insulin to its target tissues, eventually culminating in a vicious cycle. Hence, it can be concluded that insulin resistance, secondary to excess FFAs as well as endothelial dysfunction, significantly increases the risk of cardiovascular disease in metabolic syndrome.

Prothrombotic and proinflammatory states

A fundamental concept is that atherogenesis represents a state of chronic inflammation characterized by lipid-induced insult that triggers a cascade of events including invasion of macrophages and proliferation of smooth muscle cells. Within the endothelium, the secretory nature of adipose tissue, particularly that of intra-abdominal and visceral fat, is in part responsible for the proinflammatory and prothrombotic states that almost always accompany obesity. How this translates into increased risk of atherosclerotic cardiovascular disease continues to remain a bone of contention. One hypothesis that has wider acceptance is endothelial dysfunction [25] leading to enhanced atherogenicity. An interesting study by Mauras et al. [26] in obese children with no other comorbidities that could put them at a risk for metabolic syndrome showed that these children had remarkably higher levels of proinflammatory and prothrombotic markers such as hsCRP, fibrinogen, IL-6 and PAI-1. CRP, which is an acute phase reactant and an index of inflammation, has been strongly associated with CAD and acute coronary syndrome due to its ability to destabilize an atherosclerotic plaque [27]. CRP plays an essential role in the development of cardiovascular disease, particularly in metabolic syndrome. The Insulin Resistance Atherosclerosis Study (IRAS) [28] showed that even in non-diabetic populations, CRP levels were directly proportional to the incidence of metabolic syndrome [28]. Previous studies have shown that polymorphisms of CRP gene that cause higher concentrations of CRP are associated with higher risk of CVD [30]. Ridker et al. concluded that giving statins to individuals with elevated levels of hsCRP but without dyslipidemia, was associated with a significant reduction in the incidence of coronary events [31]. The association between CRP, metabolic syndrome and CVD is suggestive, but it is not clear as to how the elevations of CRP in obese individuals could lead to major coronary events. A causal relationship between elevated CRP and metabolic syndrome could not be demonstrated in a study of phenotype patterns associated with metabolic syndrome and CRP levels [32]. It must be noted that this does not rule out a causative relationship.

Multiple studies including the original Framingham study have confirmed the fact that fibrinogen is as important a risk factor for CVD as is hypertension [33,34], hyperlipidemia and smoking. PAI-1 [35], which is also released by visceral fat [36], is the principal inhibitor of fibrinolysis. PAI-1 gene knockout mice studies showed that when these mice were fed high-calorie, high-fat diet they were able to prevent obesity and insulin resistance [37]. Newer markers such as Toll-like receptor activity are being studied for their association with metabolic syndrome. Jialal et al. [38] concluded in their study that there is an increase of expression and activity of TLR-2 and TLR-4 in the monocytes of patients with metabolic syndrome and

this could contribute to increased risk for CVD and diabetes in these individuals.

Therapeutic Implications

According to ATP III, obesity is the biggest risk factor in developing cardiovascular disease in metabolic syndrome, and thus proves to be the primary target in the management of metabolic syndrome. Consequently, weight reduction and increased physical activity continue to remain the first line of therapy to effectively lower the cardiovascular risks in metabolic syndrome by reducing cholesterol levels, blood pressure, insulin resistance and increasing HDL levels. Second line therapy for management of metabolic syndrome is the use of medications, specifically targeted towards the major risk factors of metabolic syndrome such as dyslipidemia, hypertension, and insulin resistance.

Statins prove to be the most effective treatment for lowering LDL cholesterol as well as other forms of apolipoproteins. A large study involving 5 different centers using low-dose rosuvastatin in 580 patients for 12 weeks, showed significant improvement in the lipid panel from baseline. LDL and non-HDL/HDL cholesterol level ratio was reduced by 47%, non-HDL levels were down by 43%, triglyceride levels were down by 23%, and HDL levels were up by 10% [39]. However, more importantly, lipid-lowering benefits were of a similar scale in patients with metabolic syndrome in comparison to those without metabolic syndrome, proving statins to be an effective therapy for hyperlipidemia in metabolic syndrome.

Furthermore, fibrates greatly aid in lowering cardiovascular risks in metabolic syndrome, especially when used in combination with statins, by lowering pro-inflammatory markers such as CRP, fibrinogen and PAI-1 [40,41]. This is clearly demonstrated in VA-HIT trial as gemfibrozil significantly reduced the risk of developing major cardiovascular events in high-risk populations with diabetes and insulin resistance [42].

Additionally, in a recent 3-phase cross over trial [43], a patient population with metabolic syndrome diagnosed by ATPIII criteria as well as combined hyperlipidemia and hypertriglyceridemia were treated with placebo, simvastatin 10mg alone or simvastatin and fenofibrate combination. At the end of the three phases of the study, the simvastatin alone group showed a reduction of triglycerides by 23%, total cholesterol by 27%, non-HDL cholesterol by 30%, and VLDL by 36%, and an increase in HDL of 6%. Interestingly, the addition of fenofibrates had exponential effects in reducing the VLDL by an additional 36%, and increasing the HDL by another 16% as compared to the simvastatin group alone. Therefore, fibrates, especially when used in combination with statins, prove to be an effective treatment to reduce major risk factors associated with metabolic syndrome, thus reducing the incidence of cardiovascular disease in metabolic syndrome. A multicenter randomized controlled trial by Colhoun et al. [44] concluded that statin therapy is effective in reducing the risk of cardiovascular events in patients with type 2 diabetes even if the LDL levels were not elevated. Statins also have been shown to decrease inflammation by attenuating leukocyte-endothelial cell interactions [45], thereby amending ischemic injury in hypercholesterolemic mice independently of their lipid-lowering actions.

In addition to hyperlipidemia and hypertriglyceridemia, hypertension management remains an important entity to reduce cardiovascular risks associated with metabolic syndrome. Low-dose aspirin has been proved to be an effective tool, targeting prothrombotic states in the primary and secondary prevention of CAD events in patients with metabolic syndrome. In patients with a Framingham risk score of >10% aspirin has been shown to have a favorable effect. Hence, targeting proinflammatory states has been the focus of recent research aimed at reducing the cardiovascular risks associated with metabolic syndrome.

Medicine has a famous saying by Ben Franklin, "An ounce of prevention is worth a pound of cure." In the case of metabolic syndrome, proper diet and exercise prove to be an effective tool for treatment as well as prevention. As shown in the Framingham Offspring Study, diet had a significant impact on insulin resistance. Specific food types such as total fiber, cereal fiber, fruit fiber, and whole grain intakes were associated with lower insulin resistance and thus significantly reduced the risk of metabolic syndrome [46]. Lastly, pharmacologic approaches can assist in controlling major risk factors such as dyslipidemia and hypertension using statins, fibrates, niacin as well as ace-inhibitors, and thus preventing the development of metabolic syndrome.

Future Perspectives

Diagnostic

ATP III has simple current guidelines for diagnosis of metabolic syndrome, encompassing five major criteria including abdominal obesity, serum triglycerides, serum HDL, and blood pressure and fasting plasma glucose, as mentioned earlier. However, due to significantly high risk of developing CHD and CAD associated with metabolic syndrome, early detection of the disease is crucial. In addition to currently established risk factors, few other tools have been proposed to diagnose metabolic syndrome.

Several new biomarkers continue to gain importance in early detection of metabolic syndrome correlating with CVD risk, such as high leptin, elevated fasting insulin and increased hs-CRP levels as well as high uric acid levels. In addition, C-peptide may prove to be of importance in early development of CVD in metabolic syndrome [47,48].

Therapeutic

There is a growing arm of research focusing on adipokines like adiponectins, leptins, resistins, and zinc alpha-2 glycoproteinsas [49] targets of therapy, particularly as more knowledge is being gathered on the roles of different depots of fat. Another field of interest is the inhibitors of semicarbazide-sensitive amine oxidase/vascular adhesion protein-1 (SSAO/VAP-1) [50]. They have shown to exert beneficial effects on insulin in adipocytes, proving to be potential targets for management of metabolic syndrome.

Additionally, 5-HT2c receptors have been studied for a while with regards to their role in obesity management. 5-HT2c agonists, which have been considered potential drugs for treatment of obesity, include Lorcaserin, which is the only one in its class approved by the FDA specifically for treatment of obesity [51].

Genetics experts have also been targeting a specific intestinal enteropeptidase, which is involved in the digestion of dietary proteins and lipids, thereby proving to be a potential therapy for managing the primary risk factor of obesity in metabolic syndrome [52]. The LKB1/AMPK pathway is another potential target for the treatment of metabolic syndrome [53]. This pathway involves serine/threonine kinases regulating anabolic and catabolic metabolic processes, representing attractive therapeutic targets for the treatment of obesity and type II diabetes, and thus reducing cardiovascular risks in metabolic syndrome.

Furthermore, reduction of endothelial-derived nitric oxide (eNOS) is the key mechanism of insulin resistance and visceral adiposity in metabolic syndrome [54]. Thus, future pharmacologic interventions targeting eNOS regulation and increasing insulin sensitivity may prove to be beneficial in treating metabolic syndrome. Laufs et al. [55] showed that inhibition of HMG CoA reductase results in upregulation of eNOS expression by posttranscriptional mechanisms in addition to lowering of cholesterol levels.

Dipeptidyl peptidase 4 (DPP-4) inhibitors (commonly referred to as gliptins) are a novel class of oral antihyperglycemic agents with demonstrated efficacy in the treatment of type 2 diabetes mellitus as noted by Andre J Scheen. [56] Studies have indicated a possible beneficial action on blood vessels and the heart, via glucagon-like peptide effects. DPP-4 inhibition increases the concentration of many peptides with potential vasoactive and cardioprotective effects. Clinically, DPP-4 inhibitors improve several risk factors in patients with T2DM. They improve blood glucose control (mainly by reducing postprandial glycaemia), are weight neutral (or even induce modest weight loss), lower blood pressure, improve postprandial lipemia, reduce inflammatory markers, diminish oxidative stress, and improve endothelial function. Some positive effects on the heart have also been described in patients with ischemic heart disease or congestive heart failure, as indicated by Marney et al. [57] in work describing the interactive hemodynamic effects of DPP-4 inhibition and Angiotensin-converting enzyme inhibition. The actual relationship between DPP-4 inhibition and cardiovascular outcomes remains to be proven. Major prospective clinical trials with predefined cardiovascular outcomes and involving various DPP-4 inhibitors are now underway in patients with T2DM and a high-risk cardiovascular profile.

Lastly, peroxisome proliferator-activated receptors (PPARs), which have three isoforms: PPAR-α, PPAR-γ, and PPAR-δ, play a key role in regulating adipogenesis, lipid and carbohydrate metabolism, as well as insulin resistance. A trial using troglitazone demonstrated potential for effective treatment of metabolic syndrome primarily by increasing nitric oxide production via PPARγ-dependent pathway, VEGF-KDR/Flk-1-Akt-mediated eNOS-Ser1179 phosphorylation, PPARγ-independent pathway, and eNOS-Ser116 dephosphorylation [58]. In addition, another potential therapy using bezafibrate can regulate eNOS expression via PPAR-α dependent pathway.

Conclusion

Cardiovascular disease is a primary outcome of metabolic syndrome, which is defined adequately by the ATP III criteria. Abdominal obesity and insulin resistance denote the greatest risk for developing cardiovascular events in the presence of metabolic syndrome, primarily via excessive release of FFAs and impairment of endothelium function. In addition, proinflammatory markers, such as adipokines, CRP and PAI-1 play a significant role in disrupting atherosclerotic plaques, thereby leading to cardiovascular complications in metabolic syndrome.

Regardless of the risk factors involved, conservative methods for treating obesity such as diet and exercise prove to be the primary mode of treatment as well as prevention of cardiovascular disease in patients with metabolic syndrome. Pharmacologic therapy can be beneficial using statins, fibrates and aspirin to reduce the major risk factors involved in metabolic syndrome, thereby significantly lowering the risk of cardiovascular disease. Lastly, future research targeting proinflammatory markers as well as eNOS and PPARs may prove to impact the development of cardiovascular disease in metabolic syndrome.

References

1. Expert Panel on Detection, Evaluation (2001) "Executive summary of the third report of the National Cholesterol Education Program (NCEP) expert panel on Detection, Evaluation, and Treatment of high blood cholesterol in adults (Adult Treatment Panel III)." JAMA285:2486-2497.

2. Ford ES, Giles WH, Dietz WH (2002) Prevalence of the metabolic syndrome among US adults: findings from the third National Health and Nutrition Examination Survey. JAMA 287: 356-359.

3. Alexander CM, Landsman PB, Teutsch SM, Haffner SM, Third National Health and Nutrition Examination Survey (NHANES III); (2003) NCEP-defined metabolic syndrome, diabetes, and prevalence of coronary heart disease among NHANES III participants age 50 years and older. Diabetes 52: 1210-1214.

4. Ginsberg HN, Stalenhoef AF (2003) The metabolic syndrome: targeting dyslipidaemia to reduce coronary risk. J Cardiovasc Risk 10: 121-128.

5. Park YW, Zhu S, Palaniappan L, Heshka S, Carnethon MR, et al. (2003) The metabolic syndrome: prevalence and associated risk factor findings in the US population from the Third National Health and Nutrition Examination Survey, 1988-1994. Arch Intern Med 163: 427-436.

6. Girman CJ, Rhodes T, Mercuri M, Pyörälä K, Kjekshus J, et al. (2004) "The metabolic syndrome and risk of major coronary events in the Scandinavian Simvastatin Survival Study (4S) and the Air Force/Texas coronary atherosclerosis prevention study (AFCAPS/TexCAPS)." Am J cardiol 93: 136-141.

7. Haffner SM, Alexander CM, Cook TJ, Boccuzzi SJ, Musliner TA, et al. (1999) "Reduced coronary events in simvastatin-treated patients with coronary heart disease and diabetes or impaired fasting glucose levels: subgroup analyses in the Scandinavian Simvastatin Survival Study." Arch Intern Med 159: 2661-2667.

8. Steinmetz A, Fenselau S, Schrezenmeir J (2001) Treatment of dyslipoproteinemia in the metabolic syndrome. ExpClinEndocrinol Diabetes 109: S548-559.

9. Mittelman SD, Van Citters GW, Kirkman EL, Bergman RN (2002) Extreme insulin resistance of the central adipose depot in vivo. Diabetes 51: 755-761.

10. Ginsberg HN (2000) Insulin resistance and cardiovascular disease. J Clin Invest 106: 453-458.

11. Brunzell JD, Ayyobi AF (2003) Dyslipidemia in the metabolic syndrome and type 2 diabetes mellitus. Am J Med 115 Suppl 8A: 24S-28S.

12. Purnell JQ, Kahn SE, Albers JJ, Nevin DN, Brunzell JD, et al. (2000) Effect of weight loss with reduction of intra-abdominal fat on lipid metabolism in older men. J ClinEndocrinolMetab 85: 977-982.

13. McGill HC Jr, McMahan CA, Herderick EE, Zieske AW, Malcom GT, et al. (2002) Obesity accelerates the progression of coronary atherosclerosis in young men. Circulation 105: 2712-2718.

14. Grundy SM, Brewer HB Jr, Cleeman JI, Smith SC Jr, Lenfant C, et al. (2004) "Definition of metabolic syndrome report of the National Heart, Lung, and Blood Institute/American Heart Association Conference on scientific issues related to definition." ArteriosclerThrombVascBiol 109: 433-438.

15. Wilson PW, Kannel WB, Silbershatz H, D'Agostino RB (1999) Clustering of metabolic factors and coronary heart disease. Arch Intern Med 159: 1104-1109.

16. Palaniappan L, Carnethon MR, Wang Y, Hanley AJ, Fortmann SP, et al. (2004) Predictors of the incident metabolic syndrome in adults: the Insulin Resistance Atherosclerosis Study. Diabetes Care 27: 788-793.

17. Balkau B, Deanfield JE, Després JP, Bassand JP, Fox KA, et al. (2007) International Day for the Evaluation of Abdominal Obesity (IDEA): a study of waist circumference, cardiovascular disease, and diabetes mellitus in 168,000 primary care patients in 63 countries. Circulation 116: 1942-1951.

18. Dagenais, Gilles R, Qilong Yi, Johannes FE Mann, Jackie Bosch, et al. (2005) Prognostic impact of body weight and abdominal obesity in women and men with cardiovascular disease. Am Heart J 149: 54-60.

19. Reaven GM (1988) Banting lecture 1988. Role of insulin resistance in human disease. Diabetes 37: 1595-1607.

20. Bogardus C, Lillioja S, Mott DM, Hollenbeck C, Reaven G (1985) Relationship between degree of obesity and in vivo insulin action in man. Am J Physiol 248: E286-291.

21. Abbasi F, Brown BW Jr, Lamendola C, McLaughlin T, Reaven GM (2002) Relationship between obesity, insulin resistance, and coronary heart disease risk. J Am CollCardiol 40: 937-943.

22. Patel N, Taveira TH, Choudhary G, Whitlatch H, Wu WC (2012) Fasting serum C-peptide levels predict cardiovascular and overall death in nondiabetic adults. J Am Heart Assoc 1: e003152.

23. Hanson RL, Imperatore G, Bennett PH, Knowler WC (2002) Components of the "metabolic syndrome" and incidence of type 2 diabetes. Diabetes 51: 3120-3127.

24. Ford ES, Li C, Sattar N (2008) Metabolic syndrome and incident diabetes: current state of the evidence. Diabetes Care 31: 1898-1904.

25. Widlansky ME, Gokce N, Keaney JF Jr, Vita JA (2003) The clinical implications of endothelial dysfunction. J Am CollCardiol 42: 1149-1160.

26. Mauras N, Delgiorno C, Kollman C, Bird K, Morgan M, et al. (2010) Obesity without established comorbidities of the metabolic syndrome is associated with a proinflammatory and prothrombotic state, even before the onset of puberty in children. J ClinEndocrinolMetab95: 1060-1068.

27. Morrow DA, Ridker PM (2000) C-reactive protein, inflammation, and coronary risk. Med Clin North Am 84: 149-161, ix.

28. Festa A, D'Agostino R Jr, Howard G, Mykkänen L, Tracy RP, et al. (2000) Chronic subclinical inflammation as part of the insulin resistance syndrome: the Insulin Resistance Atherosclerosis Study (IRAS). Circulation 102: 42-47.

29. Zacho J, Tybjaerg-Hansen A, Jensen JS, Grande P, Sillesen H, et al. (2008) Genetically elevated C-reactive protein and ischemic vascular disease. N Engl J Med 359: 1897-1908.

30. Ridker PM, Danielson E, Fonseca FA, Genest J, Gotto AM Jr, et al. (2008) Rosuvastatin to prevent vascular events in men and women with elevated C-reactive protein. N Engl J Med 359: 2195-2207.

31. Timpson NJ, Lawlor DA, Harbord RM, Gaunt TR, Day IN, et al. (2005) C-reactive protein and its role in metabolic syndrome: mendelianrandomisation study. Lancet 366: 1954-1959.

32. Stec JJ, Silbershatz H, Tofler GH, Matheney TH, Sutherland P, et al. (2000) Association of fibrinogen with cardiovascular risk factors and cardiovascular disease in the Framingham Offspring Population. Circulation 102: 1634-1638.

33. Kannel WB, Wolf PA, Castelli WP, D'Agostino RB (1987) Fibrinogen and risk of cardiovascular disease. The Framingham Study. JAMA 258: 1183-1186.

34. Grundy SM (2002) Obesity, metabolic syndrome, and coronary atherosclerosis. Circulation 105: 2696-2698.

35. Mavri A, Alessi MC, Bastelica D, Geel-Georgelin O, Fina F, et al. (2001) Subcutaneous abdominal, but not femoral fat expression of plasminogen activator inhibitor-1 (PAI-1) is related to plasma PAI-1 levels and insulin resistance and decreases after weight loss. Diabetologia 44: 2025-2031.

36. Ma LJ, Mao SL, Taylor KL, Kanjanabuch T, Guan Y, et al. (2004) Prevention of obesity and insulin resistance in mice lacking plasminogen activator inhibitor 1. Diabetes 53: 336-346.

37. Jialal I, Huet BA, Kaur H, Chien A, Devaraj S (2012) Increased toll-like receptor activity in patients with metabolic syndrome. Diabetes Care 35: 900-904.

38. Grundy SM, Cleeman JI, Merz CN, Brewer HB Jr, Clark LT et al. (2004) Implications of recent clinical trials for the National Cholesterol Education Program Adult Treatment Panel III guidelines. Circulation 110: 227-239.

39. Bays HE, Stein EA, Shah AK, Maccubbin DL, Mitchel YB, et al. (2002) Effects of simvastatin on C-reactive protein in mixed hyperlipidemic and hypertriglyceridemic patients. Am J Cardiol 90: 942-946.

40. Cortellaro M, Cofrancesco E, Boschetti C, Cortellaro F, Mancini M et al. (2000) Effects of fluvastatin and bezafibrate combination on plasma fibrinogen, t-plasminogen activator inhibitor and C reactive protein levels in coronary artery disease patients with mixed hyperlipidaemia (FACT study). Fluvastatin Alone and in Combination Treatment." ThrombHaemost83: 549-553.

41. Robins SJ, Collins D, McNamara JR, Bloomfield HE (2008) Body weight, plasma insulin, and coronary events with gemfibrozil in the Veterans Affairs High-Density Lipoprotein Intervention Trial (VA-HIT). Atherosclerosis 196: 849-855.

42. Vega GL, Ma PT, Cater NB, Filipchuk N, Meguro S, et al. (2003) Effects of adding fenofibrate (200 mg/day) to simvastatin (10 mg/day) in patients with combined hyperlipidemia and metabolic syndrome. Am J Cardiol 91: 956-960.

43. Colhoun HM, Betteridge DJ, Durrington PN, Hitman GA, Neil HA, et al. (2004) Primary prevention of cardiovascular disease with atorvastatin in type 2 diabetes in the Collaborative Atorvastatin Diabetes Study (CARDS): multicentrerandomised placebo-controlled trial. Lancet 364: 685-696.

44. Scalia R, Gooszen ME, Jones SP, Hoffmeyer M, Rimmer DM 3rd, et al. (2001) Simvastatin exerts both anti-inflammatory and cardioprotective effects in apolipoprotein E-deficient mice. Circulation 103: 2598-2603.

45. Schulze MB, Hu FB (2004) Dietary approaches to prevent the metabolic syndrome: quality versus quantity of carbohydrates. Diabetes Care 27: 613-614.

46. Abdullah A, Hasan H, Raigangar V, Bani-Issa W (2012) C-Peptide versus insulin: relationships with risk biomarkers of cardiovascular disease in metabolic syndrome in young arab females. Int J Endocrinol 2012: 420792.

47. Nagahama K, Inoue T, Kohagura K, Ishihara A, Kinjo K, et al. (2014) Hyperuricemia predicts future metabolic syndrome: a 4-year follow-up study of a large screened cohort in Okinawa, Japan. Hypertens Res 37: 232-238.

48. Russell ST (2010) Adipokines have a role to play in the treatment of metabolic disease. Future Med Chem 2: 1721-1724.

49. Bour S, Caspar-Bauguil S, Iffiú-Soltész Z, Nibbelink M, Cousin B, et al. (2009) Semicarbazide-sensitive amine oxidase/vascular adhesion protein-1 deficiency reduces leukocyte infiltration into adipose tissue and favors fat deposition. Am J Pathol 174: 1075-1083.

50. Smith SR, Weissman NJ, Anderson CM, Sanchez M, Chuang E, et al. (2010) Multicenter, placebo-controlled trial of lorcaserin for weight management. N Engl J Med 363: 245-256.

51. Braud S, Ciufolini M, Harosh I (2010) 'Energy expenditure genes' or 'energy absorption genes': a new target for the treatment of obesity and Type II diabetes. Future Med Chem 2: 1777-1783.

52. Foretz M, Hébrard S, Leclerc J, Zarrinpashneh E, Soty M, et al. (2010) Metformin inhibits hepatic gluconeogenesis in mice independently of the LKB1/AMPK pathway via a decrease in hepatic energy state. J Clin Invest 120: 2355-2369.

53. Huang PL (2009) eNOS, metabolic syndrome and cardiovascular disease. Trends EndocrinolMetab 20: 295-302.

54. Laufs U, La Fata V, Plutzky J, Liao JK (1998) Upregulation of endothelial nitric oxide synthase by HMG CoA reductase inhibitors. Circulation 97: 1129-1135.

55. Scheen AJ (2013) Cardiovascular effects of gliptins. Nat Rev Cardiol 10: 73-84.

56. Marney A, Kunchakarra S, Byrne L, Brown NJ (2010) Interactive hemodynamic effects of dipeptidyl peptidase-IV inhibition and angiotensin-converting enzyme inhibition in humans. Hypertension 56: 728-733.

57. Cho DH, Choi YJ, Jo SA, Jo I (2004)Nitric oxide production and regulation of endothelial nitric-oxide synthase phosphorylation by prolonged treatment with troglitazone: evidence for involvement of peroxisome proliferator-activated receptor (PPAR) gamma-dependent and PPARgamma-independent signaling pathways. J BiolChem 279: 2499-2506.

58. Wang Y, Wang Y, Yang Q, Yan JT, Zhao C, et al. (2006) Effects of bezafibrate on the expression of endothelial nitric oxide synthase gene and its mechanisms in cultured bovine endothelial cells. Atherosclerosis 187: 265-273.

28

Regression of Carotid Intima Media Thickness after One Year of Atorvastatin Intervention in Dyslipidemic Obese Teenagers, a Randomized Controlled Pilot Study

Reem AL Khalifah[1,4], **Marc Girard**[2] and **Laurent Legault**[1,3*]

[1]Pediatric Endocrinology Department, McGill University, the Montreal Children's Hospital, 2300 Rue Tupper, Montreal, H3H 1P3, Canada

[2]Radiology Department, Hôpital Maisonneuve-Rosemont, 5415 Boulevard de l' Assomption, Montréal, QC H1T 2M4, Canada

[3]Pediatric Endocrinology Department, Hôpital Maisonneuve-Rosemont, 5415 Boulevard de l' Assomption, Montréal, QC H1T 2M4, Canada

[4]Pediatric Department, King Saud University, Riyadh, Saudi Arabia

*Corresponding author: Legault L, Pediatric Endocrinology Department, Montreal Children's Hospital, room C-1239, 2300 Rue Tupper, Montreal, H3H 1P3, Canada; E-mail: laurent.legault@muhc.mcgill.ca

Abstract

Objective: Metabolic syndrome in obese teenagers may contribute to future cardiovascular disease (CVD). We designed a pilot study to evaluate the effect on carotid intima media thickness (cIMT) of Atorvastatin treatment over one year in dyslipidemic obese adolescents (DLP) with metabolic syndrome markers.

Methods: We conducted a randomized double blinded control study. Adolescents 14-18 years old were recruited; 16 DLP were randomized to either 10 mg Atorvastatin or placebo. Both groups had cIMT measurements on the left and right side before and one year after the intervention. These measurements were compared to those of teenagers with familial hypercholesterolemia (FH).

Results: The average left cIMT of the DLP group was 0.582 ± 0.073 mm, and the right, 0.536 ± 0.071 mm, this compared well with measurements from FH individuals, 0.569 ± 0.947 mm and 0.548 ± 0.913 mm (right and left respectively, p=0.49). For the DLP group, the average left cIMT decreased only in the statin group to 0.509 ± 0.041 mm (p=0.04) but not on the right side 0.555 ± 0.062 (p=0.5). On average cIMT decreased by 10% in Atorvastatin treated individuals and increased by 1.6% in placebo treated ones. CIMT correlated best with the diastolic pressure but not with any of the lipid values.

Conclusion: To our knowledge this is the first pilot study that showed cIMT regression in dyslipidemic obese teenagers with features of metabolic syndrome after Atorvastatin therapy over one year. However, future long term studies should look at long term CVD risk reduction.

Keywords: Dyslipidemia; Carotid intima media thickness; Atorvastatin; Atherosclerosis; Children; Metabolic syndrome

Introduction

Childhood obesity is a worldwide health concern. Many obese teenagers show features of metabolic syndrome. There is a growing fear amongst clinicians involved in the care of obese teenagers for an eventual epidemic of early onset cardiovascular disease (CVD). This risk is based on observations from adult cohorts that metabolic syndrome markers increase the risk ratio of CVD events anywhere from 1.5-2 folds [1]. Although long-term observational studies have not been done in teenagers carrying the same risk markers, there is mounting evidence that the same might be expected of them [2]. Atherosclerosis is a continuous process that starts early in childhood, as inferred from post mortem studies clearly establishing that CVD onset starts in the pediatric age range [3]. CVD risk predictions in pediatrics are difficult as the occurrence of cardiac events is quite distant in their future. However, in adults it is clear that other surrogate markers are emerging as targets for intervention [4,5]. One of these tools, a non-invasive one, has been used more consistently to

assess the future risk of events in the CVD prevention field. Intima media thickness (IMT) measurements of the carotid artery (cIMT) have been shown to be good predictors of future cardiovascular events in at-risk individuals [6].

Regression of cIMT over time has been observed in adults, in the context of an aggressive treatment approach of familial hypercholesterolemia (FH) and produced positive cIMT changes over time [7]. Similarly, in FH children CIMT measurements are increased compared to non affected children, and treatment with statins reduces the progression of cIMT thickness over time [8,9]. Obese teenagers with features of metabolic syndrome including dyslipidemia (DLP) have comparable increased cIMT measurements and these track through adulthood [1,10,11].

HMG-CoA reductase inhibitors (Statins) are an FDA approved treatment option for children older than 10 years with familial hypercholesterolemia [12-14]. The treatment algorithm is based on LDL-C level targets [14,15]. However, up to date, no study has evaluated the effect of using statins for the treatment of dyslipidemia in obese teens with metabolic syndrome markers who do not respond to lifestyle modification [16]. In our pilot study we used cIMT measurements as a surrogate marker of atherosclerosis progression over one year to evaluate the impact of Atorvastatin therapy on obese teenagers with dyslipidemia (DLP) and metabolic syndrome features. At baseline, we also compared the cIMT measurements of a group of DLP teenagers to another with FH as this is a well known high risk group of individuals who have previously shown a potential for regression of their cIMT. Atorvastatin was chosen on the basis of its safety record, the experience gathered so far with the medication and its potential impact on Tg levels and HDL-C, lipid profile markers frequently abnormal in obese teenagers.

Methodology

Study design

We conducted a randomized double blind control trial to evaluate the effect of Atorvastatin therapy on cIMT measurements in obese post pubertal teenagers between the age of 14 and 18 years old with dyslipidemia (DLP). These teenagers were recruited from the weight management clinic in accordance with the criteria for metabolic syndrome diagnosis based on the Cardiovascular Health and Risk Reduction in Children and Adolescents Guidelines by the presence of combination of 3 or more of the following risk factors: obesity, high blood pressure, Dyslipidemia (low HDL-C<1.0 mmol/L, elevated Non-HDL-C> 3.7 mmol/L, elevated triglyceride levels of >1.7 mmol/L), impaired fasting glucose, elevated fasting insulin level [12]. Written informed consent was obtained from their parents as well as from the patients themselves. This study received Research Ethics Board approval at Hôpital Maisonneuve-Rosemont.

For the purpose of comparing cIMT measurements, a group of teenagers between the age of 14 and 18 years old diagnosed with familial hypercholesterolemia (FH) was recruited. They were selected on the basis of a Total-C>7.0 mmol/L or a LDL-C before treatment of >4.1 mmol/L, generally well accepted surrogate markers of FH in the absence of mutation analysis confirmation [17]. Those teenagers were recruited before any treatment initiation.

Clinical and biochemical assessments

Baseline assessment included; systolic and diastolic blood pressures, waist circumference measurements (WC), body mass index (BMI) and biochemical profiles. The teenagers with DLP had measurements before and after the intervention. Blood pressure was measured on the right arm with the help of an automated device (Dynamap). WC was measured by the same person at the midpoint between lower rib and iliac crest directly on the skin using a flexible tape measure. Total cholesterol (Tot-C), HDL-C and Triglyceride (Tg) levels were measured using a standard kit. The LDL-C level was calculated using the Friedewald equation. Exclusion criteria included any cause of secondary dyslipidemia including renal failure and hypothyroidism which were ruled out at the enrolment visit by measurement of creatinine and TSH levels.

All teenagers underwent an oral glucose tolerance test (OGTT) to rule out the presence of asymptomatic type 2 diabetes with insulin levels being measured at the fasting and 2 h post glucose ingestion time points. HOMA-IR scores were calculated using the formula: insulin (mcU/ml) × fasting glucose (mmol/L)/22.5. C-reactive protein (CRP) levels were also measured before and after intervention.

Carotid Intima Media Thickness (CIMT) Measurement

CIMT was measured on the right and left carotid arteries. The same ultrasonographer did all cIMT measurements. The ultrasonographer was blinded to the patient assignment group. CIMT was measured in b-mode at the level of the co mmon carotid artery, proximal to the bulb on the far wall. The images were recorded on a Video Home System (VHS) tape and sent to an outside lab for standardized measurements (Prevention concepts, Santa Monica, California); the outside lab technicians were also blinded to the patient's group assignment. The continuous video recording used by this lab allows for multiple images to be collected both sagitally and transversally, is fully computerized and automated and only showed a variability of ± 3%. The measurement technique is shown in Figure 1.

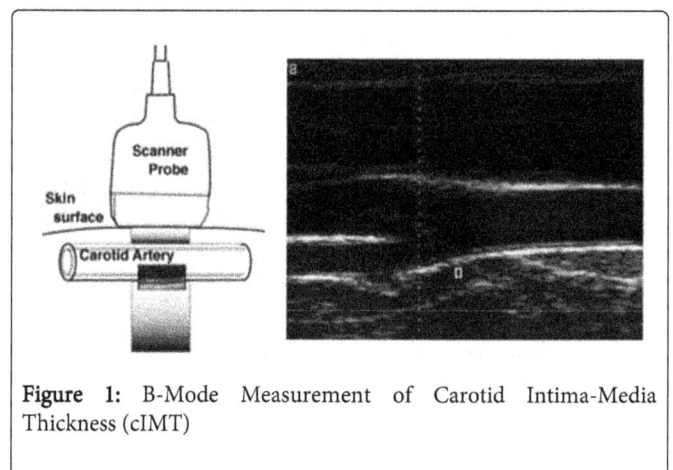

Figure 1: B-Mode Measurement of Carotid Intima-Media Thickness (cIMT)

Intervention

The DLP group was randomized through a computer generated system on a one to one basis. Accordingly, the DLP patient's either received placebo (which was manufactured by the sponsor) or Atorvastatin 10 mg according to the computer code. Patients, physicians, pharmacists and the study team were all blinded to the patient assignment group. Children of the FH group were not followed up for treatment in this trial. They were treated by their clinicians and followed up accordingly.

Lifestyle modification

All DLP groups received nutritional and exercise counselling. The diet consisted of "low-fat, low-cholesterol diet, such as the American Heart Association (AHA) Step I diet, for children with dyslipidemia that was modified to the patient's preferences and baseline diet [12]. The lifestyle protocol consisted of 4 visits with the same dietician following the initial assessment based on a food record. The initial target was 500 Kcal less than the reported intake and this was adjusted at each visit. Counselling on opportunities for increased activity, decreases in sedentary behaviour were also discussed at each session. All these teenagers were actively followed in a weight management clinic and had thus been instructed on lifestyle changes prior to the start of the study.

Study follow up

Patients in the DLP groups were followed up every 3 months. The follow up included lab evaluation for liver transaminases (ALT and

AST) as well as creatine kinase. In addition to, monitoring of side effects, compliance with medication was assessed through retrieving the pill bottles and proceeding to a pill count.

Statistical Analysis

We estimated the sample size needed to show significant difference in the thickness of the intima over one year by the reference data from the central lab to be 20 individuals (i.e. 10 in each group). IBM SPSS for Mac version 22 was used for all the statistics. Normally distributed data is presented as mean with standard deviation (SD) and non-parametric data as median with interquartile range. Within group comparisons were assessed using paired t-tests or non-parametric equivalent (Wilcoxon signed rank test). CIMT measurements of individuals were compared with normative data published by different groups. Results for boys and girls were pooled as previous studies have shown repeatedly that there are no striking sex differences before adulthood [18,19]. Comparisons were also made with FH teens at baseline. Comparisons were then made between values pre and one year post intervention for maximal, minimal and average thickness of left and right carotid arteries. Linear regression correlations were established between cIMT and blood pressure, BMI, lipid values, HOMA-IR score and fasting insulin.

Two sets of analyses were done in this study, a per protocol analysis between groups using t-tests, and for the intent to treat analysis, a paired t-tests with the last available observation carried forward used when data was missing.

Results

Baseline characteristics

Twenty six teenagers were recruited for this study, sixteen in the DLP group and ten in FH group. The baseline characteristics of both groups are shown in Table 1.

	DLP		P value	DLP N=16	FH N= 10	P value
	Placebo N= 8	Atorvastatin N=8				
Male sex, n (%)	7 (87%)	5 (62.5%)	0.2	12 (81%)	5 (50%)	0.04
Age, years	15.5 ± 1.1	15.5 ± 1.5	1	15.4 ± 1.3	15.2 ± 1.8	0.8
Weight, Kg	103.8 ± 37.3	107.2 ± 23.7	0.8	105.3 ± 29.3	77.1 ± 15.4	0.01
BMI$, kg/m^2	33.6 (29.1,43.3)	35.6 (31,4)	0.8*	38.6 ± 9.1	26.3 ± 3.7	0.001
BMI z score$^\$$	2.8 (2.3,3.7)	3.2 (2.3,3.7)	0.7*	3.1 ± 0.7	1.4 ± 1.2	<0.01*
WC, cm	113.18 ± 25.2	114.43 ± 16.1	0.9	--	--	--
Blood pressure, mm HG						
Systolic	126.2 ± 15.3	122.8 ± 12.6	0.6	124.5 ± 13.8	116.5 ± 14.1	0.1
Diastolic	70.8 ± 7.9	74.3 ± 6.5	0.3	72.6 ± 7.2	68.5 ± 7.8	0.21
Lipids, mmol/L						
TC	4.1 ± 0.4	4.7 ± 0.6	0.1	4.7 ± 0.7	6.4 ± 1.6	0.001
Triglyceride	1.7 ± 0.1	2.3 ± 0.7	0.06	2.0 ± 0.5	1.5 ± 0.6	0.04
HDL-C	0.8 ± 0.1	0.8 ± 0.1	0.5	0.9 ± 0.1	1.2 ± 0.2	0.001
LDL-C	2.6 ± 0.5	2.8 ± 0.6	0.5	2.8 ± 0.6	4.5 ± 1.5	<0.001
Tot C/ HDL-C	5.0 ± 0.7	5.3 ± 0.7	0.0	5.2 ± 0.7	5.5 ± 0.7	0.37
Non -HDL	3.4 ± 0.5	3.9 ± 0.6	0.1	3.8 ± 0.6	5.2 ± 1.3	0.001
HOMA-IR	5.8 ± 2.9	10.2 ± 3.3	0.03	--	--	--
FBG, mmol/L	4.8 ± 0.3	4.8 ± 0.3	0.8	--	--	--
Carotid intima media measurement, mm						
Mean Right	0.522 ± 0.086	0.550 ± 0.057	0.4	0.536 ± 0.071	0.548 ± 0.913	1
Mean Left	0.602 ± 0.085	0.560 ± 0.054	0.2	0.582 ± 0.073	0.552 ± 0.155	0.49

Values are given as mean ± SD or indicated otherwise. BMI, body mass index; WC, Waist circumference; HDL-C, high-density lipoprotein cholesterol; LDL-C, low-density lipoprotein cholesterol; TC, total cholesterol; CRP, C-reactive protein; HOMA-IR, homeostatic model assessment for insulin resistance; FBS, fasting blood sugar. FBS, fasting blood sugar. *Mann-Whitney U test, $Median and interquartile range 25-75

Table 1: Baseline characteristics of Dyslipidemia group (DLP) and Familial hypercholesterolemia group (FH)

Both groups were comparable at baseline except for LDL-C values, weight and BMI, as expected. Thirty percent of the DLP teenagers had high systolic blood pressure; 2 pre-hypertension and 4 hypertension. All but 1 of the DLP teens had a high HOMA score (i.e. >3.99). Only 3 were found to have a high CRP. One patient admitted to smoking.

At baseline the average cIMT measurements for the DLP and FH groups were 0.536 ± 0.071 mm and 0.548 ± 0.913 mm respectively for the right side; 0.582 ± 0.073 mm and 0.552 ± 0.155 mm for the left side. These were not significantly different as shown in Table 1. Overall, the left carotid typically showed an increased thickness as compared to the right side. The mean difference was 0.051 mm ± 0.099 mm (p=0.01). The cIMT measurements post intervention for the Atorvastatin group are presented in Table 2. The changes post intervention was significant in the maximum and average left cIMT measurements for both groups.

cIMT, mm	Pre	Post	P value$	P value*	Pre	Post	P value $	P value*
Min left	0.508 ± 0.205	0.555 ± 0.075	0.78	0.25	0.522 ± 0.071	0.467 ± 0.049	0.07	0.86
Min right	0.500 ± 0.084	0.520 ± 0.044	0.78	0.55	0.524 ± 0.63	0.469 ± 0.015	0.27	0.09
Max left	0.645 ± 0.091	0.609 ± 0.084	0.78	**0.04**	0.588 ± 0.054	0.546 ± 0.034	0.06	0.42
Max right	0.553 ± 0.086	0.585 ± 0.073	0.61	0.08	0.582 ± 0.058	0.542 ± 0.041	0.46	0.76
Average left	0.602 ± 0.086	0.579 ± 0.077	0.92	**0.03**	0.561 ± 0.054	0.509 ± 0.041	**0.049**	0.56
Average right	0.522 ± 0.086	0.555 ± 0.063	0.56	0.1	0.550 ± 0.057	0.504 ± 0.012	0.35	0.27

Values are given as mean ± SD, $Group analysis, *Paired t-tests intent to treat analysis, Bold values statistically significant

Table 2: cIMT changes pre and post intervention in dyslipidemic teenagers

CIMT showed a combined (average left and right) 1.8% progression over the study year in the placebo group, whereas the Atorvastatin treated group showed a 9% reduction. That amounts to a combined decrease of 10.8% of cIMT progression over 1 year. Again, the impact was much more pronounced on the left side (12% reduction).

There was significant correlation between Left mean cIMT measurements and diastolic blood pressure r=0.6, P<0.01. No significant correlations could be established between left cIMT and lipid values, HOMA score, waist circumference, systolic blood pressure measurements and CRP levels.

Mean lipid and lipoprotein levels at baseline and 1 year post intervention are shown in Table 3. Both Atorvastatin and placebo group had similar lipid profiles at baseline. The total cholesterol to HDL-C ratio showed significant improvement in the treatment arm, from 5.4 ± 0.8 mmol/L to 4.37 ± 0.7 mmol/L (P=0.04). None of the other biochemical marker changes over time were found to be significant.

	Placebo			Atorvastatin		
	Pre	Post	P	Pre	Post	P
Weight, kg	104.5 ± 36.3	107.5 ± 39.5	NS	107.2 ± 23.6	100.3 ± 23.15	NS
BMI, kg/m2$	33.6 (29.1, 43.3)	33.8 (28.4, 47.6)	0.72*	35.6 (31,44)	34.7 (31, 44)	0.8*
BMI z score$	2.8 (2.3, 3.7)	2.8 (2.2,4.0)	0.77*	3.16 (2.3, 3.7)	3.01 (2.46, 3.8)	0.7*
WC, cm	113.2 ± 25.2	113.5 ± 24.9	NS	116.9 ± 15.6	113.6 ± 14.4	NS
Lipid profile, mmol/L						
TC	4.3 ± 0.4	4.5 ± 1.1	NS	4.7 ± 0.6	4.1 ± 0.6	NS
Tg	1.7 ± 0.1	2.1 ± 0.9	NS	1.7 ± 0.1	2.1 ± 1.6	NS

HDL-C	0.8 ± 0.1	0.9 ± 0.1	NS	0.8 ± 0.1	0.9 ± 0.7	NS
LDL-C	2.6 ± 0.5	2.7 ± 0.8	NS	2.8 ± 0.6	2.4 ± 0.5	NS
Tot C/ HDL-C	5.1 ± 0.7	5.2 ± 1.7	NS	5.4 ± 0.8	4.3 ± 0.7*	0.04
Non-HDL	3.4 ± 0.5	3.6 ± 1.1	0.44	3.9 ± 0.6	3.4 ± 0.7	0.07
HOMA-IR	5.8 ± 2.9	3.3 ± 0.9	0.31	10.2 ± 3.3	7.6 ± 2.7	0.18
FBS, mmol/L	4.6 ± 0.3	4.8 ± 0.3	0.1	5.0 ± 0.2	4.8 ± 0.3	0.2

BMI, body mass index; WC, Waist circumference; HDL-C, high-density lipoprotein cholesterol; LDL-C, low-density lipoprotein cholesterol; TC, total cholesterol; CRP, C-reactive protein; HOMA-IR, homeostatic model assessment for insulin resistance; FBS, fasting blood sugar. Values are given as mean ± SD or indicated otherwise. *Wilcoxon Signed Rank test. $Median and interquartile range 25-75.

Table 3: Pre and post intervention clinical features and laboratory values in placebo treated (P) and statin treated (Rx) dyslipidemic teenagers

Overall the lifestyle intervention worked relatively well. Five teenagers (31%) had their BMI decrease and one saw the BMI remain the same following the counselling at one year follow up. Half recorded better waist circumference measurements and 31% an actual decrease in weight, 15% achieving more than a 5 Kg weight loss.

Safety and compliance

The overall adherence for medication uptake in the group was 86%. No significant medication associated side effects were found.

Discussion

This study, for the first time, signals potential benefit of using Atorvastatin for children with dyslipidemia and metabolic syndrome features to alter the Atherosclerosis process. The main finding of this pilot study is that the left cIMT thickness was significantly reduced over one year after Atorvastatin intervention. Hence, decrease atherosclerosis progression as we hypothesized. Interestingly, the only site where cIMT measurement is significantly changed was the left carotid artery, where the thickness is maximal. CIMT being thicker on the left side has been described in other studies; it is otherwise not well understood [1]. The fact that both the per protocol and the intent to treat analyses revealed significant changes at the left carotid artery site points towards it being a potential useful marker for monitoring impact of interventions in future studies. We may speculate this means that an aggressive treatment approach using Statins could benefit those with the highest cIMT readings.

CIMT measurements are not part of the routine follow up of teenagers at risk for future CVD and as such, there are no threshold values above which treatment is mandated. We found that the values found in our DLP group represented values more than the 95th percentile for cIMT measured in children of similar age and sex; and were comparable to values found in FH in the same age group [18-21]. This in itself could constitute a stronger argument to treat these patients since they could carry the same atherosclerotic risk based on their baseline cIMT measurements and potential for tracking. Very few studies have looked prospectively at cIMT changes in teenagers following an intervention. Positive changes were reported in FH affected individuals after a Statin intervention [7,8]. We are thus not surprised to see similar results in teenagers with DLP consequently this could translate into reduction of future CVD risk.

Only DBP correlated with cIMT in our cohort. It has been reported in adults that cIMT values correlate with age, sex and blood pressure values. There are also reports showing multiple correlations with different lipid values or markers of insulin resistance but this is not as well established in the pediatric age group [11].

In our study, the exact mechanism for the regression of cIMT measurements remains undetermined. LDL-C levels did not change significantly despite Atorvastatin therapy. In this group though, they were not considered high. However, the only biochemically significant change seen was a decrease in the total-C to HDL-C ratio. Interestingly, while the lipid profiles of the 2 groups (FH and DLP) were quite different, their total-C to HDL-C ratios was remarkably similar. This ratio has not been extensively studied in pediatrics as a marker of future CVD but may; based on adult data, also represent an important marker for future studies. Furthermore, fasting non–HDL-C levels are strongly associated with metabolic syndrome features as inferred from recent study in US youth [16,22].

Our study had many strong points that overcame many of the limitations reported in studies evaluating Statins use in FH. Our study design was a randomized controlled double-blinded study with a placebo arm; this allowed an unbiased analysis. We have shown that monitoring cIMT changes over one year is possible and may be clinically relevant. The predictive role of cIMT in pediatrics is yet to be established on a wide scale but it may play a more prominent role in the future to assess more specific individual risk and then tailor the treatment accordingly [18]. Both intensive lifestyle and Statin interventions could be monitored through cIMT, and perhaps more specifically left cIMT measurements, in at-risk individuals to determine the impact of specific interventions. Our work opens a relatively new pediatric paradigm in targeting higher risk individuals for prevention of future CVD.

We had few limitations in the pilot study, mainly, the small sample size. Unfortunately we could not recruit as many patients as needed per the sample size calculation. Nevertheless, we were able to show significant differences between groups. This will need to be replicated in a larger prospective cohort. A second limitation is that some individuals failed to complete all the analyses. This was addressed by an intention to treat analysis. While the intent to treat analysis revealed significant positive changes as well in the untreated group, the treatment group's comparisons were likely affected by using the last observation carried forward approach, which amounts to no change being seen in the group where most values are missing, in this case, the treatment group.

Conclusion

This is, to our knowledge, the first pilot study looking at treating and prospectively monitoring at risk DLP teenagers with the help of serial cIMT measurements. In this small study, we were able to show regression of cIMT over a one year period. What might be inferred from our pilot study is that dyslipidemic obese teenagers with the thickest cIMTs, expected to be at higher future risk, could see their cIMTs regress with Statin therapy over one year. The exact mechanism or biochemical marker is yet to be unravelled with larger prospective trials, although we found the ratio of total cholesterol to HDL-C correlated with these changes. We believe this study has potentially great clinical significance as it opens the door for early consideration of Statin therapy in higher risk dyslipidemic individuals when lifestyle modification fails to improve the biochemical profile and cIMT thickness over time. However, future studies should look at longer-term effects of Statins therapy on cIMT measurements and possible reduction of long term CVD risk as seen in the adult population.

Acknowledgement

This study was supported by an unrestricted grant from Pfizer Canada.

References

1. Magnussen CG, Venn A, Thomson R, Juonala M, Srinivasan SR (2009) The association of pediatric low- and high-density lipoprotein cholesterol dyslipidemia classifications and change in dyslipidemia status with carotid intima-media thickness in adulthood evidence from the cardiovascular risk in Young Finns study, the Bogalusa Heart study, and the CDAH (Childhood Determinants of Adult Health) study. J Am Coll Cardiol 53: 860-869.

2. Bleakley C, Millar A, Hamilton PK, Harbinson M, McVeigh GE (2013) Lifetime risk of cardiovascular disease: the next generation in risk prediction. Can J Cardiol 29: 147-150.

3. Berenson GS, Srinivasan SR, Bao W, Newman WP 3rd, Tracy RE, et al. (1998) Association between multiple cardiovascular risk factors and atherosclerosis in children and young adults. The Bogalusa Heart Study. N Engl J Med 338: 1650-1656.

4. Oberman A (2000) Hypertriglyceridemia and coronary heart disease. JCEM 85:2098-2105.

5. Sharma RK, Singh VN, Reddy HK (2009) Thinking beyond low-density lipoprotein cholesterol: strategies to further reduce cardiovascular risk. Vasc Health Risk Manag 5: 793-799.

6. Hodis HN, Mack WJ, LaBree L, Selzer RH, Liu CR, et al. (1998) The role of carotid arterial intima-media thickness in predicting clinical coronary events. Ann Intern Med 128: 262-269.

7. Smilde TJ, van Wissen S, Wollersheim H, Trip MD, Kastelein JJ, et al. (2001) Effect of aggressive versus conventional lipid lowering on atherosclerotic progression in familial hypercholesterolemia: a prospective, randomized, double-blind trial. Lancet 357: 577-581.

8. Virkola K, Pesonen E, Akerblom HK, Siimes MA (1997) Cholesterol and carotid artery wall in children and adolescents with familial hypercholesterolaemia: a controlled study by ultrasound. Acta Paediatr 86: 1203-1207.

9. Lavrencic A, Kosmina B, Keber I, Videcnik V, Keber D (1996) Carotid intima-media thickness in young patients with familial hypercholesterolaemia. Heart 76: 321-325.

10. Fang J, Zhang JP, Luo CX, Yu XM, Lv LQ (2010) Carotid Intima-media thickness in childhood and adolescent obesity relations to abdominal obesity, high triglyceride level and insulin resistance. Int J Med Sci 7: 278-283.

11. Dawson JD, Sonka M, Blecha MB, Lin W, Davis PH (2009) Risk factors associated with aortic and carotid intima-media thickness in adolescents and young adults: the Muscatine Offspring Study. J Am Coll Cardiol 53: 2273-2279.

12. Expert Panel on Integrated Guidelines for Cardiovascular Health and Risk Reduction in Children and Adolescents; National Heart, Lung, and Blood Institute (2011) Expert panel on integrated guidelines for cardiovascular health and risk reduction in children and adolescents: su mmary report. Pediatrics 128 Suppl 5: S213-256.

13. Lamaida N, Capuano E, Pinto L, Capuano E, Capuano R, et al. (2013) The safety of statins in children. Acta Paediatr 102: 857-862.

14. Vuorio A, Kuoppala J, Kovanen PT, Humphries SE, Strandberg T, et al. (2010) Statins for children with familial hypercholesterolemia. Cochrane Database Syst Rev : CD006401.

15. Daniels SR, Jacobson MS, McCrindle BW, Eckel RH, Sanner BM (2009) American Heart Association Childhood Obesity Research Su mmit: executive su mmary. Circulation 119: 2114-2123.

16. McCrindle BW (2004) Lipid abnormalities in children with the metabolic syndrome. Canadian Journal of Diabetes 28: 226-237.

17. Leitersdorf E, Tobin EJ, Davignon J, Hobbs HH (1990) Co mmon low-density lipoprotein receptor mutations in the French Canadian population. J Clin Invest 85: 1014-1023.

18. Slyper AH (2004) Clinical review 168: What vascular ultrasound testing has revealed about pediatric atherogenesis, and a potential clinical role for ultrasound in pediatric risk assessment. J Clin Endocrinol Metab 89: 3089-3095.

19. Sass C, Herbeth B, Chapet O, Siest G, Visvikis S, et al. (1998) Intima-media thickness and diameter of carotid and femoral arteries in children, adolescents and adults from the Stanislas cohort: effect of age, sex, anthropometry and blood pressure. J Hypertens 16: 1593-1602.

20. Doyon A, Kracht D, Bayazit AK, Deveci M, Duzova A, et al. (2013) Carotid artery intima-media thickness and distensibility in children and adolescents: reference values and role of body dimensions. Hypertension 62: 550-556.

21. Stabouli S, Kotsis V, Karagianni C, Zakopoulos N, Konstantopoulos A (2012) Blood pressure and carotid artery intima-media thickness in children and adolescents: the role of obesity. Hellenic J Cardiol 53: 41-47.

22. Li C, Ford ES, McBride PE, Kwiterovich PO, McCrindle BW, et al. (2011) Non-high-density lipoprotein cholesterol concentration is associated with the metabolic syndrome among US youth aged 12-19 years. J Pediatr 158: 201-207.

29

Multifaces of Pituitary Adenylate Cyclase-Activating Polypeptide (PACAP): From Neuroprotection and Energy Homeostasis to Respiratory and Cardiovascular Systems

Abdoulaye Diané, Geoffrey W Payne and Sarah L Gray*

Northern Medical Program, University of Northern British Columbia, Prince George, Canada

***Corresponding author:** Sarah L Gray, Northern Medical Program, University of Northern British Columbia, 3333 University Way, Prince George, BC V2N 4Z9, Canada; E-mail: Sarah.Gray@unbc.ca

Abstract

Pituitary adenylate cyclase-activating polypeptide (PACAP) belongs to the secretin/glucagon/vasoactive intestinal peptide (VIP) family and is one of the most highly conserved neuropeptides. The effects of PACAP are mediated through three G-protein coupled receptors: PAC1R, which has specific affinity for PACAP, and VPAC1 and VPAC2 that have equal affinity for both PACAP and VIP. PACAP and PAC1R are widely expressed and distributed throughout the body, including the central nervous system, the gastro-intestinal tract, the endocrine pancreas, the respiratory and cardiovascular systems. With this widespread tissue distribution, PACAP has been shown to be a pleiotropic peptide exerting a range of physiological functions. Within the body, PACAP serves as a neurotransmitter, neuromodulator, neurotrophic factor, neuroprotectant, secretagogue, and neurohormone. In this present review, we provide current insight on the role of PACAP in neuroprotection, its role in energy homeostasis and the impact PACAP may have on respiratory and cardiovascular disease. We conclude with an outlook for the future of PACAP-related research.

Keywords: PACAP; Neuroprotection; Energy homeostasis; Respiratory system; Cardiovascular system

Introduction

Pituitary adenylate cyclase-activating polypeptide (PACAP) is a neuropeptide originally isolated from ovine hypothalamic tissue by Arimura and coworkers in 1989 based on its capacity to activate adenylate cyclase to produce cyclic AMP in rat pituitary cells [1-3]. This neuropeptide belongs to the secretin/glucagon/vasoactive intestinal peptide (VIP) superfamily, and exists in two amidated forms from the same precursor, PACAP38 (38-amino acid residues) and PACAP27. Since its discovery, extensive research has been dedicated to understanding the biological role of PACAP. PACAP has been detected in all vertebrates studied so far and is one of the most highly conserved neuropeptides [4].

PACAP binds to the PACAP specific receptor 1 (PAC1R), and the receptors for VIP, VPAC1 and VPAC2. The PAC1R, of which there are at least nine variant forms, is specific for PACAP, whereas the other two receptors, VPAC1 and VPAC2, bind both PACAP and VIP [5-7]. The PAC1R belongs to the class II family of G protein-coupled receptors that trigger mainly adenylate cyclase activation through $G\alpha s$ protein subunits [8]. Alternatively, PAC1R is also capable of coupling to $G\alpha q$ proteins to activate the phospholipase C (PLC) pathways leading to increased inositol triphosphate (IP₃) turnover and a rise in intracellular calcium concentrations (Figure 1) [9,8].

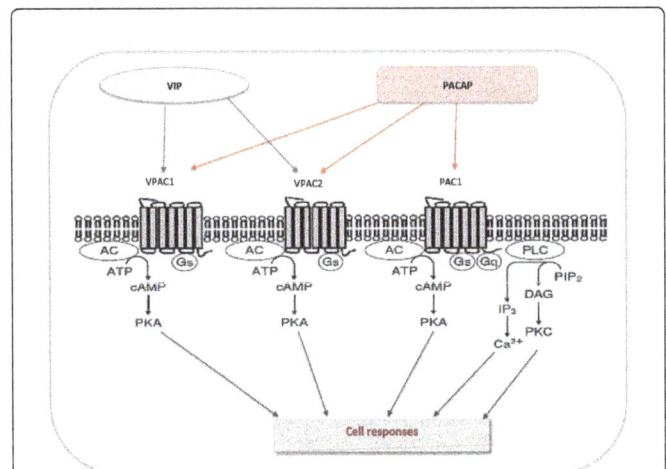

Figure 1: Schematic representation of the signal transduction pathways of VIP/PACAP receptors. Upon VIP or PACAP ligand binding to the N-terminal domain of the VIP/PACAP receptor, a cascade of transduction signals occur namely either via the adenylate cyclase or phospholipase C pathways or mobilizing intracellular calcium. VIP: Vasoactive Intestinal Peptide; PAC1: PACAP specific receptor 1; VPAC1: Receptor-1 for VIP; VPAC2: Receptor-2 for VIP; AC: Adenylyl Cyclase; DAG: Diacylglycerol; IP3: Inositol Trisphosphate; PKA: Protein-Kinase A; PKC: Protein-Kinase C; cAMP: Cyclic Adenosine Monophosphate; ATP: Adenosine Triphosphate; PIP2: Phosphatidylinositol Biphosphate.

PACAP is a neuropeptide acting as a neurotransmitter, neuromodulator, or neurotrophic factor. PACAP and its receptors are widely expressed and distributed throughout the central nervous system (CNS) and in various peripheral organs, including endocrine glands (adrenal, pancreas, ovaries, and testes), the gastro-intestinal tract, and the respiratory and cardiovascular systems [10]. Consistent with this widespread distribution, PACAP has been found to exert pleiotropic physiological functions. This review article presents an update on PACAP research and its known involvement in a variety of physiological and pathophysiological processes based on neuroprotective effects, its homeostatic control of energy metabolism and its impact on respiratory and cardiovascular systems. We conclude by discussing its possible potential for future therapeutic applications.

PACAP and its neuroprotective effects

Soon after its discovery and characterization, the distribution of PACAP in the CNS of mammals was investigated [11]. Although PACAP mRNA expression is widespread throughout the CNS, the most abundant population of PACAP-containing neurons in the brain is found in the hypothalamus [12,13]. Moreover, using *in situ* hybridization and immunocytochemistry, some extra hypothalamic regions, including the hippocampus, cerebral cortex, striatum, nucleus accumbens, amygdala and substantia nigra abundantly express both PAC1R and PACAP (Table 1) [12,14,15], suggestive of the involvement of the peptide in the neuronal functions [16].

Brain structures	mRNA
Olfactory bulb	++
Cerebral cortex	++
Amygdala	++
Hippocampal formation	+
Thalamus	++
Hypothalamus	
Arcuate nucleus	++
Mediobasal hypothalamus	++
Ventromedial nuclei	+++
Paraventricular nucleus	++
Cerebellum	–/++
Brainstem	–/++

Table 1: Localization and relative abundance of PACAP mRNA in the rat brainby in situ hybridization as denoted by: high (+++), moderate (++), low (+), very low (-).

Neurodegenerative disorders, including the most common type of dementia, Alzheimer's disease (AD), and the most frequent movement disorder, Parkinson's disease, are morphologically characterized by progressive neuronal cell death. Recently, apoptosis and inflammation, through the action of cytotoxic factors (TNF-αand IL -1), have been implicated as a general mechanism in the degeneration of selective neuronal populations [17,18]. PACAP exerts potent neuroprotective effects, through the activation of PAC1R, by reducing apoptosis, both

in vitro and *in vivo*, in rodent models of Alzheimer's, Huntington's, and Parkinson's diseases and traumatic brain and spinal cord injuries [3,16,19]. In PC12 cells, a useful cell model for neuronal differentiation, PACAP promotes cell survival by attenuating beta-amyloid-induced toxicity through reducing caspase-3 activity [20]. PACAP also protects PC12 cells from apoptosis induced by rotenone, a mitochondrial complex I inhibitor [21], known to be involved in the pathogenesis of Parkinson's disease, which is characterized by a progressive loss of dopaminergic neurons in the substantia nigra. Moreover, in a rat model of Parkinson's disease, it has been shown that pretreatment with PACAP protects 50% of dopaminergic neurons and improves behavioral deficits [22].

Another pathologiocal state associated with apoptosis and commonly found in diabetic patients is retinal neurodegeneration, the latter is also closely linked to apoptosis [23]. Diabetes-associated hyperglycemia is a key initiator of retinal damage and the mechanism of retinal cell death in diabetic retinopathy includes apoptosis. Recently, it has been demonstrated that intraocular PACAP injection markedly attenuated diabetic retinal injury by increasing the levels of several anti-apoptotic markers (p-Akt, p-ERK, p-ERK2, PKC, Bcl-2), while decreasing the levels of the pro-apoptotic markers (p-p38MAPK, caspases) [24], suggesting that PACAP mitigates diabetic retinopathy by protecting against apoptosis.

PACAP is also able to modulate the inflammatory response associated with many neurodegenerative diseases, by inhibiting both chemokine and pro-inflammatory cytokine (NFkB, TNF-a, IL-1) production [25,26]. Therefore, PACAP is able to exert anti-apoptotic, as well as anti-inflammatory effects, two mechanisms involved in the pathogenesis and the progression of neurodegenerative diseases. In addition to its protective effects on neuronal loss during neurodegenerative disorders, accumulating evidence implicates PACAP as an important regulator of neuronal cell death after ischemia [27]. Given that PACAP can cross the blood–brain barrier by a saturable mechanism [28], it has been demonstrated that intravenous injection of a very low concentration of exogenous PACAP suppresses neuronal cell death in rat global and local brain ischemia models [29-31]. However, the mechanisms underlying the neuroprotection effects of PACAP in these models are not fully elucidated. Recently, Ohtaki et al. [32] have demonstrated that after ischemia, PACAP decreases neuronal cell death by suppressing cytochrome c release. PACAP mediates such release phosphorylating extracellular signal-regulated kinase (ERK) directly and signal transducer and activator of transcription 3 (STAT 3) indirectly via IL-6 release. ERK and STAT3 increase and phosphorylate Bcl-2, an anti-apoptotic protein, suppressing cytochrome c release from the mitochondria to the cytoplasm, thereby preventing neuronal cell death.

Another example of PACAP's role as a neuroprotective peptide is the attenuation of cell apoptosis in a rat model of spinal cord injury [33]. PACAP also was found to enhance the neuroprotective ability of human mesenchymal stem cells (hMSCs) used to repair injured spinal cord tissue [34]. Additionally, administration of PACAP mitigated oxidative stress and tissue damage in a small-bowel autotransplantation model [35]. The upregulation of endogenous PACAP and its receptors and the protective effect of exogenous PACAP after the different neuronal injuries highlighted above, show the important function PACAP can play in neuronal regeneration and suggest PACAP may be a promising therapeutic agent in the treatment of neuronal injuries.

Further works to elucidate the precise mechanisms underlying the neuroprotective effects of PACAP are thus warranted. However, the therapeutic potential of PACAP for the treatment of CNS injuries or neurodegenerative diseases has many challenges including its low bioavailability. Once circulating in the blood, PACAP is subjected to rapid degradation by the endogeneous peptidase, dipeptidyl peptidase IV (DPP-IV). It has been established that the half-life of PACAP38 injected into mice or human is between 2 and 10 minutes [36,37]. This poor plasma/serum stability will hamper the therapeutic potential of PACAP. To circumvent such metabolic instability, PACAP could be injected simultaneously with a DPP-IV inhibitor, which is known to extend some of the effects of PACAP [38]. Alternatively, new strategies such as chemical modifications to increase the metabolic stability of PACAP while preserving its biological activity could be explored as new areas of pharmacological research.

PACAP regulates the stress response

In addition to its neuroprotective effects, evidence has shown PACAP as a master regulator of central and peripheral stress responses required to restore and maintain homeostasis [recently reviewed in 39,40]. PACAP has been shown to regulate catecholamine production and release and is required for sustained epinephrine release in response to metabolic stress [41]. PACAP also modulates the hypothalamic-pituitary-adrenal (HPA) axis in response to psychological stress by regulating the secretion of corticosterone [42]. Roman et al. [43] have recently demonstrated that chronic variate stress exposure in rodents increases PACAP and PAC1R transcript expression in the bed nucleus of the stria terminalis (BNST) of the limbic structure. Furthermore, acute PACAP injections can stimulate anxiety-like behavior and heightened corticosterone release while these stress-induced behavioral responses were attenuated with chronic inhibition of BNST PACAP signaling by continuous infusion with the PAC1R antagonist. Based on these findings, PACAP receptor antagonists could have therapeutic relevance in preventing hyperactivity of the HPA axis and offering protection against stress-associated behavioral and endocrine defects.

PACAP's actions on energy homeostasis

Results from a number of studies using either injection of peptides or gene deletion have highlighted a role for PACAP in the regulation of energy homeostasis including appetite, thermogenesis, body mass and endocrine parameters [44,45]. There is now strong evidence that PACAP is involved in the control of feeding behavior [46]. Hypothalamic nuclei such as ventromedial nucleus (VMN), arcuate nucleus (ARC) and paraventricular nucleus (PVN), the key feeding centers in which major peripheral energy signals are directly sensed and integrated [47] heavily express PACAP and PAC1R [48], suggesting that PACAP may be critical for the regulation of feeding behavior and body weight. Intracerebroventricular (icv) injection of PACAP into the VMN or PVN decreases food intake in rodents [44,49]. However, unlike VMN injection, only PACAP injections into the PVN affect meal patterns by producing significant reductions in meal size, duration, and total time spent eating [48]. The neurons expressing the classical feeding related neuropeptides such as proopiomelanocortin (POMC) and neuropeptide Y (NPY) express the PAC1R [50,51]. It has been reported that icv administration of PACAP to food-deprived mice causes a dose-dependent reduction of food consumption during the first 3 h post PACAP injection along with increases in energy expenditure [44,48]. One hour after PACAP administration, mRNA expression of POMC was significantly increased in the ARC, with no changes in NPY expression, indicating that hypophagia induced by central administration of PACAP is mediated, at least in part, through activation of the hypothalamic melanocortin system [44].

Based on its secretory property on exocrine and endocrine cells, PACAP induces a concentration-dependent relaxation of gastric smooth muscles [52,53], causing a decrease of gastric motility and a delay in stomach emptying [54] suggesting a satiety effect of PACAP. The satiety induced by the delay in stomach emptying could be the mechanism by which PACAP suppresses appetite. In the gastrointestinal tract, PACAP also stimulates the release of some regulatory peptides including somatostatin and PYY that may contribute to the anorexic effects of PACAP peptide.

Lower body weight and decreased fat mass under normal temperature housing conditions have been observed in PACAP null mice [55]. This reduction of body weight and adiposity was not associated with reduced food intake but instead was accompanied by a thermogenic defect [55]. Deletion of PACAP in mouse results in a temperature sensitive phenotype, whereby PACAP null pups display reduced survival at lower housing temperature with most pups dying suddenly in their second postnatal week of life [56]. Shortly thereafter it was shown that an increase in housing temperature of just three degrees (to 24°C) improved postnatal survival dramatically; suggesting PACAP plays an important role in thermoregulation [57]. Tanida et al. [58] have showed increased sympathetic nervous system (SNS) activity innervating the brown adipose tissue (BAT) and increased body temperature following a PACAP injection in rat. The thermogenic role of PACAP [59] in BAT is supported by the observation that PACAP null mice have decreased norephinephrine in this organ [57]. Despite the changes in sympathetic outflow to brown adipose tissue, the mass and histology of the interscapular BAT depot did not differ from those of the control wild-type mice [57]. Therefore, the precise underlying mechanism by which PACAP null mice are cold intolerant remains to be understood and require future studies.

In addition, Gray et al. [56] reported that PACAP null mice that died prematurely (postnatal day 7-12) showed increased lipid deposition in the liver, heart, and skeletal muscles, suggesting abnormal lipid metabolism in the PACAP null mice. The presence of PACAP mRNA and PAC1R has been detected in most endocrine glands. Furthermore, PACAP is expressed in pancreatic β cells and autonomic nerve terminals innervating the pancreas, suggesting a role for the peptide in pancreas function. As previously reviewed, PACAP seems to be much more potent than other regulatory peptides in stimulating pancreatic hormone secretion [60,61]. In vitro, PACAP potently stimulates insulin secretion from β cells, in clonal isolated mouse and rat islets as well as in the perfused rat pancreas [62,63]. Also in vivo, a clear stimulation of insulin secretion is evident from studies in mice [64]. PACAP also stimulates glucagon secretion from perfused rat pancreas [65] and in vivo in mice [66]. Of particular interest is that PACAP stimulates both insulin and glucagon secretion in humans [67]. Due to its potent insulinotropic effect, studies using PACAP receptor antagonists, mice lacking PACAP or mice with specific overexpression of PACAP in the pancreatic β cell have been undertaken to further examine the role of PACAP in islet function [60,67]. Interestingly, mice with genetic deletion of PACAP have impaired glucose-stimulated insulin secretion [68] and a PAC1R antagonist inhibits insulin secretion [69], while mice overexpressing PACAP in pancreatic β cells display increased insulin secretion in response to an oral or intraperitoneal glucose load [70]. Moreover, chronic PACAP-signaling deficiencies cause a host of carbohydrate disturbances that result in decreased insulin and blood glucose levels in fasted and fed animals under both chow and high fat/high sucrose diets [55]. However, at postnatal day 5 (P5) fasting plasma insulin levels were increased while blood glucose levels were decreased in PACAP null pups as compared to while type controls [56]. These observations reflect the important role played by PACAP in glucose and insulin homeostasis. In support of a potent insulinotropic role of this peptide, PACAP-based therapy may be a strategy for novel treatment of type 2 diabetes. However, the use of PACAP in clinic may be dampened by its stimulatory effect on glucagon secretion in human.

Effects of PACAP on the Respiratory System

Given the localization of PACAP and PAC1R to nuclei involved in the regulation of respiratory system, PACAP signaling likely plays an important role in lung function. PACAP has been localized in nerve fibers innervating the lung, is a potent bronchodilator and causes marked vasodilation of pulmonary blood vessels [71]. As mentioned above, PACAP-knockout mice appear normal at birth but show a high mortality with sudden death at ~ 2 weeks of age. Raising the ambient temperature of the room in which the mother and litter are housed can substantially decrease the mortality of PACAP deficient animals highlighting the thermoregulatory effect of PACAP. Unlike most fatal congenital abnormalities in which the highest rate of mortality is apparent immediately after birth, mortality of PACAP-deficient animals does not peak until the second week [56,57]. These phenotypic hallmarks reliably produce the spectrum and heterogeneity of traits that closely reflect the phenotype of sudden infant death syndrome (SIDS) in human. First, SIDS deaths peak during the third month of life, not immediately after birth, and secondly, thermal stress has been implicated as a causal factor in SIDS as SIDS rates are higher in winter months than summer season in northern climates [72,73]. Moreover, mutations in the PACAP gene are possible risk factors in SIDS in a subset of African– American cases [74]. Thus, PACAP-knockout mice display a SIDS-like phenotype, although the underlying physiological mechanism is unknown.

Currently, there are three tenable hypotheses for why a PACAP-signaling deficiency causes an increased susceptibility to neonatal death: (i) the metabolic hypothesis whereby PACAP-signaling deficiency causes metabolic disturbances (thermoregulatory defect) leading to wasting and death [57]; (ii) the pulmonary hypertension hypothesis whereby PACAP-signaling deficiency leads to pulmonary hypertension and right heart failure [75]: PAC1-deficient mice had abnormalities associated with pulmonary hypertension, including chronic hypoxemia, increased systolic right ventricular pressure, right ventricular enlargement, a 30% reduction in the density of the pulmonary capillary bed and an increase in wall thickness of small pulmonary arteries (an observation also made in SIDS victims; [76]; and (iii) the breathing defect hypothesis whereby PACAP-signaling deficiency causes breathing defects resulting in chronic hypoxemia and atrioventricular block [77]. It has been reported that PACAP$^{-/-}$ mice display significantly reduced ventilation during baseline breathing and show blunted responses to hypoxia [77]. Interestingly, hypoxia induced respiratory arrest in neonate PACAP$^{-/-}$ mice may be the cause of the sudden death of PACAP null mice at 2 weeks of age [78]. Endogenous PACAP plays a role as a respiratory regulator linked with the catecholaminergic system in the medulla oblongata; disruption of this system is responsible for causing the blunted

responses to hypoxia that may be involved in the SIDS-like phenotype of PACAP null mice [78]. These reports suggest that the PACAP null mouse is a good model for SIDS. Thus, information from rodent models with pathophysiological traits mimicking those found in human SIDS would be of great interest. Also, whether or not PACAP gene mutations predispose human infants to SIDS is unknown and this opens new directions for future research.

Effects of PACAP on the Cardiovascular System

The presence of PACAP and its PAC1R in cardiac tissue and blood vessels [79-81] suggests that the peptide may play an important role in the cardiovascular functions. However, one area where a role for PACAP is not well studied is its cardiovascular regulatory effect. According to recent data, the peptide is present in the cardiovascular system and has various distinct effects. PACAP has been demonstrated to exhibit protective effects against in vitro ischemia/reperfusion-induced apoptosis in cardiomyocytes [82,83] and oxidative stress-induced apoptosis in endothelial cells [84]. Intravenous injection of PACAP provokes a substantial increase in heart rate and enhances the contractile ventricular force [85,86]. In rat, PACAP knockdown-induced tachycardia is abolished by the β-adrenoreceptor antagonist propranolol, indicating that PACAP can stimulate norepinephrine release from sympathetic nerve terminals subserving the heart [87]. In addition, a report from Otto et al. [75] demonstrated that the absence of PAC1R in mice causes right heart failure after birth, demonstrating the crucial importance of PAC1-mediated signalling for the maintenance of normal cardiovascular function during early postnatal life. This in vivo finding could lead one to speculate that the increased neonatal death noticed in PAC1 deficient mice is not only related to respiratory problems but also to rapidly developing heart failure.

PACAP has also been found to stimulate the production of vascular endothelial growth factor, which plays an important role in angiogenesis [86]. During cold exposure, 60% of all energy expended by a mouse is done in BAT through high rates of oxidative metabolism that ultimately produces heat [89,90]. To allow such high rates of oxidative metabolism to be maintained during exposure to cold, BAT requires a substantial blood supply to provide adequate nutrients and oxygen and to carry away waste products and heat. This requirement for increased blood supply is met by induction of extensive angiogenesis within BAT during exposure to cold [91]. As PACAP is a known non-classic regulator of angiogenesis [92], the highly cold-sensitive phenotype of PACAP deficient mice may be related to decreased angiogenesis in their BAT.

Cold stress is also associated with cardiovascular consequences such as increased heart rate to augment energy availability to thermogenic organs such as BAT. As PACAP induces tachycardia via the SNS, it is possible that impairment of cold-induced thermogenesis in PACAP null mice relates to a decrease in heart rate that reduces the nutrient and oxygen availability to BAT. Future studies will be required to explore this hypothesis. In addition, an early report from Gray et al. [56] showed that PACAP null pups that die prematurely had increased lipid deposition in metabolically active cells, including cardiomyocytes of the heart and hepatocytes of the liver. This huge amount of lipid accumulation observed in the heart of PACAP null mice early in postnatal life suggests that PACAP may have a cardioprotective effect.

To our knowledge, there is no in vivo study looking at the role of PACAP on cardiovascular health. By using cultured vascular endothelial cells (EC) and smooth muscle cells (SMC) as model,

Chang [93] found that PACAP significantly (i) increased the production of anti-atherosclerotic substances by EC, (ii) inhibited the proliferation of SMC and (iii) reduced the production of lipid peroxide by EC and SMC in hyperlipid conditions, suggestive of anti-atherosclerotic effects of PACAP. In addition, a recent *in vitro* study has demonstrated that ApoE receptor 2 and LDL receptors expression were significantly augmented in dorsal root ganglion (DRG)-derived cells co-cultured with PACAP-treated 3T3-L1 cells [94], a finding that again supports potential anti-athersoclerotic properties of PACAP. The accumulation of lipids within arteries remains to be the initial impulse for the pathogenesis of atherosclerosis; however, both inflammation and oxidative stress are also considered to play a critical role in this process. As mentioned above, the anti-inflammatory and anti-oxidative properties of PACAP may also confer an anti-atherosclerotic effect to this peptide. Taken together, these findings and observations indicate that PACAP exerts major regulatory effects on the cardiovascular system, suggesting there may be therapeutic potential for PACAP or PAC1R agonists for the treatment of cardiovascular diseases such as heart failure and atherosclerosis.

Conclusion and Future Direction

This review provides current insight on the role of PACAP in many biological functions (summarized in Figure 2).

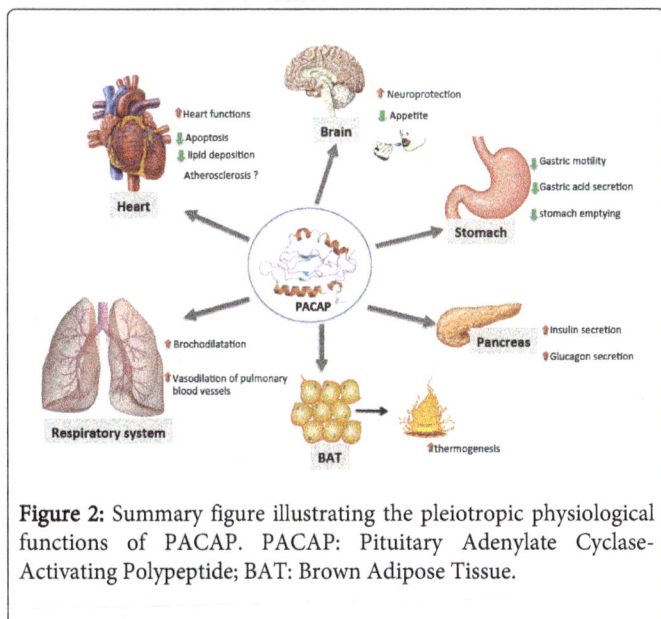

Figure 2: Summary figure illustrating the pleiotropic physiological functions of PACAP. PACAP: Pituitary Adenylate Cyclase-Activating Polypeptide; BAT: Brown Adipose Tissue.

The availability of knockout mouse models, mice with tissue-specific overexpression of PACAP and the development of PACAP agonists/antagonists have allowed for a much deeper understanding of the crucial role PACAP plays in neurodevelopment, energy metabolism, and the cardiovascular and respiratory systems. In this review, we have discussed literature that relates the role of PACAP in neuroprotection, energy metabolism, cardiovascular and respiratory systems. However, the molecular mechanisms by which PACAP exerts its effects are not completely understood. Indeed, very little is known about the role of PACAP plays in respiratory and cardiovascular diseases. Future research aimed at understanding how this highly conserved peptide regulates such diverse systems will not only enhance our understanding of PACAP biology but may also identify new therapeutic targets for the management of neurological, metabolic, respiratory or cardiovascular disease.

Acknowledgement

This work was funded by a grant from the National Sciences and Engineering Research to Council of Canada (NSERC) to Dr. Sarah Gray.

References

1. Miyata A, Arimura A, Dahl RR, Minamino N, Uehara A, et al. (1989) Isolation of a novel 38 residue-hypothalamic polypeptide which stimulates adenylate cyclase in pituitary cells. Biochem Biophys Res Commun 164: 567-574.

2. Miyata A, Jiang L, Dahl RD, Kitada C, Kubo K, et al. (1990) Isolation of a neuropeptide corresponding to the N-terminal 27 residues of the pituitary adenylate cyclase activating polypeptide with 38 residues (PACAP38). Biochem Biophys Res Commun 170: 643-648.

3. Vaudry D, Falluel-Morel A, Bourgault S, Basille M, Burel D, et al. (2009) Pituitary adenylate cyclase-activating polypeptide and its receptors: 20 years after the discovery. Pharmacol Rev 61: 283-357.

4. Sherwood NM, Krueckl SL, McRory JE (2000) The origin and function of the pituitary adenylate cyclase-activating polypeptide (PACAP)/glucagon superfamily. Endocr Rev 21: 619-670.

5. Harmar AJ, Arimura A, Gozes I, Journot L, Laburthe M, et al. (1998) International Union of Pharmacology. XVIII. Nomenclature of receptors for vasoactive intestinal peptide and pituitary adenylate cyclase-activating polypeptide. Pharmacol Rev 50: 265-270.

6. Laburthe M, Couvineau A (2002) Molecular pharmacology and structure of VPAC Receptors for VIP and PACAP. Regul Pept 108: 165-173.

7. Dickson L, Finlayson K (2009) VPAC and PAC receptors: From ligands to function. Pharmacol Ther 121: 294-316.

8. Siu FK, Lam IP, Chu JY, Chow BK (2006) Signaling mechanisms of secretin receptor. Regul Pept 137: 95-104.

9. McCulloch DA, Lutz EM, Johnson MS, Robertson DN, MacKenzie CJ, et al. (2001) ADP-ribosylation factor-dependent phospholipase D activation by VPAC receptors and a PAC(1) receptor splice variant. Mol Pharmacol 59: 1523-1532.

10. Vaudry D, Gonzalez BJ, Basille M, Yon L, Fournier A, et al. (2000) Pituitary adenylate cyclase-activating polypeptide and its receptors: from structure to functions. Pharmacol Rev 52: 269-324.

11. Arimura A, Somogyvári-Vigh A, Miyata A, Mizuno K, Coy DH, et al. (1991) Tissue distribution of PACAP as determined by RIA: highly abundant in the rat brain and testes. Endocrinology 129: 2787-2789.

12. Vigh S, Arimura A, Köves K, Somogyvári-Vigh A, Sitton J, et al. (1991) Immunohistochemical localization of the neuropeptide, pituitary adenylate cyclase activating polypeptide (PACAP), in human and primate hypothalamus. Peptides 12: 313-318.

13. Shioda S, Nakai Y, Nakajo S, Nakaya K, Arimura A (1996) Pituitary adenylate cyclase-activating polypeptide and its type I receptors in the rat hypothalamus: neuroendocrine interactions. Ann N Y Acad Sci 805: 670-676.

14. Köves K, Arimura A, Görcs TG, Somogyvári-Vigh A (1991) Comparative distribution of immunoreactive pituitary adenylate cyclase activating polypeptide and vasoactive intestinal polypeptide in rat forebrain. Neuroendocrinology 54: 159-169.

15. Kivipelto L, Absood A, Arimura A, Sundler F, Håkanson R, et al. (1992) The distribution of pituitary adenylate cyclase-activating polypeptide-like immunoreactivity is distinct from helodermin- and helospectin-like immunoreactivities in the rat brain. J Chem Neuroanat 5: 85-94.

16. Dejda A, Jolivel V, Bourgault S, Seaborn T, Fournier A, et al. (2008) Inhibitory effect of PACAP on caspase activity in neuronal apoptosis: a better understanding towards therapeutic applications in neurodegenerative diseases. J Mol Neurosci 36: 26-37.

17. Reed JC, Tomaselli KJ (2000) Drug discovery opportunities from apoptosis research. Curr Opin Biotechnol 11: 586-592.

18. Friedlander RM (2003) Apoptosis and caspases in neurodegenerative diseases. N Engl J Med 348: 1365-1375.

19. Bourgault S, Vaudry D, Dejda A, Doan ND, Vaudry H, et al. (2009) Pituitary adenylate cyclase-activating polypeptide: focus on structure-activity relationships of a neuroprotective Peptide. Curr Med Chem 16: 4462-4480.

20. Onoue S, Endo K, Ohshima K, Yajima T, Kashimoto K (2002) The neuropeptide PACAP attenuates beta-amyloid (1-42)-induced toxicity in PC12 cells. Peptides 23: 1471-1478.

21. Wang G, Qi C, Fan GH, Zhou HY, Chen SD (2005) PACAP protects neuronal differentiated PC12 cells against the neurotoxicity induced by a mitochondrial complex I inhibitor, rotenone. FEBS Lett 579: 4005-4011.

22. Reglodi D, Lubics A, Tamás A, Szalontay L, Lengvári I (2004) Pituitary adenylate cyclase activating polypeptide protects dopaminergic neurons and improves behavioral deficits in a rat model of Parkinson's disease. Behav Brain Res 151:303-312.

23. Abu El-Asrar AM, Dralands L, Missotten L, Geboes K (2007) Expression of antiapoptotic and proapoptotic molecules in diabetic retinas. Eye (Lond) 21: 238-245.

24. Szabadfi K, Szabo A2, Kiss P3, Reglodi D3, Setalo G Jr4, et al. (2014) PACAP promotes neuron survival in early experimental diabetic retinopathy. Neurochem Int 64: 84-91.

25. Delgado M (2002) Vasoactive intestinal peptide and pituitary adenylate cyclase-activating polypeptide inhibit CBP-NF-kappaB interaction in activated microglia. Biochem Biophys Res Commun 297: 1181-1185.

26. Ohtaki H, Nakamachi T, Dohi K, Shioda S (2008) Role of PACAP in ischemic neural death. J Mol Neurosci 36: 16-25.

27. Banks WA, Uchida D, Arimura A, Somogyvári-Vigh A, Shioda S (1996) Transport of pituitary adenylate cyclase-activating polypeptide across the blood-brain barrier and the prevention of ischemia-induced death of hippocampal neurons. nn N Y Acad Sci 805:270-277.

28. Uchida D, Arimura A, Somogyvári-Vigh A, Shioda S, Banks WA (1996) Prevention of ischemia-induced death of hippocampal neurons by pituitary adenylate cyclase activating polypeptide. Brain Res 736: 280-286.

29. Dohi K, Mizushima H, Nakajo S, Ohtaki H, Matsunaga S, et al. (2002) Pituitary adenylate cyclase-activating polypeptide (PACAP) prevents hippocampal neurons from apoptosis by inhibiting JNK/SAPK and p38 signal transduction pathways. Regul Pept 109: 83-88.

30. Reglodi D, Tamás A, Somogyvári-Vigh A, Szántó Z, Kertes E, et al. (2002) Effects of pretreatment with PACAP on the infarct size and functional outcome in rat permanent focal cerebral ischemia. Peptides 23: 2227-2234.

31. Ohtaki H, Nakamachi T, Dohi K, Aizawa Y, Takaki A, et al. (2006) Pituitary adenylate cyclase-activating polypeptide (PACAP) decreases ischemic neuronal cell death in association with IL-6. Proc Natl Acad Sci U S A 103: 7488-7493.

32. Chen WH, Tzeng SF (2005) Pituitary adenylate cyclase-activating polypeptide prevents cell death in the spinal cord with traumatic injury. Neurosci Lett 384: 117-121.

33. Fang KM, Chen JK, Hung SC, Chen MC, Wu YT, et al. (2010) Effects of combinatorial treatment with pituitary adenylate cyclase activating peptide and human mesenchymal stem cells on spinal cord tissue repair. PLoS One 5: e15299.

34. Ferencz A, Racz B, Tamas A, Reglodi D, Lubics A, et al. (2009) Influence of PACAP on oxidative stress and tissue injury following small-bowel autotransplantation. J Mol Neurosci 37: 168-176.

35. Zhu L, Tamvakopoulos C, Xie D, Dragovic J, Shen X, et al. (2003) The role of dipeptidyl peptidase IV in the cleavage of glucagon family peptides: in vivo metabolism of pituitary adenylate cyclase activating polypeptide-(1-38). J Biol Chem 278: 22418-22423.

36. Li M, Maderdrut JL, Lertora JJ, Batuman V (2007) Intravenous infusion of pituitary adenylate cyclase-activating polypeptide (PACAP) in a patient with multiple myeloma and myeloma kidney: a case study. Peptides 28: 1891-1895.

37. Ahrén B, Hughes TE (2005) Inhibition of dipeptidyl peptidase-4 augments insulin secretion in response to exogenously administered glucagon-like peptide-, glucose-dependent insulinotropic polypeptide, pituitary adenylate cyclase-activating polypeptide, and gastrin-releasing peptide in mice. Endocrinology 146: 2055-2059.

38. Mustafa T (2013) Pituitary adenylate cyclase-activating polypeptide (PACAP): a master regulator in central and peripheral stress responses. Adv Pharmacol 68: 445-457.

39. Hashimoto H, Shintani N, Tanida M, Hayata A, Hashimoto R, et al. (2011) PACAP is implicated in the stress axes. Curr Pharm Des 17: 985-989.

40. Hamelink C, Tjurmina O, Damadzic R, Young WS, Weihe E, et al. (2002) Pituitary adenylate cyclase-activating polypeptide is a sympathoadrenal neurotransmitter involved in catecholamine regulation and glucohomeostasis. Proc Natl Acad Sci U S A 99: 461-466.

41. Lehmann ML, Mustafa T, Eiden AM, Herkenham M, Eiden LE (2013) PACAP-deficient mice show attenuated corticosterone secretion and fail to develop depressive behavior during chronic social defeat stress. Psychoneuroendocrinology 38: 702-715.

42. Roman CW, Lezak KR2, Hartsock MJ2, Falls WA2, Braas KM, et al. (2014) PAC1 receptor antagonism in the bed nucleus of the stria terminalis (BNST) attenuates the endocrine and behavioral consequences of chronic stress. Psychoneuroendocrinology 47: 151-165.

43. Mounien L, Do Rego JC, Bizet P, Boutelet I, Gourcerol G, et al. (2009) Pituitary adenylate cyclase-activating polypeptide inhibits food intake in mice through activation of the hypothalamic melanocortin system. Neuropsychopharmacology 34: 424-435.

44. Inglott MA, Farnham MM, Pilowsky PM (2011) Intrathecal PACAP-38 causes prolonged widespread sympathoexcitation via a spinally mediated mechanism and increases in basal metabolic rate in anesthetized rat. Am J Physiol Heart Circ Physiol 300:2300-2307.

45. Matsuda K, Maruyama K (2007) Regulation of feeding behavior by pituitary adenylate cyclase-activating polypeptide (PACAP) and vasoactive intestinal polypeptide (VIP) in vertebrates. Peptides 28: 1761-1766.

46. Kohno D, Yada T (2012) Arcuate NPY neurons sense and integrate peripheral metabolic signals to control feeding. Neuropeptides 46: 315-319.

47. Resch JM, Maunze B, Gerhardt AK, Magnuson SK, Phillips KA, et al. (2013) Intrahypothalamic pituitary adenylate cyclase-activating polypeptide regulates energy balance via site-specific actions on feeding and metabolism. Am J Physiol Endocrinol Metab 305: E1452-1463.

48. Morley JE, Horowitz M, Morley PM, Flood JF (1992) Pituitary adenylate cyclase activating polypeptide (PACAP) reduces food intake in mice. Peptides 13: 1133-1135.

49. Mounien L, Bizet P, Boutelet I, Gourcerol G, Basille M, et al. (2006) Expression of PACAP receptor mRNAs by neuropeptide Y neurons in the rat arcuate nucleus. Ann N Y Acad Sci 1070: 457-461.

50. Mounien L, Bizet P, Boutelet I, Gourcerol G, Fournier A, et al. (2006) Pituitary adenylate cyclase-activating polypeptide directly modulates the activity of proopiomelanocortin neurons in the rat arcuate nucleus. Neuroscience 143: 155-163.

51. Katsoulis S, Schmidt WE (1996) Role of PACAP in the regulation of gastrointestinal motility. Ann N Y Acad Sci 805: 364-378.

52. Mukai K, Takeuchi T, Toyoshima M, Satoh Y, Fujita A, et al. (2006) PACAP- and PHI-mediated sustained relaxation in circular muscle of gastric fundus: findings obtained in PACAP knockout mice. Regul Pept 133: 54-61.

53. Ozawa M, Aono M, Moriga M (1999) Central effects of pituitary adenylate cyclase activating polypeptide (PACAP) on gastric motility and emptying in rats. Dig Dis Sci 44: 735-743.

54. Adams BA, Gray SL, Isaac ER, Bianco AC, Vidal-Puig AJ, et al. (2008) Feeding and metabolism in mice lacking pituitary adenylate cyclase-activating polypeptide. Endocrinology 149: 1571-1580.

55. Gray SL, Cummings KJ, Jirik FR, Sherwood NM (2001) Targeted disruption of the pituitary adenylate cyclase-activating polypeptide gene

results in early postnatal death associated with dysfunction of lipid and carbohydrate metabolism. Mol Endocrinol 15: 1739-1747.

56. Gray SL, Yamaguchi N, Vencová P, Sherwood NM (2002) Temperature-sensitive phenotype in mice lacking pituitary adenylate cyclase-activating polypeptide. Endocrinology 143: 3946-3954.

57. Tanida M, Shintani N, Hashimoto H (2011) The melanocortin system is involved in regulating autonomic nerve activity through central pituitary adenylate cyclase-activating polypeptide. Neurosci Res 70: 55-61.

58. Arimura A (2002) Impaired adaptive thermogenesis in pituitary adenylate cyclase-activating polypeptide-deficient mice. Endocrinology 143: 3715-3716.

59. Winzell MS, Ahrén B (2007) Role of VIP and PACAP in islet function. Peptides 28: 1805-1813.

60. Ahrén B (2008) Role of pituitary adenylate cyclase-activating polypeptide in the pancreatic endocrine system. Ann N Y Acad Sci 1144: 28-35.

61. Portela-Gomes GM, Lukinius A, Ljungberg O, Efendic S, Ahrén B, et al. (2003) PACAP is expressed in secretory granules of insulin and glucagon cells in human and rodent pancreas. Evidence for generation of cAMP compartments uncoupled from hormone release in diabetic islets. Regul Pept 113: 31-39.

62. Nakata M, Yada T (2007) PACAP in the glucose and energy homeostasis: physiological role and therapeutic potential. Curr Pharm Des 13: 1105-1112.

63. Persson-Sjögren S, Forsgren S, Lindström P (2006) Vasoactive intestinal polypeptide and pituitary adenylate cyclase activating polypeptide: effects on insulin release in isolated mouse islets in relation to metabolic status and age. Neuropeptides 40: 283-290.

64. Bertrand G, Puech R, Maisonnasse Y, Bockaert J, Loubatières-Mariani MM (1996) Comparative effects of PACAP and VIP on pancreatic endocrine secretions and vascular resistance in rat. Br J Pharmacol 117: 764-770.

65. Fridolf T, Sundler F, Ahrén B (1992) Pituitary adenylate cyclase-activating polypeptide (PACAP): occurrence in rodent pancreas and effects on insulin and glucagon secretion in the mouse. Cell Tissue Res 269: 275-279.

66. Filipsson K, Tornøe K, Holst J, Ahrén B (1997) Pituitary adenylate cyclase-activating polypeptide stimulates insulin and glucagon secretion in humans. J Clin Endocrinol Metab 82: 3093-3098.

67. Shintani N, Tomimoto S, Hashimoto H, Kawaguchi C, Baba A (2003) Functional roles of the neuropeptide PACAP in brain and pancreas. Life Sci 74: 337-343.

68. Filipsson K, Holst JJ, Ahrén B (2000) PACAP contributes to insulin secretion after gastric glucose gavage in mice. Am J Physiol Regul Integr Comp Physiol 279: R424-432.

69. Yamamoto K, Hashimoto H, Tomimoto S, Shintani N, Miyazaki J, et al. (2003) Overexpression of PACAP in transgenic mouse pancreatic beta-cells enhances insulin secretion and ameliorates streptozotocin-induced diabetes. Diabetes 52: 1155-1162.

70. Kinhult J, Andersson JA, Uddman R, Stjärne P, Cardell LO (2000) Pituitary adenylate cyclase-activating peptide 38 a potent endogenously produced dilator of human airways. Eur Respir J 15: 243-247.

71. Sawczenko A, Fleming PJ (1996) Thermal stress, sleeping position, and the sudden infant death syndrome. Sleep 19: S267-270.

72. Mitchell EA, Clements M, Williams SM, Stewart AW, Cheng A, et al. (1999) Seasonal differences in risk factors for sudden infant death syndrome. The New Zealand Cot Death Study Group. Acta Paediatr 88: 253-258.

73. Cummings KJ, Klotz C, Liu WQ, Weese-Mayer DE, Marazita ML, et al. (2009) Sudden infant death syndrome (SIDS) in African Americans: polymorphisms in the gene encoding the stress peptide pituitary adenylate cyclase-activating polypeptide (PACAP). Acta Paediatr 98: 482-489.

74. Otto C, Hein L, Brede M, Jahns R, Engelhardt S, et al. (2004) Pulmonary hypertension and right heart failure in pituitary adenylate cyclase-

75. activating polypeptide type I receptor-deficient mice. Circulation 110: 3245-3251.

75. Prandota J (2004) Possible pathomechanisms of sudden infant death syndrome: key role of chronic hypoxia, infection/inflammation states, cytokine irregularities, and metabolic trauma in genetically predisposed infants. Am J Ther 11: 517-546.

76. Cummings KJ, Pendlebury JD, Sherwood NM, Wilson RJ (2004) Sudden neonatal death in PACAP-deficient mice is associated with reduced respiratory chemoresponse and susceptibility to apnoea. J Physiol 555: 15-26.

77. Arata S, Nakamachi T, Onimaru H, Hashimoto H, Shioda S (2013) Impaired response to hypoxia in the respiratory center is a major cause of neonatal death of the PACAP-knockout mouse. Eur J Neurosci 37: 407-416.

78. Hoover DB, Girard BM, Hoover JL, Parsons RL (2013) PACâ, receptors mediate positive chronotropic responses to PACAP-27 and VIP in isolated mouse atria. Eur J Pharmacol 713: 25-30.

79. Merriam LA, Baran CN, Girard BM, Hardwick JC, May V, et al. (2013) Pituitary adenylate cyclase 1 receptor internalization and endosomal signaling mediate the pituitary adenylate cyclase activating polypeptide-induced increase in guinea pig cardiac neuron excitability. J Neurosci 33: 4614-4622.

80. Nandha KA, Benito-Orfila MA, Smith DM, Ghatei MA, Bloom SR (1991) Action of pituitary adenylate cyclase-activating polypeptide and vasoactive intestinal polypeptide on the rat vascular system: effects on blood pressure and receptor binding. J Endocrinol 129:69-73.

81. Gasz B, Rácz B, Roth E, Borsiczky B, Ferencz A, et al. (2006) Pituitary adenylate cyclase activating polypeptide protects cardiomyocytes against oxidative stress-induced apoptosis. Peptides 27: 87-94.

82. Roth E, Wéber G, Kiss P, Horváth G, Tóth G, et al. (2009) Effects of PACAP and preconditioning against ischemia/reperfusion-induced cardiomyocyte apoptosis in vitro. Ann N Y Acad Sci 1163: 512-516.

83. Rácz B, Gasz B, Borsiczky B, Gallyas F Jr, Tamás A, et al. (2007) Protective effects of pituitary adenylate cyclase activating polypeptide in endothelial cells against oxidative stress-induced apoptosis. Gen Comp Endocrinol 153: 115-123.

84. Minkes RK, McMahon TJ, Hood JS, Murphy WA, Coy DH, et al. (1992) Differential effects of PACAP and VIP on the pulmonary and hindquarters vascular beds of the cat. J Appl Physiol (1985) 72: 1212-1217.

85. Birk S, Sitarz JT, Petersen KA, Oturai PS, Kruuse C, et al. (2007) The effect of intravenous PACAP38 on cerebral hemodynamics in healthy volunteers. Regul Pept 140: 185-191.

86. Whalen EJ, Johnson AK, Lewis SJ (1999) Tachyphylaxis to PACAP-27 after inhibition of NO synthesis: a loss of adenylate cyclase activation. Am J Physiol 277: R1453-1461.

87. Gloddek J, Pagotto U, Paez Pereda M, Arzt E, Stalla GK, et al. (1999) Pituitary adenylate cyclase-activating polypeptide, interleukin-6 and glucocorticoids regulate the release of vascular endothelial growth factor in pituitary folliculostellate cells. J Endocrinol 160:483-490.

88. Golozoubova V, Gullberg H, Matthias A, Cannon B, Vennström B, et al. (2004) Depressed thermogenesis but competent brown adipose tissue recruitment in mice devoid of all hormone-binding thyroid hormone receptors. Mol Endocrinol 18: 384-401.

89. Cannon B, Nedergaard J (2011) Nonshivering thermogenesis and its adequate measurement in metabolic studies. J Exp Biol 214: 242-253.

90. Xue Y, Petrovic N, Cao R, Larsson O, Lim S, et al. (2009) Hypoxia-independent angiogenesis in adipose tissues during cold acclimation. Cell Metab 9: 99-109.

91. Castorina A, Giunta S, Mazzone V, Cardile V, D'Agata V (2010) Effects of PACAP and VIP on hyperglycemia-induced proliferation in murine microvascular endothelial cells. Peptides 31: 2276-2283.

92. Chang Q (1997) [Experimental study of the effects of pituitary adenylate cyclase-activating polypeptide (PACAP) and its mechanism on the vascular cell components--the possible relationship between PACAP and atherosclerosis]. Sheng Li Ke Xue Jin Zhan 28: 132-135.

30

Metabolic Syndrome is Associated with Increased Severity of Diabetic Retinopathy

Anand CR[1], Sandeep Saxena[1*], Khushboo Srivastav[1], Poonam Kishore[1], Shashi K Bhaskar[1], Arvind Misra[2], Shankar M Natu[3], Abbas A Mahdi[4] and Vinay K Khanna[5]

[1]Department of Ophthalmology, King George's Medical University, Lucknow, India

[2]Department of Medicine, King George's Medical University, Lucknow, India

[3]Department of Pathology, King George's Medical University, Lucknow, India

[4]Department of Biochemistry, King George's Medical University, Lucknow, India

[5]Indian Institute of Toxicology and Research, Lucknow, India

*Corresponding author: Sandeep Saxena, Department of Ophthalmology, King George's Medical University, Lucknow, 226003, India;
E-mail: sandeepsaxena2020@yahoo.com

Abstract

Purpose: To study the association of metabolic syndrome with severity of diabetic retinopathy.

Materials and method: Seventy-one consecutive cases of type 2 diabetes mellitus of more than 10 years duration aged 38 to 82 years were included. Metabolic syndrome was identified as per American Heart Association-National Cholesterol Education Programme Adult Treatment Panel III (AHA-NCEP ATP III) criteria. All the cases were assessed for log MAR visual acuity, intraocular pressure (IOP) and seven field fundus photography. The photographs were scored for 16 diabetic lesions. A single severity level (identical to the ETDRS Interim Scale) was calculated for each eye by using the Vanderbilt Classification System. Data was analysed using paired t-test.

Results: Of the 71 cases, 47 cases fulfilled at least 3 of the ATP III criteria for metabolic syndrome. Among the cases of metabolic syndrome, 18 cases fulfilled 3 criteria, 28 cases fulfilled 4 criteria and 1 case fulfilled all the 5 criteria. The analyses of the mean Vanderbilt score for severity of retinopathy showed significantly higher score (more severe retinopathy) in cases of metabolic syndrome (p<0.001). Higher IOP was observed in cases of metabolic syndrome (p<0.001). LogMAR visual acuity deteriorated (p<0.01), severity of retinopathy and intraocular pressure increased (p<0.001, p<0.001, respectively) with an increase in the number of components of metabolic syndrome. Triglyceride levels showed positive correlation with severity of retinopathy (p<0.001) and IOP (p<0.001). High density lipoprotein (HDL) levels also showed positive correlation with vision (p<0.001), severity of retinopathy (p<0.001) and IOP (p<0.001).

Conclusion: Metabolic syndrome is significantly associated with increased severity of diabetic retinopathy, decreased visual acuity and increased IOP.

Keywords: Metabolic syndrome; Diabetes mellitus; Diabetic retinopathy; Intraocular pressure

Introduction

Metabolic syndrome has become increasingly common in the developed world and now even in the developing countries. It is known under various other names, such as Syndrome X, insulin resistance syndrome, Reaven's syndrome or CHAOS (Coronary artery disease, Hypertension, Atherosclerosis, Obesity, and Stroke) and Deadly quartet [1-3].

It has been estimated that about 20–25 percent of US adults are affected by metabolic syndrome [4,5]. However, the prevalence of metabolic syndrome in people with type 2 diabetes mellitus in Central India was found to be 45.8 percent as per Adult Treatment Panel-III criteria [6].

American Heart Association (AHA) modified Third Report of the National Cholesterol Education Program (NCEP) Expert Panel on Detection, Evaluation, and Treatment of High Blood Cholesterol in Adults (Adult Treatment Panel III) criteria is the most current and widely used one [7]. More over in this definition, presence of type 2 diabetes does not exclude a diagnosis of metabolic syndrome.

According to the AHA-NCEP ATP III criteria, the metabolic syndrome is identified by the presence of three or more of the following components: Elevated waist circumference, elevated triglycerides, reduced High density lipoprotein (HDL) cholesterol, elevated blood pressure and elevated fasting glucose.

In this definition, treatment for diabetes or hypertension forms one of the criteria unlike in other definitions which use blood glucose value (fasting or glucose tolerance test values) or blood pressure as one of the criteria. Diabetic cases with metabolic syndrome are at high risk for developing various diseases primarily coronary artery disease [8,9]. Type 2 diabetes mellitus individuals with metabolic syndrome seemingly are also susceptible to polycystic ovary syndrome, fatty liver, cholesterol gallstones, asthma, sleep disturbances, and some forms of cancer [9-13].

It is not yet known whether type 2 diabetes individuals with metabolic syndrome are at a high risk for ocular changes when compared with type 2 diabetes individuals without metabolic syndrome. Hence, a tertiary care center-based study was undertaken to evaluate the association of change in visual acuity, intraocular pressure (IOP) and severity of retinopathy by using the Vanderbilt Classification System [14] in metabolic syndrome.

Material and Methods

Our study had institutional review board clearance and was performed in accordance to the tenets of the Helsinki declaration. Seventy-one consecutive cases of type 2 diabetic mellitus with more than 10 years duration, aged 38 to 82 years, attending diabetes and retina clinic of our tertiary care centre were included. Exclusion criteria included cases having media haze (corneal, lenticular, and vitreous), which was hampering complete retina evaluation. Patients who had undergone laser or surgery for glaucoma, retinopathy or retinal detachment were excluded. Patients already on treatment for dry eye or glaucoma or with pre-existent ocular illness like Stevens Johnson syndrome and other retinal vascular disorders were also excluded. Patients who were not willing or with poor general condition were not enrolled.

The duration of illness was defined as the duration from the time of the diagnosis of diabetes mellitus given by the participant until the time of the examination. Current age was defined as the age at the time of the examination.

The examination consisted of an explanation of the study, measurement of the blood pressure, refraction and assessment of the logMAR best corrected visual acuity (LogMAR is expressed as decadic logarithm of minimum angle of resolution with 20/20 line equivalent to LogMAR 0.00 and the 20/200 line to LogMAR 1.0) and slit-lamp biomicroscopy of the anterior segment. Measurement of the intraocular pressure using applanation tonometry was done. Cases having intraocular pressure (IOP) greater than 21 mm of Hg or showing optic disc changes were subjected to automated perimetry using Humphrey's automated visual field analyzer (Carl Zeiss Humphrey Field Analyser 750i, Dublin, CA, USA). Gonioscopic evaluation of the angle of anterior chamber was done using Goldmann three mirror lens. Fundus examination was done by slit lamp biomicroscopy with a 90-diopter lens and indirect ophthalmoscopy. Seven field fundus photography was done in all cases using Zeiss fundus camera FF 450 Plus with pixel width of 0.0054 and image size 2588 x 1958. Cases showing retinal changes were subjected to fundus fluoresce in angiography.

The seven field fundus photographs were scored for retinopathy. The photographs were scored for 16 diabetic lesions. A single severity level (identical to the ETDRS Interim Scale) was calculated for each eye by using, the Vanderbilt Classification System (Table 1) [14]. This method has been proven to give quantitative data (numeric values) and evaluate incremental changes in an accurate, reproducible manner and is highly reliable between graders. The person scoring the photographs did not know the history or reports of the investigations of the case while scoring the photographs for severity to avoid bias. This scoring system gave a retinopathy score from 10 to 75, higher scores indicating more severity.

	Ma and all other lesions absent
14	HE, SE, or IRMA definite, Ma absent
15	RH definite, Ma absent
20	Ma definite, no other lesions present
30	Ma plus SE, IRMA, or VB questionable; Ret.Hem. present, H/Ma < 5/1*; or HE definite Levels 41 and above require Ma s: 3/1
41	IRMA a 3/1-3; or SE a 3/1-3
45	IRMA 2= 3/4-5; or SE s 3/4-5; or VB definite; or H/Ma a 5/1-3
51	H/Ma a 5/4-5; or VB > definite/2-3; or Combination of SE a 4/4-5, IRMA a 3/2-3, and H/Ma > 5/1
55	IRMA a= 4/2-3; or VB a def/2-3, plus 2 other P2 lesions; or 4 P2 lesions; or H/Ma a 5/4-5 plus 2 other P2 lesions
61	FPE, or FPD definite, NVE or NVD absent; or NVE definite
65	Either NVE s 4/1; or NVD a 3/1; or VH or PRH a 3/1, plus NVE > 3/1
71	VH or PRH > 4/1; or NVE a 4/1, and VH or PRH a 3/1; or NVD a 3/1, and VH or PRH > 3/1; or NVD a 4/1
75	NVD > 4/1, and VH or PRH a 3/1

Table 1: Vanderbilt classification system for scoring of diabetic retinopathy lesions, Ma=Micro Aneurysms; HE=Hard Exudates; SE=Soft Exudates; IRMA=Intraretinal Micro Vascular Abnormalities; RH=Retinal Hemorrhage; VB=Venous Beading; FPE=Fibrous Proliferation Elsewhere; FPD=Fibrous Proliferation on Disc; NVE=Neovascularization Elsewhere; NVD=Neovascularization on Disc; VH=Vitreous Hemorrhage; PRH=Preretinal Hemorrhage.

Numbers indicate summary scores of maximum grade/number of fields with maximum.
P2 lesions=SE >/= 3/2-3;

IRMA >/= 3/2-3; VB >/= 3/2-3; H/Ma >/= 5/1.

Clinically significant macular edema (CSME) global grading scores were: 1=no evidence; 2=questionable; 3=definitely present. (For this study, the definition of CSME, as defined by the ETDRS was used). CSME scores were added to the score thus obtained and final score obtained.

Fasting and post prandial blood glucose, serum levels of high density lipoprotein (HDL), triglycerides and glycosylated hemoglobin was estimated as per standard protocol.

Statistical significance of mean values was assessed using two-sample t test. By linear regression analysis best corrected visual activity, severity of retinopathy and IOP were compared with the number of components of metabolic syndrome, triglyceride levels and HDL level.

Results

A total of 141 eyes were evaluated in the study. One eye with phthisis bulbi was excluded. Of the 71 cases, 47 cases fulfilled at least 3 of the ATP III criteria for metabolic syndrome. Among the cases of metabolic syndrome, 18 cases fulfilled 3 criteria, 28 cases fulfilled 4 criteria and 1 case fulfilled all the 5 criteria's.

The mean age of the cases included in the study was 53.54+12.41 years in cases of diabetes without metabolic syndrome. Among the cases of diabetes with metabolic syndrome, mean age of the cases was 55.91+9.91years. No statistically significant difference in the ages of cases in the two groups was observed (p=0.22).

Among the cases of diabetes with metabolic syndrome, 27 were men and 20 were women. In cases of diabetes without metabolic syndrome, 17 were men and 7 were women. No statistically significant difference in the gender distribution of cases in the two groups was observed (x^2=0.71, p=0.40).

The mean duration of diabetes in patients of diabetes without metabolic syndrome was 13.43+2.31 years and with metabolic syndrome was 12.26+2.32 years. A statistically significant difference was observed (p=0.52).

Mean Vanderbilt score for severity of retinopathy was 26.17+10.86 for cases of diabetes without metabolic syndrome. For the metabolic syndrome cases, the mean score was 46.94+14.36 (Figure 1). A statistically significant difference was observed (t=8.81, p<0.001).

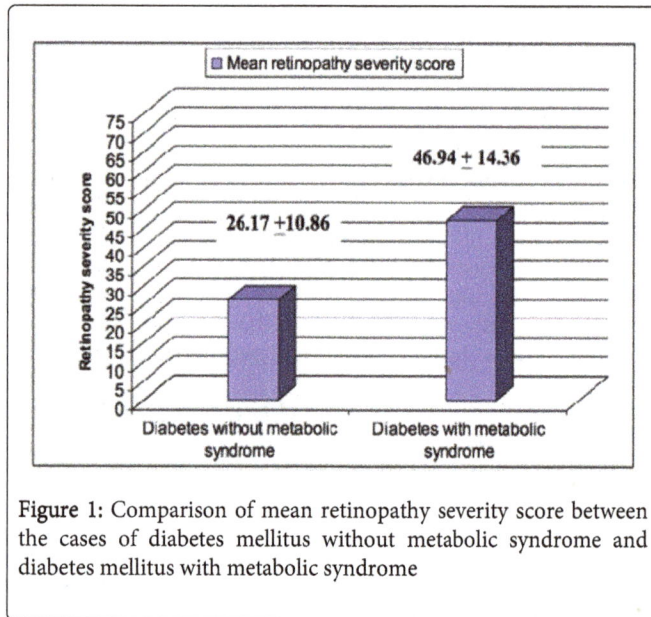

Figure 1: Comparison of mean retinopathy severity score between the cases of diabetes mellitus without metabolic syndrome and diabetes mellitus with metabolic syndrome

Mean IOP (in mm Hg) of the diabetes cases without metabolic syndrome was 14.20+2.20 mm Hg and in diabetes cases with metabolic syndrome, it was 18.44+5.10 mm Hg. A statistically significant difference was observed (t=6.47, p<0.001).

The cases were subdivided into 4 groups according to the number of components of metabolic syndrome present. The first group had diabetes only while the subsequent groups had additional 1, 2 or 3 components with diabetes being the common factor. There was a linear increase in the fall in visual acuity, severity of retinopathy and intraocular pressure with increase in number of components of metabolic syndrome. It was observed that the visual acuity deteriorated with an increase in the number of components of metabolic syndrome (p<0.01). It was seen that the severity of retinopathy (p<0.001) and IOP (p<0.001) increased with increase in number of components of metabolic syndrome (Table 2).

No. of components	No. of eyes	Best corrected visual acuity (mean logMAR value)	Mean Retinopathy score	Mean intraocular pressure
Diabetes only	24	-0.33 ± 0.31	23.52 ± 11.09	13.26 ± 1.86
Diabetes+1 component*	24	-0.35 ± 0.37	28.71 ± 10.23	13.58 ± 2.70
Diabetes+2 components*	36	-0.69 ± 0.59	42.20 ± 14.76	15.26 ± 4.20
Diabetes+3 components*	56	-0.81 ± 0.74	50.20 ± 13.55	20.34 ± 4.25

Table 2: Correlation of number of components of metabolic syndrome with vision, retinopathy score and intraocular pressure of metabolic syndrome

The change was not very significant if the number of components of metabolic syndrome varied by only 1 component. If the number of components of metabolic syndrome varied by more than 1 component, the groups had a significant change in best corrected visual acuity, mean retinopathy score and mean IOP (Table 3).

$	Best corrected visual acuity		Retinopathy score		Intraocular pressure	
	t	P	t	P	t	P
Diabetes only Vs Diabetes+1 component*	0.2	0.8	1.69	0.1	0.4	0.7
Diabetes only Vs Diabetes+2 components*	2.74	<0.01	5.28	<0.001	2.19	<0.05
Diabetes only Vs Diabetes+3 components*	3.06	<0.01	8.49	<0.001	7.82	<0.001
Diabetes+1 component* Vs Diabetes+2 components*	2.51	<0.05	3.89	<0.001	1.73	0.1
Diabetes+1 component* Vs Diabetes+3 components*	2.88	<0.01	6.95	<0.001	7.18	<0.001
Diabetes+2 component* Vs Diabetes+3 components*	0.82	0.4	2.67	<0.01	5.62	<0.001

Table 3: Linear regression analysis among best corrected visual acuity, retinopathy score and intraocular syndrome of metabolic syndrome

Triglyceride level showed strong correlation with severity of retinopathy (p<0.001) (Figure 2) and IOP (p<0.001). HDL showed positive correlation with vision (the higher the HDL the better the vision) but negative correlation with severity of retinopathy (Figure 3) and IOP (the higher HDL, the less severe diabetic retinopathy and less severe increase in the IOP).

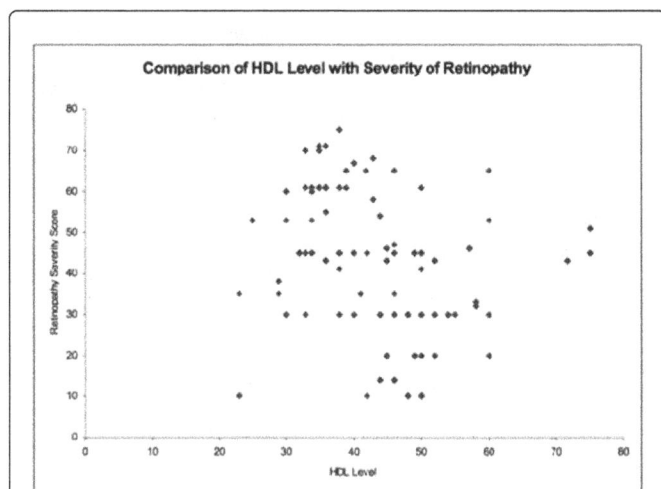

Figure 2: Comparison of HDL levels with severity of retinopathy

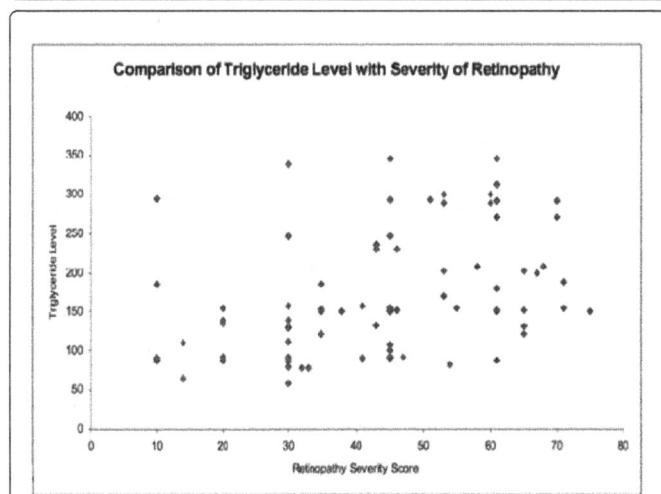

Figure 3: Comparison of triglyceride Level with severity of retinopathy

Discussion

Increased severity of retinopathy was observed with increasing components of metabolic syndrome. Previous study by Corrêa et al. [15] found that the severity of diabetic retinopathy appeared to be associated with risk factors such as duration of disease. In our study, no statistically significant difference in duration of disease was found in the two groups.

When the ocular parameters such as best corrected visual acuity, retinopathy severity score and intraocular pressure were compared in the cases, significantly worse visual status and significantly higher score (more severe retinopathy) in diabetes cases with metabolic syndrome was found. A previous study done by Malik et al. [16] had showed that retinopathy lesions similar to diabetic retinopathy can be seen in cases of metabolic syndrome even if they were not suffering from diabetes signifying that there retinopathy lesions may be caused by other components of metabolic syndrome. This could probably

explain the higher mean Vanderbilt scores for severity of retinopathy among cases of diabetes with metabolic syndrome.

Significantly higher intraocular pressure in eyes of diabetes cases with metabolic syndrome was found. This correlated with findings of Oh et al. [17] who also found that intraocular pressure was higher in participants with metabolic syndrome, as compared to those who did not have metabolic syndrome.

It was observed that the visual acuity deteriorated whereas severity of retinopathy and intraocular pressure increased with an increase in the number of components of metabolic syndrome. If the number of components varied by more than 1 component, the groups had a significant change in best corrected visual acuity, mean retinopathy score and mean intraocular pressure.

Our findings correlated with the findings of Oh et al. [17] who also found that the mean intraocular pressure tends to increase linearly with the presence of increasing numbers of components for metabolic syndrome.

Searches for previous studies correlating number of components of metabolic syndrome with mean retinopathy severity score and mean intraocular pressure have not yielded any result.

Conclusions

Cases of diabetes mellitus with metabolic syndrome have significantly poor visual acuity, increased severity of retinopathy and higher IOP than cases of diabetes mellitus who do not have metabolic syndrome. Also, it was observed that as the number of components increased by more than 1 component, the groups showed significant change in the above mentioned parameters.

References

1. Reaven GM (1988) Banting lecture 1988. Role of insulin resistance in human disease. Diabetes 37: 1595-1607.

2. Reynisdottir S, Ellerfeldt K, Wahrenberg H, Lithell H, Arner P (1994) Multiple lipolysis defects in the insulin resistance (metabolic) syndrome. J Clin Invest 93: 2590-2599.

3. Sirdah MM, Al Laham NA, Abu Ghali AS (2011) Prevalence of metabolic syndrome and associated socioeconomic and demographic factors among Palestinian adults (20-65 years) at the Gaza Strip. Diabetes Metab Syndr 5: 93-97.

4. Ford ES, Giles WH, Dietz WH (2002) Prevalence of the metabolic syndrome among US adults: findings from the third National Health and Nutrition Examination Survey. JAMA 287: 356-359.

5. Beltrán-Sánchez H, Harhay MO, Harhay MM, McElligott S (2013) Prevalence and trends of metabolic syndrome in the adult U.S. population, 1999-2010. J Am Coll Cardiol 62: 697-703.

6. Yadav D, Mahajan S, Subramanian SK, Bisen PS, Chung CH, et al. (2013) Prevalence of metabolic syndrome in type 2 diabetes mellitus using NCEP-ATPIII, IDF and WHO definition and its agreement in Gwalior Chambal region of Central India. Glob J Health Sci 5: 142-155.

7. Grundy SM, Brewer HB, Cleeman JI, Smith SC, Lenfant D (2004) Definition of metabolic syndrome: report of the National, Heart, Lung, and Blood Institute/American Heart Association conference on scientific issues related to definition. Circulation 109: 433-38.

8. Tsai JC, Chang DM, Chung FM, Wu JC, Shin SJ, et al. (2004) The association of silent coronary artery disease and metabolic syndrome in Chinese with type 2 diabetes mellitus. Rev Diabet Stud 1: 18-28.

9. Monteiro J, Leslie M, Moghadasian MH, Arendt BM, Allard JP, et al. (2014) The role of n - 6 and n - 3 polyunsaturated fatty acids in the

manifestation of the metabolic syndrome in cardiovascular disease and non-alcoholic fatty liver disease. Food Funct 5: 426-435.

10. Elizondo-Montemayor L, Ugalde-Casas PA, Lam-Franco L, Bustamante-Careaga H, Serrano-González M, et al. (2014) Association of ALT and the metabolic syndrome among Mexican children. Obes Res Clin Pract 8: e79-87.

11. Chen LY, Qiao QH, Zhang SC, Chen YH, Chao GQ, et al. (2012) Metabolic syndrome and gallstone disease. World J Gastroenterol 18: 4215-4220.

12. **Ersan F, Arslan E, Esmer AÇ, Aydın S, Gedikbaşı A, et al. (2012) Prediction of metabolic syndrome in women with polycystic ovary syndrome. J Turk Ger Gynecol Assoc 13: 178-183.**

13. Nandi A, Chen Z, Patel R, Poretsky L (2014) Polycystic ovary syndrome. Endocrinol Metab Clin North Am 43: 123-147.

14. Feman SS, Leonard-Martin TC, Andrews JS, Armbruster CC, Burdge TL, et al. (1995) A quantitative system to evaluate diabetic retinopathy from fundus photographs. Invest Ophthalmol Vis Sci 36: 174-181.

15. Corrêa ZM, Freitas AM, Marcon IM (2003) Risk factors related to the severity of diabetic retinopathy. Arq Bras Oftalmol 66: 739-43.

16. Malik S, Wong ND, Franklin SS, Kamath TV, L'Italien GJ, et al. (2004) Impact of the metabolic syndrome on mortality from coronary heart disease, cardiovascular disease, and all causes in United States adults. Circulation 110: 1245-1250.

17. Oh SW, Lee S, Park C, Kim DJ (2005) Elevated intraocular pressure is associated with insulin resistance and metabolic syndrome. Diabetes Metab Res Rev 21: 434-440.

31

Pregnancy in PCOS Women and their History of Diabetes

Mette Viftrup-Lund, Melina Gade and Finn F Lauszus*

Department of Gynecology and Obstetrics, Herning Hospital, Denmark

*Corresponding author: Finn Friis Lauszus, Senior Consultant, Department of Gynecology and Obstetrics, Herning Hospital, Gl. Landevej 61, DK-7400 Herning, Denmark; E-mail: finlau@rm.dk

Abstract

Objective: Evaluation of the incidence of gestational diabetes in PCOS women treated with metformin before and during early pregnancy and to ascertain their family history of diabetes.

Design: Follow-up on all women with PCOS and infertility who received treatment with metformin prior to pregnancy (=index pregnancy) during 10 years. Data on diabetes was retrieved by questionnaire and hospital charts. Main outcome measures: Incidence of gestational diabetes, pregnancy outcome, and fetal size

Results: In 18 % of the women GDM was diagnosed at some stage. The clinical and obstetrical outcome of the women showed no association with family history of diabetes or GDM. No neonatal anthropometric feature was different with respect to family history of diabetes or GDM and no fetal malformations were found

Conclusion: GDM and family history of diabetes seem not to be associated with unfavourable pregnancy outcome in PCOS women.

Keywords: Metformin; Pregnancy; Pregnancy loss; Malformation; Polycystic ovarian syndrome

Abbreviations:

DHAS: Dihydroepiandrosterone sulphate; GDM: Gestational diabetes; PCOS: Polycystic ovary syndrome; SHBG: Sexual hormone binding globulin; FAI: Calculated free androgen index; IUI: Intrauterin insemination; IVF: *In-vitro* fertilization

Introduction

Polycystic ovarian syndrome (PCOS) is the most common endocrine disorder in women of fertile age with an estimated prevalence of up to 5-10%. Hyperandrogenism and insulin resistance are cornerstones of PCOS, even though not mandatory according to the consensus criteria [1]. Metformin improves metabolic, endocrine, and ovulatory parameters, probably improving fertility in women with PCOS. Pregnancy and PCOS are variably associated with higher risk of developing gestational diabetes (GDM), pregnancy-induced hypertension, preeclampsia, and preterm birth; however, the contribution of obesity to the prevalence of obstetrical morbidity is unresolved [2]. Several retrospective and non-randomized studies have reported beneficial effects of metformin on pregnancy complications, but this is not supported by a randomized, double-blinded controlled trial [3].

In this study we sought to evaluate the incidence of gestational diabetes, pregnancy outcome, and fetal size in women treated with metformin before and during early pregnancy and to ascertain their family history of diabetes.

Materials and Methods

We examined the records of all women with PCOS and infertility who received treatment with metformin prior to pregnancy (=index pregnancy). They were referred to the Department of Gynecology at Herning and Holstebro Hospital, Denmark, during from 1999 to 2010. We defined our PCOS inclusion criteria as presence of amenorrhea, oligomenorrhea or irregular menstruation with anovulation and concomitant elevated plasma-testosterone (>1.8 nmol/l). Oligomenorrhea was defined as cycle duration between 35 days and 6 months and amenorrhea as the absence of menstruation for more than 6 months. Exclusion criteria were type 1 and 2 diabetes mellitus. A total of 117 women fulfilled our criteria. The study was approved by the Danish Data Protection Agency (no. 2013-41-1998) and conducted in accordance with the Helsinki Declaration and the guidelines for Good Clinical Practice. Questionnaires do not need approval by the Danish Ethical Committee system according to its regulatory law.

Through our records we obtained information about age, BMI, former pregnancies, former infertility treatment, and menstrual cycle pattern as well as information about conception method and consumption of medicine, tobacco, and alcohol. Our records also included plasma levels of LH, FSH, testosterone, dihydroepiandrosterone sulphate (DHAS), sexual hormone binding globulin (SHBG), thyroid stimulating hormone, prolactin (measured in early follicular phase or at random in amenorrhic women), progesterone (measured one week before expected menstruation or at random in amenorrhic women), and a calculated free androgen index (FAI = testosterone/SHBG). A physical examination was performed at first visit including a gynecological examination and vaginal ultrasound.

We supplemented our data with a questionnaire mailed to the women; we ascertained hereby information about the first pregnancy outcome associated with metformin use, neonatal weight and height, neonatal malformations, gestational age at birth, pregnancy complications like gestational diabetes and preeclampsia, smoking and alcohol use, medication taken during pregnancy, family history of diabetes, cardiovascular and endocrine disease, cholesterol and genetic disorders. These data in the responding women were supplemented and compared with the medical records of mother and infant. The non-responding women's data charts were scrutinized for relevant, historical obstetrical data and compared with the responders where appropriate.

The women received metformin treatment at standard dosage 850 mg twice a day. The fertility treatment consisted of first line clomiphene for six months followed by three months of intrauterine insemination (IUI). If no pregnancy was achieved the couple was referred to in-vitro fertilization (IVF) treatment. Heterologue insemination was discussed if oligospermia was found in two sperm samples. If sterility (tubal occlusion or azoospermia) was present further treatment was at the IVF clinic. If the couple had no child they were eligible for free IVF treatment. The women were told to continue with metformin treatment for no longer than the 7th gestational week where the first ultrasound could verify a viable fetus.

For statistical calculations of proportions the χ^2-test with Yates' correction for discontinuity was applied. If the expected number was less than five, Fisher's Exact test was used. For continuous variables Student's t-test, Mann-Whitney's U–test, and Wilcoxon's Signed Rank test was used when appropriate. ANOVA was performed between group variables. Post-hoc test with Newman-Keul's test was performed between group pairs. The level of significance was 0.05. IBM SPSS Statistics 20 was used as the statistical software.

Results

A total of 117 PCOS women with pregnancies and periconceptional metformin were included in the study and questionnaires were mailed to them; hereof 76 (65 %) responded. The initial blood sample was drawn on day 3 or 4 in cycle; if she had oligo-/amenorrhea testing was performed on the same day (Table 1).

	The 76 included women		In 41 non-responding women	
	Before metformin treatment	3-6 months after treatment (n=59)	Before metformin treatment	3-6 months after treatment (n=27)
Age at treatment (yrs)	29 ± 4		29 ± 4	
Weight kg	88 ± 21 (59,139)		83 ± 26 (47,150)	
BMI kg/m^2	31 ± 7 (18,47)		29 ± 8 (17,51)	
Testosterone (nmol/l)	2.93 ± 1.0 (1.91, 6.74) §	1.74 ± 0.7 (0.52,3.74) **	2.60 ± 0.5 (1.81,4.32)	1.63 ± 0.6 (0.57,3.32)
Testosterone > 2.4 (no.(%))	47 (62)	7 (12) **	25 (61)	0 **
DHAS(nmol/l)	5934 ± 3084 (837,15000)	4921 ± 2357 (1680,11000)	5256 ± 2151 (1956,12131)	5251 ± 2040 (2290,9828) **
SHBG(nmol/l)	44 ± 25 (9,132)	49 ± 27 (13,137) *	45 ± 27 (18,134)	56 ± 46 (16,229) **
FAI (%)	9.0 ± 6.3 (2.2,26.9)	4.7 ± 3.2 (0.9,17.0)**	7.4 ± 4.3 (1.6,24)	5.0 ± 4.1 (1.1,21) **
FAI above 97.5 percentile (FAI=7%) (no. (%))	35 (46)	9 (16) **	18 (44)	4 (15) **
FSH(IE/l)	5.6 ± 6.4 (0.4,55.9)	4.7 ± 1.8 (0.8,8.6)	4.7 ± 1.8 (1.2,8)	4.9 ± 1.8 (1.2,8.9)
LH (IE/l)	12.4 ± 7.3 (1.0,44.0)	9.3 ± 5.7 (1.6,29.6) **	11.3 ± 6.1 (1.2,27.9)	9.1 ± 6.2 (1.3,24.3)
HbA1c (%)	5.4 ± 0.3 (4.8,5.9)	5.4 ± 0.3 (5,6.3)	5.2 ± 0.5 (4.4,6.6)	5.2 ± 0.6 (4,6)
Fasting blood glucose (mmol/l)	5.2 ± 0.6 (4.0,6.1) §§	5.2 ± 0.5 (4.4,6.6)	4.6 ± 0.6 (4,5.5)	5.0 ± 0.7 (4,6)

Table 1: Paraclinical data before and after metformin treatment in 117 women (mean ± SD (range)).

We found after 3-6 months of treatment a significant drop in LH, total testosterone levels and more so in its relative level of bioavailability, the free androgen index, FAI. The non-responding women showed similar trends. The paraclinical values were similarly available in the non-responding women and differed only slightly (Table 1). The results showed no difference in any of the paraclinical results in repect to GDM or diabetes in the family history. Fifty-three of the 117 women had a BMI ≥ 30 kg/m^2 at first visit. In all, 86 (74 %) had a clinical check-up 3- 6 months after the initial visit.

Before vs. after treatment: *: p<0.05, **: p<0.01. Paired, non-parametric and t-test when appropriate, Difference between included and non-responding women: § p<0.05, §§. p<0.01

The follow-up by questionnaire in the 76 responding women was performed 5 ± 2 years after the first visit at which time the women's weight and BMI had significantly decreased (88 ± 21 to 85 ± 20 kg and 31 ± 7 to 30 ± 7 kg/m^2, p<0.02, paired, non-parametric test). Twenty-three percent had managed to decrease their BMI<30 kg/m^2.

Pregnancies

At first visit, 47 women were nulligravidae and 29 women had 50 various previous pregnancy outcomes. These historic pregnancies consisted of 26 live births, 17 spontaneous abortion, 6 induced abortions, and one extrauterine pregnancy. Further, in the index pregnancy the women were treated with metformin only, ovarian stimulation, IUI, and IVF in 22, 38, 8, and 8 of the cases, respectively. This resulted in 66 live deliveries (eight twins and 58 singletons), nine abortions and one legal abortion. The clinical results of the singleton pregnancies are shown in Table 2.

	GDM in history	No GDM in history	All	No GDM or family history of DM	Family history of DM/GDM
No.	14	62	76§	34	42
Nulligravidae	8	39	47	23	24
Metformin only	2	20	22	10	12
Ovulation induction	8	30	38	18	20
IUI	2	6	8	4	4
IVF	2	6	8	2	6
Preeclampsia	2	2	4	2	2
Family history of diabetes	8	28	42	0	42
Spontaneous abortions previously/in index pregnancy	3/2	8/7	11/9	4/3	7/6
Twins	0	8	8	6	2
Hypothyroidism pregravid	-	2	2	-	2
Hypertension at follow up	1	3	4	3	1
Singleton birth weight (n=58) (g)#	3658 ± 478	3569 ± 612	3571 ± 592	3714 ± 655	3488 ± 517
Singleton length (cm)#	52 ± 2	52 ± 2	52 ± 2.3	53 ± 3*	52 ± 2
Singleton ponderal index (g/dm3)#	27 ± 4	25 ± 3	25.2 ± 2.8	25 ± 2	25 ± 3
GDM in history	14	-	14	8	6

Table 2: The clinical data by history of GDM in 76 responding of PCOS women, § one woman had a legal, induced abortion, #: Excluding eight twins, nine abortions, and one extra-uterine pregnancy, *: $p<0.03$ Mann-Whitney U-test: PCOS women with DM history vs. no DM or GDM in history

In 11 of 66 deliveries GDM was diagnosed in the responding group of PCOS women and further two of 29 deliveries in the non-responding group. Three of the women who had abortions had gestational diabetes in either the previous or subsequent pregnancy; thus, at follow-up 14 % of the study group had had GDM at some stage. The clinical and obstetrical outcome of the women showed no association with family history of diabetes or GDM (Tables 2 and 3).

Five women had preeclampsia; one of these women had prepregnancy hypertension. Two women had concomitantly hypothyroidism and one woman hypertension; both conditions were diagnosed and treated before pregnancy. No neonatal anthropometric feature was different with respect to family history of diabetes or GDM and no fetal malformations were found; neither in hospital charts nor in the questionnaire.

	Spontaneous abortion	Singleton delivery	Twin deliveries	Induced abortion	Extra-uterine pregnancy
No.	20	85	10**	1	1
Nulligravidae	8	50	6	0	1
Metformin only	11	27	0		0
Ovulation induction	4	36	7	1	1
IUI	4	12	3		0
IVF	1	10	0		0

Preeclampsia	-	3	1		
Family history of diabetes	6	28	2	0	0
GDM*	2	11	0	1	0
Hypothyroidism pregravid	-	2			
Hypertension at follow up	2	1	1		

Table 3: Fertility treatment and maternal morbidity by pregnancy outcome in all 117 women, *: 2 women with spontaneous abortions had subsequently a pregnancy with gestational diabetes; the woman with induced abortion had previously had gestational diabetes, **: one triplet pregnancy

Discussion

We find no association of clinical outcome with history of diabetes and GDM despite the pregravid improvement of androgen status by metformin treatment. In this study metformin is only administered preconceptional and during early pregnancy. In contrast, Glueck et el. found decreased early pregnancy loss and gestational weight gain, less GDM and decreased androgen indices in pregnancy with a study design of prospective intervention and retrospective pregnancy loss data [4,5].

A Cochrane review on this subject concludes that concomitant metformin treatment improves clinical pregnancy rates when given in the time before and the immediate beginning of pregnancy with and without fertility treatment [6]. The credit for beneficial effect is given to the improvement of insulin sensitivity markers, which is expressed in general lower blood glucose, LH, and testosterone and an increase of SHBG [7-10]. Our women improve in similar insulin resistance markers.

The obvious bias of our study is that women are treated with different ovarian stimulation regimens, which will improve success rates given that each of the regimens increases the pregnancy rate. On the other hand, if insulin resistance affects pregnancy outcome in PCOS negatively, the dose of metformin would be decisive and not the ovarian stimulation. This was indicated by Khattab et al. who discontinued metformin after conception in a control group of PCOS women [11]. The PCOS women who continued with metformin throughout reduced their incidence of GDM to an OR of 0.17 compared to the control group. Similar the women are highly motivated and may seek a healthier lifestyle, which could include un-reported smoking cessation, diet, and weight reduction, all of which also improves insulin resistance.

Metformin intake throughout pregnancy has no androgen lowering effect and, if hyperandrogenism increase risk of GDM, metformin will not likely decrease the risk by this mechanism [2,3]. The reported incidence of GDM is variable in PCOS and potential prophylaxis with metformin is, thus, questionable. Glintborg et al. show no effect of metformin in increased inflammatory markers associated with diabetes and metabolic syndrome in PCOS women [12]. Although we screened for hyperglycemia in the pre-pregnancy period we found higher rate of GDM than in the background population. This may be due to the biochemical inclusion criteria together with other potential bias like obesity, age, and diabetes family history. If diabetogenic factors were involved in the etiology of miscarriages and pregnancy outcome of PCOS women, we find the family history or the likeliness of GDM itself seem not to herald increased risk. Thus, the glucose and

HbA1c values at first visit were similar with respect to subsequent GDM and diabetes history. Randomized studies of treatment effects of metformin in early pregnancy showed that obese PCOS have more benefit of treatment; this is suggestive for environmental factors' causative effect, i.e. body weight as well as the pregnancy's insulin resistant milieu [10].

To be included in our study group only the first two of the consensus criteria had to be fulfilled, namely oligo- and or an ovulation and clinical and/or biochemical signs of hyperandrogenism, excluding women diagnosed due to polycystic ovaries only [1]. Thus, our inclusion criteria were stricter and perhaps only included the most severe case of PCOS. Similarly, women with ovaries of polycystic morphology (PCO), without any other features of PCOS, show no effect of metformin treatment in a randomized study [13]. We, therefore, recommend the careful selection of study population, as it should limit some of the clinical heterogeneity of PCOS regarding disease phenotype like the ultrasound appearance of ovaries, obesity, hyperandrogenemia, and glycemia.

The varying association of PCOS with GDM depends on the population studied due to genetic factors where the metabolic syndrome in parents and their siblings seems to be fundamental to the pathogenesis of PCOS [14,15]. Franks et al. conclude that PCOS is inherited on an oligogenic basis and the co-morbidity and phenotype are due to the interaction of a small number of key genes with environmental and nutritional factors [16].

Selection bias of those who participated in the questionnaire part of the study is not likely as the non-responding women had comparable BMI, testosterone, and HbA1c as to the responding women. Nearly half of women (45%) in our study are obese and 47 % had a family history of diabetes mellitus. Further, our incidence of GDM in 14 % of the women seems reasonable compared with other studies in similar populations [2,3,15].

We have no reason to believe that the women were disfavored by commencing on metformin. On the contrary, we even find that the women lost weight since the initial visit five years previously which suggests that the women are motivated and have focus on the weight issue after pregnancy. Whether metformin has any long-term effect on diabetes prevention, weight reduction, and hyperandrogenism in PCOS remains unsolved.

To date only sparse data are available regarding the effect of metformin on a large scale when administered throughout the pregnancy [17]. Vanky et al. show in their randomized study that metformin administered from third month and throughout pregnancy is not associated with any improved outcome in terms of neonatal and maternal complications, i.e. GDM; preeclampsia, preterm delivery [3].

In conclusion, GDM and family history of diabetes is not associated with unfavorable pregnancy outcome in PCOS women.

References

1. Rotterdam ESHRE/ASRM-Sponsored PCOS Consensus Workshop Group (2004) Revised 2003 consensus on diagnostic criteria and long-term health risks related to polycystic ovary syndrome (PCOS). Hum Reprod 19: 19-25.

2. Vanky E, Carlsen SM (2012) Androgens and antimüllerian hormone in mothers with polycystic ovary syndrome and their newborns. Fertil Steril 97: 509-515.

3. Vanky E, Stridsklev S, Heimstad R, Romundstad P, Skogøy K, et al. (2010) Metformin versus placebo from first trimester to delivery in polycystic ovary syndrome: a randomized, controlled multicenter study. J Clin Endocrinol Metab 95: E448-455.

4. Glueck CJ, Wang P, Goldenberg N, Sieve-Smith L (2002) Pregnancy outcomes among women with polycystic ovary syndrome treated with metformin. Hum Reprod 17: 2858-2864.

5. Glueck CJ, Bornovali S, Pranikoff J, Goldenberg N, Dharashivkar S, et al. (2004) Metformin, pre-eclampsia, and pregnancy outcomes in women with polycystic ovary syndrome. Diabet Med 21: 829-836.

6. Tang T, Lord JM, Norman RJ, Yasmin E, Balen AH (2010) Insulin-sensitising drugs (metformin, rosiglitazone, pioglitazone, D-chiro-inositol) for women with polycystic ovary syndrome, oligo amenorrhoea and subfertility. Cochrane Database Syst Rev CD003053.

7. Jakubowicz DJ, Iuorno MJ, Jakubowicz S, Roberts KA, Nestler JE (2002) Effects of metformin on early pregnancy loss in the polycystic ovary syndrome. J Clin Endocrinol Metab 87: 524-529.

8. Palomba S, Falbo A, Orio F Jr, Zullo F (2009) Effect of preconceptional metformin on abortion risk in polycystic ovary syndrome: a systematic review and meta-analysis of randomized controlled trials. Fertil Steril 92: 1646-1658.

9. Boomsma CM, Eijkemans MJ, Hughes EG, Visser GH, Fauser BC, et al. (2006) A meta-analysis of pregnancy outcomes in women with polycystic ovary syndrome. Hum Reprod Update 12: 673-683.

10. Morin-Papunen L, Rantala AS, Unkila-Kallio L, Tiitinen A, Hippeläinen M, et al. (2012) Metformin improves pregnancy and live-birth rates in women with polycystic ovary syndrome (PCOS): a multicenter, double-blind, placebo-controlled randomized trial. J Clin Endocrinol Metab 97: 1492-1500.

11. Khattab S, Mohsen IA, Aboul Foutouh I, Ashmawi HS, Mohsen MN, et al. (2011) Can metformin reduce the incidence of gestational diabetes mellitus in pregnant women with polycystic ovary syndrome? Prospective cohort study. Gynecol Endocrinol 27: 789-793.

12. Glintborg D, Mumm H, Altinok ML, Richelsen B, Bruun JM, et al. (2014) Adiponectin, interleukin-6, monocyte chemoattractant protein-, and regional fat mass during 12-month randomized treatment with metformin and/or oral contraceptives in polycystic ovary syndrome. J Endocrinol Invest (In press).

13. Swanton A, Lighten A, Granne I, McVeigh E, Lavery S, et al. (2011) Do women with ovaries of polycystic morphology without any other features of PCOS benefit from short-term metformin co-treatment during IVF? A double-blind, placebo-controlled, randomized trial. Hum Reprod 26: 2178-2184.

14. Leibel NI, Baumann EE, Kocherginsky M, Rosenfield RL (2006) Relationship of adolescent polycystic ovary syndrome to parental metabolic syndrome. J Clin Endocrinol Metab 91: 1275-1283.

15. Helseth R, Vanky E, Salvesen O, Carlsen SM (2013) Gestational diabetes mellitus among Norwegian women with polycystic ovary syndrome: prevalence and risk factors according to the WHO and the modified IADPSG criteria. Eur J Endocrinol 169: 65-72.

16. Franks S, Gharani N, Waterworth D, Batty S, White D, et al. (1997) The genetic basis of polycystic ovary syndrome. Hum Reprod 12: 2641-2648.

17. Ekpebegh CO, Coetzee EJ, van der Merwe L, Levitt NS (2007) A 10-year retrospective analysis of pregnancy outcome in pregestational Type 2 diabetes: comparison of insulin and oral glucose-lowering agents. Diabet Med 24: 253-258.

32

Metabolic Syndrome Prevalence and Risk in the United States based on NHANES 2001-2012 Data

Brian Miller[1,2*] **and Mark Fridline**[3]

[1]School of Sport Science and Wellness Education, The University of Akron, Akron, OH, USA

[2]Health Education and Promotion, School of Health Sciences, Kent State University, Kent, OH, USA

[3]Department of Statistics, The University of Akron, Akron, OH, USA

[*]**Corresponding author:** Brian Miller, The University of Akron, School of Sport Science and Wellness Education, InfoCision Stadium 317, Akron OH, USA; E-mail: bm25@zips.uakron.edu

Abstract

Purpose: The purpose of the current investigation was to assess Metabolic Syndrome prevalence and risk estimates using United States nationally representative data.

Methods: Study sample was derived from 6 National Health and Nutrition Examination Survey (NHANES) cohorts from 2001-2012, N = 9,326 (male: n = 4,814; female: n = 4,512) including ages 18-59 presenting as fasted for 12 hours prior to laboratories collection. Variables included AHA/NHBLI Metabolic Syndrome classification criteria as well as additional cardiometabolic measures. Prevalence of Metabolic Syndrome and risk factors across cohorts as well as relative risk estimates were derived. Estimates were adjusted for age, race, and sex.

Results: There was no statistically significant difference between Metabolic Syndrome prevalence across cohorts. The order of Metabolic Syndrome criteria from highest to lowest risk were waist circumference, triglycerides, HDL, fasting plasma glucose, and blood pressure for the total sample and across sex, with women presenting with larger risk estimates than men. Women had larger prevalence of waist circumference, HDL, and blood pressure risk factors compared to men who had a larger prevalence of triglyceride and fasting plasma glucose risk factors. Those presenting with Metabolic Syndrome were twice as likely to have a cardiovascular event.

Conclusion: Waist circumference and triglycerides were the Metabolic Syndrome risk factors with the highest prevalence and associated risk of developing Metabolic Syndrome. Those with Metabolic Syndrome were at increased risk of having a cardiovascular event.

Keywords: Cardiovascular disease; Metabolic syndrome; Waist circumference; NHANES; Risk

Introduction

Metabolic Syndrome (MetS) is a constellation of cardio-metabolic risk factors that, when present in tandem, increase cardiovascular morbidity and/or mortality [1-3]. The high prevalence of cardiometabolic risk factors in MetS threatens to undermine all recent gains to prevent and control related chronic disease [4]. Originally described in 1988 by Gerald Reaven as Syndrome X, MetS was classified by the interrelationship between inflammation, impaired fibrinolysis, hypertension, atherogenic dyslipidemia, visceral obesity, and dysglycemia and their association with developing chronic diseases including cardiovascular disease (CVD), insulin resistance (IR), and hypertension (HTN) [5]. The prevalence and complications associated with MetS have remained a major health concern in the US [5,6].

The classification of MetS is based on the presence of 3 of 5 risk factors including dyslipidemia characterized by increased triglycerides (TG) and decreased HDL-cholesterol (HDL-C), hypertension, hyperglycemia, and central obesity. Current classification models [National Health Lung and Blood Institute (AHA/NHLBI), National Cholesterol Education Program (NCEP), and International Diabetes Federation (IDF)] have been limited in their usefulness given that each is only able to identify the presence or absence of MetS rather than identifying changes in risk of developing MetS [7-11] and related cardiovascular mortality [12]. Presently, the National Health Lung and Blood Institute (AHA/NHLBI) classification criteria are the accepted classification protocol for MetS. (Table 1) [1].

Given the limitations of the MetS classification and the dynamic nature of cardio-metabolic disease research, current nationally representative risk estimates based on the current MetS classification criteria and additional cardiometabolic risk factors are necessary to inform future research and clinical practice. To date, there have been numerous reports on the prevalence and associated risk of MetS [2,12,13]. However these systematic reviews present risk and prevalence statistics using antiquated data. Numerous studies have presented MetS prevalence statistics derived from multiple classification criteria using data from the National Health and Nutrition Examination Survey (NHANES), (Table 1). However, these studies were based on limited amounts of data utilizing few representative cohorts with Beltrán-Sánchez et al. utilizing the most NHANES cohorts [14-18].

Study	Cohort Years	Classification Criteria	MetS Prevalence
Mozumdar and Liguori [15]	NHANES III	NCEP	27.9% NHANES III
	NHANES 1999-2006		34.1% NHANES 1999-2006
Beltrán-Sanchez et al. [14]*	NHANES 1999-2010	IDF	25.5-22.9%
Ford et al. [16]*	NHANES III NHANES 1999-2000	NCEP	23.1% NHANES III
			26.7% NHANES 1999-2000
Ford et al. [3]	NHANES 2003-2006	NCEP	34.10%
Miller and Fridline [17]	NHANES 2009-2010	NCEP	33.10%
*Age-Adjusted			

Table 1: Select MetS Publications Reporting Prevalence using NHANES data.

The purpose of the current investigation was to develop MetS prevalence and risk estimates using a nationally representative data from NHANES 2001-2012 cohorts. This study was guided by 2 aims. The first aim was to identify the prevalence of MetS in the United States general population using NHANES data from 2001-2012. The second aim was to identify MetS risk based on AHA/NHLBI classification criteria, sex, and cardiovascular events.

Methods

Data management

The study sample was derived from National Health and Nutrition Examination Survey (NHANES) data made publically available by the Centers for Disease Control and Prevention which included cohorts. Data was collected from 2001-2012 in 2 year intervals resulting in a total of 6 cohorts. The data was arranged in a column-wise format with each subject given a sequence identifier. Data management was performed using dataset merging and data subset functions using SPSS version 22 (SPSS Inc., Chicago, IL).

The inclusion criteria were based on the following parameters: Age range of 18-59 years, 12 hour fasting protocol for laboratory values, abstinence from alcohol and/or tobacco use prior to laboratories, and a negative exam for pregnancy for females. The age criteria was chosen based on Ford Li, and Zhao where the highest prevalence of MetS was exhibited after 59 years of age [3]. Inclusion of ages beyond 59 resulted in inflation of risk estimates. The MetS classification was defined as the presence of 3 of 5 risk factors based on the clinical classification model proposed by the AHA/NHLBI (Table 2) [1] Subjects with missing criteria were excluded from the analysis unless the criteria present were adequate to make a MetS classification. This decision was made in order to control for the inability to make a complete classification. Blood pressure readings were the average of 4 blood pressure collections per subject. The presence of each MetS classification criteria was dichotomized with ≥3 of 5 criteria classified as MetS. The final sample size for inclusion was N = 9,326 (male: n = 4,814; female: n =

4,512). The current investigation was approved by the Institutional Review Board of the University of Akron.

Measure	Defining Cut-off Points
Elevated Waist Circumference[1]	
Male	>94 cm
Female	>80 cm
Elevated Triglycerides[2]	≥ 150 mg/dl
HDL Cholesterol[2]	
Male	<40 mg/dl
Female	<50 mg/dl
Blood Pressure[2]	≥130 mmHg Systolic and/or ≥80 mmHg Diastolic
Fasting Plasma Glucose[2]	≥100 mg/dl
[1]Values based on lowered AHA/NHLBI Guidelines (Alberit)	
[2]Drug therapy for dyslipidemia, hypertension, and/or hyperglycemia were alternate indicators meeting the criteria for MetS for that risk factor	

Table 2: National Health Lung & Blood Institute Metabolic Syndrome Classification Criteria.

In addition to the AHA/NHLBI MetS classification criteria, indicators of cardio-metabolic morbidity included: a binary indicator of cardiovascular events built off of the presence of 1 of 5 cardiovascular events including congestive heart failure, coronary heart disease, angina, heart attack, and/or stroke [19]. Descriptive statistics included the above mentioned measure were presented as M ± SD in addition to the following measures: HOMA-IR, an indicator of insulin resistance defined as [Insulin (uU/dl) x FPG(mg/dl)/405] [6,18,19], cardio-metabolic risk factors [total cholesterol (TC), LDL cholesterol, and C-Reactive Protein (CRP) - systemic inflammatory marker [20], anthropometrics [height(cm), weight(kg), and Body Mass Index (BMI) (kg/m^2) [8,21]; and socioeconomic status measured via Family Poverty to Income ratio (PIR) a measure of adjusted family income to relative poverty threshold based on house size [22].

Sample adjustment

Sample weights were created in NHANES to account for the complex sample design when capturing participant data. This sample design included survey non response, post-stratification, and oversampling certain demographic groups. When a sample is weighted using NHANES data, the results are representative of the U.S. Census civilian non-institutionalized population. A sample weight is assigned to each person in the sample, where it measures the frequency of people in the population represented by that sample individual. It is important to utilize the weights to ensure that the calculated parameter estimates are truly representative of our population. To account for the complex survey design, statistical results were calculated according to NHANES guidelines [23]. The SPSS Complex Sampling module was used to take into account the NHANES complex survey design.

Statistical analysis

A Chi-Squared (X^2) test of goodness of fit was employed to indentify differences in the prevalence of MetS by NHANES cohort year. Additionally in cases where the X^2 test reached statistical significance, post hoc tests were performed using the standardized residuals (SR) with SR>2 indicating significant deviations. Risk estimates [relative risk (RR) accompanied with 95% confidence intervals] were produced for each MetS classification criteria as well as

Cardiovascular Events and Sex in relation to MetS. All statistical analysis were performed using SPSS version 22 (IBM, Chicago, IL, 2013) with statistical significance for all tests set at p ≤ 0.05 (Table 3).

Variable	Sample	No MetS			MetS		
		n	M	SD	n	M	SD
Age (years)	Male	3543	33.05	12.09	1931	42.48	11.11
	Female	3570	34.41	11.87	1595	43.23	11.31
Family PIR	Male	3278	2.55	1.63	1806	2.69	1.67
	Female	3285	2.53	1.68	1460	2.35	1.64
Height (cm)	Male	3542	175.57	7.77	1931	175.79	7.72
	Female	3570	162.43	6.96	1592	161.71	7.02
BMI	Male	3542	25.83	4.83	1931	31.37	5.65
	Female	3570	26.54	6.25	1592	33.13	7.57
CRP(mg/dL)	Male	3003	0.25	0.72	1645	0.41	0.77
	Female	3027	0.36	68.00%	1357	0.72	0.97
TC (mg/dL)	Male	3543	186.22	3928.00%	1931	205.24	45
	Female	3570	186.46	37.6	1595	204.27	45.07
LDL-C (mg/dL)	Male	3462	113.67	34.55	1729	123.55	36.22
	Female	3512	108.52	31.87	1512	122.15	36.89
WC (cm)	Male	3543	90.78	13.32	1931	107.89	13.85
	Female	3570	88.24	14.3	1595	104.93	15.42
TG (mg/dL)	Male	3543	105.17	68.16	1931	224.58	212.46
	Female	3570	87.23	40.54	1595	178.77	144.36
HDL-C (mg/dL)	Male	3543	51.7	13.37	1931	40.86	10.59
	Female	3570	60.39	14.59	1595	47.74	13.36
SBP (mmHg)	Male	3543	117.68	11.59	1931	126.54	15.03
	Female	3570	110.92	12.26	1595	123.38	17.7
DBP (mmHg)	Male	3543	69.35	11.08	1931	77.04	11.67
	Female	3570	67.34	9.55	1595	73.79	11.24
FPG (mg/dL)	Male	3543	96.51	18.47	1931	118.46	47.53
	Female	3570	91.73	14.3	1595	114.9	43.92
HOMA-IR	Male	3500	2.37	2.08	1917	5.96	8.49
	Female	3530	2.29	1.72	1577	5.45	5.48
Descriptive statistics presented as Mean ± Standard Deviation (M ± SD) for unadjusted NHANES data							

Table 3: Descriptive Statistics for Total NHANES Cohort and by Sex.

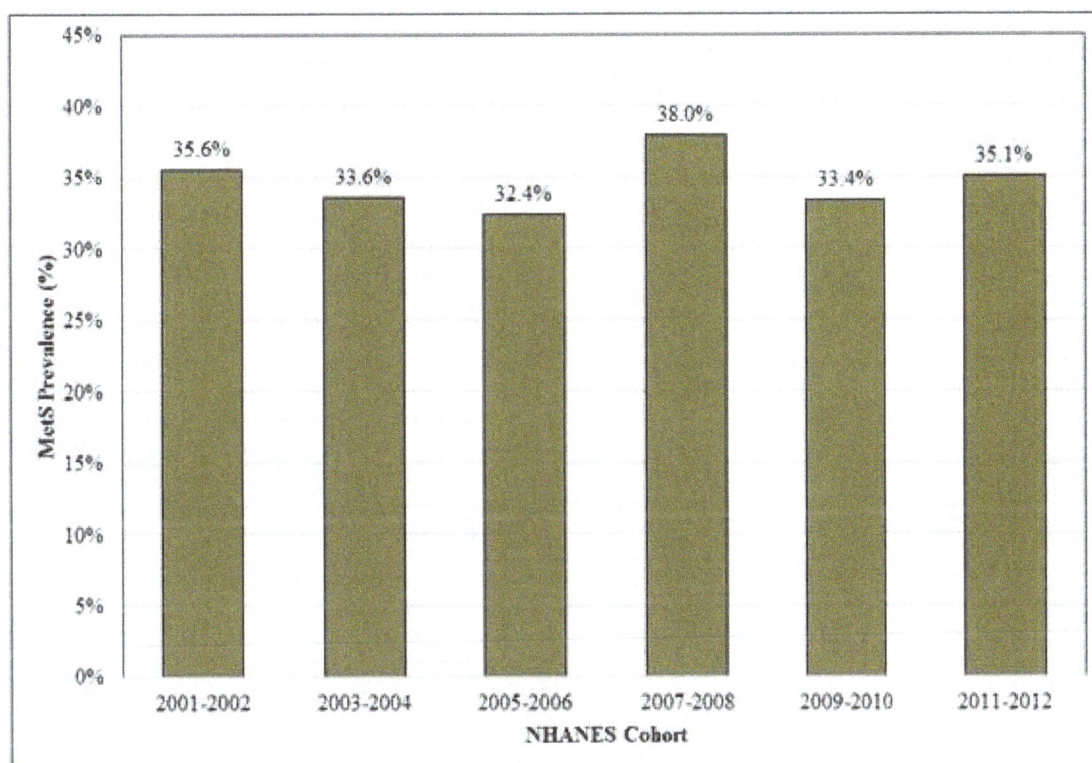

Figure 1: Prevalence of MetS classified by AHA/NHLBI criteria for each NHANES cohort year.

Results

Prevalence of MetS

Table 3 depicts the sample characteristics by MetS and no-MetS. There was not a statistically significant difference in prevalence of MetS by NHANES cohort year, $\chi^2(6) = 13.83$, $p = 0.257$.

The average prevalence of MetS in the total cohort was 34.7 ± 1.4%. Figure 1 for MetS prevalence by NHANES cohort year.

Based on the indicators of MetS risk based on the presence of each risk factor (see Table 4 for total cohort and by sex), the order of highest to lowest risk were WC, TG, HDL, FPG, and BP for the total sample and across sex, respectively. However, females had larger risks than men for all MetS risk factors. The risk factor with the largest difference by sex was WC with women being on average 14.11 times more likely to develop MetS compare to men; RR = 23.8 (14.58-38.77) compared to RR = 9.69 (7.93-11.86) for men and women respectively. Women had a larger prevalence of risk WC, HDL, and BP risk factors compared to men who had a larger prevalence of TG and FPG risk factors. Specifically the risk factor with the largest prevalence was WC representing 77% of women and 61% men. There was a 2 fold increase in risk of a cardiovascular event given the presence of metabolic syndrome for the total sample [RR = 2.02 (1.83-2.23)] with a higher risk for men [RR = 1.81 (1.54, 2.13)] compared to women [RR = 2.32 (2.01-2.68)].

Discussion

Metabolic Syndrome is a constellation of cardiometabolic risk factors that when present in tandem increase the risk morbidity and mortality [1,3]. The current investigation was guided by 2 aims. The first aim explored the prevalence of MetS by NHANES cohort year from 2001-2012. Differences in prevalence rates of the current investigation compared to other studies is likely based on differences in MetS classification criteria, subject inclusion criteria, and adjustments made for age. The MetS prevalence of this study (34.7%) approximates the prevalence of MetS for Ford et al. = 34.1%, Miller and Fridline = 33.1%, and Mozumdar and Liguori = 34.1%. Beltrán-Sánchez et al. reported an average prevalance of MetS using NHANES data at 25.5% in 1999 and 22.9% in 2010. However this article used an age-adjustment and did not restrict age.

The second aim was to identify MetS risk based on AHA/NHLBI classification criteria, sex, and history of cardiovascular events. The risk factor with the largest risk of MetS was WC with a larger impact for men than women. This results corroborates with Miller et al. who found WC as the strongest predictor of MetS using a decision tree algorithm. Additionally, Beltrán-Sánchez et al. reported an increase in abdominal obesity, with a more drastic increase among women. Increased WC has been used as a screening phenotype to identify those at high risk of MetS [24]. This study identified TG as the second strongest indicator of MetS risk with 32%, 38%, and 25% for the total cohort, male, and female presenting with this risk factor, respectively.

Miller and Fridline and Worachartcheewan et al. both identified that the TG criteria resulted in the highest risk of MetS. However based on risk estimates of the currefnt investigation, TG and HDL had less risk than WC. Dyslipidemia in MetS, defined as high serum TG and low HDL-C, have been demonstrated as effective markers for the presence of cardio-metabolic abnormalities [24]. An analysis of NHANES 2003-2006 data showed that 31% of adults exhibit hypertriglyceridemia (>150 mg/dl) [3]. Beltrán-Sánchez et al. reported an increase in dyslipidemia, hyperglycemia, and waist circumference from 1999-2010 with a decrease prevalence in hyper tension.

Variable	Sample	Proportion	RR	95% Confidence Interval
WC	Total	0.68	9.69	7.93 – 11.86
	Male	0.61	8.68	6.97 – 10.82
	Female	0.77	23.8	14.58 – 38.77
TG	Total	0.32	5.69	5.29 – 6.12
	Male	0.38	5.14	4.62 – 5.70
	Female	0.25	6.38	5.71 – 7.13
HDL	Total	0.35	4.93	4.59 – 5.29
	Male	0.33	4.3	3.93 – 4.71
	Female	0.37	6.31	5.50 – 7.24
FPG	Total	0.37	4	3.69 – 4.34
	Male	0.45	3.34	2.99 – 3.72
	Female	0.28	4.88	4.35 – 5.49
BP	Total	0.28	3.58	3.36 – 3.81
	Male	0.32	3.15	2.87 – 3.45
	Female	0.24	4.1	3.78 – 4.46
CE	Total	0.04	2.02	1.83 – 2.25
	Male	0.04	1.81	1.54 – 2.13
	Female	0.03	2.32	2.01 – 2.68

WC = Waist Circumference, TG = Triglycerides, HDL =HDL Cholesterol, BP = Blood Pressure, FPG = Fasting Plasma Glucose, CE = Cardiovascular Event, and RR = Relative Risk, Proportion = proportion of sample presenting with criterion

Table 4: Adjusted MetS Risk Statistics for the Total Cohort and by Sex

Després et al. found that a tandem increase of TG above 2 mmol/L with a WC greater than 90 cm showed a greater than 80% increase in risk of developing MetS. Although there was not a large difference in MetS risk by sex, the order of risk contribution for each MetS criteria to MetS risk were different. This supports the need for future investigation to consider differences in cardio-metabolic risk by sex as well as the clustering interaction of MetS risk factors. Specific to cardiovascular risk in the current investigation was approximately 2 times greater for those with MetS. This finding corroborates with Mottillo et al. who found that MetS was associated with a 2-fold increase risk of cardiovascular events in addition to a 1.5 fold increase in all-cause mortality.

The results of this study are meant to provide risk estimates for MetS across multiple cardiometabolic risk factors and differences by sex.

Future investigation should employ these estimates to guide future investigation for MetS risk factors investigated. The predominant finding of the current investigation was the drastic risk increase of MetS based on presenting with WC risk factor. Furthermore there was a large disparity for women compared to men based on presenting with the WC risk factor. The results of this article in tandem with recommendations from Beltrán-Sánchez et al., Miller and Fridline and Miller et al. emphasizes the urgency of recognizing abdominal obesity as a healthcare priority.

This study had numerous strengths which included the use of large amounts of nationally representative data and described contributions to MetS risk. Beltran-Sanchez et al. utilized data from the 1999-2010 NHANES cohorts to explore the prevalence of the MetS classification criteria across race, age, and sex. However this study did not investigate the contribution of cardio-metabolic risk factors to overall MetS risk. The current investigation study also had limitations. This study did not employ an age-adjustment to describe prevalence and risk of MetS but rather an adjustment across sex and race. This study also relied on secondary, observational data where differences in data collection and analysis were not accounted for.

In summary, the purpose of this study was to explore differences in MetS prevalence across 6 NHANES cohorts and MetS risk for MetS classification criteria and additional cardio-metabolic risk factors. There were differing levels MetS risk for each of the cardiometabolic risk factors for the total sample and by sex. The risk factor with the highest proportion and risk for the total sample and by sex was WC. Women had a higher prevalence of WC, HDL, and BP risk factors compared to men who had a higher prevalence of TG and FPG. Presenting with the WC risk factor had the largest associated risk with MetS with a larger risk for women compared to mean. Future research should utilize these findings to guide experimental research considering MetS risk [25,26].

Conflict of Interest

The author of this study declared no conflict of interest.

References

1. Alberti KGMM, Eckel RH, GrundySM, Zimmet PZ, CleemanJI, et al. (2009) Harmonizing the metabolic syndrome: A joint interim statement of the international diabetes federation task force on epidemiology and prevention; national heart, lung, and blood institute; american heart association; world heart federation; international atherosclerosis society; and international association for the study of obesity. Circulation 120: 1640-1645.

2. Eberly LE, Prineas R, Cohen JD, Vazquez G, Zhi X, et al. (2006) Metabolic syndrome risk factor distribution and 18-year mortality in the Multiple Risk Factor Intervention Trial. Diabetes Care 29: 123-130.

3. Ford ES, Li C, Zhao G (2010) Prevalence and correlates of metabolic syndrome based on a harmonious definition among adults in the US. J Diabetes 2: 180-193.

4. Eckel RH, Grundy SM, Zimmet PZ (2005) The metabolic syndrome. The Lancet 365: 1415-1428.

5. Grundy SM (2011) The metabolic syndrome. Atlas of atherosclerosis and metabolic syndrome (5th edn), NY: Springer, New York.

6. Wilson PW, D'Agostino RB, Parise H, Sullivan L, Meigs JB (2005) Metabolic syndrome as a precursor of cardiovascular disease and type 2 diabetes mellitus. Circulation 112: 3066-3072.

7. Alberti KG, Zimmet P, Shaw J; IDF Epidemiology Task Force Consensus Group (2005) The metabolic syndrome-a new worldwide definition. Lancet 366: 1059-1062.

8. Arnlov J, Ingelsson E, Sundström J, Lind L (2010) Response to letters regarding article,"The impact of body mass index and the metabolic syndrome on the risk of cardiovascular disease and death in middle-aged men". Circulation 122: e457-e457.

9. Boudreau DM, Malone DC, Raebel MA, Fishman PA, Nichols GA, et al. (2009) Health care utilization and costs by metabolic syndrome risk factors. Metab Syndr Relat Disord 7: 305-314.

10. Kassi E, Pervanidou P, Kaltsas G, Chrousos G (2011) Metabolic syndrome: definitions and controversies. BMC Med 9: 48.

11. Miller B, Fridline M, Liu PY, Marino D (2014) Use of CHAID decision trees to formulate pathways for the early detection of metabolic syndrome in young adults. Computational and mathematical methods in medicine.

12. Mottillo S, Filion KB, Genest J, Joseph L, Pilote L, et al. (2010) The metabolic syndrome and cardiovascular risk a systematic review and meta-analysis. J Am Coll Cardiol 56: 1113-1132.

13. Gami AS, Witt BJ, Howard DE, Erwin PJ, Gami LA, et al. (2007). Metabolic syndrome and risk of incident cardiovascular events and death: a systematic review and meta-analysis of longitudinal studies. Journal of the American College of Cardiology 49: 403-414.

14. Beltrán-Sánchez H, Harhay MO, Harhay MM, McElligott S (2013) Prevalence and trends of metabolic syndrome in the adult U.S. population, 1999-2010. J Am Coll Cardiol 62: 697-703.

15. Mozumdar A, Liguori G (2011) Persistent increase of prevalence of metabolic syndrome among U.S. adults: NHANES III to NHANES 1999-2006. Diabetes Care 34: 216-219.

16. Ford ES, Giles WH, Mokdad AH (2004) Increasing prevalence of the metabolic syndrome among u.s. Adults. Diabetes Care 27: 2444-2449.

17. Miller B, Fridline M (2015) Development and Validation of Metabolic Syndrome Prediction and Classification-Pathways using Decision Trees. J Metabol Synd 4: 2167-0943.

18. Angelico F, Burattin M, Alessandri C, Del Ben M, Lirussi F (2007) Drugs improving insulin resistance for non-alcoholic fatty liver disease and/or non-alcoholic steatohepatitis. The Cochrane Library.

19. Ninomiya JK, L'Italien G, Criqui MH, Whyte JL, Gamst A, et al. (2004). Association of the metabolic syndrome with history of myocardial infarction and stroke in the third national health and nutrition examination survey. Circulation 109: 42-46.

20. Nayak BS, Teelucksingh S, Jagessar A, Maharaj S, Maharaj N (2013) A cross sectional study comparing traditional risk factors with N-terminal pro-BNP in high risk groups for cardiovascular disease in Trinidad, West Indies. Diabetes & Metabolic Syndrome: Clinical Research & Reviews 7: 8-11.

21. Camhi SM, Bray GA, Bouchard C, Greenway FL, Johnson WD, et al. (2011) The relationship of waist circumference and BMI to visceral, subcutaneous, and total body fat: sex and race differences. Obesity (Silver Spring) 19: 402-408.

22. Matthews KA, Räikkönen K, Gallo L, Kuller LH (2008) Association between socioeconomic status and metabolic syndrome in women: testing the reserve capacity model. Health Psychology 27: 576.

23. National Center for Health Statistics (2008) Specifying Weighting Parameters. Atlanta, GA:Centers for Disease Control and Prevention, NCHS.

24. Roger VL, Go AS, Lloyd-Jones DM, Adams RJ, Berry JD, et al. (2011) Heart disease and stroke statistics—2011 update a report from the American Heart Association. Circulation 123: e18-e209.

25. Worachartcheewan A, Dansethakul P, Nantasenamat C, Pidetcha P, Prachayasittikul V (2012) Determining the optimal cutoff points for waist circumference and body mass index for identification of metabolic abnormalities and metabolic syndrome in urban Thai population. Diabetes Research and Clinical Practice 98: e16-e21.

26. Despres JP, Lemieux I, Bergeron J, Pibarot P, Mathieu P, et al. (2008) Abdominal obesity and the metabolic syndrome: Contribution to global cardiometabolic risk. Arterioscler Thromb Vasc Biol 28: 1039-1049.

33

Stimulating Effect of Ethanol on Erythropoietin Production in the Liver Cells

Kazuhiko Nishimura*, Hideaki Katuyama, Hiroshi Nakagawa and SaburoMatuo

Laboratory of Bioenvironmental Sciences, Course of Veterinary Science, Graduate School of Life and Environmental Sciences, Osaka Prefecture University,Osaka, Japan

*Corresponding author: Kazuhiko Nishimura, Laboratory of Bioenvironmental Sciences, Course of Veterinary Science, Graduate School of Life and Environmental Sciences, Osaka Prefecture University, 1-58 RinkuOhrai-Kita, Izumisano, Osaka 598-8531, Japan; E-mail: nisimura@vet.osakafu-u.ac.jp

Abstract

Increased erythropoietin (EPO) production is important for erythropoiesis as well as cell viability. The most effective factor for promoting EPO production is hypoxia, which alters the redox state and produces a reducing environment in the cell. In this study, we examined the influence of ethanol on EPO production in HepG2 cells to investigate the effect of increasing the free NADH/NAD+ ratio in the cytosol during normoxia. Ethanol treatment increased the lactate/pyruvate ratio, an index of the cytosolic redox state, in a dose-dependent manner, with maximal promotion of EPO production observed at 300 µM ethanol. These results suggest that altering the cytosolic NADH/NAD+ redox state to the same degree as hypoxia is effective in promoting EPO production. Ethanol (300 µM) increased mRNA expression and protein levels of sirtuin1, which is a transcription factor, related to both hypoxia inducible factor and cytosolic redox state, whereas 2000 µM ethanol did not produce these effects. Although the sirtuin1 inhibitorEX-527 did not affect the lactate/pyruvate ratio, EX-527 inhibited the induction of EPO mRNA expression by 300 µM ethanol. In rat primary hepatocytes and kidney cells, 300 µM ethanol increased sirtuin1 and EPO mRNA expression, as well as EPO concentrations in media. In conclusion, we showed low concentrations of ethanol promote EPO production by increasing sirtuin1 in HepG2 cells, as well as primary liver and kidney cells. The use of ethanol represents a hypoxia-independent method to promote EPO production.

Keywords: Erythropoietin; Ethanol; Redox state

Introduction

Erythropoietin (EPO) is a hematopoietic cytokine that is best known for its role in promoting red blood cell formation and survival [1-4]. EPO is an indispensable factor for regulation of mammalian erythropoiesis, and increasing EPO production is important in recovery from anemia. In adults, EPO is mainly produced by the kidneys and the liver produces EPO when stimulated with moderate to severe hypoxia.

EPO production is regulated by hypoxia inducible factor (HIF), which is a heterodimer consisting of HIF-α and β subunits [5,6]. Both HIF-1 and 2 promote EPO production, and the role of each HIF subtype in EPO production differs according to cell type and the duration of exposure [7,8]. HIF-α levels are regulated by prolyl hydroxylases (PHDs), which are oxygen-dependent enzymes that hydrolyze HIF-α [9]. Hypoxia increases the content of HIF-1α and/or 2α by reducing the activity of PHDs, which hydrolyze HIF-α, and increases transcription of EPO mRNA in the nucleus [9]. PHDsmaintain HIF-α at low levels during normoxia and consequently EPO production is low. Hypoxia, caused by anemia or relocation to mountainous elevations, decreases PHD activity and increases HIF-α content, resulting in elevated EPO production [5,10].

EPO mRNA expression has also been detected in the brain, lung, heart, bone marrow, spleen, hair follicles, osteoblasts, and the reproductive tract [3,4]. EPO production by these cells is more likely to act locally and modulate cellular viability and function related to cytoprotective effects [11-15]. EPO has emerged as a major tissue-protective survival factor in various non-haematopoietic organs [16].

Elevation of EPO production is important for erythropoiesis as well as cell viability and overall health. The most effective factor for increasing EPO production is hypoxia. [5,6]. However, hypoxia is toxic for various organs and induces neuronal apoptosis [17,18]. Therefore, it is thought that using hypoxia to increase EPO production in therapeutic settings is a flawed concept. However, inducing EPO production under normoxic conditions is difficult. There are reports that cobalt and quercetin are capable of increasing HIF levels and thereby increasing EPO production [6,9,19]. Monitoring increases in HIF levels are frequently targeted in the development of drugs that promote EPO production under normoxic conditions [20,21]; however, this is not a practical approach for this objective.

Hypoxia also influences the cellular redox state. Hypoxia-induced glycolysis produces a reducing environment within the cell. Mikko et al [22] reported that the reducing environment leads to increased stability of HIF. It is reported that the interaction of the regulatory factor sirtuin1 (SIRT1) with HIF is dependent on the cytosolic redox state [23]. Moreover, Gambini et al [24] reported that an increase in cytosolic NADH / NAD+ ratio by ethanol addition promoted SIRT1 mRNA expression. SIRT1 activity is increased in a NAD+-dependent manner and stabilizes HIF-1 by deacetylation [25]. However, it is not clear that changes in the cytosolic redox state during normoxia influences EPO production. Changes in the cytosolic redox state similar to those produced by hypoxia may promote EPO production under normoxic conditions.

Ethanol is a substance that produces a reducing environment in cells. Ethanol is metabolized to acetaldehyde in the cytosol by alcohol dehydrogenase. This reaction produces NADH, primarily in the liver and kidneys, and acetaldehyde is immediately metabolized to acetic acid thereafter [26-28]. In this study, to clarify whether increased EPO production results from a reduction in the cytosolic redox state during normoxia, we examined the influence of ethanol on EPO production in HepG2 cells, which have an EPO-producing ability.

Materials and methods

Materials

HepG2 cells were provided by RIKEN BRC through the National Bio-Resource Project of MEXT, Japan. Primers for real-time reverse transcription-polymerase chain reaction (RT-PCR) were purchased from Genedesign Co. (Osaka, Japan). Dulbecco's modified Eagle's medium (DMEM) was purchased from Nissui Pharmaceuticals Co. (Tokyo, Japan). Glucose and pyruvate free DMEM was purchased from Sigma-Aldrich (St. Louis, MO) and 2.5 mM glucose with or without 1.25 mM sodium pyruvate was added. The SIRT1 inhibitor EX-527 was purchased from Sigma-Aldrich. Standard laboratory chemicals and reagents were purchased from Wako Pure Chemical Co. (Osaka, Japan). To amplify human mRNA, we designed the following pairs of primers: 5'- ATGTGGATAAAGCCGTCAGTGG-3' and 5'- GACGAGGTGAGGCTTGTTAGT-3' for EPO mRNA, spanning positions 543 to 662 [29]; 5'-GTCTGTTTCATGTGGAATACCTGACT -3' and 5'-GTCTACAGCAAGGCGAGCATAA -3' for SIRT1 mRNA, spanning positions 845 to 911 [30]. To amplify rat mRNA, we designed the following pairs of primers: 5'- GCTCAGAAGGAATTGATGTCGC-3' and 5'- TTGGAGTAGACCCGGAAGAGCT-3' for EPO mRNA, spanning positions 492 to 592 [31]; 5'- TCCAAGGCCACGGATAGG -3' and 5'- GGATCGGTGCCAATCATGAG -3' for SIRT1 mRNA, spanning positions 483 to 545 (accession number, XM_003751934). The primers 5'-CACCACCAACTGCTTAGCCC-3' and 5'-TCTGAGTGGCAGTGATGGCA-3' were selected for amplification of human and rat glyceraldehyde phosphate dehydrogenase (GAPDH) mRNA both, spanning positions 343 to 443 in rat GAPDH mRNA [32].

Animals

Male Wistar rats (7-week-old) were purchased from Nippon SLC Co. (Shizuoka, Japan). The experimental design and methods for animal care were pre-approved according to the guideline for animal experimentation of the animal care committee of Osaka Prefecture University. Liver and kidney cells of 9-week-old rats were harvested by tissue perfusion with 0.05% collagenase in Ringer's solution. Liver and kidney cells were seeded at a concentration of 2.0×10^5 cells/ml in DMEM containing 10% fetal bovine serum.

Cell culture

HepG2 cells were sub-cultured in DMEM containing 10% fetal bovine serum in 95% air and 5% CO_2 at 37°C. When HepG2 cells reached a concentration of 10^6 cells/ml, they were used for culture experiments. Cells used for experimentation had >95% viability as determined by trypan blue-exclusion assay. In culture experiments, 1 ml of HepG2, liver, and kidney cells (final concentration of 2.0×10^5 cells/ml) were sub-cultured for 24 h in 5% CO_2 at 37°C. Sub-cultured cells were incubated in the presence of various concentrations of ethanol and other chemicals and cultured for an additional 6 h. Hypoxic conditions were produced by culturing in 5% O_2, 90% N_2, and 5% CO_2 at 37°C for 6 h. Cells were collected for measurement of mRNA concentrations by RT-PCR and protein levels of HIF-1α, HIF-2α and SIRT1. All samples were tested in duplicate.

Determination of mRNA levels

RNA was collected from whole cultured cells using a Gen Elute Mammalian total RNA kit (Sigma-Aldrich). The relative levels of specific mRNAs were determined by RT-PCR using a PowerSYBR Green RNA-to-C_T 1-Step Kit (Applied Biosystems, Foster City, CA) on an ABI StepOnePlus Real-Time PCR System (Applied Biosystems, Carlsbad, CA). The following PCR program was used: 48°C for 30 min, 95°C for 10 min; 40 cycles of 95°C for 15 sec and 60°C for 60 sec. After PCR, dissociation curves were constructed to confirm the amplification of uniform products. Quantification of mRNA was performed using the comparative delta CT method. GAPDH mRNA was used as the control, and the ratio of each experimental mRNA to GAPDH was calculated. The values of mRNAs are provided as values relative to the value of untreated cells. Each mRNA sample was measured twice and the levels of EPO, HIF-α and GAPDH were measured from the same samples.

Determination of metabolites and erythropoietin

Lactate and pyruvate contents in HepG2 cell were measured spectrophotometrically with an enzymatic assay [33]. HepG2 cells were washed twice with ice-cold phosphate buffered saline, and washed cells terminated by the addition of 1 ml of 5% (v/v) $HClO_4$. Each sample was neutralized by K_2CO_3 and collected supernatant by centrifuging for assay. Ethanol concentrations in the culture media were measured fluorescence spectrophotometrically using an enzymatic assay [34]. Concentrations of erythropoietin in culture media were determined using an ELISA kit (ABnova, Taipei, Taiwan).

Western blot analysis

For the identification of HIF-1α and 2α protein levels, proteins were extracted from whole cell lysates in RIPA buffer and were separated by 10% SDS-PAGE before being transferred onto polyvinyl difluoride membranes (Biorad, Hercules, CA). After blocking with 5% skim milk, the membranes were incubated with anti-HIF-1α, 2α and total PHDs (PHD1,2,3) monoclonal antibodies (1:2,000; Novus Biologicals, Littleton, CO), or anti-β-actin monoclonal antibody (1:40,000; Sigma-Aldrich) overnight at 4°C. After incubation with an HRP-labeled secondary antibody (1:20,000; MP Biomedicals, Solon, OH) for 1 h at room temperature, reactive proteins were detected using a LAS-3000 (Fujifilm, Tokyo, Japan) after enhancement with a chemiluminescence detection kit (Millipore, Billerica, MA). β-actin was used as the control, and the values for HIF-1α or 2α were calculated relative to β-actin. The protein data are given as values relative those of untreated cells.

Statistical analysis

Statistical significance was determined using the Tukey-Kramer method.

Results

Figure 1 shows the effects of ethanol on EPO mRNA expression in normoxic HepG2 cells. Ethanol at 300 μM increased EPO mRNA expression; however, the EPO levels decreased at ethanol concentrations greater than 300 μM and were not significantly elevated at concentrations greater than 1000 μM.

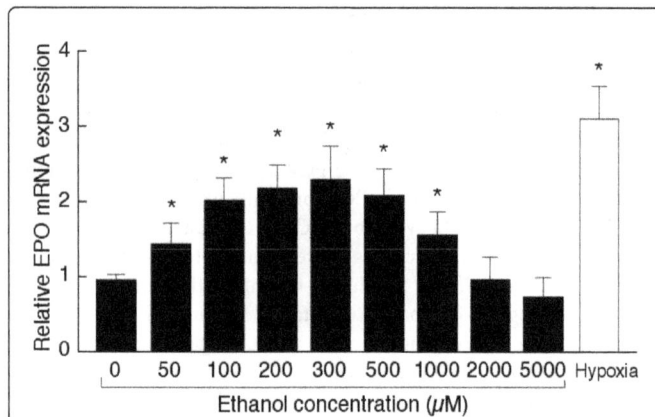

Figure 1: Effect of ethanol on erythropoietin mRNA expression in HepG2 cells. HepG2 cells were cultured in 5% CO2 at 37°C for 6 h in the absence or presence of ethanol and EPO mRNA levels were normalized to expression in the absence of ethanol, with GAPDH mRNA used as the control. Hypoxic condition involved culturing in 5% O_2, 90% N_2, and 5% CO2 at 37°C for 6 h. Each mRNA sample was measured twice. Values represent the mean ± S.D. (n = 4). Asterisks indicate significant differences as compared with the values for 0 μM of ethanol (p<0.05).

Hypoxia increased EPO mRNA levels three-fold relative to normoxia. Ethanol treatment, at all concentrations, did not affect cell viability as determined by trypan blue staining (data not shown). Ethanol concentration in the culture media decreased in a time-dependent manner, and did not significantly decrease up to 6 h after the addition of 2000 μM ethanol (Table 1).

Time after addition (hour)	Ethanol addition	
	300 μM	2000 μM
0	309.0 ± 13.7	1990 ± 58
2	265.9 ± 19.8	1920 ± 69
4	202.5 ± 15.3*	1890 ± 78
6	162.2 ± 11.6*	1850 ± 75
8	115.9 ± 10.5*	1820 ± 81*
10	75.0 ± 8.9*	1790 ± 84*
12	35.7 ± 5.9*	1750 ± 94*

Table 1: Changes of ethanol concentration in culture media, Values represent the mean ± S.D. (n = 4). Asterisks indicate significant differences as compared with the values for 0 hour of ethanol addition (p<0.05).

Ethanol metabolism by alcohol dehydrogenase produces reducing equivalents and affects the cellular redox state. The ratio of lactate to pyruvate is shown in Figure 2A as an index of the cytosolic redox state. The ratio of lactate to pyruvate significantly increased in an ethanol dose-dependent fashion. Hypoxia also increased the ratio of lactate to pyruvate to the same degree as 300 μM ethanol (Figure 2A).

Since the effect of ethanol on EPO mRNA expression was not observed at high ethanol concentrations, the effects of 2000 μM ethanol were compared to 300 μM ethanol, which showed increased EPO mRNA expression. The lactate concentration was increased at 1 h after addition of 300 and 2000 μM ethanol and remained stable for up to 6 h after addition (Figure 2B). The pyruvate concentration was increased temporally by 300 μM ethanol and decreased by 2000 μM ethanol (Figure 2C).

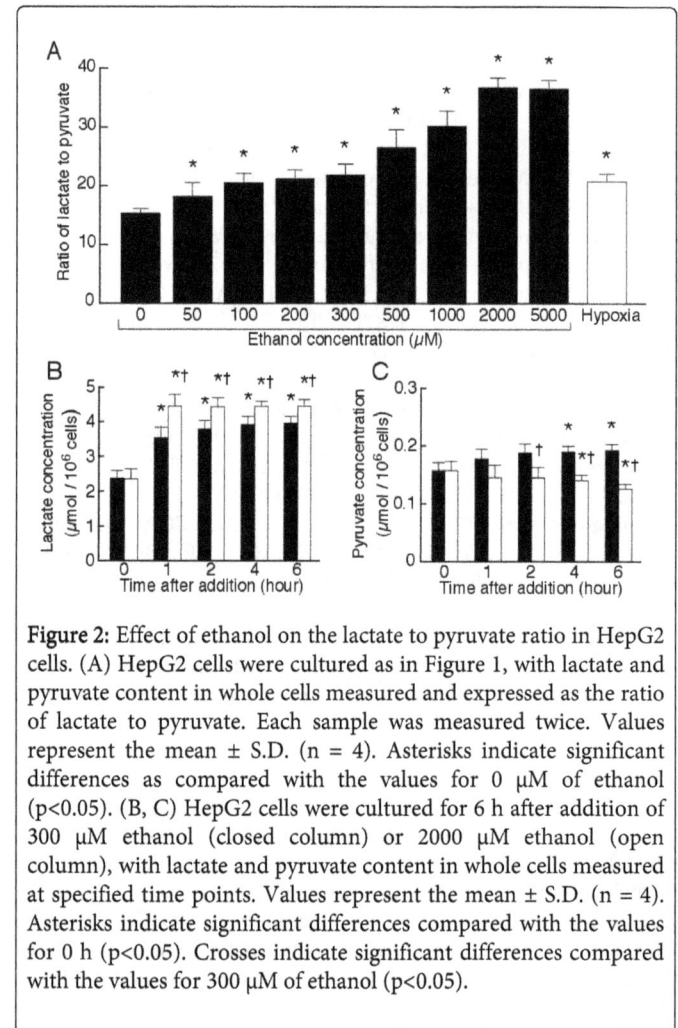

Figure 2: Effect of ethanol on the lactate to pyruvate ratio in HepG2 cells. (A) HepG2 cells were cultured as in Figure 1, with lactate and pyruvate content in whole cells measured and expressed as the ratio of lactate to pyruvate. Each sample was measured twice. Values represent the mean ± S.D. (n = 4). Asterisks indicate significant differences as compared with the values for 0 μM of ethanol (p<0.05). (B, C) HepG2 cells were cultured for 6 h after addition of 300 μM ethanol (closed column) or 2000 μM ethanol (open column), with lactate and pyruvate content in whole cells measured at specified time points. Values represent the mean ± S.D. (n = 4). Asterisks indicate significant differences compared with the values for 0 h (p<0.05). Crosses indicate significant differences compared with the values for 300 μM of ethanol (p<0.05).

To clarify whether the effect of 300 μM ethanol on promoting EPO mRNA expression is due to the influence of the ethanol metabolite acetate, the effect of equivalent concentrations of acetate was examined. Acetate alone did not alter either EPO mRNA expression (Figure 3A) or the ratio of lactate to pyruvate (Figure 3B). In the presence of pyruvate-free DMEM, increases in the ratio of lactate to pyruvate by 300 μM ethanol were elevated in comparison with normal DMEM, while ethanol-induced EPO mRNA expression was inhibited (Figure 3). Methanol, which like ethanol produces NADH, increased EPO mRNA expression at a concentration of 300 μM; however, no change was observed with 2000 μM methanol.

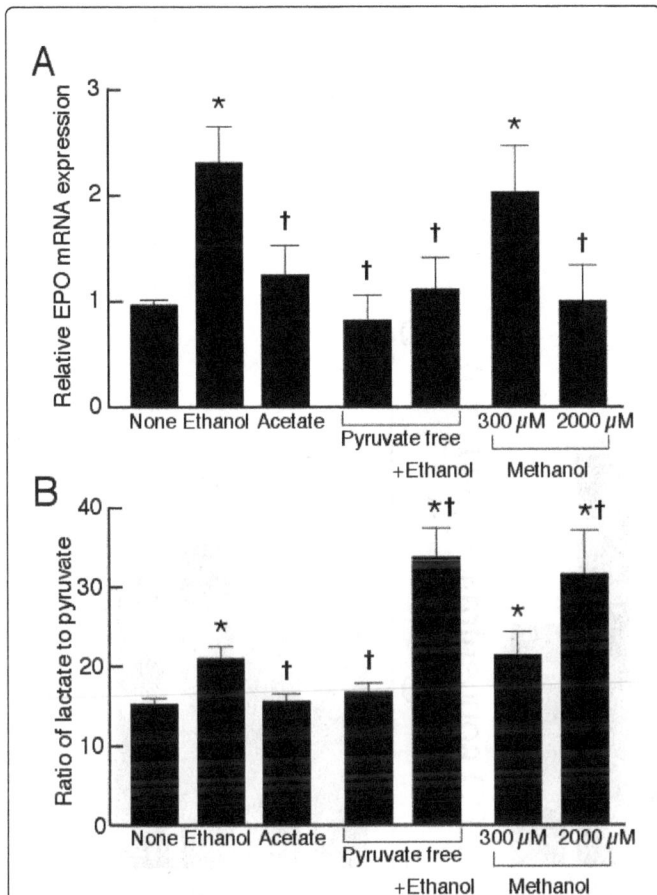

Figure 3: Effect of acetate and the absence of pyruvate on EPO mRNA expression and the lactate to pyruvate ratio in HepG2 cells. HepG2 cells were cultured in 5% CO2 at 37°C for 6 h in the absence and presence of 300 μM ethanol, 300 μM acetate, in the absence of pyruvate (± ethanol), or 300 μM and 2000 μM methanol. After 6 h, cells were harvested and EPO mRNA expression and whole cell lactate and pyruvate contents were determined. Each sample was measured twice. Values represent the mean ± S.D. (n = 4). Asterisks indicate significant differences as compared with the values for none (0 μM of ethanol) (p<0.05). Crosses indicate significant differences as compared with the values for 300 μM of ethanol (p<0.05).

Figure 4 shows the effects of 300 μM and 2000 μM ethanol on HIF in HepG2 cells. Levels of both HIF-1α and HIF-2α mRNA were increased in the presence of 300 μM ethanol, while no changes were observed in the presence of 2000 μM ethanol. Similarly, cellular HIF-1α and HIF-2α contents were also increased by 300 μM ethanol only. Total PHD content was not changed by treatment with either 300 or 2000 μM ethanol (data not shown).

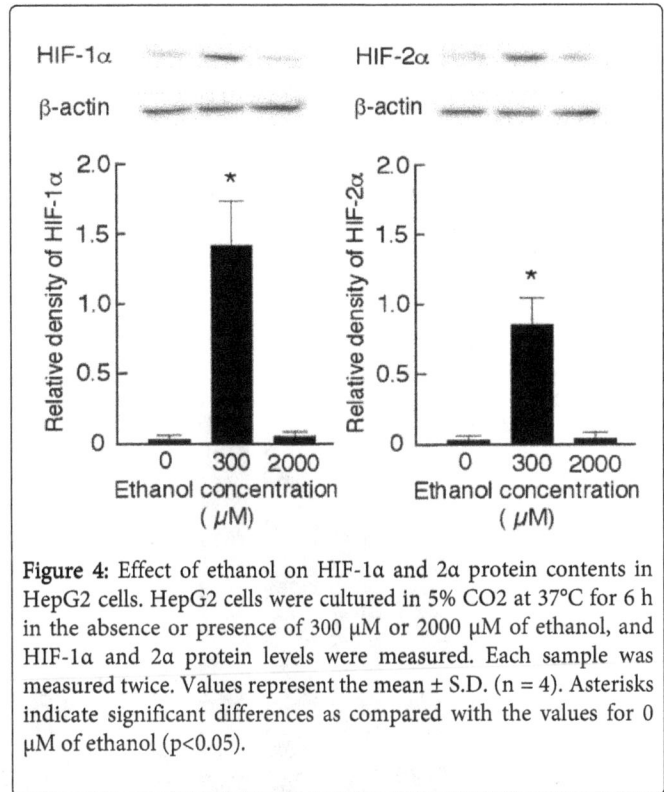

Figure 4: Effect of ethanol on HIF-1α and 2α protein contents in HepG2 cells. HepG2 cells were cultured in 5% CO2 at 37°C for 6 h in the absence or presence of 300 μM or 2000 μM of ethanol, and HIF-1α and 2α protein levels were measured. Each sample was measured twice. Values represent the mean ± S.D. (n = 4). Asterisks indicate significant differences as compared with the values for 0 μM of ethanol (p<0.05).

SIRT-1 is a transcriptional factor related to both HIF and cytosolic redox state. Because redox dependent SIRT1 activity influences the quantity of HIF [35,36] the effect of ethanol on SIRT1 was examined. Figure 5 shows the effects of 300 μM and 2000 μM ethanol on SIRT1 mRNA expression and cellular SIRT1 content. At 300 μM, ethanol increased SIRT1 mRNA expression, while 2000 μM ethanol had no effect. Cellular SIRT1 content was also increased at 300 μM ethanol only.

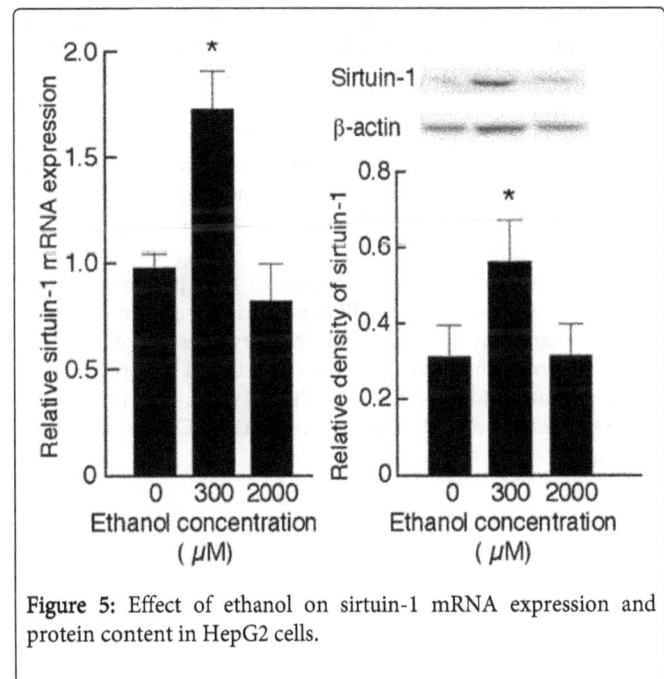

Figure 5: Effect of ethanol on sirtuin-1 mRNA expression and protein content in HepG2 cells.

HepG2 cells were cultured as in Figure 4 and sirtuin-1 mRNA expression and protein content were measured. Each sample was measured twice. Values represent the mean ± S.D. (n = 4). Asterisks indicate significant differences as compared with the values for 0 μM of ethanol (p<0.05).

To confirm that SIRT1 regulates EPO production, the effect of the SIRT1 inhibitor EX-527 on EPO production was measured (Figure 6).

EX-527 treatment inhibited the elevation in EPO mRNA expression produced by 300 μM ethanol. EX-527 also inhibited the increases in HIF-1α and 2α by300 μM ethanol (data not shown). However, EX-527 did not affect the ratio of lactate to pyruvate (Figure 6A).

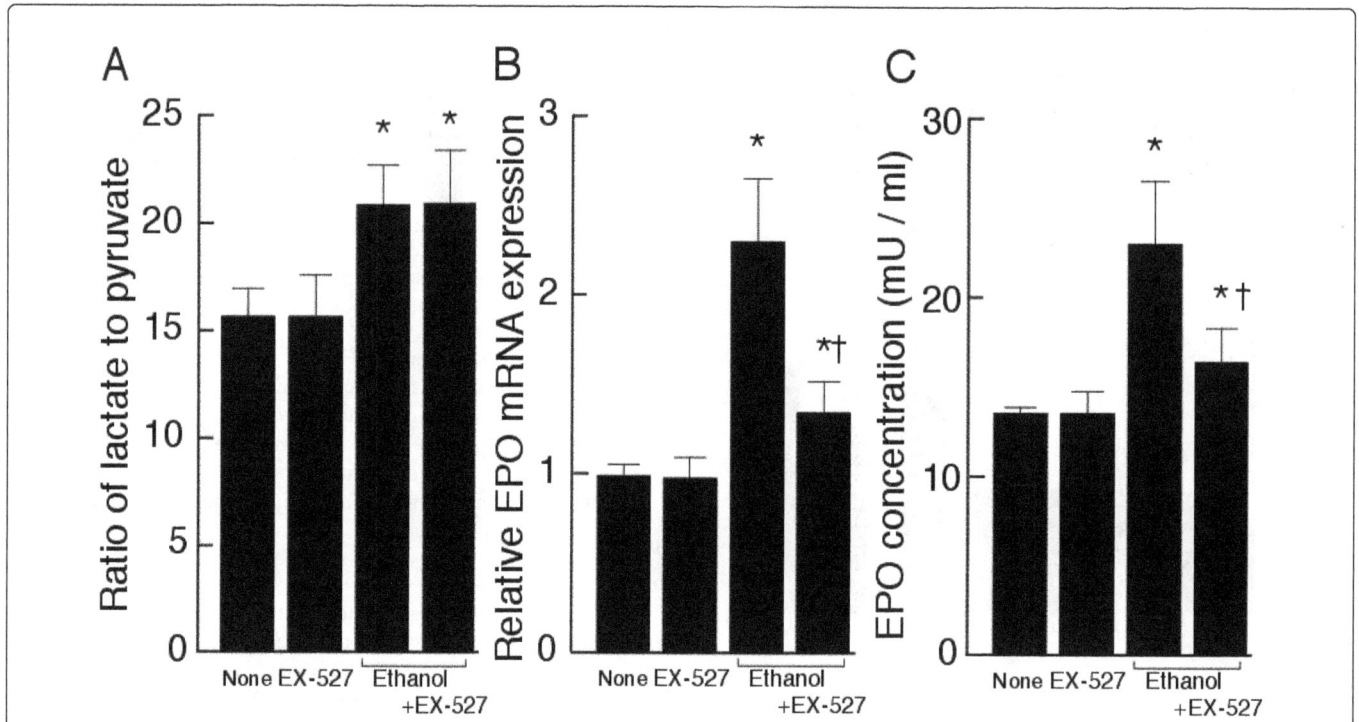

Figure 6: Effect of EX-527 on EPO production by 300 μM ethanol in HepG2 cells.

HepG2 cells were cultured in 5% CO_2 at 37°C in the absence or presence of 300 μM ethanol and/or 300 μM EX-527 for 6 h to determine the ratio of lactate to pyruvate (A) and EPO mRNA expression (B) or for 24 h to determine EPO production (C). Each sample was measured twice. Values represent the mean ± S.D. (n = 4). Asterisks indicate significant differences as compared with the values for 0 μM of ethanol (p<0.05). Crosses indicate significant differences as compared with the values for 300 μM of ethanol (p<0.05).

To examine the influence of ethanol on EPO production in the kidneys and liver, which are the EPO-producing organs in adults, the effect of ethanol on liver and kidneyprimary cells was determined. Figure 7 shows the effect of 300 μM ethanol on rat primary hepatocytes and kidney cells. In both cell types, 300 μM ethanol increased SIRT1 and EPO mRNA expression and EPO concentration in media.

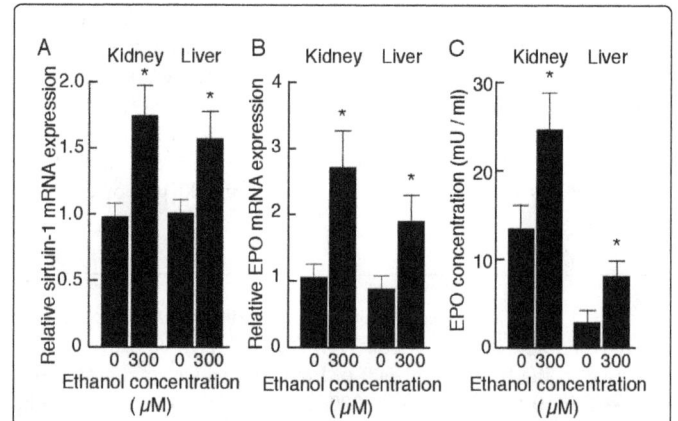

Figure 7: Effect of ethanol on EPO production in rat primary liver and kidney cells.

Liver and kidney cells were cultured in 5% CO_2 at 37°C with 100 μM ethanolfor 6h to determine sirtuin-1 (A) and EPO (B) mRNA expression or for 24 hrs to determine EPO production (C). Each sample was measured twice. Values represent the mean ± S.D. (n = 4).

Asterisks indicate significant differences as compared with the values for 0 μM of ethanol (p<0.05).

Discussion

We showed that low concentrations of ethanol increased EPO production in HepG2 cells and rat primary hepatocytes or kidney cells. It is generally known that acetaldehyde produced by ethanol metabolism is hepatotoxic. Many studies on ethanol-induced liver toxicity have been performed, however, most cytotoxicity experiments have used ethanol more than 10 mM [26,27,37,38]. Acetaldehyde produced at low ethanol concentrations (300 μM) is immediately metabolized to acetic acid [26-28], and it is thought that the majority of the toxicity is avoided. Acetic acid is a substrate for various metabolic pathways, including the TCA cycle. Because increased EPO mRNA expression in response to acetic acid was not observed, it was hypothesized that ethanol-induced reducing equivalent, produced by ethanol metabolism, was involved in promoting EPO production.

Highly concentrated ethanol greatly increased the ratio of lactate to pyruvate and committed the cells to a reducing environment, thereby eliminating the effect of ethanol on increasing EPO production. In the absence of pyruvate, 300 μM ethanol increased the ratio of lactate to pyruvate to a greater extent than hypoxia, whereas EPO mRNA expression did not increase. These results suggest that a change in cytosolic redox state to the same extent as hypoxia was effective in promoting EPO production.

Gambini et al. [24] reported that an ethanol addition promoted SIRT1 mRNA expression. However, because they used 10 mM ethanol, it is unclear whether the mechanism is the same as in our experiment.

Because the effect of 300 μM ethanol on EPO production was greatly inhibited by the SIRT1 inhibitor EX527, it was thought that the promotion of EPO production with 300 μM ethanol was dependent on SIRT1. In fact, addition of 2000 μM ethanol decreased NAD+ content and did not alter the levels of SIRT1 mRNA and SIRT1 protein, resulting in no change in EPO production. It is reported that SIRT1 interacts with HIF [35,36]. SIRT1 inhibits the inactivation of HIF-α by PHD via deacetylation of HIF-α and enhances the effects of HIF [35,36]. In this study, both HIF-1α and 2α levels were increased by 300 μM ethanol. Therefore, it was thought that increased SIRT1 activity, induced by the addition of low ethanol concentrations, promotes EPO production by activation of HIF. In this study, the effects of ethanol on HIF-1α and 2α expression were similar, and differences in the role of HIF1 and 2 in ethanol-induced EPO production are not clear. On the other hand, it has been reported that HIF influences SIRT1 [39]. Because EX-527 inhibited HIF induction and EPO production induced by 300 μM ethanol, it was thought that regulation of SIRT1 by HIF was minimal. It has also been reported that reducing conditions in cells induces HIF [22,24]. These reports are consistent with the results of the present study.

Promotion of EPO production by low ethanol concentrations was observed with HepG2 cells as well as cultured primary liver and kidney cells. Therefore, it is expected that low ethanol concentrations will promote *in vivo* EPO production. It is well known that chronic liver damage is a consequence of ethanol toxicity [26-28,38]. It is reported that chronic ethanol exposure affects HIF [40,41]. In this study, single ethanol treatments were utilized, which did not influence cell viability. Therefore, it is thought that ethanol toxicity was not a confounding factor in the present study. Generally, in the stages of ethanol

intoxication, 0.1-0.5 mg/ml blood (about 2-11 mmol/l blood) is considered subclinical. An ethanol concentration of 300 μM, which was observed to promote EPO production, is approximately 1/7-1/30 of the subclinical level and is only 0.015 promille. Therefore, it is thought that a blood concentration representative of that used experimentally is accomplished by slight alcohol intake.

In conclusion, we showed that low concentrations of ethanol promote EPO production by increasing SIRT1 in HepG2 cells and primary liver and kidney cells. The use of ethanol represents a hypoxia-independent method to promote EPO production.

References

1. Krantz SB (1991) Erythropoietin. Blood 77: 419-434.
2. Lacombe C, Mayeux P (1998) Biology of erythropoietin. Haematologica 83: 724-732.
3. Jelkmann W (2007) Erythropoietin after a century of research: younger than ever. Eur J Haematol 78: 183-205.
4. Haase VH (2013) Regulation of erythropoiesis by hypoxia-inducible factors. Blood Rev 27: 41-53.
5. Webb JD, Coleman ML, Pugh CW (2009) Hypoxia, hypoxia-inducible factors (HIF), HIF hydroxylases and oxygen sensing. Cell Mol Life Sci 66: 3539-3554.
6. Haase VH (2010) Hypoxic regulation of erythropoiesis and iron metabolism. Am J Physiol Renal Physiol 299: F1-13.
7. Yeo EJ, Cho YS, Kim MS, Park JW (2008) Contribution of HIF-1alpha or HIF-2alpha to erythropoietin expression: in vivo evidence based on chromatin immunoprecipitation. Ann Hematol 87: 11-17.
8. Ramadori P, Sheikh N, Ahmad G, Dudas J, Ramadori G (2010) Hepatic changes of erythropoietin gene expression in a rat model of acute-phase response. Liver Int 30: 55-64.
9. Jelkmann W (2011) Regulation of erythropoietin production. J Physiol 589: 1251-1258.
10. Haase VH (2013) Mechanisms of hypoxia responses in renal tissue. J Am Soc Nephrol 24: 537-541.
11. Katavetin P, Tungsanga K, Eiam-Ong S, Nangaku M (2007) Antioxidative effects of erythropoietin. Kidney Int Suppl : S10-15.
12. Maiese K, Chong ZZ, Hou J, Shang YC (2008) Enhanced tolerance against early and late apoptotic oxidative stress in mammalian neurons through nicotinamidase and sirtuin mediated pathways. Curr Neurovasc Res 5: 125-142.
13. Chong ZZ, Li F, Maiese K (2005) Erythropoietin requires NF-kappaB and its nuclear translocation to prevent early and late apoptotic neuronal injury during beta-amyloid toxicity. Curr Neurovasc Res 2: 387-399.
14. Li Y, Lu Z, Keogh CL, Yu SP, Wei L (2007) Erythropoietin-induced neurovascular protection, angiogenesis, and cerebral blood flow restoration after focal ischemia in mice. J Cereb Blood Flow Metab 27. 1043-1054.
15. Chateauvieux S, Grigorakaki C, Morceau F, Dicato M, Diederich M (2011) Erythropoietin, erythropoiesis and beyond. Biochem Pharmacol 82: 1291-1303.
16. Arcasoy MO (2008) The non-haematopoietic biological effects of erythropoietin. Br J Haematol 141: 14-31.
17. Chen A, Xiong LJ, Tong Y, Mao M (2013) The neuroprotective roles of BDNF in hypoxic ischemic brain injury. Biomed Rep 1: 167-176.
18. Marti HH (2004) Erythropoietin and the hypoxic brain. J Exp Biol 207: 3233-3242.
19. Radreau P, Rhodes JD, Mithen RF, Kroon PA, Sanderson J (2009) Hypoxia-inducible factor-1 (HIF-1) pathway activation by quercetin in human lens epithelial cells. Exp Eye Res 89: 995-1002.
20. Hong YR, Kim HT, Lee SC, Ro S, Cho JM, et al. (2013) [(4-Hydroxyl-benzo[4,5]thieno[3,2-c]pyridine-3-carbonyl)-amino]-acetic acid

derivatives; HIF prolyl 4-hydroxylase inhibitors as oral erythropoietin secretagogues. Bioorg Med Chem Lett 23: 5953-5957.

21. Laitala A, Aro E, Walkinshaw G, Mäki JM, Rossi M, et al. (2012) Transmembraneprolyl 4-hydroxylase is a fourth prolyl 4-hydroxylase regulating EPO production and erythropoiesis. Blood 120: 3336-3344.

22. Nikinmaa M, Pursiheimo S, Soitamo AJ (2004) Redox state regulates HIF-1alpha and its DNA binding and phosphorylation in salmonid cells. J Cell Sci 117: 3201-3206.

23. Leiser SF, Kaeberlein M (2010) A role for SIRT1 in the hypoxic response. Mol Cell 38: 779-780.

24. Gambini J, Gomez-Cabrera MC, Borras C, Valles SL, Lopez-Grueso R, et al. (2011) Free [NADH]/[NAD(+)] regulates sirtuin expression. Arch Biochem Biophys 512: 24-29.

25. Caito S, Rajendrasozhan S, Cook S, Chung S, Yao H, et al. (2010) SIRT1 is a redox-sensitive deacetylase that is post-translationally modified by oxidants and carbonyl stress. FASEB J 24: 3145-3159.

26. Majchrowicz E (1975) Metabolic correlates of ethanol, acetaldehyde, acetate and methanol in humans and animals. Adv Exp Med Biol 56: 111-156.

27. Henzel K, Thorborg C, Hofmann M, Zimmer G, Leuschner U (2004) Toxicity of ethanol and acetaldehyde in hepatocytes treated with ursodeoxycholic or tauroursodeoxycholic acid. Biochim Biophys Acta 1644: 37-45.

28. FarfánLabonne BE, Gutiérrez M, Gómez-Quiroz LE, Konigsberg Fainstein M, Bucio L, et al. (2009) Acetaldehyde-induced mitochondrial dysfunction sensitizes hepatocytes to oxidative damage. Cell Biol Toxicol 25: 599-609.

29. Watkins PC, Eddy R, Hoffman N, Stanislovitis P, Beck AK, et al. (1986) Regional assignment of the erythropoietin gene to human chromosome region 7pter----q22. Cytogenet Cell Genet 42: 214-218.

30. Frye RA (1999) Characterization of five human cDNAs with homology to the yeast SIR2 gene: Sir2-like proteins (sirtuins) metabolize NAD and may have protein ADP-ribosyltransferase activity. Biochem Biophys Res Commun 260: 273-279.

31. Nagao M, Suga H, Okano M, Masuda S, Narita H, et al. (1992) Nucleotide sequence of rat erythropoietin. Biochim Biophys Acta 1171: 99-102.

32. Tajima H, Tsuchiya K, Yamada M, Kondo K, Katsube N, et al. (1999) Over-expression of GAPDH induces apoptosis in COS-7 cells transfected with cloned GAPDH cDNAs. Neuroreport 10: 2029-2033.

33. Rosenberg JC, Rush BF (1966) An enzymatic-spectrophotometric determination of pyruvic and lactic acid in blood. Methodologic aspects. Clin Chem 12: 299-307.

34. Perez VJ, Cicero TJ, Bahn BA (1971) Ethanol in brain, as assayed by microfluorometry. Clin Chem 17: 307-310.

35. Dioum EM, Chen R, Alexander MS, Zhang Q, Hogg RT, et al. (2009) Regulation of hypoxia-inducible factor 2alpha signaling by the stress-responsive deacetylasesirtuin 1. Science 324: 1289-1293.

36. Geng H, Liu Q, Xue C, David LL, Beer TM, et al. (2012) HIF1α protein stability is increased by acetylation at lysine 709. J Biol Chem 287: 35496-35505.

37. Senthil Kumar KJ, Liao JW, Xiao JH, Gokila Vani M, Wang SY (2012) Hepatoprotective effect of lucidone against alcohol-induced oxidative stress in human hepatic HepG2 cells through the up-regulation of HO-1/Nrf-2 antioxidant genes. Toxicol In Vitro 26: 700-708.

38. Uemura T, Tanaka Y, Higashi K, Miyamori D, Takasaka T, et al. (2013) Acetaldehyde-induced cytotoxicity involves induction of spermine oxidase at the transcriptional level. Toxicology 310: 1-7.

39. Chen R, Dioum EM, Hogg RT, Gerard RD, Garcia JA (2011) Hypoxia increases sirtuin 1 expression in a hypoxia-inducible factor-dependent manner. J Biol Chem 286: 13869-13878.

40. Wang X, Wu D, Yang L, Gan L, Cederbaum AI (2013) Cytochrome P450 2E1 potentiates ethanol induction of hypoxia and HIF1α in vivo. Free Radic Biol Med 63: 175-186.

41. Tajima M, Kurashima Y, Sugiyama K, Ogura T, Sakagami H (2009) The redox state of glutathione regulates the hypoxic induction of HIF-1. Eur J Pharmacol 606: 45-49.

34

The Metabolic Syndrome in Rural UAE: The Effect of Gender, Ethnicity and the Environment in its Prevalence

Rodhan Khthir* and Felyn Luz Espina

Marshall university-school of medicine, Huntington, West Virginia, USA

*Corresponding author: Rodhan Abass khthir, Marshall university-school of medicine, Huntington, West Virginia, USA; E-mail: khthir@marshall.edu

Abstract

Objective: The purpose of this study was to examine the prevalence of the metabolic syndrome and its individual components among multiethnic population in a rural area in the Western region of Abu Dhabi in The United Arab Emirates (UAE)

Methods: The analytic sample consisted of 575 adults (males: 309, females: 266), between the age of 22 and 65 years. The National Cholesterol Education Program's Adult Treatment Panel III (NCEP/ATP III) guidelines (with race specific abdominal circumference cutoff level) were used to identify adults who met their criteria for metabolic syndrome with. Prevalence estimates were calculated for each component of the metabolic syndrome in addition to the overall prevalence of metabolic syndrome. Prevalence estimates were analyzed by sex, ethnicity and working hours.

Results: Approximately 22% of adults met the criteria for metabolic syndrome. The prevalence was 26% in Males and 14% in females, P. Value <0.01. The prevalence was 16% among South East Asians (SEA), 20% among Arabs (ARB) and 26% among South Asians (SA), with P value of 0. 523, 0.075 and <0.05 for ARB versus SEA, ARB versus SA, and SA vs SEA respectively. The prevalence of the metabolic syndrome among night shift workers was 25% in comparison to 19% among daytime workers (P value 0.1). The prevalence of the different components of the metabolic syndrome varied by race and ethnicity

Conclusions: These results demonstrate that metabolic syndrome is less prevalent in rural area than inner city population in UAE which was reported to be around 40% in previous studies possibly because of lifestyle differences. The prevalence varied significantly by race and ethnicity and gender. Night shift work was associated with higher prevalence of the metabolic syndrome in our study but this was not statistically significant.

Keywords Metabolic syndrome; Abdominal obesity; Blood pressure; Diabetes

Introduction

The metabolic syndrome is the co-occurrence of multiple metabolic abnormalities (abdominal obesity, hyperglycemia, dyslipidemia, and hypertension). These metabolic abnormalities are considered metabolic risk factors for both type 2 diabetes and cardiovascular disease. Prospective observational studies demonstrate a strong association between the metabolic syndrome and the risk for subsequent development of type 2 diabetes [1-5]. The metabolic syndrome increased the relative risk (RR) for incident diabetes by 2.1-fold with the ATP III definition and 3.6-fold using the WHO definition.

Three meta-analyses, found that the metabolic syndrome increases also the risk for cardiovascular disease (CVD) (RRs ranging from 1.53 to 2.18) and all cause mortality (RRs 1.27 to 1.60) [6-8].

Current ATP III criteria define the metabolic syndrome as the presence of any three of the following five traits [9,10]:

• Abdominal obesity, defined as a waist circumference in men ≥ 102 cm (40 in) and in women ≥ 88 cm (35 in)

• Serum triglycerides ≥ 150 mg/dL (1.7 mmol/L) or drug treatment for elevated triglycerides

• Serum HDL cholesterol <40 mg/dL (1 mmol/L) in men and <50 mg/dL (1.3 mmol/L) in women or drug treatment for low HDL-C

• Blood pressure ≥ 130/85 mmHg or drug treatment for elevated blood pressure

• Fasting plasma glucose (FPG) ≥ 100 mg/dL (5.6 mmol/L) or drug treatment for elevated blood glucose

According to ATP III, a diagnosis of the metabolic syndrome is made when three or more of the risk factors. In 2009, a new cut point was suggested for South Asians and South East Asians (Chinese/Japanese population) [11].

The metabolic syndrome is becoming increasingly common. Using data from the National Health and Nutrition Examination Survey 1999 to 2002 database, 34.5 percent of participants met ATP III criteria for the metabolic syndrome compared with 22 percent in NHANES III (1988 to 1994) [12,13]. Racial and gender discrepancy in the prevalence of the metabolic syndrome was described previously. For example, the prevalence of the metabolic syndrome, as defined by the 2001 ATP III criteria, was evaluated in 8814 adults in the United States participating in the third National Health and Nutrition Examination Survey (NHANES III, 1988 to 1994) [12]. Mexican-Americans had the highest age-adjusted prevalence (31.9 percent). Among African-Americans and Mexican-Americans, the prevalence was higher in women than in men (57 and 26 percent higher, respectively).

The prevalence of the metabolic syndrome in the United Arab Emirates (UAE) was estimated to be around 40% based on a single prevalence study done in two big cities. [14]. UAE has a very high prevalence of diabetes and obesity and also has very racially diverse population.

The purpose of this study was to examine the prevalence of the metabolic syndrome in the rural part of the UAE and to study the racial and gender discrepancy in the prevalence of the metabolic syndrome and its different components among multiethnic population in a rural area in the Western region of Abu Dhabi-UAE. The study examined also the association between the metabolic syndrome prevalence and night shift work one of the potential risk factor for the metabolic syndrome and other metabolic disorders.

Methods

Subjects

The study is a cross-sectional prevalence study conducted over a period of 4 weeks at Madinat Zayed hospital, a secondary care rural hospital in the Western region of Abu Dhabi. The study population consisted of hospital employees and the study was done during the annual employee health campaign. The surveillance process included healthcare questionnaire, measurement of weight, Height, BMI and abdominal circumference, health examination and laboratory test in fasting state for glucose and lipids.

Height, weight, and waist circumference were all measured using standardized techniques and calibrated equipment. A certified phlebotomist drew fasting morning blood samples from the examinee's arm for the lipid and glucose assays. Standardized techniques were used to obtain the blood pressure measurements. Abdominal circumference was measured at standing position with a measurement tape at the level of the upper border of the anterior superior iliac crest. Weight and height measurement were done by standard electronic machines that computed the BMI directly.

Pregnant females and participants with incomplete data were deleted from the analytic sample. The final analytic sample consisted of 575 adults (males: 309, females: 266), between the age of 22 and 65 years.

Definition of metabolic syndrome

The NCEP/ATP III revised guidelines (see introduction) were used to identify adults in the analytic sample who had metabolic syndrome. In addition, individuals who reported currently taking antihypertensive medication were classified as having high blood pressure and individuals currently taking insulin or an oral diabetic medication were classified as having diabetes. According to these guidelines, metabolic syndrome is defined as the presence of three or more of these risk factors.

BP above 130/85 was confirmed after 5 minutes. The averages of the two systolic and diastolic blood pressure readings were used for the analysis.

Regarding the cutoff level for the waist circumference used, we used 88 cm for Arab females, 102 cm for Arab males, and 80 cm for non-Arab females and 90 cm for non-Arab Males based on the updates 2009 NCEP-ATP 3 definition [11].

Data analyses

The prevalence of the metabolic syndrome in the whole group was evaluated and stratified by ethnicity, gender, BMI and work shift. The prevalence of the individual component of the metabolic syndrome was reported as well by ethnicity and gender.

BMI was categorized into three groups. These categories were: >25 kg/m^2, 25-30 kg/m^2, and >30 kg/m^2.

Results are reported for self-identified Arabs (AR), South Asians (SA) (mainly from India, Pakistan and Bangladish) and South East Asian (SEA) (mainly from the Philippines and Indonesia).

BMI measures relative weight for height. BMI was calculated by dividing weight by height squared (kg/m^2). Weight categories were created based on the National Heart, Lung, and Blood Institute's classification system. The underweight and normal weight categories were combined as well as the obese and extremely obese categories because of limited sample sizes. The three categories used in this analysis were underweight and normal weight (BMI less than 25), overweight (BMI 25–29.9), and obese and extremely obese (BMI 30 or greater).

Differences in continuous data between the two groups were evaluated using the t-test. Differences between categorical data were compared using chi-square test. P value <0.05 was considered statistically significant. Statistical analysis was performed using QI Macros 2012.

Results

The Study population consisted of 309 males and 266 females with 269 South Asians, 195 Arabs and 112 South East Asians. The average age of the study population is 37.96. The average age for males is 37.1, female 38.66 (p=0.03). The average age for Arabs is 41.16, South East Asians is 38.77, and Asians: 34.59 (P value was <0.5 for all comparisons).

The average age for shift workers is 37.21 and for non-shift workers is 38.75 (p value 0.046).

The weight distribution varied between Arabs and other groups, with 75% of Arabs were either overweight or obese versus 35% in South Asians (p<0.01) and 39% in South East Asians (p<0.01) Figure 1. The prevalence of overweight and obesity were similar between males and females (51% in both groups) but the prevalence of abdominal obesity was 76% in females versus 34% in Males (p<0.01).

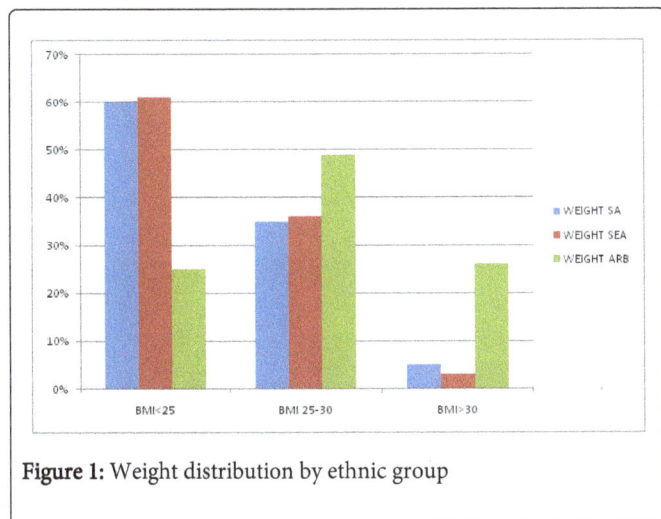

Figure 1: Weight distribution by ethnic group

Approximately 22% (124/575) of adults met the criteria for metabolic syndrome. Abdominal obesity (53%), low HDL (34%), high triglyceride (21%) and hyperglycemia (20%) were the most frequently occurring risk factors for metabolic syndrome (Figure 2).

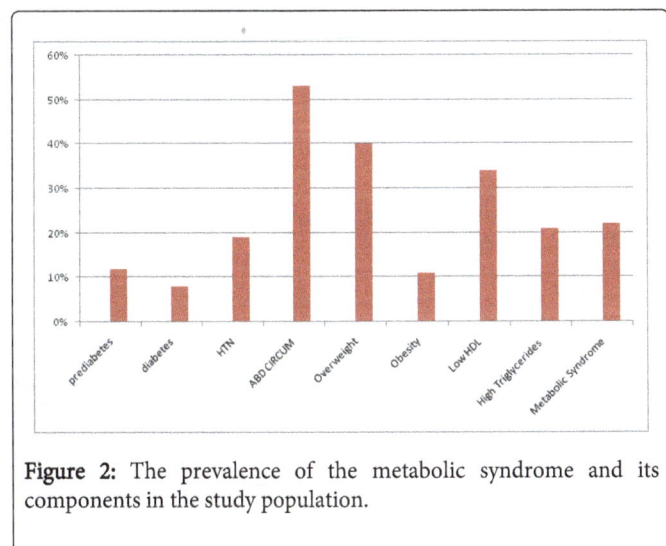

Figure 2: The prevalence of the metabolic syndrome and its components in the study population.

The prevalence of the metabolic syndrome was 26% in Males (81/309) and 14% in females (36/266), P. Value <0.01. The prevalence was 16% (18/112) among South East Asians, 20% (37/195) among Arabs and 26% (69/269) among South Asians. (P value 0.523, 0.075 and <0.05 for ARB versus SEA, ARB versus SA, and SA versus SEA respectively).

The prevalence of hyperglycemia was 15% (17/112) in Southeast Asians, 26% (52/195) among Arabs and 18% (47/265) among South Asian. The prevalence of HTN was 16% (18/112) in Southeast Asians, 8% (16/195) among Arabs and 28% (75/265) among South Asian. The prevalence of abdominal obesity was 63% (71/112) in Southeast Asians, 51% (100/195) among Arabs and 51% (136/265) among South Asian. For HDL abnormality, the prevalence was 20% (22/112) in Southeast Asians, 34% (67/195) among Arabs and 40% (105/265) among South Asian and the prevalence of hypertriglyceridemia was 18% (20/112) in Southeast Asians, 18% (36/195) among Arabs and 23% (62/265) among South Asians. There was a statistically significant

difference between the groups except for hypertriglyceridemia (Table 1).

	South East Asians (SEA)	Arabs (ARB)	South Asians (SA)	P value SEA vs ARB	P value SEA vs SA	P value SA vs ARB
Hyperglycemia	15 %	26 %	18 %	0.02	0.02	0.5
HTN	16 %	8 %	28 %	0.049	0.015	<0.001
Abdominal obesity	63 %	51 %	51 %	0.039	0.031	0.99
Low HDL	20 %	34 %	40 %	0.006	<0.001	0.248
High Triglycerides	18 %	18 %	23 %	0.89	0.233	0.2

Table 1: Racial discrepancy in the prevalence of the different component of the metabolic syndrome (statistical analysis)

The prevalence of the metabolic syndrome among night shift workers was 25% (54/215) in comparison to 19% (70/360) among daytime workers. P value didn't reach statistical significance.

Discussion

Based on the NCEP/ATP III guidelines, a little more than 20% of the adults in the study group could be characterized as having metabolic syndrome. These results demonstrate that metabolic syndrome is less prevalent in rural area than inner city population in UAE which was reported to be around 40% in previous studies possibly because of life style differences. The prevalence of metabolic syndrome varied by race and ethnicity with the highest prevalence was among South Asians in spite of having a lower prevalence of obesity than Arab population and similar weight distribution to South East Asians. This paradox is most likely related to genetic and environmental factors that predispose South Asians to higher prevalence of hypertension, hypertriglyceridemia and low HDL level at lower BMI. In our study the prevalence of the metabolic syndrome was 10% in South Asians with BMI of <23 kg/m² reaching to 58% in the same group as BMI increase in the obesity range (>30) kg/m² while in Arabs the prevalence of the metabolic syndrome in normal weight population was 3%, reaching only to 36% in obese population.

It should be noted that the mean age of South Asians was lower than other Ethnic groups and this should have predicted lower prevalence rate as there is a positive association between age and the prevalence of the metabolic syndrome.

The sharp increase in the prevalence of the metabolic syndrome in obese South Asians and the relatively high prevalence at normal BMI need further studies in a larger cohort and further evaluation of the current BMI cut-off levels in that population (Figure 3).

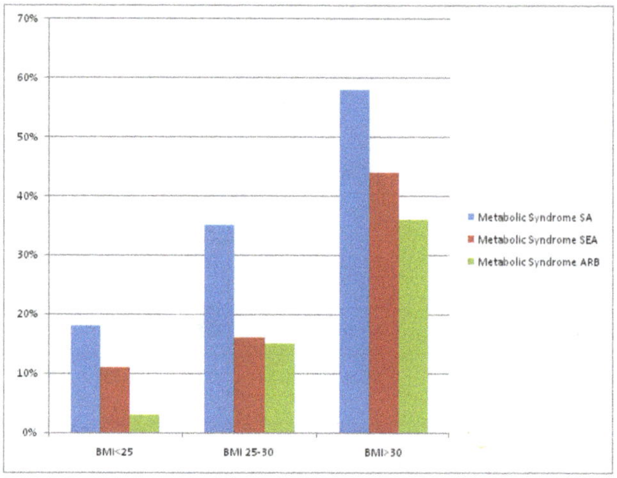

Figure 3: The prevalence of the metabolic syndrome among different ethnicities according to the weight category

The prevalence varied significantly also by sex with significantly lower prevalence among females in spite of the very high prevalence of abdominal obesity among females and in spite of having higher mean age than males. The very high prevalence of abdominal obesity in certain racial group didn't predict higher prevalence of the metabolic syndrome (Figure 4).

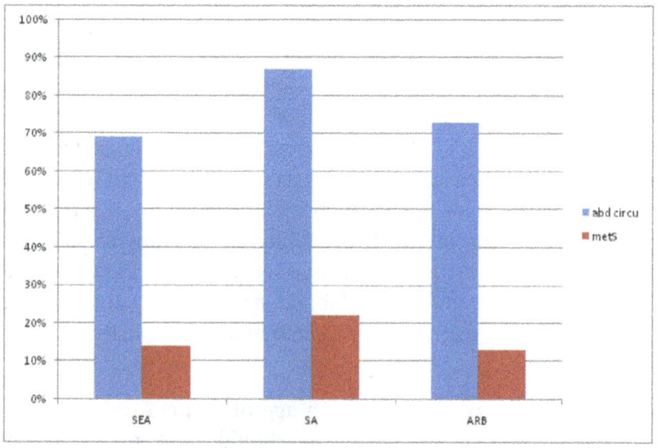

Figure 4: Abdominal Circumference and the Metabolic Syndrome in Females

This may suggest that the current race based cut-off level need to be re-examined. While in males the correlation between prevalence of abdominal obesity and the metabolic syndrome was stronger especially in South Asians (Figure 5).

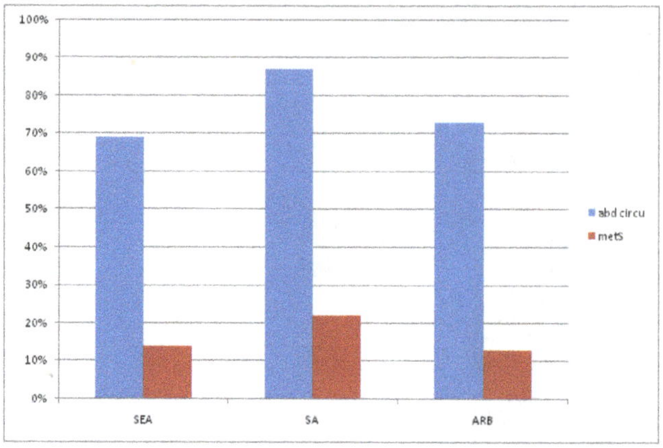

Figure 5: Abdominal Circumference and the Metabolic Syndrome in Males

Finally, Night shift work was associated with higher prevalence of the metabolic syndrome in our study but this didn't reach statistical significance. It should be noted that shift workers has lower mean age. Our study was not powered to detect such difference and more research is needed to explore the importance of night shift work as a potential risk factor for metabolic abnormalities.

References

1. Hanson RL, Imperatore G, Bennett PH, Knowler WC (2002) Components of the "metabolic syndrome" and incidence of type 2 diabetes. Diabetes 51: 3120-3127.

2. Resnick HE, Jones K, Ruotolo G, Jain AK, Henderson J, et al. (2003) Insulin resistance, the metabolic syndrome, and risk of incident cardiovascular disease in nondiabetic american indians: the Strong Heart Study. Diabetes Care 26: 861-867.

3. Klein BE, Klein R, Lee KE (2002) Components of the metabolic syndrome and risk of cardiovascular disease and diabetes in Beaver Dam. Diabetes Care 25: 1790-1794.

4. Sattar N, Gaw A, Scherbakova O, Ford I, O'Reilly DS, et al. (2003) Metabolic syndrome with and without C-reactive protein as a predictor of coronary heart disease and diabetes in the West of Scotland Coronary Prevention Study. Circulation 108: 414-419.

5. Sattar N, McConnachie A, Shaper AG, Blauw GJ, Buckley BM, et al. (2008) Can metabolic syndrome usefully predict cardiovascular disease and diabetes? Outcome data from two prospective studies. Lancet 371: 1927-1935.

6. Ford ES (2005) Risks for all-cause mortality, cardiovascular disease, and diabetes associated with the metabolic syndrome: a summary of the evidence. Diabetes Care 28: 1769-1778.

7. Galassi A, Reynolds K, He J (2006) Metabolic syndrome and risk of cardiovascular disease: a meta-analysis. Am J Med 119: 812-819.

8. Gami AS, Witt BJ, Howard DE, Erwin PJ, Gami LA, et al. (2007) Metabolic syndrome and risk of incident cardiovascular events and death: a systematic review and meta-analysis of longitudinal studies. J Am Coll Cardiol 49: 403-414.

9. Expert Panel on Detection, Evaluation, and Treatment of High Blood Cholesterol in Adults (2001) Executive Summary of The Third Report of The National Cholesterol Education Program (NCEP) Expert Panel on Detection, Evaluation, And Treatment of High Blood Cholesterol In Adults (Adult Treatment Panel III). JAMA 285: 2486-2497.

10. Grundy SM, Cleeman JI, Daniels SR, Donato KA, Eckel RH, et al. (2005) Diagnosis and management of the metabolic syndrome: an American

Heart Association/National Heart, Lung, and Blood Institute Scientific Statement. Circulation 112: 2735-2752.

11. Alberti KG, Eckel RH, Grundy SM, (2009) Harmonizing the metabolic syndrome: a joint interim statement of the International Diabetes Federation Task Force on Epidemiology and Prevention; National Heart, Lung, and Blood Institute; American Heart Association; World Heart Federation; International Atherosclerosis Society; and International Association for the Study of Obesity. Circulation 120:1640

12. Ford ES, Giles WH, Dietz WH (2002) Prevalence of the metabolic syndrome among US adults: findings from the third National Health and Nutrition Examination Survey. JAMA 287: 356-359.

13. Ford ES (2005) Prevalence of the metabolic syndrome defined by the International Diabetes Federation among adults in the U.S. Diabetes Care 28: 2745-2749.

14. Malik M, Razig SA (2008) The prevalence of the metabolic syndrome among the multiethnic population of the United Arab Emirates: a report of a national survey. Metab Syndr Relat Disord 6: 177-186.

35

Stroke in Severity of Sickle Cell Diseases

Mehmet Rami Helvaci[1*] , **Ramazan Davran**[2], **Akin Aydogan**[3], **Seckin Akkucuk**[3], **Mustafa Ugu**[3], and **Cem Oruc**[3]

[1] *Department of Internal Medicine, Medical Faculty of Mustafa Kemal University, Antakya, Turkey*

[2] *Department of Radiology, Medical Faculty of Mustafa Kemal University, Antakya, Turkey*

[3] *Department of General Surgery, Medical Faculty of the Mustafa Kemal University, Antakya, Turkey*

Corresponding author: Mehmet Rami Helvaci, Medical Faculty of the Mustafa Kemal University, 31100, Serinyol, Antakya, Hatay, Turkey; E-mail: mramihelvaci@hotmail.com

Abstract

Background: Sickle cell diseases (SCDs) are chronic inflammatory process on capillary level. We tried to understand whether or not there are some positive correlations between stroke and severity of SCDs.

Methods: All patients with SCDs were taken into the study.

Results: The study included 343 patients (169 females and 174 males). There were 30 cases (8.7%) with stroke. The mean ages were similar in both groups (32.5 versus 29.1 years in the stroke group and other, respectively, $p>0.05$). The female ratios were similar in both groups, too (43.3% versus 49.8%, respectively, $p>0.05$). Prevalences of associated thalassemia minors were also similar in them (73.3% versus 65.1%, respectively, $p>0.05$). Smoking was higher among the stroke cases (26.6% versus 13.0%, $p<0.05$). Mean white blood cell count, hematocrit value, and mean platelet count of the peripheric blood were similar in both groups ($p>0.05$ for all). On the other hand, although the painful crises per year, tonsilectomy, priapism, ileus, pulmonary hypertension, chronic obstructive pulmonary disease, coronary heart disease, chronic renal disease, rheumatic heart disease, avascular necrosis of bones, cirrhosis, and mortality were all higher in the stroke group, the differences were only significant for digital clubbing, leg ulcers, and acute chest syndrome ($p<0.05$ for all), probably due to the small sample size of the stroke group.

Conclusion: SCDs are chronic destructive process on capillaries iniatiating at birth, and terminate with early organ failures in life. Probably stroke is one of the terminal consequences of the inflammatory process that may indicate shortened survival in such cases.

Keywords: Sickle cell diseases; Stroke; Chronic capillary inflammation; Atherosclerosis

Introduction

Atherosclerosis may be the most significant underlying cause of aging by inducing prolonged cellular hypoxia all over the body. As an example for the hypothesis, cardiac cirrhosis develops due to the prolonged hepatic hypoxia in patients with pulmonary and/or cardiac diseases. Whole afferent vasculature including capillaries is probably involved in atherosclerosis. Some of the currently known accelerators of the systemic process are smoking, physical inactivity, and overweight for the development of terminal consequences including obesity, hypertension (HT), diabetes mellitus (DM), peripheric artery disease, chronic obstructive pulmonary disease (COPD), chronic renal disease (CRD), coronary heart disease (CHD), cirrhosis, mesenteric ischemia, osteoporosis, stroke, and aging, all of which are researched under the title of metabolic syndrome in the literature, extensively [1-3]. Similarly, sickle cell diseases (SCDs) are chronic destructive process mainly affecting capillaries. Hemoglobin S (Hb S) causes loss of elastic and biconcave disc shaped structures of red blood cells (RBCs). Probably, loss of elasticity instead of shapes of RBCs is the major problem, since sickling is rare in the peripheral blood samples of SCDs patients with associated thalassemias, and human survival is not

so affected in hereditary elliptocytosis or spherocytosis. Loss of elasticity is probably present in whole life, but it is exaggerated with stressful conditions. The hard RBCs may take their normal elastic natures after normalization of the stresses, but they become hard bodies in time, permanently. The hard cells induced prolonged endothelial inflammation, edema, and fibrosis at capillaries, and tissue ischemia and infarcts are the terminal consequences [4,5]. On the other hand, obvious vascular occlusions may not develop in greater vasculature due to the transport instead of distribution functions of them. We tried to understand whether or not there are some positive correlations between stroke and severity of SCDs.

Material and Methods

The study was performed in the Medical Faculty of the Mustafa Kemal University between March 2007 and November 2014. All cases with SCDs were taken into the study. The SCDs are diagnosed by the hemoglobin electrophoresis performed via high performance liquid chromatography (HPLC). Patients' medical histories including smoking habit, regular alcohol consumption, painful crises per year, operations, priapism, leg ulcers, and stroke were learnt. Cases with a history of one pack-year were accepted as smokers, and one drink a day for one year were accepted as drinkers. A checkup procedure including serum iron, total iron binding capacity, ferritin, creatinine, hepatic function tests, markers of hepatitis viruses A, B, and C and human immunodeficiency virus, a posterior-anterior chest X-ray film, an electrocardiogram, a Doppler echocardiogram both to evaluate cardiac walls and valves and to measure the systolic blood pressure (BP) of pulmonary artery, an abdominal ultrasonography, a Doppler ultrasonography to evaluate the portal blood flow in required cases, a computed tomography of brain, and a magnetic resonance imaging (MRI) of hips was performed. Other bones for avascular necrosis were scanned according to the patients' complaints. So avascular necrosis of bones was diagnosed via MRI [6]. Cases with acute painful crises or any other inflammatory event were treated at first, and then the laboratory tests and clinical measurements were performed on the silent phase. Stroke is diagnosed by the computed tomography of brain. Acute chest syndrome (ACS) is diagnosed clinically with the presence of new infiltrates on chest X-ray film, fever, cough, sputum production, dyspnea, or hypoxia in such patients [7]. An X-ray film of abdomen in upright position was taken just in cases with abdominal distention and discomfort, vomiting, obstipation, and lack of bowel movement. The criterion for diagnosis of COPD is post-bronchodilator forced expiratory volume in 1 second/forced vital capacity of less than 70% [8]. Systolic BP of the pulmonary artery of 40 mmHg or higher during the silent phase is accepted as pulmonary hypertension [9]. CRD is diagnosed with a serum creatinine level of 1.3 mg/dL or higher in males and 1.2 mg/dL or higher in females during the silent phase. Cirrhosis is diagnosed with hepatic function tests, ultrasonographic findings, and histologic procedure in case of indication. Digital clubbing is diagnosed with the ratio of distal phalangeal diameter to interphalangeal diameter which is greater than 1.0, and with the presence of Schamroth's sign [10,11]. Associated thalassemia minors are detected by serum iron, total iron binding capacity, ferritin, and hemoglobin electrophoresis performed via HPLC. A stress electrocardiography is performed for cases with an abnormal electrocardiogram and/or angina pectoris. A coronary angiography is taken for the stress electrocardiography positive cases. So CHD was diagnosed either angiographically or with the Doppler echocardiographic findings as the movement disorders in the cardiac walls. Rheumatic heart disease is diagnosed with the echocardiographic findings, too. Ileus was diagnosed by the General Surgeons with the consultations in case of indication. Eventually, cases with stroke and without were collected into the two groups, and they were compared in between. Mann-Whitney U test, Independent-Samples t test, and comparison of proportions were used as the methods of statistical analyses.

Results

The study included 343 patients with the SCDs (169 females and 174 males). There were 30 cases (8.7%) with stroke. The mean ages were similar in both groups (32.5 versus 29.1 years in the stroke group and other, respectively, p>0.05). The female ratios were similar in both groups, too (43.3% versus 49.8%, respectively, p>0.05). Prevalences of associated thalassemia minors were also similar in them (73.3% versus 65.1%, respectively, p>0.05). As a different result, smoking was higher among the stroke cases (26.6% versus 13.0%, p<0.05) (Table 1).

Variables	Cases with stroke	p-value	Cases without stroke
Prevalence	8.7% (30)		91.2% (313)
Female ratio	43.3% (13)	Ns*	49.8% (156)
Mean age (year)	32.5 ± 11.8 (9-56)	Ns	29.1 ± 9.7 (5-59)
Thalassemia minors	73.3% (22)	Ns	65.1% (204)
Smoking	26.6% (8)	<0.05	13.0% (41)
*Nonsignificant (p>0.05)			

Table 1: Characteristic features of the study cases.

The mean white blood cell (WBC) count, hematocrit (Hct) value, and the mean platelet (PLT) count of the peripheric blood were similar in both groups (p>0.05 for all) (Table 2).

Variables	Cases with stroke	p-value	Cases without stroke
Mean WBC* counts (μL)	14.292 ± 4.861 (7.310-26.020)	Ns†	15.151 ± 6.581 (1.580-39.200)
Mean Hct‡ value (%)	23.2 ± 5.0 (12-36)	Ns	23.7 ± 4.9 (11-42)
Mean PLT§ counts (μL)	383.070 ± 176.318 (114.000-955.000)	Ns	460.030 ± 232.897 (48.000-1.827.000)
*White blood cell †Nonsignificant (p>0.05) ‡Hematocrit §Platelet			

Table 2: Peripheric blood values of the study cases.

On the other hand, although the painful crises per year, tonsilectomy, priapism, ileus, pulmonary hypertension, COPD, CHD, CRD, rheumatic heart disease, avascular necrosis of bones, cirrhosis, and mortality were all higher in the stroke group, the differences were only significant for digital clubbing, leg ulcers, and ACS (p<0.05 for all), probably due to the small sample size of the stroke group (Table 3).

Variables	Cases with stroke	p-value	Cases without stroke
Painful crises per year	7.4 ± 11.4 (0-36)	Ns*	4.8 ± 7.6 (0-52)
Tonsilectomy	6.6% (2)	Ns	4.7% (15)
Priapism	3.3% (1)	Ns	2.5% (8)
Ileus	6.6% (2)	Ns	1.9% (6)
Digital clubbing	26.6% (8)	<0.001	7.9% (25)
Leg ulcers	26.6% (8)	<0.05	13.0% (41)
Pulmonary hypertension	20.0% (6)	Ns	10.5% (33)
COPD†	20.0% (6)	Ns	13.4% (42)
CHD‡	6.6% (2)	Ns	6.3% (20)
CRD§	10.0% (3)	Ns	7.9% (25)
Rheumatic heart disease	10.0% (3)	Ns	6.3% (20)
Avascular necrosis of bones	23.3% (7)	Ns	20.7% (65)
Cirrhosis	6.6% (2)	Ns	4.1% (13)
ACS¶	13.3% (4)	<0.01	3.5% (11)
Mortality	6.6% (2)	Ns	4.4% (14)
*Nonsignificant (p>0.05) †Chronic obstructive pulmonary disease ‡Coronary heart disease §Chronic renal disease ¶Acute chest syndrome			

Table 3: Associated pathologies of the study cases.

Additionally, there were four patients with regular alcohol consumption who are not cirrhotic at the moment. Although antiHCV was positive in seven of the cirrhotics, HCV RNA was detected as positive just in one by polymerase chain reaction method.

Discussion

It is obvious that atherosclerosis is the most common type of vasculitis all over the world, and it is the leading cause of morbidity and mortality particularly in elderlies. Probably whole afferent vasculatures including capillaries are affected in the body. Chronic endothelial injury and inflammation due to the much higher BP of afferent vasculature may be the major underlying cause, and efferent vessels are probably protected due to the much lower BP in them. Vascular walls become thickened due to the chronic endothelial injury, inflammation, edema, and fibrosis, and they lose their elastic structures which can reduce the blood flow and increase BP further. In the SCDs, the hard RBCs induced chronic endothelial injury, inflammation, edema, and fibrosis mainly at the capillary level build up prototype of an advanced atherosclerosis even in younger ages.

SCDs are life-threatening genetic disorders affecting nearly 100.000 individuals in the United States [12]. They keep vascular endothelium mainly at the capillary level [13], since the capillary system is the main distributor of the hard RBCs to cells. Due to microvascular nature of the SCDs, as in microvascular complications of DM, complete healing of leg ulcers can usually be achieved with hydroxyurea in children and adolescents, but it may be difficult due to the excessive fibrosis on the vascular walls later in life. In other words, SCDs are mainly chronic inflammatory instead of obstructive disorders, and the major problem is probably endothelial injury, inflammation, edema, and fibrosis rather than the hard RBCs induced occlusions in the capillary lumen. As a result, the lifespans of females and males with the SCDs were 48 and 42 years in the literature [14], whereas they were 33.3 and 29.9 years in the present study, respectively. The great differences may be secondary to initiation of hydroxyurea therapy much earlier in developed countries. On the other hand, the prolonged lifespan of females with SCDs and longer overall survival of females in the world cannot be explained by the atherosclerotic effects of smoking alone, instead it may be explained by more physical power requiring role of male sex in life [15,16].

Stroke is the third most common cause of death in Western countries, and thromboembolism due to atherosclerosis is the most common cause of the stroke. Similar to atherosclerosis, aging, male sex, smoking, DM, HT, dyslipidemia, and excess weight are the major accelerator factors of the stroke. Cerebral emboli usually come from atheromas in extracranial vessels or from thrombi in a damaged heart. Large atheromas usually affect the common carotid and vertebral arteries at their origins, but the cervical bifurcation of the common carotid artery is the most common site giving rise to emboli that cause stroke. Main trunk of the middle cerebral artery and its branches are the most common sites of intracranial thrombosis. Stroke is also a traumatic complication of the SCDs [17,18]. The incidence of stroke is higher in sickle cell anemia (Hb SS) [19], and a higher WBC count is associated with a higher incidence [20]. It is attributed to sickling induced endothelial injury, WBC, PLT, and coagulation activation, hemolysis, and subsequent chronic endothelial inflammation, edema, remodeling, and fibrosis [21]. Probably, stroke is a complex and terminal event in the SCDs. All stroke episodes do not have a macrovascular origin, and disseminated capillary inflammation and endothelial edema may be important. Infections and other stressful conditions may precipitate the stroke, since the increased metabolic rate during such episodes may accelerate sickling, disseminated capillary injury, endothelial edema, and fibrosis. A preliminary result from the Multi-Institutional study of Hydroxyurea in the SCDs indicating a significant reduction of stroke in those on hydroxyurea [22] suggests that a significant proportion of strokes are secondary to the increased WBC and PLT counts induced disseminated capillary endothelial injury [13].

RBC transfusions are the most significant preventive approach for stroke in the SCDs [29,30]. They decrease sickle cell concentrations in blood, suppress their production in bone marrow, and prevent sickling induced endothelial injury, inflammation, edema, and fibrosis in brain, lungs, liver, bones, kidneys, and other organs [23,24]. Since the main pathology is disseminated and prolonged tissue ischemia in the SCDs [2], simple and repeated RBCs transfusions are highly effective to restore tissue oxygenation. Ileus is also a common pathology in the SCDs' patients probably due to their atherosclerotic natures [31], and all of the ileus cases were able to be treated with simple and repeated RBCs transfusions in the present study. But transfusions have to be given early in ileus and other clinically severe conditions rather than too late when the patient is clearly comatose. According to our experiences, simple and repeated RBC transfusions are superior to RBC exchange in the SCDs. First of all, simplicity of preparation of RBC suspensions in a short period of time provides advantages to clinicians. Secondly, preparation of one or two units of RBC suspension in each time rather than preparation of several units provides time to clinicians to prepare more units by preventing sudden death of such patients. Thirdly, transfusion of RBC suspensions in secondary health centers can prevent some deaths developed during transport to tertiary centers for exchange.

Painful crises are nearly pathognomonic for the SCDs, and they are precipitated by infection, operation, depression, and traumas. Although these painful crises are not life-threatening directly [25], crises induced increased metabolic rate may cause multiorgan failures on the chronic inflammatory background of the SCDs [26]. The severe pain is probably caused by the exaggerated inflammation of capillary endothelium all over the body, and the increased WBC and PLT counts and decreased Hct values even in silent periods may show the chronic inflammatory process during whole their lives in such cases. Similar to the present study, increased WBC counts even during the silent periods may be an independent predictor of severity [27], and it was associated with an increased risk of stroke by inducing disseminated capillary endothelial inflammation, edema, and fibrosis even in the brain [28]. According to our experiences, simple and repeated RBC transfusions according to the requirement are also effective during the severe painful crises both to relieve pain and to prevent sudden death which may develop secondary to the multiorgan failures on the chronic inflammatory background of the SCDs.

Two disease-modifying therapies, hydroxyurea daily and RBC transfusions in severe clinical conditions are underused [32]. Hydroxyurea is safe and highly effective for the SCDs [13]. It is an oral and cheap drug that blocks cell division by suppressing formation of deoxyribonucleotides which are building blocks of DNA. Although the action way of hydroxyurea is thought to be the increase of gamma globin synthesis for fetal hemoglobin (Hb F) [33], its main action may be suppression of hyperproliferative WBCs and PLTs in the SCDs. Although presence of a continuous damage of hard RBCs on capillary endothelium, severity of the destructive process is probably exaggerated by the patients' own WBCs and PLTs. So mechanism of tissue destruction of the SCDs may mimic autoimmune disorders, and suppression of excessive proliferation of patients' own WBCs and PLTs by the drug may limit the capillary endothelial injury, inflammation, edema, and fibrosis induced disseminated tissue ischemia and infarcts all over the body. Similarly, lower neutrophil counts were associated with lower crises rates, and if a tissue infarction occurs, lower neutrophil counts may decrease severity of pain and tissue damage [34]. Furthermore, final Hb F levels did not differ with hydroxyurea therapy [34]. Due to the same reason, hydroxyurea is also used to suppress hyperproliferative cells in chronic myeloproliferative disorders and psoriasis, effectively. According to our practices during the eight-year period, the only side effect of hydroxyurea is a deep anemia. Although hydroxyurea increases Hct level in smaller doses, it may cause a deep anemia when used as a dose of 35 mg/kg/day. But this effect is usually harmless, and Hct level increases rapidly by decreasing the daily dose if the patient is clinically silent.

As a conclusion, SCDs are chronic destructive process on capillaries iniatiating at birth, and terminate with early organ failures in life. Probably stroke is one of the terminal consequences of the inflammatory process that may indicate shortened survival in such cases.

References

1. Eckel RH, Grundy SM, Zimmet PZ (2005) The metabolic syndrome. Lancet 365: 1415-1428.

2. Helvaci MR, Aydin LY, Aydin Y (2012) Chronic obstructive pulmonary disease may be one of the terminal end points of metabolic syndrome. Pak J Med Sci 28: 376-379.

3. Stojanovic OI, Lazovic M, Lazovic M, Vuceljic M (2011) Association between atherosclerosis and osteoporosis, the role of vitamin D. Arch Med Sci 7: 179-188.

4. Helvaci MR, Sevinc A, Camci C, Keskin A (2014) Atherosclerotic background of cirrhosis in sickle cell patients. Pren Med Argent 100: 127-133.

5. Helvaci MR, Acipayam C, Davran R (2014) Autosplenectomy in severity of sickle cell diseases. Int J Clin Exp Med 7: 1404-1409.

6. Mankad VN, Williams JP, Harpen MD, Manci E, Longenecker G, et al. (1990) Magnetic resonance imaging of bone marrow in sickle cell disease: clinical, hematologic, and pathologic correlations. Blood 75: 274-283.

7. Castro O, Brambilla DJ, Thorington B, Reindorf CA, Scott RB, et al. (1994) The acute chest syndrome in sickle cell disease: incidence and risk factors. The Cooperative Study of Sickle Cell Disease. Blood 84: 643-649.

8. Global strategy for the diagnosis, management and prevention of chronic obstructive pulmonary disease (2010). Global initiative for chronic obstructive lung disease.

9. Fisher MR, Forfia PR, Chamera E, Housten-Harris T, Champion HC, et al. (2009) Accuracy of Doppler echocardiography in the hemodynamic assessment of pulmonary hypertension. Am J Respir Crit Care Med 179: 615-621.

10. Vandemergel X, Renneboog B (2008) Prevalence Aetiologies and significance of clubbing in a department of general internal medicine. Eur J Intern Med; 19: 325-329.

11. Schamroth L (1976) Personal experience. S Afr Med J 50: 297-300.

12. Yawn BP, Buchanan GR, Afenyi-Annan AN, Ballas S, Hassell KL, et al. (2014) Management of sickle cell disease: summary of the 2014 evidence-based report by expert panel members. JAMA 312: 1033-1048.

13. Helvaci MR, Aydin Y, Ayyildiz O (2013) Hydroxyurea may prolong survival of sickle cell patients by decreasing frequency of painful crises. HealthMED 7: 2327-2332.

14. Platt OS, Brambilla DJ, Rosse WF, Milner PF, Castro O, et al. (1994) Mortality in sickle cell disease. Life expectancy and risk factors for early death. N Engl J Med 330: 1639-1644.

15. Mathers CD, Sadana R, Salomon JA, Murray CJ, Lopez AD (2001) Healthy life expectancy in 191 countries, 1999. Lancet 357: 1685-1691.

16. Rami Helvaci M, Ayyildiz O, Gundogdu M (2013) Gender differences in severity of sickle cell diseases in non-smokers. Pak J Med Sci 29: 1050-1054.

17. DeBaun MR, Gordon M, McKinstry RC, Noetzel MJ, White DA, et al. (2014) Controlled trial of transfusions for silent cerebral infarcts in sickle cell anemia. N Engl J Med 371: 699-710.

18. Gueguen A, Mahevas M, Nzouakou R, Hosseini H, Habibi A, et al. (2014) Sickle-cell disease stroke throughout life: a retrospective study in an adult referral center. Am J Hematol 89: 267-272.

19. Majumdar S, Miller M, Khan M, Gordon C, Forsythe A, et al. (2014) Outcome of overt stroke in sickle cell anaemia, a single institution's experience. Br J Haematol 165: 707-713.

20. Helvaci MR, Aydogan F, Sevinc A, Camci C, Dilek I (2014) Platelet and white blood cell counts in severity of sickle cell diseases. Pren Med Argent 100: 49-56. Spanish.

21. Kossorotoff M, Grevent D, de Montalembert M (2014) [Cerebral vasculopathy in pediatric sickle-cell anemia]. Arch Pediatr 21: 404-414.

22. Charache S, Terrin ML, Moore RD, Dover GJ, Barton FB, et al. (1995) Effect of hydroxyurea on the frequency of painful crises in sickle cell anemia. Investigators of the Multicenter Study of Hydroxyurea in Sickle Cell Anemia. N Engl J Med 332: 1317-1322.

23. Charache S, Scott JC, Charache P (1979) "Acute chest syndrome" in adults with sickle cell anemia. Microbiology, treatment, and prevention. Arch Intern Med 139: 67-69.

24. Davies SC, Luce PJ, Win AA, Riordan JF, Brozovic M (1984) Acute chest syndrome in sickle-cell disease. Lancet 1: 36-38.

25. Parfrey NA, Moore W, Hutchins GM (1985) Is pain crisis a cause of death in sickle cell disease? Am J Clin Pathol 84: 209-212.

26. Helvaci MR, Gokce C. Painful crises and survival of sickle cell patients. HealthMED 2014; 8: 598-602.

27. Miller ST, Sleeper LA, Pegelow CH, Enos LE, Wang WC, et al. (2000) Prediction of adverse outcomes in children with sickle cell disease. N Engl J Med 342: 83-89.

28. Balkaran B, Char G, Morris JS, Thomas PW, Serjeant BE, et al. (1992) Stroke in a cohort of patients with homozygous sickle cell disease. J Pediatr 120: 360-366.

29. Switzer JA, Hess DC, Nichols FT, Adams RJ (2006) Pathophysiology and treatment of stroke in sickle-cell disease: present and future. Lancet Neurol 5: 501-512.

30. Gebreyohanns M1, Adams RJ (2004) Sickle cell disease: primary stroke prevention. CNS Spectr 9: 445-449.

31. Helvaci MR1, Aydogan A1, Akkucuk S1, Oruc C1, Ugur M1 (2014) Sickle cell diseases and ileus. Int J Clin Exp Med 7: 2871-2876.

32. Kurantsin-Mills J, Jacobs HM, Lessin LS (1987) Sickle cell vaso-occlusion in an animal model; intravital microscopy and radionuclide imaging of selective sequestration of dense cells. Prog Clin Biol Res 240: 313-327.

33. Miller BA1, Platt O, Hope S, Dover G, Nathan DG (1987) Influence of hydroxyurea on fetal hemoglobin production in vitro. Blood 70: 1824-1829.

34. Charache S (1997) Mechanism of action of hydroxyurea in the management of sickle cell anemia in adults. Semin Hematol 34: 15-21.

36

The Association between Periodontal Disease and Obesity among Middle-aged Adults Periodontitis and Obesity

Pejcic Ana[1], Mirkovic Dimitrije[2], Minic Ivan[1*] and Stojanovic Mariola[3]

[1]Department of Periodontology and Oral Medicine, University of Nis, Serbia

[2]Private Practice – "Smile-Dent", Nis, Serbia

[3]Institute for Public Health, University of Nis, Serbia

*Corresponding author: Dr. Ivan M, Medical Faculty, Periodontology and Oral Medicine, University of Nis, Serbia; E-mail: Ivanminic@yahoo.com

Abstract

Objective: Obesity is characterized by the abnormal or excessive deposition of fat in the adipose tissue. Besides being a risk factor for cardiovascular diseases, certain cancers and type II diabetes, obesity has been suggested to be a risk factor for periodontitis. A number of epidemiological studies have studied the association between obesity and periodontitis. The aim of this study was to determine the relationship between periodontitis and overweight/obesity in subjects aged 28-55 years.

Study design: A representative sample of the population, which was enrolled in a study, was examined. A total of 300 chronic periodontitis subjects had a clinical periodontal examination and their weight and height were recorded. Periodontal parameters were: probing pocket depth, clinical attachment level, bleeding on probing, gingival inflammation and presence of visible plaque. In the control group there were 100 periodontal healthy subjects. Moderate periodontitis was identified when teeth had attachment loss of <6 mm and a pocket depth<5 mm, and severe periodontitis with attachment loss ≥ 6 mm and pocket depth ≥ 5 mm. Body weight was measured using body mass index.

Results: Researchers have found a significant association between obesity and prevalence of periodontal disease, among the population aged 28-55. Obesity was associated with periodontitis after adjustment for confounders. Greatest association was found between BMI and severe periodontitis measured by periodontal parameters.

Conclusion: The data suggest that obesity is associated with periodontitis. Obese individuals might be at risk for initiation and progression of periodontitis.

Keywords: BMI; Obesity; Moderate periodontitis; Severe periodontitis; Periodontal parameters

Introduction

Over the past few decades, obesity has become a significant worldwide health problem. The most recent data from the indicated that 32% of adults were obese in 2004 [1]. In the , the prevalence of obesity among adults almost tripled between 1980 and 2002 [2]. The incidence of obesity and elevated body mass index (BMI) has dramatically increased in most industrialized countries. Obesity is now recognized as a chronic disease with a multifactorial etiology that develops from an interaction of genotype and the environment. Obesity has been associated with many serious, life–treating medical conditions. Besides being a risk factor for cardiovascular diseases, type II diabetes [3] and certain cancers [4], obesity has also been suggested to be risk factor for periodontitis. A number of studies have evaluated the relationship between obesity and gum disease. It has become clear that genetic and environmental factors and socioeconomic and behavioral influences leading to excess caloric intake decreased physical activity, and metabolic and endocrine abnormalities are likely important factors [5,6].

The mechanism of how obesity affects the periodontium is currently poorly understood. It is known that obesity has several harmful biological effects that might be related to the pathogenesis of periodontitis. The high prevalence of both obesity and periodontal disease (PD) poses a substantial public health risk [7-10]. Dental providers should anticipate a higher incidence of gum disease among this patient population.

Although obesity is becoming a worldwide problem, in Serbia there is a small number of works devoted to this problem, especially about the relationship between obesity and periodontal disease.

The aim of the current study was to investigate whether there were associations between obesity and periodontal status in population aged 28-55 years.

Materials and Methods

The study population comprised persons aged 28 to 55 years living in . The first group comprised periodontitis free subjects (n=100) or having periodontitis-with evidence of attachment loss (n=300). The subjects were enrolled in the Department of Periodontology at the Dental Clinic in and were selected for study. All subjects provided signed informed consent. The Ethics Committee of the Faculty of medicine University of Nis, Serbia approved the study protocol (No: 01-2800-5). The data for this research were collected by taking the anamnestic data and clinical oral examinations.

One calibrated dentist performed clinical oral examinations in a dental chair using a headlamp, mouth mirror and a WHO periodontal probe (Michigan 0). The clinical oral examinations included assessment of the condition of periodontium.

Exclusion criteria for all subjects included: periodontal or antibiotic therapy in the previous 6 months; any systemic condition which might have influenced the course of periodontal disease or treatment (e.g. diabetes and cardiovascular disease); any systemic condition which required antibiotic coverage for routine periodontal procedures. Diabetic patients were excluded because interrelations between obesity and diabetes, which depend on the type and the severity of the diabetes, can be complex and prevent accurate control.

Each subject completed a questionnaire, which gathered information on their demographic and socio-economic status (SES). Socio-demographic variables included gender, marital status, years of education, occupational activity and tobacco consumption. The analyses were carried out to all participants. Education was categorized into two categories, <12 years (low) and >12 years (high). Smokers were divided into current smokers or non-smokers. Socio-economic status was categorized as good or bad according to the statements of the respondents. Occupational activity was categorized as moderate or active (once a week or four times a week).

In addition to clinical measurements, subjects were measured for height and weight. The BMI is calculated by dividing the body weight (in kilograms) by the height (in meters) squared (BMI = weight/height^2). The BMI measured was categorized using the World Health Organization: normal weight (<24.9 kg/m^2), overweight (25-29.9 kg/m^2) and obesity (>30 kg/m^2) [11].

In this study, only baseline clinical periodontal measurements were used and they included: plaque accumulation (PLI), gingival inflammation (GI), bleeding on probing (BOP), periodontal pocket depth (PPD) and clinical attachment loss (CAL) [12,13]. These clinical parameters were measured at six sites per tooth (mesiobuccal, buccal, distobuccal distolingual, lingual and mesiolingual) in all teeth excluding third molars [14].

Periodontal status was determined in all subjects. The proportions of individuals were compared in the periodontal health and periodontitis group according to periodontal status. Periodontal subjects had PPD<5 mm and CAL<6 mm (moderate periodontitis) or PPD ≥ 5 mm and CAL ≥ 6 mm (severe periodontitis). Periodontal pocket depths were measured from the gingival margin to the base of the clinical pocket with the probe tip parallel to the long axis of the tooth. Clinical attachment loss was recorded as the distance from the cement-enamel junction to the base of the clinical pocket.

Statistical Analysis

Tests of general parameters, except the BMI t-test, between the periodontitis patients and control group were done with χ^2 test. Testing of the mean age was done by ANOVA test. Furthermore, 50 respondents were classified by BMI category into 3 groups. This groups and the control group also crafted the χ^2 test to compare the distribution of general parameters. As for clinical parameters, the same tests were applied for all four groups.

Results

A total of 300 individuals 28 to 55 years old, with periodontitis, participated in this study. Of these, 54% were men and 46% women (Table 1). Likewise, significantly more individuals had less than 12 years of education (64%). The number of smokers was also less (38%) in periodontitis group compared to the control group (32% and 40%). The subjects of these two groups differ significantly in education, socioeconomic status, and BMI. The majority of respondents were poorer (66%) in periodontitis group. In the control group there were more affluent people (68%).

Variable	Periodontitis group (n=300)	Control group (n=100)	p value
Gender			
Male	162 (54 %)	28 (28 %)	χ^2=3.64
Female	138 (46%)	72 (72%)	p>0.05
Age (years), mean ± SD	48.76 ± 15.83	42.80 ± 5.76	t=1.799
Age range	28-55	31-51	p>0.05
Years of education, No, %			
<12 year	192 (64%)	32 (32 %)	χ^2=6.86
>12 year	108 (36%)	68 (68 %)	p<0.005
Socioeconomic status, No, %			
Bad	198 (66%)	32 (32%)	χ^2=9.67
Good	102 (34%)	68 (68%)	p<0.005
Smoking, No, %			
Yes	114 (38%)	40 (40%)	χ^2=0.03
No	186 (62%)	60 (60%)	p>0.05
Physical activity, No, %			
Active	90 (30%)	24 (24%)	χ^2=0.30
Moderate	210 (70%)	76 (76%)	p>0.05
BMI, kg/cm^2 Mean ± SD	26 .04 ± 3.38	22.08 ± 4.10	t=4.387
	19.0-33.5	17.8-35.9	p<0.05

Table 1: Basic characteristics of the study population.

In terms of physical activity, there were more respondents who declared themselves to be moderately physically active (70%) than active (30%). BMI was higher in the periodontitis-affected group (26.04 ± 3.38) compared to the periodontitis-free group (22.08 ± 4.10). Results of BMI compared to the basic characteristics of the study population are shown in Table 2. The number of overweight subjects (24 subjects, 46%) was larger than the number of normal-weight subjects (19 subjects, 40%). A very small number of the subjects was obese (7 subjects, 14%), as they exhibited a mean BMI of ≥30 kg/m^2. In the Serbian population, the number of obese persons was small.

Variable	Normal <24.9 (n=108)	Overweight 25 – 29.9 (n=134)	Obese ≥30 (n=58)	Control (n=100)	p value
Gender					
Male	31 (28.7%)	95 (70.89%)	35 (60.34%)	28 (28%)	$\chi^2=8.361$
Female	77 (71.3%)	39 (29.11%)	23 (39.66%)	72 (72%)	$p<0.05$
Age(years) mean ± SD	35.37 ± 6.48	56.96 ± 13.05	64.14 ± 12.80	42.80 ± 5.76	F=27.269
Age range	28 - 36	36 - 55	40 - 55	31 - 51	$p<0.001$
Years of education, No, %					
<12 year	82 (75.93%)	99 (73.88%)	33 (56.9%)	32 (32%)	$\chi^2=7.063$
>12 year	26 (24.07%)	35 (26.12%)	25 (43.1%)	68 (68%)	$p>0.05$
Socioeconomic status, No, %					
Bad	69 (63.9%)	90 (67.16%)	33 (56.9)%	28 (28%)	$\chi^2=10.177$
Good	39 (36.1%)	44 (32.84%)	25 (43.1)%	72 (72%)	$p<0.05$
Smoking, No, %					
Yes	73 (67.6%)	40 (29.85%)		40 (40%)	$\chi^2=10.151$
No	35 (32.4%)	94 (70.15%)	58 (100%)	60 (60%)	$p<0.05$
Physical activity, No, %					
Active	46 (42.6%)	34 (25.37%)	11 (18.97%)	24 (24%)	$\chi^2=2.834$
Moderate	62 (57.4%)	100(74.63%)	47 (81.03%)	76 (76%)	$p>0.05$

Table 2: BMI according to the basic characteristics of the study population

Among the overweight and obese subjects there were more males non-smokers. Overweight and obese individuals were older, less educated, and with bad SES. Physical activity was more moderate in overweight and obese subjects. The mean clinical periodontal parameters were compared in subjects according to BMI categories (Table 3). There was a strong association between BMI and periodontal status. Clinical periodontal parameters were compared among subjects according to BMI. There were a larger number of overweight and obese subjects in the group with severe periodontitis compared to the group with moderate periodontitis.

The subjects with periodontitis exhibited significant differences in clinical parameters among BMI categories. The values of periodontal parameters increased along with the increase in body weight of respondents. The highest values for all parameters were reported in the group of obese persons. Table 3 also shows that the severity of periodontal attachment loss and pocket depth increased proportionally with increasing BMI. Plaque index was 1.52, 1.70, and 1.71 to BMI status. Gingival inflammation was 1.68, 170, and 1.85. Bleeding on probing was 1.73, 1.75, and 1.85.

Subjects who had the highest BMI had a deeper pocket (6.92 mm) than those with the lowest BMI (5.13 mm). Individuals who were overweight or obese were more likely to have severe periodontitis than

subjects with normal BMI. Similar results were obtained with respect to the values for the attachment level. In obese subjects CAL was 8.05 mm, and in subjects with normal weight CAL was 6.15 mm. The analysis indicated that BMI was significantly associated with periodontal status even after adjusting for gender, age, socioeconomic status and smoking.

Discussion

The main finding of this study was that obesity in Serbian population was associated with a significantly increased prevalence of periodontitis but much lower than overweight, too. The relationship was much stronger in individuals with severe periodontitis than in the subjects with moderate periodontitis. This was in keeping with a number of studies which have suggested that obesity is associated with oral diseases, particularly periodontitis [15,16]. The first report on the relationship between obesity and periodontal disease was written in 1977, when Perlstein et al. [15] observed histopathological changes in the periodontium in hereditary obese Zucker rats. Also, it seemed that under healthy oral conditions, obesity *per se* does not promote pathological periodontal alterations; however, in response to bacterial plaque accumulation, periodontal inflammation and destruction were more severe in obese animals.

Periodontal variable	Normal <24.9 (n=108)	Overweight 25 – 29.9 (n=134)	Obese ≥30 (n=58)	Control (n=100)	p value
Plaque index (PLI)	1.526 ± 0.612	1.708 ± 0.464	1.714 ± 0.488	0.520 ± 0.420	F=29.036 p<0.0001
Gingival inflammation (GI)	1.684 ± 0.478	1.708 ± 0.464	1.857 ± 0.378	0.400 ± 0.382	F=51.491 p<0.0001
Bleeding on probing (BOP)	1.737 ± 0.452	1.750 ± 0.442	1.857 ± 0.378	0.400 ± 0.382	F=58.321 p<0.0001
Periodontal pocket depth (PPD) - mm, mean ± SD	4.24 ± 0.83	4.79 ± 0.98	5.48 ± 1.68	1.90 ± 0.55	F=55.280 p<0.001
PPD > 5 mm	29 (26.85%)	46 (33.3%)	34 (58.62%)		χ^2=13.776
PPD ≤ 5 mm	79 (73.15%)	92 (66.7%)	24 (41.38%)	100 (100%)	p<0.005
Clinical attachment level (CAL) - mm, mean ± SD	5,38 ± 0.83	5.91 ± 0.97	5.95 ± 1.13	1.90 ± 0.55	F=119.073 p<0.0001
CAL>6 mm	29 (26.85%)	44 (33.3%)	34 (58.62%)		χ^2=13.776
CAL ≤ 6 mm	79 (73.15%)	92 (66.7%)	24 (41.38%)	100 (100%)	p<0.005

Table 3: Presents BMI (normal, overweight or obese) according to periodontal parameters.

Later on, the hypothesis of obesity as a risk factor for periodontal disease was supported by epidemiological study [17]. There are studies in which obesity is not significantly associated with severe periodontitis [18].

Obesity is a complex disease, and its relationship with oral status has been realized by the scientific community in the recent years. Various cross-sectional and case-control studies found a strong association between obesity and periodontal disease. Body mass index (BMI) was calculated as the body weight/height^2 (kg/h^2). The BMI measured was categorized using the World Health Organization (2000) classification: normal weight equated to BMI<25 kg/m^2, overweight 25 – 29.9 kg/m^2 and obese ≥ 30 kg/m^2.

In this study, obesity measured by BMI, was related to periodontal status in terms of health versus periodontitis after adjusting for age, gender, smoking and socioeconomic status. Clinical parameters, including the presence of plaque, gingival inflammation, BOP, mean PPD and mean CAL were also related to BMI status. These data are in accord with the findings of other studies [19,20].

They found that total body weight was associated with an increased risk for periodontitis in the older subjects (17-21 years), but not in the younger subjects (13-16 years). Gender also had an impact on the relationship between obesity and periodontitis. In this study, there were significantly higher proportions of normal BMI subjects in both normal and overgrowth females compared with male subjects in the same clinical groups (Table 4).

Statistical analysis shows that there was an association between BMI and periodontitis. Obese people with BMI ≥ 30 had an adjusted odds ratio of 7.659 for having periodontitis. In the study in Japanese subjects indicated that both smoking and obesity were independent risk factors

for periodontitis. One of the most important confounders in this context is smoking, which is considered to be a risk factor for periodontitis. Smoking most probably confounds the association between body weight and periodontal infection [21].

In our study, there were fewer smokers in all groups. Thus, smoking had smaller impact on the results. In our study, overweight and obese patients are characterized by worse periodontal status when compared to the subjects with normal BMI. Variations in the strength of the association between obesity and periodontitis reported in studies on different populations may reflect a lack of uniformity in the case definitions used for periodontal disease. The average PPD was significantly higher in obese subjects (p<0.001) when compared with that among participants with BMI<25 kg/m^2. The average CAL was significantly higher (p<0.001) in both overweight and obese participants when compared to normal weight participants. This finding was consistent with the findings of the study conducted by Khader et al. [20] who reported that CAL and PPD, as indicators of periodontal disease, were correlated with increased BMI.

In case of periodontitis with periodontal pockets of 5 mm or deeper BMI increases. This analysis showed a positive association between BMI and periodontal pockets (5 mm or more). This finding could be interpreted that body weight has an effect on the extent of periodontal infection among subjects with periodontal infection. In our study, moderate periodontitis was relatively common affecting 90% of the population with normal weight, which is similar to periodontitis-free group. Severe periodontitis was identified only in 10% of the population examined in the group with normal weight, in 60% in group with overgrowth subjects and in 86% in the obese subjects.

In general, the obese subjects had different risk factors, such as lower SES, fewer years of education. All three factors have been associated with an increased risk of periodontitis; however, it is possible that there are other confounders that were not controlled in the analysis. The mechanisms how obesity has effects on periodontium are not known, but there are several possible biological explanations.

Plum	Mean ± SD	Wald	Significance
Level – 0[a]:1[b]	4.55 ± 2.55	3.179	0.075
Level - 1[b]:2[c]	7.309 ± 2.641	7.659	0.006
Gender	-0.16 ± 0.52	0.090	0.764
Age (years)	-0.002 ± 0.02	0.738	0.390
Education	-0.38 ± 0.51	0.546	0.460
Social status	-1.62 ± 0.55	8.572	0.003
Smoking	-0.29 ± 0.53	0.297	0.586
Physical activity	0.87 ± 0.56	2.444	0.118
BMI	0.35 ± 0.08	16.597	0.000
Level - 0[a]:1[b]	25.96 ± 8.27	9.858	0.002
Level - 1[b]:2[c]	49.74 ± 15.58	10.196	0.001
PLI[d]	-0.13 ± 2.27	0.003	0.954
GI[e]	9.94 ± 49.86	0.040	0.842
BOP[f]	-12.48 ± 50.11	0.062	0.803
PPD[g]	2.18 ± 2.77	0.619	0.431
CAL[h]	7.22 ± 3.21	5.056	0.025

Table 4: PLUM-ordinal regression analysis for periodontal healthy.

Obesity is a risk factor for several chronic diseases, most notably hypertension, type 2 diabetes dyslipidemia and coronary heart disease [22,23]. According to the current knowledge, the adverse effects of obesity on the periodontium might be mediated through impaired glucose tolerance, dyslipidemia or through increased levels of various bioactive substances secreted by adipose tissue. Its consequences go far beyond adverse metabolic effects on health, causing an increase in oxidative stress, which leads not only to endothelial dysfunction but also to negative effects in relation to periodontitis, because of the increase in pro-inflammatory cytokines [24,25].

The adipose tissue actively secretes a variety of cytokines and hormones that are involved in inflammatory processes, pointing toward similar pathways involved in the pathophysiology of obesity, periodontitis and related inflammatory diseases. Adipocytes appear to secrete pro-inflammatory cytokines which may be the molecules linking the pathogenesis of these diseases. For example, it has been well established that inflammation is an essential component in the development of atherosclerosis, and observational studies showed that periodontitis is associated with a moderately, but significantly higher risk of coronary heart disease [26].

Inflammatory diseases like periodontitis induce the production of proinflammatory cytokines such as TNF-α, IL-1 and IL-6. It has been suggested that the secretion of TNF-α by adipose tissue triggered by LPS from periodontal gram-negative bacteria promotes hepatic dyslipidemia and decreases insulin that may enhance periodontal degradation [27]. Systemic inflammation, defined by increased circulating IL-6, is associated with obesity and periodontitis and has been proposed as a mechanism for the connection between these conditions [28]. For example, poor diet and physical inactivity could be such factors. The possibility that these mechanisms might act simultaneously is not excluded either [29].

Pro-inflammatory cytokines may be a multidirectional link among periodontitis, obesity and other chronic diseases. The adipose tissue is a large reservoir of biologically active mediators. Studies have demonstrated a close involvement of the adipokines –such as leptin and adiponectin - in inflammatory processes [30]. However, their role in periodontal inflammation has yet to be defined. Whether the relationship between obesity and periodontitis is causal needs to be assessed in future studies

In future, if obesity is to be acknowledged as a multiple-risk-factor syndrome for overall and oral health, general and oral risk assessment in the dental office should include the evaluation of body mass index on a regular basis.

To truly clarify the direction of the association between body weight and periodontal infection, longitudinal studies are needed. The link between obesity and periodontitis is inflammation. Since it is impossible to have a direct impact on a patients' BMI, it is possible to eliminate or control the inflammatory contribution of periodontitis by intervening and treating this chronic inflammation. Obesity may be the link between periodontitis and other diseases. For example, obesity is a risk factor for atherosclerotic cardiovascular disease and, due to its associations with periodontitis, it is a potential confounder in the association between periodontitis and atherosclerotic cardiovascular disease.

Conclusion

The results of this study indicate that overweight and obesity are potential confounders and significant predictors of periodontal disease. These results indicate that obesity increases the risk of periodontitis, and suggest that people exhibiting several components of obesity should be encouraged to undergo a periodontal therapy.

References

1. Ogden CL, Carroll MD, Curtin LR, McDowell MA, Tabak CJ, et al. (2006) Prevalence of overweight and obesity in the United States, 1999-2004. JAMA 295: 1549-1555.

2. Rennie KL, Jebb SA (2005) Prevalence of obesity in Great Britain. Obes Rev 6: 11-12.

3. Wilson PW, Bozeman SR, Burton TM, Hoaglin DC, Ben-Joseph R, et al. (2008) Prediction of first events of coronary heart disease and stroke with consideration of adiposity. Circulation 118: 124-130.

4. Calle EE, Rodriguez C, Walker-Thurmond K, Thun MJ (2003) Overweight, obesity, and mortality from cancer in a prospectively studied cohort of U.S. adults. N Engl J Med 348: 1625-1638.

5. Han DH, Lim SY, Sun BC, Paek DM, Kim HD (2010) Visceral fat area-defined obesity and periodontitis among Koreans. J Clin Periodontol 37: 172-179.

6. Linden G, Patterson C, Evans A, Kee F (2007) Obesity and periodontitis in 60-70-year-old men. J Clin Periodontol 34: 461-466.

7. Genco RJ, Grossi SG, Ho A, Nishimura F, Murayama Y (2005) A proposed model linking inflammation to obesity, diabetes, and periodontal infections. J Periodontol 76: 2075-2084.

8. Vecchia CFD, Susin C, Rösing CK, Oppermann RV, Albandar JM (2005) Overweight and obesity as risk indicators for periodontitis in adults. J Periodontol 76: 1721-1728.

9.   WHO (2000) Obesity: preventing and managing the global epidemic. Report of a WHO consultation. World Health Organ Tech Rep Ser 894: 1-253.

10. Silness J, Loe H (1964) Periodontal Disease in Pregnancy. II. Correlation between Oral Hygiene and Periodontal Condition. Acta Odontol Scand 22: 121-135.

11. Löe H (1967) The Gingival Index, the Plaque Index and the Retention Index Systems. J Periodontol 38: 610-616.

12. Carranca AF, Newman GM: Clinical periodontology (8th Edn) Epidemiology of gingiva and periodontal disease. W.B. Saunders Company, United States.

13. Ylostalo P, Suominen-Taipale L, Reunen A, Knuuttila M (2008) Association between body weight and periodontal infection. J Clin Periodontol 35: 297-304.

14. Haffajee AD, Socransky SS (2009) Relation of body mass index, periodontitis and Tannerella forsythia. J Clin Periodontol 36: 89-99.

15. Perlstein MI, Bissada NF (1977) Influence of obesity and hypertension on the severity of periodontitis in rats. Oral Surg Oral Med Oral Pathol 43: 707-719.

16. Kim EJ, Jin BH, Bae KH (2011) Periodontitis and obesity: a study of the Fourth Korean National Health and Nutrition Examination Survey. J Periodontol 82: 533-542.

17. Al-Zahrani MS, Bissada NF, Borawskit EA (2003) Obesity and periodontal disease in young, middle-aged, and older adults. J Periodontol 74: 610-615.

18. Reeves AF, Rees JM, Schiff M, Hujoel P (2006) Total body weight and waist circumference associated with chronic periodontitis among adolescents in the United States. Arch Pediatr Adolesc Med 160: 894-899.

19. Chaffee BW, Weston SJ (2010) Association between chronic periodontal disease and obesity: a systematic review and meta-analysis. J Periodontol 81: 1708-1724.

20. Khader YS, Bawadi HA, Haroun TF, Alomari M, Tayyem RF (2009) The association between periodontal disease and obesity among adults in Jordan. J Clin Periodontol 36: 18-24.

21. Haslam DW, James WP (2005) Obesity. Lancet 366: 1197-1209.

22. Stumvoll M, Goldstein BJ, van Haeften TW (2005) Type 2 diabetes: principles of pathogenesis and therapy. Lancet 365: 1333-1346.

23. Pischon N, Heng N, Bernimoulin JP, Kleber BM, Willich SN, et al. (2007) Obesity, inflammation, and periodontal disease. J Dent Res 86: 400-409.

24. Saito T, Shimazaki Y (2007) Metabolic disorders related to obesity and periodontal disease. Periodontol 2000 43: 254-266.

25. Jagannathachary S, Kamaraj D (2010) Obesity and periodontal disease. J Indian Soc Periodontol 14: 96-100.

26. Beck JD, Offenbacher S (2005) Systemic effects of periodontitis: epidemiology of periodontal disease and cardiovascular disease. J Periodontol 76: 2089-2100.

27. Saxlin T, Suominen-Taipale L, Leiviskä J, Jula A, Knuuttila M, et al. (2009) Role of serum cytokines tumour necrosis factor-alpha and interleukin-6 in the association between body weight and periodontal infection. J Clin Periodontol 36: 100-105.

28. Yudkin JS, Kumari M, Humphries SE, Mohamed-Ali V (2000) Inflammation, obesity, stress and coronary heart disease: is interleukin-6 the link? Atherosclerosis 148: 209-214.

29. Dietrich T, Garcia RI (2005) Associations between periodontal disease and systemic disease: evaluating the strength of the evidence. J Periodontol 76: 2175-2184.

30. Mattila KJ, Pussinen PJ, Paju S (2005) Dental infections and cardiovascular diseases: a review. J Periodontol 76: 2085-2088.

37

The Metabolic Syndrome and Cardiovascular Diseases: An Update of Medical Treatment

Markolf Hanefeld[1], Frank Pistrosch[1], Jan Schulze[2] and Ulrike Rothe[3*]

[1]GWT-TUD GmbH, Study center Prof. Hanefeld, Dresden, Germany

[2]Saxonian Chamber of Physicians, Dresden, Germany

[3]Health Sciences/Public Health, Faculty of Medicine, TU Dresden, Germany

*Corresponding author: Ulrike Rothe, Health Sciences/Public Health, Faculty of Medicine Carl Gustav Carus, Technische Universität Dresden, Fetscherstrabe 74, D-01307 Dresden, Germany; E-mail: ulrike.rothe@tu-dresden.de

Abstract

The metabolic syndrome represents a cluster of closely connected premorbid risk factors or diseases with visceral obesity, prediabetes or type 2 diabetes, hypertension and low dyslipidemia as established traits affecting about 20 % of adults in developed countries. This syndrome develops on a common soil with overnutrition, low physical activity and psychosocial stress as major components. Common comorbidities are fatty liver, sleep apnoe and gout with cardiovascular complications, nephropathy and type 2 diabetes as 'endstage' diseases. The term metabolic vascular syndrome was proposed to signal premorbid cardiovascular state and increased cardiovascular morbidity. Thus, a rational diagnostic is needed to elucidate the complex cluster of diseases as basis for an integrated therapy. There is a clear priority for life style intervention however most diseases of the metabolic syndrome need medical treatment. Medical treatment of single traits has to take into account possible pleiotropic or adverse effects on the other traits. Here we present the pros and cons of major medical interventions in type 2 diabetes, hypertension, dyslipidemia and hypercoagulation in the context with the metabolic syndrome.

Keywords: Actigraphy; Sleep disorders; Attention deficit and hyperactivity disorder; Pediatric population

Introduction and Definition

Pre-diabetes or type 2 diabetes, hypertension and dyslipidemia are core components (Table1). Moreover, clinical manifestations include increased risk of non-alcoholic fatty liver (NAFLD), gout, sleep apnoe, depression cancer and sexual dysfunction. It is mainly caused by overeating together with low level of physical and socio-cultural activity in societies with a rapid transition to western life style and aging populations. The relationship between type 2 diabetes, hypertension and gout was first described by Maranon and Kylin [2] J. Vague in 1956 linked visceral (masculine) obesity to glucose intolerance and dyslipidemia what was later described as 'plurimetabolic syndrome' by G. Crepaldi [3,4]. In 1981 we gave a first definition of the metabolic syndrome: "By this term, we understand the simultaneous occurrence of obesity, hyper- and dyslipoproteinemia, maturity onset diabetes (type 2), gout, and hypertension, associated with an elevated incidence of atherosclerotic vascular diseases, fatty liver, and gallstones in overfed, physically inactive and genetically predisposed people" [5]. The rise of the metabolic syndrome into one of the most cited syndromes however started when G. Reaven presented insulin resistance as the common soil for type 2 diabetes, hypertension and dyslipidemia in his 1988 Banting Lecture and called it syndrome X, more or less as synonym for insulin resistance syndrome [6,7].With a rapid change in life-style around the globe a pandemic of the diseases of the metabolic syndrome was observed affecting 20 to 50 % of the adult population [8]. A first world-wide definition was published by the International Diabetes Federation (IDF) in 2006 [9] (Table 1) with the American Heart Association (AHA) /National Cholesterol Education Program III (NCEPIII) criteria as one of the most frequently used competitor which better meets cardiovascular risk [10]. To overcome confusion by too many competing definitions a unifying definition was developed in 2009 (Table 1) [11].

	AHA/ NCEP III	IDF	Consensus statement
Central obesity/waist	>102 cm (m) >88 cm (w)	≥ 94 cm (m, European) ≥ 90 cm (m, Asian) ≥ 80 cm (w)	Population and country specific increased waist circumference
Blood pressure (mmHg)	≥ 130/85 or treated for hypertension	≥ 130/85 or treated for hypertension	≥ 130/85 or treated for hypertension
Triglycerides (mmol/l)	≥ 1.7	≥ 1.7 or treatment	≥ 1.7 or treatment
HDL-cholesterol (mmol/l)	<1.03 (m), <1.29 (w)	<1.03 (m), <1.29 (w)	<1.03 (m), <1.29 (w) or treatment

		or treatment	
Fasting plasma glucose (mmol/l)	≥ 5.6	≥ 5.6 or diagnosed with diabetes mellitus	≥ 5.6 or drug treatment for elevated glucose

Table 1: Definition of the metabolic syndrome, AHA: American Heart Association, NCEP: National Cholesterol Education Program, IDF: International Diabetes Federation

Here we consider the metabolic syndrome as a cluster of premorbid risk factors and/or developed diseases with a common soil in malnutrition, lifestyle factors, socio-economic conditions and genetic predisposition. These conditions not only affect diseases of the metabolic syndrome but also interact with classical risk factors such as smoking and low-densitiy lipoprotein (LDL)-cholesterol. Recently increased inflammatory activity and endothelial dysfunction could be identified as components of the metabolic syndrome [12]. Therefore the term metabolic vascular syndrome was proposed to signal premorbid cardiovascular state and increased cardiovascular morbidity [13]. Type 2 diabetes and cardiovascular diseases thus may be considered as 'end stage' sickness of the metabolic syndrome [14]. With this in mind the metabolic syndrome provides an integrated approach for rational diagnostic and prevention of a broad spectrum of intricately connected diseases.

Pathophysiology

The metabolic syndrome rose to increased clinical consideration and scrutiny together with the worldwide epidemic of obesity and diabetes. However the pathophysiological mechanisms leading to this cluster of metabolic diseases and eventually cardiovascular complications are not completely understood [15]. Although insulin resistance is a core abnormality of individuals with metabolic syndrome [16], there is no sufficient evidence for a causal link between the two [17]. The most promising hypothesis for a single causal link between the development of the different traits of the metabolic syndrome and atherosclerosis is chronic low grade inflammation, particularly in dysfunctional adipose tissue [18]. The onset of abdominal obesity is central to the alteration of normal adipose tissue function with decreased glucose uptake, increased storage of fat as well as increased release of non esterified fatty acids (FFA) into the circulation. In obesity adipose tissue is infiltrated by macrophages which influence its cytokine production. There is an increased release of interleukin 6, tumor necrosis factor α (TNFα), monocyte chemo attractant protein 1 (MCP1) or C-reactive protein (CRP) whereas release of adiponectine is decreased. Whether the inflammatory response of the visceral adipose tissue is primarily induced by intracellular fat accumulation or by infiltration of activated macrophages is still a matter of debate [19]. Thus, the impact of changes in visceral adipose tissue can be summarized as a state of systemic lipotoxicity and low grade inflammation. Inflammatory cytokines are involved in the induction of endothelial dysfunction and insulin resistance [20]. Furthermore the insulin resistant state of obesity is characterised by increased plasma levels of free fatty acids that have cardiotoxic effects and impair the production of endothelial vasodilators [2,22].

In addition to these systemic effects of visceral obesity there is a local impairment of cardiac and vascular function by dysfunctional perivascular adipose tissue (PVAT) [23]. Under normal conditions PVAT produces different cytokines and hormones which contribute to vascular relaxation. In the obese state PVAT mass, like visceral adipose mass is increased and its anticontractile effects are diminished. Therefore PVAT in obesity may contribute to endothelial function and hence atherosclerosis and plays a key role in the development of vascular insulin resistance [24,25] .

A common hypothesis describes metabolic susceptibility as central factor for the development of the metabolic syndrome. This metabolic susceptibility is determined by polygenic variability of individuals [26] but also gene-environment interactions [20,27]. Once a sedentary lifestyle with decreased physical activity and high caloric intake leads to the acquisition of body fat and development of overweight and obesity, a susceptible individual is at high risk to develop the metabolic syndrome and cardiovascular consequences. Genome wide association studies have identified a lot of potential genetic variants that may contribute to development of metabolic syndrome, however, the complexity of its different single traits with their own genetic determinants is a major challenge for the genetic studies [28]. Despite this complex pathophysiology as soil for the metabolic syndrome and associated diseases, we also have to keep in mind the strong impact of lifestyle and environment which lead to epigenetic regulation such as the methylation of desoxyribonucleinacids (DNA) nucleotides and the modification of histone proteins surrounding the DNA double helix. These mechanisms as key regulators of gene expression can explain inter-individual variation of phenotypes [29]. Recent studies demonstrated a close relationship between intrauterine growth retardation and metabolic disease in adulthood. Low birth weight has also been associated with hypertension and susceptibility to cardiovascular diseases [30]. In addition to heritable regulation of the epigenome, there is also evidence of lifestyle-related modification of genes in adulthood [31].

A completely new area of metabolic and genetic research is the so called intestinal microbiome. Intestinal bacteria can influence immunological and inflammatory processes as well as gene expression within the intestinal wall. Animal studies demonstrated that gut microbiota can transfer metabolic diseases between individuals [32].

As a conclusion, there are several genetic and environmental factors which contribute to the development of both metabolic disorders which are summarized as metabolic syndrome and cardiovascular disease. It is conceivable that metabolic and cardiovascular disorders develop in parallel and and eventually interact in a vicious cycle. Therefore, the term metabolic vascular syndrome might be the most comprehensive description of this cluster of diseases [13].

Comorbidities and related cardiovascular risk factors

In the majority of cases which meet the criteria of the unifying definition or NCEPIII criteria we find comorbidities and cardiovascular risk factors which are summarized in Table 2. Among these broad spectrum NAFLD and albuminuria have been identified as major risk factors for both type 2 diabetes and cardiovascular disease

[33,34]. Therefore abdominal palpitation and ultrasound measurement of the liver and measurement of liver enzymes is good clinical practice in cases with metabolic vascular syndrome. The same applies for measurement of albumin to creatinine ratio in urine. However there don´t exist any specific complication or comorbidity. The majority of related risk factors can be linked to visceral obesity or ectopic fat but also can be found in single diseases such as hypertension or dyslipidemia. For example hypertriglyceridemia is associated with an increase in highly atherogenic small dense LDL. Risk scores (e.g. Prospective cardiovascular Muenster [PROCAM]-Score) are useful to support physician's decision making [13].

Fatty liver (NAFLD)
Hyperuricaemia/gout
Hypercoagulation/impaired fibrinolysis
Endothelial dysfunction , insulin resistance
Osteoporosis
Late hypogonadism
Sleep apnoe

Table 2: Frequent comorbidities and associated risk factors of the metabolic syndrome

Consequences for an integrated prevention of 'end-stage diseases'

Lifestyle intervention

From a clinical viewpoint type 2 diabetes and cardiovascular disease such as coronary heart disease, cerebrovascular disease and peripheral arterial disease can be considered as end-stage diseases developing on the complex prodiabetic and proatherogenic soil of the metabolic vascular syndrome. The rational of this concept is essential for lifestyle intervention and improving socio-economic conditions, avoiding stress exposure and as guide for regulation of food production and trade. This is a challenge for the whole society.

So far best evidence for modifiable risk factors for prevention of the metabolic vascular syndrome is available for changes in nutrition and increased physical activity to reduce overweight and insulin resistance. There exists now a bulk of evidence that with effective lifestyle intervention the incidence of type 2 diabetes can be reduced by about 50 % [35,36]. Lifestyle intervention trials with similar integrated approach including psychosomatic treatment tools – have also successfully been performed for the prevention, primary and secondary, of cardiovascular diseases [37-39].

Medical intervention balance – antihypertensive drugs

Subjects with the metabolic vascular syndrome are at high risk for development of cardiovascular events according to the Systematic Coronary Risk Evaluation (SCORE) model even if they have grade 1 hypertension [40]. International guidelines recommend systolic blood pressure control to a level <140 mmHg and diastolic blood pressure control to < 90 mmHg depending on age, individual risk and comorbidities with focus on kidney disease [13,41]. To reach this treatment goal 4 classes of antihypertensive drugs are recommended as first line treatment by the European Society of Hypertension/

European Society of Cardiology (ESH/ESC) guidelines: angiotensin converting enzyme (ACE) inhibitors/angiotensin II receptor (ARB) blockers, calcium channel blockers, beta blockers and diuretics. While blood pressure lowering effect and cardiovascular benefit is similar for these 4 classes of antihypertensive agents there are some differences in metabolic effects which should be considered in patients with the metabolic vascular syndrome. Beta blocker can increase body weight and – in combination with diuretics – the incidence of type 2 diabetes [13,42,43] however, newer beta blocker e.g. nebivolol and carvedilol did not affect insulin sensitivity and should therefore be preferred in patients with the metabolic vascular syndrome [44,45]. The ACCOMPLISH (Avoiding cardiovascular events in combination therapy in patients living with systolic hypertension) trial demonstrated a higher rate of cardiovascular events in patients receiving a combination therapy of a thiazide diuretic and an ACE inhibitor compared to patients with an ACE inhibitor/calcium channel blocker [46]. So far other randomized trials confirmed this superiority of calcium channel blocker over a diuretic treatment [41]. The use of thiazide diuretics can induce hypokalemia which may worsen glucose tolerance and provoke cardiac arrhythmias [47]. Due to their unfavourable metabolic effects beta blocker and diuretics should only be considered as additional blood pressure lowering drugs in metabolic syndrome in particular if free of vascular disease. If thiazide diuretics are used the addition of a potassium sparing diuretic agents could reduce the risk of hypokalemia [48].

ACE-inhibitor or ARB and calcium channel blocker should be preferred for the treatment of hypertension in patients with the metabolic vascular syndrome because they have no negative effect on insulin sensitivity or body weight. ACE-inhibitors/ARB are most effective in reducing proteinuria and preventing the progression of diabetic nephropathy whereas calcium channel blocker are the best choice for the prevention of stroke [49,50]. There is no evidence of an additional benefit of the newer ARB compared to ACE -inhibitors in patients with the metabolic vascular syndrome.

In the ONTARGET (Ongoing telmisartan alone and in combination with ramipril global endpoint) trial ARB telmisartan was associated with a significantly higher incidence of diabetes while no effect on primary objectives – major cardiovascular events was achieved [51]. In the HOPE (Heart outcomes prevention evaluation) study however with ACE inhibitor ramipril fewer patients were diagnosed with diabetes at the end of the study as in the placebo group 52. This could not be confirmed in the DREAM (Diabetes reduction assessment with ramipril and rosiglitazone medication) trial in people with impaired glucose tolerance where ramipril had no effect on the incidence of diabetes as a primary objective [53]. The same applies for ARB valsartan in the NAVIGATOR (Nateglinid and valsartan in impaired glucose tolerance outcomes research) trial – a prospective primary prevention study with cardiovascular complications as primary objective and diabetes as secondary objective [54].

To achieve blood pressure goals most patients need a combination therapy of 2 or more antihypertensive drugs. As recently recommended by the ESH/ESC Guidelines the initiation of a combination therapy instead of a monotherapy should be considered in patients with >160 mmHg systolic and/or >100 mmHg diastolic blood pressure. With combinations a prompter response in a larger number of patients to reach target blood pressure and a higher adherence of patients to the therapy was achieved [41]. Preferred drug combinations for initial treatment are that between ACE-inhibitor or ARB and calcium channel blocker whereas a combination of beta blocker and thiazide diuretic is not recommended as initial treatment for patients with the metabolic vascular syndrome [42].

In conclusion national and international guidelines recommend in patients with the metabolic vascular syndrome an individualized approach with age, comorbidities and presence or absence of end stage diseases as guide to decision.

Antidiabetic drugs

Evidence with antidiabetic drugs for the prevention of type 2 diabetes in people with abnormal glucose tolerance is available only for metformin [55], acarbose [56] and thiazolidinediones [57-59].

Metformin has consistent evidence to prevent progression of impaired glucose tolerance (IGT)/impaired fasting glucose (IFG) to type 2 diabetes. In the DPP Diabetes prevention program) sStudy the reduction in incidence of diabetes was 31% vs. 58% with lifestyle intervention alone [55]. The reduction of newly diagnosed diabetes in the STOP NIDDM (Study to prevent non-insulin-dependent diabetes mellitus) trial with α glucosidase inhibitor acarbose was in the same range if the same diagnostic criteria were used as in the DPP [56]. Despite glitazones were very effective to reduce incidence of newly diagnosed diabetes and had pleiotropic effects on blood pressure, biomarkers of inflammation and endothelial dysfunction [60-62] they cannot be recommended because of serious adverse effects such as edema, congestive heart failure and bone fractures for primary prevention of diseases of the metabolic vascular syndrome [63]. Orlistat, a weight reducing intestinal lipase inhibitor reduced incidence of diabetes in obese subjects with abnormal glucose tolerance by ~ 31 % [64]. Metformin in addition had beneficial effects on weight and minor effects on blood lipids, but did not affect blood pressure in the DPP 64 and BIGPRO (Treatment with metformin of non-diabetic men with hypertension, hypertriglyceridaemia and central fat distribution) trial [66]. However, none of the primary prevention trials with metformin has shown an effect on major cardiovascular events, even in the long term follow-up after termination of the studies [65]. Acarbose so far is the only antidiabetic drug with a significant pleiotropic effect on elevated blood pressure [67]. It significantly reduced body weight, postprandial hyperinsulinemia, biomarkers of inflammation and hypertriglyceridemia [68,69]. Predefined cardiovascular events were secondary objectives in the STOP-NIDDM trial. In this trial a significant reduction in the incidence of myocardial infarction and of overall predefined cardiovascular events was registered [67]. Furthermore, 36% less newly diagnosed cases of hypertension were observed. Of notice stable IGT or remission to NGT (normal glucose tolerance) was associated with a lower incidence of hypertension compared to progresses to type 2 diabetes [69]. In subjects with metabolic vascular syndrome the number needed to treat to prevent one case of diabetes was 5.8 versus ~16.5 in people without diabetes 71 (Figure 1). Intervention with basal insulin glargine in prediabetic subjects was evaluated in the ORIGIN (Outcome reduction with initial glargine intervention) trial. Reduction of newly diagnosed diabetes after 3 months stop of insulin treatment was 20 %. There was however no effect on major cardiovascular events achieved [72]. In conclusion, except for acarbose no evidence is available for glucose lowering treatment in subjects with prediabetes to prevent cardiovascular end stage diseases.

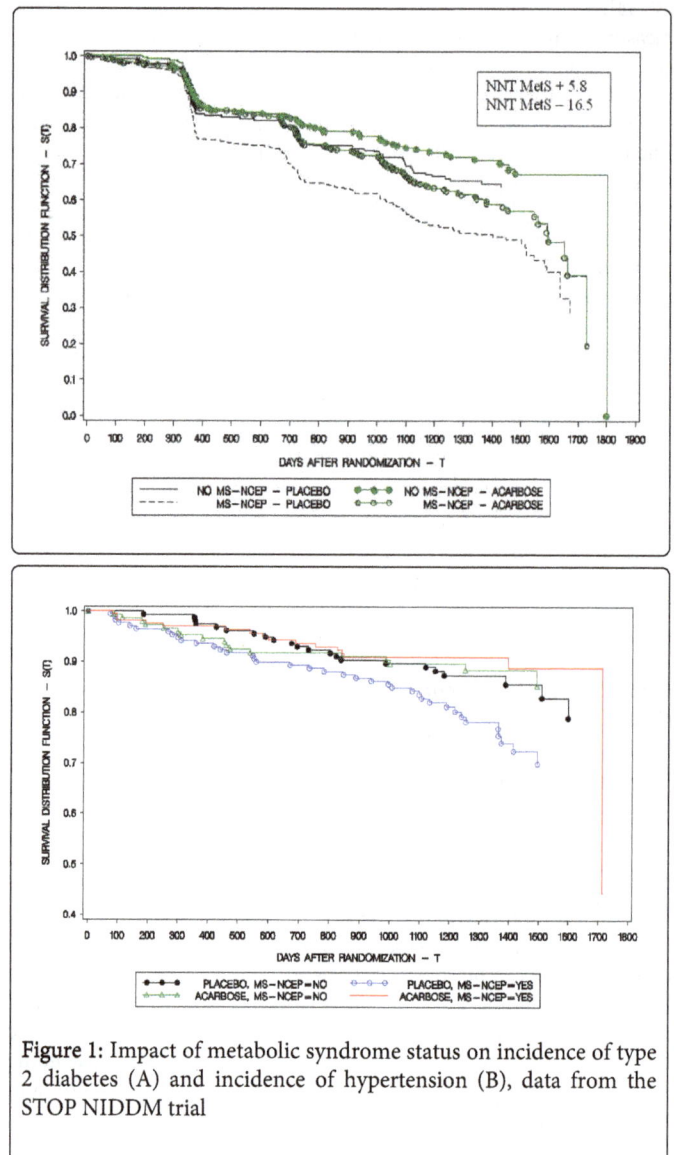

Figure 1: Impact of metabolic syndrome status on incidence of type 2 diabetes (A) and incidence of hypertension (B), data from the STOP NIDDM trial

Lipid lowering drugs

Dyslipidemia with hypertriglyceridemia and low high density lipoprotein (HDL) is in the majority of cases associated with an increase in small dense LDL, a lipoprotein subfraction with high atherogenic potential which is intricately connected with insulin resistance and low grade inflammation (Figure 2) [73]. This lipid triad together with high cardiovascular risk provides a rational pathophysiological basis for the use of statins as first line drug. Statins have a grade I evidence for primary [74,75] and secondary [76,77] prevention of cardiovascular disease. In the case of dyslipidemia with hypertriglyceridemia/low HDL they can be used in combination with fibrates. In the ACCORD (Action to Control Cardiovascular Risk in Diabetes) trial [78] and FIELD (Fenofibrate Intervention and Event Lowering in Diabetes) [79] in patients with hypertriglyceridemia fenofibrate had an additional beneficial effect on cardiovascular outcome when used in combination with statins. As shown in a metaanalysis of data from 170000 participants with intensive statin treatment reduction of cardiovascular events was mainly due to LDL-cholesterol lowering efficacy [80]. However in the JUPITER

(Justification for the use of statin in prevention: an intervention trial evaluating rosuvastatin) study in patients with elevated high sensitive C-reactive protein (hsCRP) but LDL-cholesterol in the normal range rosuvastatin, one of the strong statins, reduced major cardiovascular events versus placebo [81]. Beneficial effects on the lipid triad in patients with the metabolic vascular syndrome have been documented for atorvastatin and rosuvastatin [8,83]. In long term studies, however, statins increased the risk of newly diagnosed diabetes [83]. This is far outweighted by the cardiovascular benefit. In a metaanalysis intensive dose statin therapy had a number needed to harm for one case of new onset diabetes of 498 versus a number needed to prevent one case of major cardiovascular events of 155 per year [84]. In addition statin treatment has a small but significant beneficial effect on blood pressure [85].

Fibrates have been shown to reduce cardiovascular events in patients with the metabolic vascular syndrome and type 2 diabetes [78,79]. The Helsinki Heart Study (HHS) and VAHIT (Veterans Affairs High-Density Lipoprotein Cholesterol Intervention Trial) study have demonstrated a significant reduction of cardiovascular events in patients with dyslipidemia and metabolic vascular syndrome treated with gemfibrozil versus placebo [86-88]. Gemfibrozil, however, is contraindicated for combination with statins because of high rates of myopathies and increased risk of rhabdomyolysis [89]. Low HDL is an established trait of the metabolic syndrome in all definitions (Table 1). However the concept to increase HDL-cholesterol to protect the vessel wall was not supported by recently published trials with nicotinic acid [90] and cholesteryl ester transfer protein (CETP) inhibitors [91,92] showing increased rates of serious adverse events but no benefit for primary objectives. Therefore, ESC Guidelines no longer support drug interventions to increase HDL-cholesterol [92].

The ESH recommends are careful diagnostic of all parameters of the metabolic vascular syndrome in all patients with hypertension. In these individuals premorbid risk factors of the metabolic vascular syndrome are common inclusive the lipid triad, albuminurea and elevated hsCRP. This clustering of risk factors can be used as a guide to prescription of statins [41].

Anticoagulatory treatment

Patients with a metabolic vascular syndrome have a complex pathophysiology of cellular and humoral coagulation with activated platelet aggregation, impaired fibrinolysis and elevated factors of the coagulation cascade as major components. This is particularly critical in patients with type 2 diabetes [94,95]. Subjects with diabetes have a higher rate of major cardiovascular events but inferior outcomes and effects of intervention after acute coronary syndrome [96]. This can be at least partially explained by harmful alterations in the coagulation associated with the metabolic syndrome. According to this critical weight of atherothrombogenic risk factors randomised trials and meta analysis revealed a greater benefit of anticoagulatory prevention for patients with diabetes and metabolic vascular syndrome.

Acetyl salicylic acid (aspirin) is widely used for secondary prevention in type 2 diabetes. Recently published metaanalysis however reveal no significant impact on mortality while bleeding episodes are significantly increased [97,98]. No positive outcome data on primary prevention are available for aspirin and the new platelet aggregation inhibitors such as clopidogrel, prasugrel and ticagrelor. The benefit of low dose aspirin (75-100 mg/d) for secondary prevention is well documented for patients with type 2 diabetes [97]. In the CAPRIE (Clopidogrel versus aspirin in patients at risk of ischaemic events) study clopidogrel 74 mg was significantly more effective in patients with type 2 diabetes compared to aspirin [99]. Incidence of major cardiovascular events (MACE) with clopidogrel was 5.32 %, with aspirin 5.83 % (RR 8.7 %, p=0.043). Benefit of clopidogrel was even higher in patients with peripheral arterial disease. Therefore, the American Diabetes Association (ADA) recommends clopidogrel in very high risk groups with type 2 diabetes. This could be applied in general for type 2 diabetes with metabolic vascular syndrome. New platelet aggregation inhibitors prasugrel and ticagrelor have shown a significantly higher benefit in acute coronary syndrome versus clopidogrel [100], however, large outcome trials in patients with stable atherosclerotic disease are not yet published. Diabetes is an independent risk factor for atrial fibrillation and thrombolic complications. Therefore, risk scores for stroke and systemic embolism result in an indication for anticoagulant therapy with vitamin K antagonists (cumarins) or direct-acting oral anticoagulants (apixaban, dabigatran, rivaroxaban). No data from controlled prospective trials are available in diabetes comparing old and new anticoagulants.

Conclusion

In conclusion, a rational diagnostic is needed to elucidate the complex cluster of diseases as basis for an integrated therapy by using synergistic and pleiotropic effects to avoid polypharmacy which is written down in the new German Guideline Metabolic Vascular Syndrome [13].

Future directions

In the process of globalization with a rapid transition from traditional life habits to westernized life style in developing countries and aging societies in developed countries we will see a further increase in patients with the metabolic vascular syndrome. There is a common soil of malnutrition and inertia which gives a priority to life style intervention for the whole society. The components of the metabolic vascular syndrome and associated risk factors can be used as a simple guide for an individualized medical treatment approach to use synergistic effects of drugs and avoid counterproductive adverse effects.

Acknowledgements

We will gratefully acknowledge all authors of the Guideline Metabolic Vascular Syndrome and the Chamber of Physicians in Saxony (Sächsische Landes-ärztekammer, Fachkommission Diabetes) for their input.

References

1. Maranon G (1922) Über Hypertonie und Zuckerkrankheit. Z Inn Med. 43: 169-176.

2. Kylin O (1923) Studien ueber das Hypertonie-Hyperglykaemie-Hyperurikaemiesyndrom. Zentralblatt Inn Med 44: 105-127.

3. VAGUE J (1956) The degree of masculine differentiation of obesities: a factor determining predisposition to diabetes, atherosclerosis, gout, and uric calculous disease. Am J Clin Nutr 4: 20-34.

4. Avagaro P, Nadin C (1967) Association of hyperlipidemia, diabetes mellitus and obesity. Acta Diabetol Let. 4: 572-590.

5. Hanefeld M, Leonhardt W (1981) Das Metabolische Syndrom. Deutsche Gesundheit Wesen 36: 545-552.

6.   Reaven GM (1988) Banting lecture 1988. Role of insulin resistance in human disease. Diabetes 37: 1595-1607.

7.   Ferrannini E (1997) Insulin resistance is central to the burden of diabetes. Diabetes Metab Rev 13: 81-86.

8.   Hu G, Qiao Q, Tuomilehto J, Balkau B, Borch-Johnsen K, et al. (2004) Prevalence of the metabolic syndrome and its relation to all-cause and cardiovascular mortality in nondiabetic European men and women. Arch Intern Med 164: 1066-1076.

9.   Alberti KG, Zimmet P, Shaw J (2006) Metabolic syndrome--a new worldwide definition. A Consensus Statement from the International Diabetes Federation. Diabet Med 23: 469-480.

10.   Expert Panel on Detection, Evaluation, and Treatment of High Blood Cholesterol in Adults (2001) Executive Summary of The Third Report of The National Cholesterol Education Program (NCEP) Expert Panel on Detection, Evaluation, And Treatment of High Blood Cholesterol In Adults (Adult Treatment Panel III). JAMA 285: 2486-2497.

11.   Alberti KG, Eckel RH, Grundy SM (2009) Harmonizing the metabolic syndrome: a joint interim statement of the International Diabetes Federation Task Force on Epidemiology and Prevention; National Heart, Lung, and Blood Institute; American Heart Association; World Heart Federation; International Atherosclerosis Society; and International Association for the Study of Obesity. Circulation 120: 1640-1645.

12.   Huang JW, Yang CY, Wu HY, Liu KL, Su CT, et al. (2013) Metabolic syndrome and abdominal fat are associated with inflammation, but not with clinical outcomes, in peritoneal dialysis patients. Cardiovasc Diabetol 12: 86.

13.   Hanefeld M, Rothe U, Fischer S, Scholz GH, Schulze J, et al. (2007) The German Guideline Metabolic Vascular Syndrome. TUD and Academia for Health Saxonia (AGS) (in press).

14.   Hanefeld M, Koehler C, Gallo S, et al. (2007) Impact of the individual components of the metabolic syndrome and their different combinations on the prevalence of atherosclerotic vascular disease in type 2 diabetes: the Diabetes in Germany (DIG) study. Cardiovasc Diabetol. 6: 13.

15.   Grundy SM (2007) Metabolic syndrome: a multiplex cardiovascular risk factor. J Clin Endocrinol Metab 92: 399-404.

16.   Reaven GM (1993) Role of insulin resistance in human disease (syndrome X): an expanded definition. Annu Rev Med 44: 121-131.

17.   Cornier MA, Dabelea D, Hernandez TL, Lindstrom RC, Steig AJ, et al. (2008) The metabolic syndrome. Endocr Rev 29: 777-822.

18.   Hotamisligil GS (2006) Inflammation and metabolic disorders. Nature 444: 860-867.

19.   Bouloumié A, Casteilla L, Lafontan M (2008) Adipose tissue lymphocytes and macrophages in obesity and insulin resistance: makers or markers, and which comes first? Arterioscler Thromb Vasc Biol 28: 1211-1213.

20.   Du X, Edelstein D, Obici S, Higham N, Zou MH, et al. (2006) Insulin resistance reduces arterial prostacyclin synthase and eNOS activities by increasing endothelial fatty acid oxidation. J Clin Invest 116: 1071-1080.

21.   Rutter MK, Parise H, Benjamin EJ, Levy D, Larson MG, et al. (2003) Impact of glucose intolerance and insulin resistance on cardiac structure and function: sex-related differences in the Framingham Heart Study. Circulation 107: 448-454.

22.   Lehman SJ, Massaro JM, Schlett CL, O'Donnell CJ, Hoffmann U, et al. (2010) Peri-aortic fat, cardiovascular disease risk factors, and aortic calcification: the Framingham Heart Study. Atherosclerosis 210: 656-661.

23.   Payne GA, Borbouse L, Kumar S (2010) Epicardial perivascular adipose-derived leptin exacerbates coronary endothelial dysfunction in metabolic syndrome via a protein kinase C-beta pathway. Arterioscler Thromb Vasc Biol 30: 1711-1717.

24.   Meijer RI, Bakker W, Alta CL, Sipkema P, Yudkin JS, et al. (2013) Perivascular adipose tissue control of insulin-induced vasoreactivity in muscle is impaired in db/db mice. Diabetes 62: 590-598.

25.   Dastani Z, Hivert MF, Timpson N, Perry JR, Yuan X, et al. (2012) Novel loci for adiponectin levels and their influence on type 2 diabetes and metabolic traits: a multi-ethnic meta-analysis of 45,891 individuals. PLoS Genet 8: e1002607.

26.   Neeland IJ, Turer AT, Ayers CR, Powell-Wiley TM, Vega GL, et al. (2012) Dysfunctional adiposity and the risk of prediabetes and type 2 diabetes in obese adults. JAMA 308: 1150-1159.

27.   Sookoian S, Pirola CJ (2011) Metabolic syndrome: from the genetics to the pathophysiology. Curr Hypertens Rep. 13: 149-57.

28.   Fraga MF, Ballestar E, Paz MF et al. (2005) Epigenetic differences arise during the lifetime of monozygotic twins. Proc Natl Acad Sci. U.S.A 102:10604-09.

29.   Luyckx VA, Bertram JF, Brenner BM, Fall C, Hoy WE, et al. (2013) Effect of fetal and child health on kidney development and long-term risk of hypertension and kidney disease. Lancet 382: 273-283.

30.   Barrès R, Yan J, Egan B, Treebak JT, Rasmussen M, et al. (2012) Acute exercise remodels promoter methylation in human skeletal muscle. Cell Metab 15: 405-411.

31.   Burcelin R, Serino M, Chabo C, Blasco-Baque V, Amar J (2011) Gut microbiota and diabetes: from pathogenesis to therapeutic perspective. Acta Diabetol 48: 257-273.

32.   Asrih M, Jornayvaz FR (2013) Inflammation as a potential link between nonalcoholic fatty liver disease and insulin resistance. J Endocrinol 218: R25-36.

33.   Wall BM (2010) Cardiorenal risk factors. Am J Med Sci 340: 25-29.

34.   Tuomilehto J, Lindström J, Eriksson JG, Valle TT, Hämäläinen H, et al. (2001) Prevention of type 2 diabetes mellitus by changes in lifestyle among subjects with impaired glucose tolerance. N Engl J Med 344: 1343-1350.

35.   Grundy SM (2012) Pre-diabetes, metabolic syndrome, and cardiovascular risk. J Am Coll Cardiol 59: 635-643.

36.   Estruch R, Ros E, Salas-Salvadó J, Covas MI, Corella D, et al. (2013) Primary prevention of cardiovascular disease with a Mediterranean diet. N Engl J Med 368: 1279-1290.

37.   Ornish D, Brown SE, Scherwitz LW, Billings JH, Armstrong WT, et al. (1990) Can lifestyle changes reverse coronary heart disease? The Lifestyle Heart Trial. 336: 129-133.

38.   Ornish D, Brown SE, Scherwitz LW, Billings JH, Armstrong WT, et al. (1990) Can lifestyle changes reverse coronary heart disease? The Lifestyle Heart Trial. Lancet 336: 129-133.

39.   Mente A, de Koning L, Shannon HS, Anand SS (2009) A systematic review of the evidence supporting a causal link between dietary factors and coronary heart disease. Arch Intern Med 169: 659-669.

40.   Conroy RM, Pyörälä K, Fitzgerald AP, Sans S, Menotti A, et al. (2003) Estimation of ten-year risk of fatal cardiovascular disease in Europe: the SCORE project. Eur Heart J 24: 987-1003.

41.   Mancia G, Fagard R, Narkiewicz K, (2013) 2013 ESH/ESC Guidelines for the management of arterial hypertension: the Task Force for the management of arterial hypertension of the European Society of Hypertension (ESH) and of the European Society of Cardiology (ESC). J Hypertens. 31: 1281-1357.

42.   Sharma AM, Pischon T, Hardt S, Kunz I, Luft FC (2001) Hypothesis: Beta-adrenergic receptor blockers and weight gain: A systematic analysis. Hypertension 37: 250-254.

43.   Elliott WJ, Meyer PM (2007) Incident diabetes in clinical trials of antihypertensive drugs: a network meta-analysis. Lancet 369: 201-207.

44.   Bakris GL, Fonseca V, Katholi RE, McGill JB, Messerli FH, et al. (2004) Metabolic effects of carvedilol vs metoprolol in patients with type 2 diabetes mellitus and hypertension: a randomized controlled trial. JAMA 292: 2227-2236.

45.   Celik T, Iyisoy A, Kursaklioglu H, Kardesoglu E, Kilic S, et al. (2006) Comparative effects of nebivolol and metoprolol on oxidative stress, insulin resistance, plasma adiponectin and soluble P-selectin levels in hypertensive patients. J Hypertens 24: 591-596.

46.   Jamerson K, Weber MA, Bakris GL (2008) Benazepril plus amlodipine or hydrochlorothiazide for hypertension in high-risk patients. N Engl J Med 359:2417-2428.

47. Shafi T, Appel LJ, Miller ER 3rd, Klag MJ, Parekh RS (2008) Changes in serum potassium mediate thiazide-induced diabetes. Hypertension 52: 1022-1029.

48. Stears AJ, Woods SH, Watts MM, Burton TJ, Graggaber J, et al. (2012) A double-blind, placebo-controlled, crossover trial comparing the effects of amiloride and hydrochlorothiazide on glucose tolerance in patients with essential hypertension. Hypertension 59: 934-942.

49. Verdecchia P, Reboldi G, Angeli F, Gattobigio R, Bentivoglio M, et al. (2005) Angiotensin-converting enzyme inhibitors and calcium channel blockers for coronary heart disease and stroke prevention. Hypertension 46: 386-392.

50. Bakris GL, Sarafidis PA, Weir MR (2010) Renal outcomes with different fixed-dose combination therapies in patients with hypertension at high risk for cardiovascular events (ACCOMPLISH): a prespecified secondary analysis of a randomised controlled trial. Lancet 375: 1173-1181.

51. Yusuf S, Teo KK, Pogue J (2008) Telmisartan, ramipril, or both in patients at high risk for vascular events. N Engl J Med 358:1547-59.

52. Yusuf S, Sleight P, Pogue J (2000) Effects of an angiotensin-converting-enzyme inhibitor, ramipril, on cardiovascular events in high-risk patients. The Heart Outcomes Prevention Evaluation Study Investigators. N Engl J Med 342: 145-153.

53. DREAM Trial Investigators, Bosch J, Yusuf S, Gerstein HC, Pogue J, et al. (2006) Effect of ramipril on the incidence of diabetes. N Engl J Med 355: 1551-1562.

54. NAVIGATOR Study Group, McMurray JJ, Holman RR, Haffner SM, Bethel MA, et al. (2010) Effect of valsartan on the incidence of diabetes and cardiovascular events. N Engl J Med 362: 1477-1490.

55. Knowler WC, Barrett-Connor E, Fowler SE, et al. (2002) Reduction in the incidence of type 2 diabetes with lifestyle intervention or metformin. N Engl J Med 346: 393-403.

56. Chiasson JL, Josse RG, Gomis R, Hanefeld M, Karasik A, et al. (2002) Acarbose for prevention of type 2 diabetes mellitus: the STOP-NIDDM randomised trial. Lancet 359: 2072-2077.

57. DREAM On (Diabetes Reduction Assessment with Ramipril and Rosiglitazone Medication Ongoing Follow-up) Investigators, Gerstein HC, Mohan V, Avezum A, Bergenstal RM, et al. (2011) Long-term effect of rosiglitazone and/or ramipril on the incidence of diabetes. Diabetologia 54: 487-495.

58. Defronzo RA, Tripathy D, Schwenke DC, Banerji M, Bray GA, et al. (2013) Prevention of diabetes with pioglitazone in ACT NOW: physiologic correlates. Diabetes 62: 3920-3926.

59. Zinman B, Harris SB, Neuman J, Gerstein HC, Retnakaran RR, et al. (2010) Low-dose combination therapy with rosiglitazone and metformin to prevent type 2 diabetes mellitus (CANOE trial): a double-blind randomised controlled study. Lancet 376: 103-111.

60. Hanefeld M, Marx N, Pfützner A, Baurecht W, Lübben G, et al. (2007) Anti-inflammatory effects of pioglitazone and/or simvastatin in high cardiovascular risk patients with elevated high sensitivity C-reactive protein: the PIOSTAT Study. J Am Coll Cardiol 49: 290-297.

61. Pistrosch F, Passauer J, Herbrig K, Schwanebeck U, Gross P, et al. (2012) Effect of thiazolidinedione treatment on proteinuria and renal hemodynamic in type 2 diabetic patients with overt nephropathy. Horm Metab Res 44: 914-918.

62. Pistrosch F, Passauer J, Fischer S, Fuecker K, Hanefeld M, et al. (2004) In type 2 diabetes, rosiglitazone therapy for insulin resistance ameliorates endothelial dysfunction independent of glucose control. Diabetes Care 27: 484-490.

63. Kung J, Henry RR (2012) Thiazolidinedione safety. Expert Opin Drug Saf 11: 565-579.

64. Torgerson JS, Hauptman J, Boldrin MN, Sjöström L (2004) XENical in the prevention of diabetes in obese subjects (XENDOS) study: a randomized study of orlistat as an adjunct to lifestyle changes for the prevention of type 2 diabetes in obese patients. Diabetes Care 27: 155-161.

65. Diabetes Prevention Program Outcomes Study Research Group, Orchard TJ, Temprosa M, Barrett-Connor E, Fowler SE, et al. (2013) Long-term effects of the Diabetes Prevention Program interventions on cardiovascular risk factors: a report from the DPP Outcomes Study. Diabet Med 30: 46-55.

66. Charles MA, Eschwège E, Grandmottet P, Isnard F, Cohen JM, et al. (2000) Treatment with metformin of non-diabetic men with hypertension, hypertriglyceridaemia and central fat distribution: the BIGPRO 1.2 trial. Diabetes Metab Res Rev 16: 2-7.

67. Chiasson JL, Josse RG, Gomis R, Hanefeld M, Karasik A, et al. (2003) Acarbose treatment and the risk of cardiovascular disease and hypertension in patients with impaired glucose tolerance: the STOP-NIDDM trial. JAMA 290: 486-494.

68. Rudofsky G Jr, Reismann P, Schiekofer S, Petrov D, von Eynatten M, et al. (2004) Reduction of postprandial hyperglycemia in patients with type 2 diabetes reduces NF-kappaB activation in PBMCs. Horm Metab Res 36: 630-638.

69. Hanefeld M, Cagatay M, Petrowitsch T, Neuser D, Petzinna D, et al. (2004) Acarbose reduces the risk for myocardial infarction in type 2 diabetic patients: meta-analysis of seven long-term studies. Eur Heart J 25: 10-16.

70. Hanefeld M, Pistrosch F, Koehler C, Chiasson JL (2012) Conversion of IGT to type 2 diabetes mellitus is associated with incident cases of hypertension: a post-hoc analysis of the STOP-NIDDM trial. J Hypertens 30: 1440-1443.

71. Hanefeld M, Karasik A, Koehler C, Westermeier T, Chiasson JL (2009) Metabolic syndrome and its single traits as risk factors for diabetes in people with impaired glucose tolerance: the STOP-NIDDM trial. Diab Vasc Dis Res 6: 32-37.

72. ORIGIN Trial Investigators, Gerstein HC, Bosch J, Dagenais GR, Díaz R, et al. (2012) Basal insulin and cardiovascular and other outcomes in dysglycemia. N Engl J Med 367: 319-328.

73. Terán-García M, Bouchard C (2007) Genetics of the metabolic syndrome. Appl Physiol Nutr Metab 32: 89-114.

74. Taylor F, Huffman MD, Macedo AF, Moore TH, Burke M, et al. (2013) Statins for the primary prevention of cardiovascular disease. Cochrane Database Syst Rev 1: CD004816.

75. Tonelli M, Lloyd A, Clement F, Conly J, Husereau D, et al. (2011) Efficacy of statins for primary prevention in people at low cardiovascular risk: a meta-analysis. CMAJ 183: E1189-1202.

76. Yusuf S, Islam S, Chow CK, Rangarajan S, Dagenais G, et al. (2011) Use of secondary prevention drugs for cardiovascular disease in the community in high-income, middle-income, and low-income countries (the PURE Study): a prospective epidemiological survey. Lancet 378: 1231-1243.

77. Spector R, Snapinn SM (2011) Statins for secondary prevention of cardiovascular disease: the right dose. Pharmacology 87: 63-69.

78. Tonkin AM, Chen L (2010) Effects of combination lipid therapy in the management of patients with type 2 diabetes mellitus in the Action to Control Cardiovascular Risk in Diabetes (ACCORD) trial. Circulation 122: 850-852.

79. Burgess DC, Hunt D, Li L, Zannino D, Williamson E, et al. (2010) Incidence and predictors of silent myocardial infarction in type 2 diabetes and the effect of fenofibrate: an analysis from the Fenofibrate Intervention and Event Lowering in Diabetes (FIELD) study. Eur Heart J 31: 92-99.

80. Cholesterol Treatment Trialistsa™ (CTT) Collaboration, Baigent C, Blackwell L, Emberson J, Holland LE, et al. (2010) Efficacy and safety of more intensive lowering of LDL cholesterol: a meta-analysis of data from 170,000 participants in 26 randomised trials. Lancet 376: 1670-1681.

81. Ridker PM, Danielson E, Fonseca FA.(2008) Rosuvastatin to prevent vascular events in men and women with elevated C-reactive protein. N.Engl.J.Med 359:2195-207.

82. Ooi EM, Watts GF, Chan DC, Chen MM, Nestel PJ, et al. (2008) Dose-dependent effect of rosuvastatin on VLDL-apolipoprotein C-III kinetics in the metabolic syndrome. Diabetes Care 31: 1656-1661.

83. Rosenson RS, Otvos JD, Hsia J (2009) Effects of rosuvastatin and atorvastatin on LDL and HDL particle concentrations in patients with

metabolic syndrome: a randomized, double-blind, controlled study. Diabetes Care 32: 1087-1091.

84. Preiss D, Seshasai SR, Welsh P, Murphy SA, Ho JE, et al. (2011) Risk of incident diabetes with intensive-dose compared with moderate-dose statin therapy: a meta-analysis. JAMA 305: 2556-2564.

85. Strazzullo P, Kerry SM, Barbato A, Versiero M, D'Elia L, et al. (2007) Do statins reduce blood pressure?: a meta-analysis of randomized, controlled trials. Hypertension 49: 792-798.

86. Tenkanen L, Mänttäri M, Kovanen PT, Virkkunen H, Manninen V (2006) Gemfibrozil in the treatment of dyslipidemia: an 18-year mortality follow-up of the Helsinki Heart Study. Arch Intern Med 166: 743-748.

87. Frick MH, Elo O, Haapa K, Heinonen OP, Heinsalmi P, et al. (1987) Helsinki Heart Study: primary-prevention trial with gemfibrozil in middle-aged men with dyslipidemia. Safety of treatment, changes in risk factors, and incidence of coronary heart disease. N Engl J Med 317: 1237-1245.

88. Rubins HB, Robins SJ, Collins D (1999) Gemfibrozil for the secondary prevention of coronary heart disease in men with low levels of high-density lipoprotein cholesterol. Veterans Affairs High-Density Lipoprotein Cholesterol Intervention Trial Study Group. N Engl J Med 341: 410-418.

89. Davidson MH, Armani A, McKenney JM, Jacobson TA (2007) Safety considerations with fibrate therapy. Am J Cardiol 99: 3C-18C.

90. AIM-HIGH Investigators, Boden WE, Probstfield JL, Anderson T, Chaitman BR, et al. (2011) Niacin in patients with low HDL cholesterol levels receiving intensive statin therapy. N Engl J Med 365: 2255-2267.

91. Schwartz GG, Olsson AG, Abt M, Ballantyne CM, Barter PJ, et al. (2012) Effects of dalcetrapib in patients with a recent acute coronary syndrome. N Engl J Med 367: 2089-2099.

92. Barter PJ, Caulfield M, Eriksson M, Grundy SM, Kastelein JJ, et al. (2007) Effects of torcetrapib in patients at high risk for coronary events. N Engl J Med 357: 2109-2122.

93. Catapano AL, Reiner Z, De Backer G, Graham I, Taskinen MR, et al. (2011) ESC/EAS Guidelines for the management of dyslipidaemias The Task Force for the management of dyslipidaemias of the European Society of Cardiology (ESC) and the European Atherosclerosis Society (EAS). Atherosclerosis 217: 3-46.

94. Gawaz M, Langer H, May AE (2005) Platelets in inflammation and atherogenesis. J Clin Invest 115: 3378-3384.

95. Randriamboavonjy V, Fleming I (2012) Platelet function and signaling in diabetes mellitus. Curr Vasc Pharmacol 10: 532-538.

96. Donahoe SM, Stewart GC, McCabe CH, Mohanavelu S, Murphy SA, et al. (2007) Diabetes and mortality following acute coronary syndromes. JAMA 298: 765-775.

97. Antithrombotic Trialists' (ATT) Collaboration, Baigent C, Blackwell L, Collins R, Emberson J, et al. (2009) Aspirin in the primary and secondary prevention of vascular disease: collaborative meta-analysis of individual participant data from randomised trials. Lancet 373: 1849-1860.

98. Seshasai SR, Wijesuriya S, Sivakumaran R, Nethercott S, Erqou S, et al. (2012) Effect of aspirin on vascular and nonvascular outcomes: meta-analysis of randomized controlled trials. Arch Intern Med 172: 209-216.

99. Bhatt DL, Marso SP, Hirsch AT, Ringleb PA, Hacke W, et al. (2002) Amplified benefit of clopidogrel versus aspirin in patients with diabetes mellitus. Am J Cardiol 90: 625-628.

100. Wallentin L, Becker RC, Budaj A, Cannon CP, Emanuelsson H, et al. (2009) Ticagrelor versus clopidogrel in patients with acute coronary syndromes. N Engl J Med 361: 1045-1057.

38

Stimulation of Glycolysis in the Lens by Pyruvate: Implications in Protection against Oxidative Stress

Kavita R Hegde[1,3*] and Sambhu D Varma[1,2]

[1]Department of Ophthalmology and Visual Sciences, University of Maryland School of Medicine, Baltimore, USA

[2]Department of Biochemistry and Molecular Biology, University of Maryland School of Medicine, Baltimore, USA

[3]Department of Natural Sciences, Coppin State University, Baltimore, USA

*Corresponding author: Kavita Hegde, Associate Professor, Department of Natural Sciences, Coppin State University, West North Avenue, Baltimore, United States; E-mail: khegde@coppin.edu

Abstract

Objective: We have previously demonstrated that pyruvate protects the lens against oxidative stress *in vitro* as well as prevents cataract formation *in vivo* induced by oxidative stress. The effects have been attributed to its property of scavenging various reactive oxygen species (ROS). Additionally we hypothesize that the preventive effect is also due to its effect of stimulating glycolysis.

Methods: This has been tested as follows: freshly isolated mice lenses were incubated for 4 hours in Tyrode medium containing 5-^{3}H-glucose as a tracer in the presence and absence of 2 mM sodium pyruvate and determining generation of ^3H2O and ^3H-lactate separated by column chromatography in succession through homemade anion exchange column followed by the phenylboronate and formate mini-columns.

Results: the concentration of ^3H_2O in the medium at the end of incubation was 95 µM in the controls incubated without pyruvate. In the presence of pyruvate (2 mM) added to the medium, the concentration of ^3H_2O attained in the medium was 152 µM. The corresponding value expressed on the basis of lens weight was 46 nanomoles/lens in the control group vs. 88 nanomoles/lens with 2 mM pyruvate.

Conclusion: As hypothesized, pyruvate was found to stimulate glycolysis in the lens as indicated by the enhanced generation of both ^3H_2O and ^3H-lactate in lenses incubated in its presence as compared to controls. The observed metabolic stimulation is attributed to recycling of NAD generated during the reduction of pyruvate to lactate, NAD being the required cofactor in the oxidation of glyceraldehyde-3-phosphate to 1,3-diphosphoglycerate. That such stimulation is involved in its protective effect is also apparent by our previous reports showing higher ATP levels in the lenses cultured in medium generating ROS in the presence of pyruvate than in its absence, the primary source of ATP in lens being glycolysis.

Keywords Glycolysis; Tritiated glucose; Tritiated lactate; Tritiated water; Pyruvate; Oxidative stress; Ion exchange chromatography; Phenylboronate column; NAD/NADH

Introduction

Generation of reactive oxygen species (ROS) in aqueous humor and lens is well-known to induce oxidative stress to the tissue and consequent cataract formation [1,2]. Such species are also implicated in the pathogenesis of many other aging diseases. Although ROS can be generated by several ambient oxidation reactions such as the metal catalyzed auto-oxidation of ascorbate and –SH containing proteins and glutathione, as well as the leakage of electrons during their transport through the cytochrome chain and its capture by molecular oxygen, the process is significantly augmented in the eye by several photochemically induced pseudocatalytic reactions [3]. Hence, continued penetration of light into the eye, though necessary for vision, has an unwanted side effect of causing aberrant oxidations that lead to many subsequent adverse physiologic and metabolic consequences. Such an effect assumes a greater significance at higher light intensities, especially of the UV frequencies. The visible

frequencies can also initiate ROS generation by activation of various redox susceptible components that have absorption maxima in the visible range, such as kynurenine and flavins.

Oxidative stress is known to induce damage not only to lipids and enzymatic and non-enzymatic proteins, but also to DNA. It has been shown that expression of DNA repair genes is altered in lens epithelial cells of age-related cataracts [4]. Cataractous lenses have also been demonstrated to have decrease in the levels of glutathione and thioredoxin, with concomitant decrease in the activities of thioredoxin reductase, thiol transferase and glutathione reductase [5]. Several studies with lens organ culture system as well as with experimental animals have shown that the formation of cataracts can indeed be inhibited by administration of certain oxyradical scavengers such as ascorbate, Vitamin E, and bioflavonoids, to name a few [6-9]. However, the effectiveness of such nutraceuticals can become limited because of their instability due to their spontaneous oxidation, especially by the photochemical reactions initiated in the eye during photopic vision. The products of such oxidation, especially the carbonyls from ascorbate and tocopherols have been suggested to act as potential protein cross linking agents [10,11]. They also can become pro-oxidant in presence of certain metal ions. Ascorbate has been shown to glycate lens proteins with eventual formation of advanced glycated end products known to be associated with lens aging and cataract formation [12]. Additionally, since ascorbate and tocopherols are not of endogenous nature, they are required to be continuously supplemented in the diet. Epidemiological studies investigating the association of antioxidant vitamins and a lowered incidence of cataracts have yielded results that are yet equivocal [13-15]. Hence we considered the desirability of studying the anti-cataractogenic potential of certain endogenously derived ROS scavengers such as pyruvate, a keto acid metabolite well- known to scavenge various ROS, with rate constants of reaction reaching the diffusion limit [16,17]. This is especially true with respect to hydroxyl radical [18]. That pyruvate could be effective against oxidative stress was first suggestible by its effectiveness in prolonging the life of bacteria when exposed to excessive oxygen, the latter being lethal [19]. Such lethality is decreased by pyruvate. It has also been shown to protect the ocular lens against ROS induced damage [20]. Lenses when cultured in media generating ROS by direct addition of hydrogen peroxide, xanthine-xanthine oxidase or by photochemical reactions undergo significant physiological damage. This is initially reflected by an inhibition of active cation transport, depletion of GSH, generation of protein carbonyls, lipid peroxidation and loss of ATP [20,21]. Addition of pyruvate to the medium has been shown to be highly protective, the cation transport as well as the biochemistry of the tissue being well maintained. We have hypothesized that the protective effect of pyruvate against ROS induced damage to the lens in vitro and its anti-cataractogenic effect in vivo is due, in addition to its action as a ROS scavenger, to its action of stimulating tissue metabolism, particularly glycolysis, the main source of ATP in this tissue. The aim of this investigation was hence to further ascertain this possibility. We investigated this hypothesis by culturing mice lenses in presence of 5-^{3}H-glucose and determining the formation ^{3}H$_2$O and ^{3}H-lactate.

Materials and Methods

All the chemicals used were obtained from Sigma Chemical Company (St. Louis, MO). Ion exchange (AG1-X8, 200-400 mesh, OH form, Catalog #143-2446) and phenylboronate (Affi-Gel, Catalog #153-6103) resins were obtained from Bio-rad laboratories (Hercules, CA). Mice (CD-1, 25-30g.) were obtained from Harlan Laboratories. Animal handling procedures were according to the guidelines prescribed by the Institutional Animal Care and Use Committee and the ARVO statement for the use of animals in research.

Freshly isolated lenses were incubated in 0.5 ml of Tyrode buffer containing 26 mM sodium bicarbonate, 1mM glucose and trace amounts of 5-^{3}H-glucose, without (Controls) and with (Experimentals) the addition of pyruvate (2 mM). The specific activity of 5-^{3}H-glucose was ~1400 CPM/nanomole. Incubations were done in a humidified incubator maintained at 37°C and gassed with 5% carbon dioxide in air. At the end of 4 hours, aliquots of the medium were analyzed chromatographically for the contents of ^{3}H$_2$O as well as ^{3}H-lactate generated during incubation, as follows:

Determination of ^{3}H$_2$O [22,23] this was done by loading 50 μl of the medium on a homemade anion exchange column (4 × 0.5 cm, AG1X8-OH) piggybacked on a home-made phenylboronate column (3 × 0.5 cm). The radioactive glucose and the charged intermediates of glycolysis including the lactate and the glucose present in the medium remained bound to the anion exchange portion of the combined column. Any glucose remaining unbound by the above column gets

bound and trapped to the phenylboronate column. The final effluent of the combined column thus contained the ^{3}H$_2$O generated during the incubation. This was determined by liquid scintillation counting.

Determination of ^{3}H-lactate produced: An aliquot of the medium was loaded on a phenylboronate column (which binds glucose) piggybacked on a formate column. The boronate column retains the free glucose including the 5-^{3}H-glucose. The formate column retains lactate and other charged components of the glycolysis, including some glucose leaked out of the boronate column. The columns were then eluted with dH$_2$O to get rid of the ^{3}H$_2$O as well as any free glucose that might have been unbound on the column. The boronate column was then detached, and lactate including ^{3}H-lactate generated during incubation was recovered by elution with 0.1M formic acid and quantified by liquid scintillation counting.

Results

Several previous investigations on lens metabolism have assessed the status of glycolysis by incubating the tissue in various media and determining change in medium lactate [24,25]. A decrease in medium lactate with time of incubation, relative to a control is taken as an index of the inhibition of glycolysis. Since glycolysis includes several reactions representing the Embden-Myerhoff pathway, such measurement of lactate provides only limited information on the status of overall process of glycolysis, unless lactate determination is combined with the determinations of several other substrates generated over the specific period of experiment. Quantitation of lactate actually produced during incubation also needs to be corrected for the endogenous lactate that pre-exists in the lens prior to incubation [26]. In the present investigations, it was hypothesized that the beneficial effect of pyruvate in protecting the lens against oxidative stress could also be due to metabolic stimulation caused by recycling of NAD generated during the reduction of pyruvate to lactate, NAD being the required co-substrate in the oxidation of glyceraldehyde-3-phosphate to 1,3-diphosphoglycerate. The reaction is also accompanied with ATP generation by substrate phosphorylation and simultaneous generation of 3-phosphoglycerate. The intra-molecular dismutation of the latter produces 2-phosphoglycerate, which generates water and phosphoenol pyruvic acid, another major high-energy compound generating ATP as well as pyruvate. The stimulation of glucose metabolism via glycolysis caused by exogenously added pyruvate in the medium was hence hypothesized to be associated with generation of water. This was conceived to be reflected by an increase in the amount of ^{3}H$_2$O starting with 5-^{3}H glucose. That has been found to be true.

As shown in Figure 1, the concentration of ^{3}H$_2$O in the medium at the end of incubation was 95 μM in the controls incubated without pyruvate. The corresponding value expressed on the basis of lens weight was 46 nanomoles/ lens Figure 2. In the presence of pyruvate (2 mM) added to the medium, the concentration of ^{3}H$_2$O attained in the medium was 152 μM. Expressed on the basis of lens weight, ^{3}H$_2$O produced was 88 nanomoles/lens. Hence, formation of ^{3}H$_2$O is substantially higher when the lenses were incubated with pyruvate, expressed as its concentration in the medium as well as when calculated on the basis of lens weight. The results therefore provide convincing evidence of the possibility that pyruvate offers protection to the lens under stress situations by accelerating glycolysis, in addition to its oxyradical scavenging function.

This possibility was examined further by measuring the formation of ^{3}H-lactate. As shown in Figure 3 concentration of the ^{3}H-lactate derived from 5-^{3}H glucose was 8.6 μM. The amount expressed on the per lens basis was 4.3nanomoles/lens Figure 4. In experiments where incubations were done with pyruvate, the medium lactate concentration rose to ~13 μM. The value on the per lens basis was 6.5 nanomoles. Hence it was about 1.5 times more than that in the absence of pyruvate. These results hence further prove the stimulation of glycolysis by exogenous enrichment with this compound.

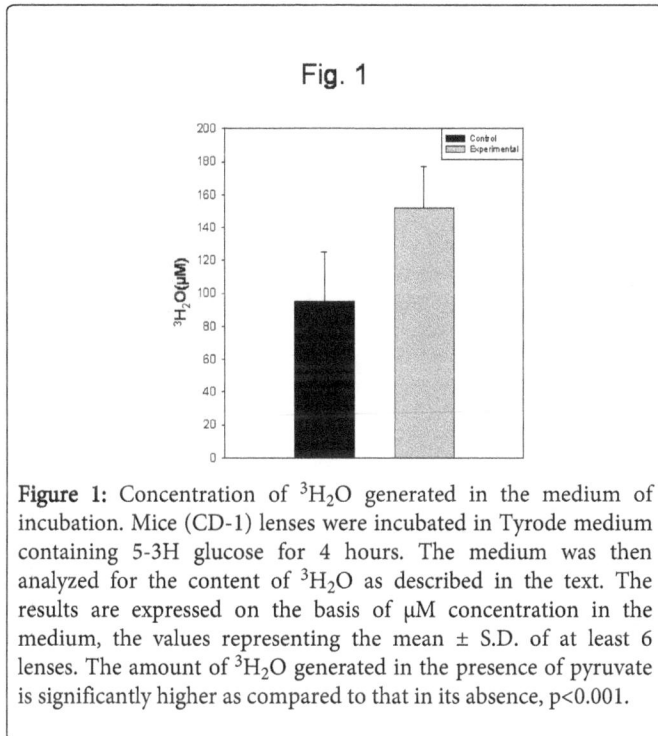

Figure 3: Concentration of ^{3}H-lactate in the incubation medium: CD-1 mice lenses were incubated in Tyrode medium containing 5-^{3}H-glucose in the absence (Control) and presence (Experimental) of 2 mM pyruvate for 4 hours. The post-incubation medium was analyzed for the content of lactate following its elution from a formate column and liquid scintillation counting, as described in the text. The results are expressed as the mean ± S.D. of at least 6 lenses; p<0.001 between control and experimental.

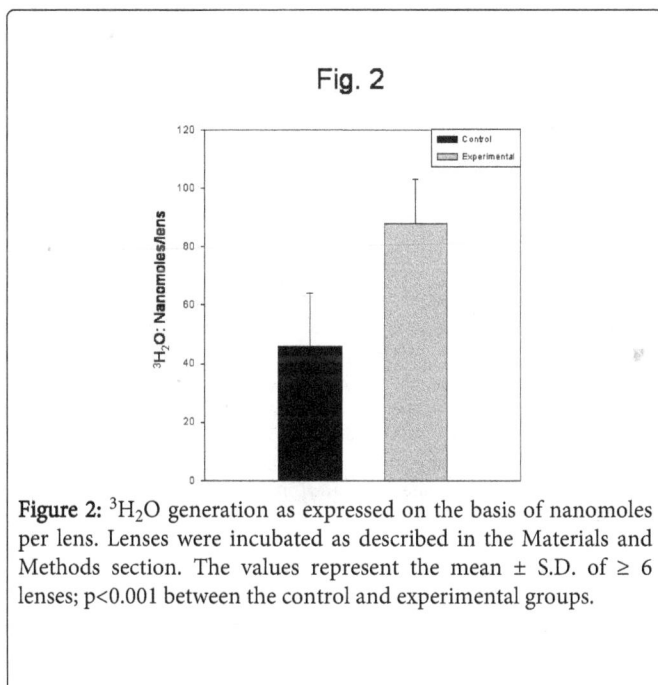

Figure 1: Concentration of ^{3}H$_2$O generated in the medium of incubation. Mice (CD-1) lenses were incubated in Tyrode medium containing 5-3H glucose for 4 hours. The medium was then analyzed for the content of ^{3}H$_2$O as described in the text. The results are expressed on the basis of μM concentration in the medium, the values representing the mean ± S.D. of at least 6 lenses. The amount of ^{3}H$_2$O generated in the presence of pyruvate is significantly higher as compared to that in its absence, p<0.001.

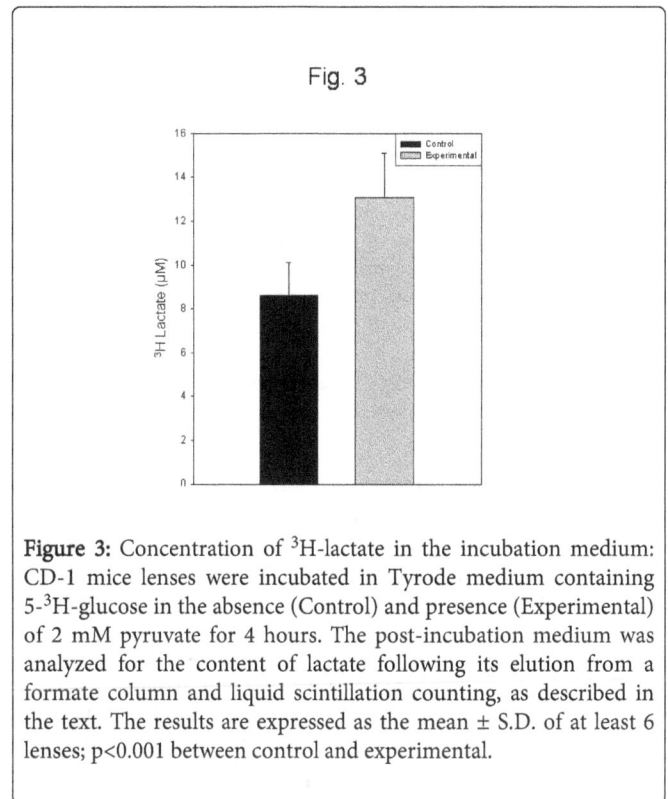

Figure 2: ^{3}H$_2$O generation as expressed on the basis of nanomoles per lens. Lenses were incubated as described in the Materials and Methods section. The values represent the mean ± S.D. of ≥ 6 lenses; p<0.001 between the control and experimental groups.

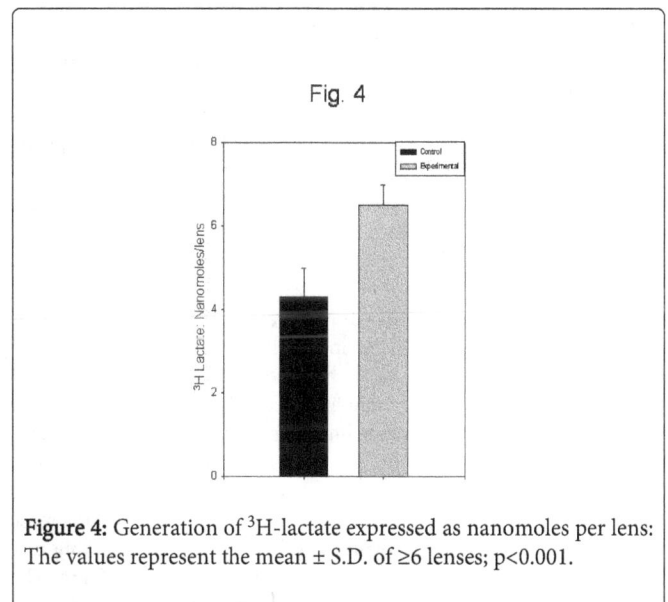

Figure 4: Generation of ^{3}H-lactate expressed as nanomoles per lens: The values represent the mean ± S.D. of ≥6 lenses; p<0.001.

Discussion

Previous studies have shown that the bioenergetic support to the lens is primarily provided by glycolysis. A number of such studies have shown that this pathway becomes sluggish with aging as well as with certain diseases including diabetes and galactosemia. This is reflected by decreases in the contents of lens lactate as well as ATP. In addition, decrease in the activity of glyceraldehyde-3-phosphate dehydrogenase has also been shown to occur in aging and cataractous lenses [5]. Comparison of metabolomic profiles of normal and cataractous lenses using high-frequency nuclear magnetic resonance (NMR) and high-performance liquid chromatography with high-resolution mass-spectrometric detection (LC-MS) methods has revealed a lowered metabolic activity in cataractous lenses, as suggested by decrease in the levels of almost all metabolites in the cataractous lens vs. normal lens [27].

Inactivation of glyceraldehyde-3-phosphate dehydrogenase, a key glycolytic enzyme, as well as others is highly likely to cause inhibition of tissue glycolysis and other metabolic pathways. Such inactivation can be induced by oxidation of several enzymes by oxyradicals generated during photochemical oxidation of certain lens constituents, as well as during many metal ion dependent auto-oxidative reactions that proceed ambiently. Hence inhibition of cataract formation would require the presence of oxyradical scavengers as a first line of defense. A second line of defense would be to use compounds that have the ability to overcome the accompanying metabolic inhibitions, by acting as metabolic substrates. Previous studies have demonstrated that pyruvate inhibits the cataractogenic process in diabetic animals [28-30]. It is quite likely that it provides the lens a first line of defense via its oxyradical scavenging properties and a second line of defense by stimulating glycolysis. It is conceived that it can potentially do the latter by maintaining a consistent supply of NAD generated by various NADH dependent dehydrogenation reactions, including NADH dependent reduction of the exogenously supplied pyruvate. That its conversion to lactate is a favorable reaction is also apparent from its ΔG values of -6 kcal/mole [31]. Hence the possibility that increasing the amount of pyruvate would enhance NAD generation is feasible thermodynamically also. Additional generation of NAD is expected to stimulate glycolysis by driving the glyceraldehyde-3-phosphate dehydrogenase reaction in the direction of oxidation, converting glyceraldehyde-3-phosphate to 1,3-diphosphoglycerate with eventual stimulation of ATP formation. The possibility that pyruvate can indeed accomplish such enhancement of glycolysis is convincingly demonstrable by incubation of the lenses with 5-^{3}H glucose and determining the formation of titrated water chromatographically as described above. Passage of the incubation medium through anion exchange column in tandem with the boronate column removes most of the expected glycolytic metabolites and unused glucose, ensuring that the radioactivity in the final eluate is due to the water simultaneously generated in the enolase-catalyzed reaction that converts 2-phosphoglycerate to phosphoenolpyruvate. Hence measurement of the amount of ^{3}H$_2$O and its increase or decrease under various conditions provides a strong means of detecting any alteration in the glycolytic activity of a tissue under examination. The increase in the formation of ^{3}H$_2$O by the lenses incubated with 5-^{3}H glucose in the presence of pyruvate, especially associated also with the increase in the contents of ^{3}H-lactate, therefore provides a more convincing evidence of enhancement in the glycolytic activity of the lens than the measurement of lactate alone from pyruvate, which can be reduced to lactate by NADH and NADPH generated from several glycolytic as well as non-glycolytic reactions. Mechanistically, formation of water during the conversion of 2-phoshoglycerate (2-PGA) to phosphoenolpyruvate requires the formation of an initial Mg^{2+} enolase complex. Combination of this complex with 2-PGA then causes dissociation of an acidic proton from C-2. This combines with the nucleophilic –OH base of –CH$_2$OH at C-3 of 2-PGA, to be followed by the splitting of a water molecule with simultaneous generation of phosphoenolpyruvate. The free energy change of this reaction is reasonably small (~1 kcal), so that the reaction can proceed at physiological temperature without any thermodynamic hindrance. The results obtained showing an increase in the ^{3}H$_2$O from 5-^{3}H glucose in presence of pyruvate is also strongly supported by the isotopic exchange studies [32], as well as by crystal structure of the enzyme-Mg^{2+}complex [33]. Mg^{2+} is a well-known essential cofactor required for the activity of enolase.

The results therefore strongly suggest that the protective effect of pyruvate against cataract formation induced by ROS generation as well as by diabetic conditions is attributable to its action as a metabolic agonist, supporting glycolysis. This is in addition to its effectiveness in scavenging ROS. Unlike many other scavengers of ROS, the products of the reaction of pyruvate with ROS are not toxic. The possibility that it may have other beneficial effects such as competitive inhibition of polyol synthesis and protein glycation has also been shown before.

Acknowledgements

The authors are thankful to NEI, NIH, and Research to Prevent Blindness Inc., for their financial support, and to Svitlana Kovtun for technical assistance.

References

1. Varma SD, Ets TK, Richards RD (1977) Protection against superoxide radicals in rat lens. Ophthalmic Res 9: 421-431.

2. Zigler JS Jr, Goosey JD (1984) Singlet oxygen as a possible factor in human senile nuclear cataract. Curr Eye Res 3: 39-45.

3. Varma SD, Kumar S, Richards RD (1979) Light induced damage to ocular lens cation pump. Prevention by Vitamin C. Proc Natl Acad Sci 76: 3504-3506.

4. Li F, Wang Y, Zhang G, Zhou J, Yang L, et al. (2014) Expression and methylation of DNA repair genes in lens epithelium cells of age-related cataract. Mutat Res. 766-767: 31-36.

5. Wei M, Xing KY, Fan YC, Libondi T, Lou MF (2014) Loss of thiol repair systems in human cataractous lenses. Invest Ophthalmol Vis Sci 56: 598-605.

6. Hegde KR, Varma SD (2004) Protective effect of ascorbate against oxidative stress in the mouse lens. Biochim Biophys Acta 1670: 12-18.

7. Trevithick JR, Linklater HA, Mitton KP, Dzialoszynski T, Sanford SE (1989) Modeling cortical cataractogenesis: IX. Activity of vitamin E and esters in preventing cataracts and gamma-crystallin leakage from lenses in diabetic rats. Ann N Y Acad Sci 570: 358-371.

8. Ayala MN, Söderberg PG (2004) Vitamin E can protect against ultraviolet radiation-induced cataract in albino rats. Ophthalmic Res 36: 264-269.

9. Varma SD, Mizuno A, Kinoshita JH (1977) Diabetic cataracts and flavonoids. Science 195: 205-206.

10. Nagaraj RH, Monnier VM (1992) Isolation and characterization of a blue fluorophore from human eye lens crystallins: in vitro formation from Maillard reaction with ascorbate and ribose. Biochim Biophys Acta 1116: 34-42.

11. Cheng R, Lin B, Lee KW, Ortwerth BJ (2001) Similarity of the yellow chromophores isolated from human cataracts with those from ascorbic acid-modified calf lens proteins: evidence for ascorbic acid glycation during cataract formation. Biochim Biophys Acta 1537: 14-26.

12. Smuda M, Henning C, Raghavan CT, Johar K, Vasavada AR, et al. (2015) Comprehensive analysis of maillard protein modifications in human lenses: effect of age and cataract. Biochemistry 54: 2500-2507.

13. Leske MC, Chylack LT Jr, He Q, Wu SY, Schoenfeld E, et al. (1998) Antioxidant vitamins and nuclear opacities: the longitudinal study of cataract. Ophthalmology 105: 831-836.

14. Jacques PF, Hartz SC, Chylack LT Jr, McGandy RB, Sadowski JA (1988) Nutritional status in persons with and without senile cataracts: blood vitamin and mineral levels. Am J Clin Nutr 48: 152-158.

15. Taylor A, Jacques PF, Chylack LT Jr, Hankinson SE, Khu PM, et al. (2002) Long-term intake of vitamins and carotenoids and odds of early age-related cortical and posterior subcapsular lens opacities. Am J Clin Nutr 75: 540-549.

16. Fenton HJH, Jones HO (1900) Oxidation of organic acids in presence of ferrous iron, Part I. J Chem Soc Trans 77: 69-76.

17. Holleman AF (1904) Note on the action of oxygenated water on alpha-keto acids and 1,2 dicetones. Recl Tran Chi Pays Bas Belq 23: 169-172.

18. Ervens B, Gligorovski S, Herrmann H (2003) Temperature dependent rate constants for hydroxyl radical reactions with organic compounds in aqueous solutions. Phys Chem Chem Phys 5: 1811-1824.

19. Sevag MG, Maiweg L (1934) The respiration mechanism of pneumococcus III. J Exp Med 60: 95-105.

20. Varma SD, Morris SM (1988) Peroxide damage to the eye lens in vitro prevention by pyruvate. Free Rad Res Comm 4: 283-290.

21. Varma SD, Hegde K, Henein M (2003) Oxidative damage to mouse lens in culture. Protective effect of pyruvate. Biochim Biophys Acta 1621: 246-252.

22. Clark DG, Rongstad R and Katz J (1973). Isotopic evidence of futile cycles in liver cells. Biochem Biophys Res Comm 54: 1141-1148.

23. Allard MF, Schönekess BO, Henning SL, English DR, Lopaschuk GD (1994) Contribution of oxidative metabolism and glycolysis to ATP production in the hypertrophied heart. Am J Physiol Heart Circ Physiol 267: H742-H750.

24. Van Heyningen R (1965) The metabolism of glucose by rabbit lens in the presence and absence of oxygen. Biochem J 96: 419-431.

25. Hightower KR and Harrison SE (1987) The influence of calcium on glucose metabolism in the rabbit lens. Invest Ophthalmol Vis Sci 28: 1433-1436.

26. Gillis KM, Chylack LT Jr, Cheng HM (1981) Age and the control of glycolysis in the rat lens. Invest Ophthalmol Vis Sci 20: 457-466.

27. Tsentalovich YP, Verkhovod TD, Yanshole VV, Kiryutin AS, Yanshole LV, et al. (2015) Metabolomic composition of normal aged and cataractous human lenses. Exp Eye Res 134: 15-23.

28. Varma SD, Ramachandran S, Devamanoharan PS, Morris SM, Ali AH (1995) Prevention of oxidative damage to rat lens by pyruvate in vitro: possible attenuation in vivo. Curr Eye Res 14: 643-649.

29. Zhao W, Devamanoharan PS, Henein M, Ali AH, Varma SD (2000) Diabetes-induced biochemical changes in rat lens: attenuation of cataractogenesis by pyruvate. Diabetes Obes Metab 2: 165-174.

30. Hegde KR, Varma SD (2005) Prevention of cataract by pyruvate in experimentally diabetic mice. Mol Cell Biochem 269: 115-120.

31. West ES, Todd WR, Mason HS, Van Bruggen JT (1970) Textbook of Biochemistry. The Macmillan Company, London.

32. Dinovo EC, Boyer PD (1971) Isotopic Probes of the Enolase Reaction Mechanism. J Biol Chem 246: 4586-4593.

33. Lebioda L, Stec B (1991) Mechanism of enolase: the crystal structure of enolase-Mg2(+)2phosphoglycerate/phosphoenolpyruvate complex at 2.2-A resolution 30: 2817-2822.

39

The Role of Actigraphy to Identify Sleep Disorders in Children with ADHD

Checa-Ros Ana[1,2*], Vargas-Pérez M[2], Muñoz-Gallego A[3], Molina-Carballo A[2], Uberos-Fernández J[2] and Muñoz-Hoyos A[2]

[1]School of Medicine of Granada, San Cecilio University Hospital, Spain

[2]Department of Pediatrics, University of Granada, San Cecilio Hospital, Spain

[3]Department of Language and Computer Science, University of Málaga, Spain

*Corresponding author: Checa Ros Ana, paediatric resident at San Cecilio University Hospital, Doctor Oloriz Street, 1, Granada-18012, Spain; E-mail: anaxeca@hotmail.com

Abstract

Currently sleep disorders are one of the most prevalent problems in children, with an estimated prevalence of 15-20% and a highly variable clinical spectrum. One of the pathologies in which sleep disorders achieve special relevance is in attention-deficit and hyperactivity disorder (ADHD), because the complex association between these two phenomena can largely determine the therapeutic handling and prognosis of these patients. Nowadays, the number of research articles that makes unquestionable the relation between ADHD and sleep disorders is increasing, as well as studies in which actigraphy acquires increasingly validity as a tool to asses sleep in the paediatric population, with a good correlation with polysomnography, considered the "gold standard" in sleep medicine. Our review aims to highlight the positive impact that the use of actigraphy as a screening tool for the detection of sleep problems in ADHD may have on the quality of life of these children and their families. After an exhaustive review of the most recent published literature on this topic, we suggest a set of recommendations which are summarized in that the actigraphy allows us to study longer periods of sleep-wake in an stable way, avoiding the difficulties of polysomnographic studies in children. All this makes it an ideal screening element in the initial assessment of patients with ADHD who report sleep problems.

Keywords: Actigraphy; Sleep disorders; Attention deficit and hyperactivity disorder; Pediatric population

Introduction

According to recent data, sleep disorders in children are one of the most prevalent problems found by paediatricians in their daily clinical practice, accounting for 15-20% of the general population and with an apparently growing incidence according to different references. Generally, in children under the age of 5, it is estimated that 30% have sleep disturbances of various kinds [1], and a review of several studies shows that between 13 and 27% of parents of children from 4 to 12 years relate the presence of sleep difficulties of varying magnitude. Most of these difficulties corresponding to poor sleep hygiene, bedtime resistance, anxiety at the time of going to sleep, delayed sleep onset, reactive co-sleeping, snoring , enuresis, nocturnal awakenings, parasomnias, nightmares, night terrors, sleepwalking, early morning awakening and excessive daytime sleepiness [1].

These problems are usually stable throughout childhood, so that a child with sleep difficulties at 8 months probably will still display at 3 years, and those who exhibited them at 2 years will follow present in adolescence. Among the long-term consequences of disturbed sleep patterns have been included physical stunting, behavioural and performance problems in school, family and social disruption, etc. [2], problems that must be related in some way to the maturation of central nervous system. Any disturbance of the normal sleep development could lead to neurodevelopmental disorders [3].

Despite this, there are relatively few longitudinal studies that examine sleep development in children within their own home environment [4], since most studies are conducted in sleep laboratories, only during night periods [5]. In this sense, actigraphy provides an useful tool over other methods of evaluation of sleep/wake cycle that allows a continuous noninvasive evaluation and that can be used for extended periods of time in the child's environment [6].

Over the last two decades, actigraphy has become one of the main tools in sleep medicine, as can be seen in the growing number of publications including actigraphy compared to them that include polysomnography (PSG) (ratio 1:10 actigraphy-PSG in 1991 compared to a ratio of 1:4 in 2009) [7]. The recent reviews and clinical guidelines introduced by the American Sleep Disorders Association (ASDA) have established actigraphy as a method of valid and reliable assessment in specific domains of research in sleep medicine [8,9].

One of the fields of child neurology where sleep disorders acquires a great interest is in attention-deficit and hyperactivity disorder (ADHD), which is one of the most common childhood behavioural disorders, with an estimated prevalence of 5% in school children [10]. In these patients, complaints about sleep problems are very common, reaching up to 55% of cases according to Corkum et al. [11].

Fortunately, the relationship between ADHD and sleep disorders has recovered interest in the last 5-10 years, after having been overlooked for years by researchers and clinicians in this field. Progress in this knowledge area can have a great impact on the daily clinical practice: 1). On the one hand, the management of sleep problems in children with ADHD could significantly reduce the severity of behavioural symptoms and improve quality of life for these children and their families [12]. 2). On the other hand, take into consideration sleep disturbances may also be critical in the evaluation and treatment of children who are sent for consultation with problems of inattention, hyperactivity and/or impulsivity but do not meet diagnostic criteria for ADHD according to DSM -IV.

In fact, it has been pointed out that any sleep disturbance resulting in inadequate duration, interrupted or fragmented sleep, or excessive daytime sleepiness can lead or contribute to behaviour or attention problems [12]. Thereby at least in one sample of patients with inattention, hyperactivity and/or impulsivity, these symptoms can be improved or even eliminated after the primary sleep problem has been corrected.

Material and Methods

Our purpose is to outline, through a literature review, the importance of actigraphy as an essential tool for the study of sleep medicine, both in adults and especially in children, and its value not only diagnostic but also therapeutic and prognostic.

For that we have consulted databases "PubMed", "ScienceDirect" and "Scopus". Using keywords as "actigraphy", "sleep disorders", "attention deficit and hyperactivity disorder" and "pediatric population", we have selected the most current articles about this issue.

In this article we review the role of actigraphy in sleep medicine and particularly in paediatric settings, its applicability for detecting altered patterns of sleep/wake in children with ADHD and the implication that this may have on treatment, monitoring and the final prognosis of these patients.

Fundaments of actigraphy

Actigraphy is a technique that consists in recording the movements. It is based on the employ of similar devices to a wristwatch usually placed on the non-dominant wrist (although they can also be placed in ankle or the trunk). This device monitors the movements for extended periods time, so that scores or scales of activity obtained (in periods of 1 minute, for example) are transferred to scales of sleep/wake based on computerized algorithms. The latest models of actigraphs incorporate other complementary registration procedures, as a photometric system, which quantifies the amount of existing light, or a thermometric system, which allows studying the temperature fluctuations and their correlation with activity, being a parameter for chronobiological studies.

Actimeters are connected by a suitable interface to a computer with the appropriate signal treatment programs, allowing the display of records, analysis and reproduction by printer. There are several models on the market, each one has its own characteristics and requires appropriate measurement algorithms for categorizing sleep/wake and validation studies [7]. There may be artefacts that alter the results of actigraph in the determinations of the sleep/wake cycle, such as a failure to record the movements, postures that block arm movements, the breathing movements themselves and the external movement caused by the normal use of vehicles.

Reliability and validity of actigraph

The reliability and validity of actigraphy to detect the sleep-wake cycle has been established by previous studies, especially in a normal population of children and adults [8]. However, this is less clear in research on specific populations or specific devices [13,14], in which some authors conclude that the very low ability of actigraph to detect awakenings questions its validity for measuring sleep quality in clinical

populations with interrupted sleep. For example, Sitnick et al. [14] compared minute by minute the sleep-wake scores based on actigraphy and videosomnography in young people, collecting an percentage of agreement of 94%, a sensitivity of 97% (percentage of sleep minutes identified by PSG which are collected as such by actigraphy) and a specificity of 24% (rate of wake minutes collected by PSG which are identified as such by actigraphy). De Souza et al. [15] also provided relatively low percentages of specificity (34-44%). On the other hand, the review of Tryon [16] illustrated that the validity of actigraphy is acceptable compared to many other medical tests. He also indicated that the discrepancy PSG-actigraphy should be attributed to the accuracy of PSG, being part thereof predictable and correctable.

Recent studies in the context of the child population, such as Gnidovec and Hyde ones [17,18], reflect low percentages of specificity (between 39.4 and 68.9%). However they conclude that actigraphy is a reliable method for the assessment of sleep in children. This validity is also present in the case of children with intellectual and motor deficits [19].

Another aspect that requires attention in the validation studies of actigraphy compared to PSG is that these studies are based, almost without exception, in the period of "time in bed" (usually in sleep laboratories). However the main advantage of actigraphy is its ability to document sleep-wake patterns continuously over a 24 hour period over days. Therefore, the validation studies should also allow a comparison of long periods in and out of the bed with long periods of wakefulness [7].

There is a frequent comparison between data provided by actigraphy and data provided by subjective measures, such as daily sleep records reported by parents and caregivers. So et al. [6] compared the two methods in a sample of 20 infants during the first year of life. They found a good relationship between both methods, although the data from parental sleep diaries overestimated the nocturnal sleep time compared with actigraphy. Similar results have been reported in other studies that have worked with an older child population [20]. Another interesting issue is the stability of actigraphic measurements over time, both in adult and paediatric population. According to this, Sadeh et al. [21] confirmed a significant stability of actigraphic measures which were compared annually during early adolescence, despite the maturational changes in sleep patterns that occur in this age period.

Regarding data analysis, a new approach to modern actigraphy has been introduced by Sazonov et al. [22]. In their study, the device was placed in the diaper collecting similar rates of validity in comparison to those who placed the device in the ankle. Enomoto et al. [23] also provided similar results with the placement of a new device on the wrist. Chae et al. [24] have reevaluated specific criteria for sleep onset detected by actigraphy. They define it as 5 minutes of inactivity to achieve a better correlation between PSG and actigraphy in the data referring to sleep onset latency (SOL), total sleep time (TST) and wake after sleep onset (WASO). This is a change with regard to the criteria used previously (e.g., 10 or 15 minutes of immobility).

Actigraphic detection of sleep disorders

Regarding the assessment of insomnia, several studies have concluded that actigraphy is a sensitive tool to detect differences between groups of individuals with insomnia and control population. However, the discrepancies found between actigraphy and subjective assessments of patients could be attributed, among other factors, to the fact that actigraphy overestimates sleep time, because of the efforts of patients with insomnia for remaining immobile in bed during long periods of time [25,26].

One of recent applications of actigraphy has been the detection of periodic limb movements during sleep (PLMS) using a high-resolution model (e.g. every 5 seconds), and comparing data of electromyography (EMG) with data derived from a simultaneous study PSG-actigraphy. Sforza et al [27] showed the highest correlation between actigraphy and PSG in detecting movements, although actigraphy underestimated electromyographic activity of legs. This problem could be partially solved with the use of a new device designed especially for detection of periodic limb movements during sleep with a high time resolution [28]. However, the application in children ages 4 to 12 years [29] has not demonstrated acceptable validity.

As regards sleep-disordered breathing (SDB), results indicate that the estimated total sleep time provided by actigraph improved the validity of apnea-hypopnea index (AHI) compared to the results based on the simple polygraph [30]. In addition, actigraphy can also be used to assess efficacy of treatment with nasal continuous positive airway pressure (nCPAP) [31].

Although less common, actigraphy can also help in the diagnosis of narcolepsy, apart from detecting the behavioural changes induced by sleep deprivation as an essential part in the evaluation of patients with narcolepsy [32].

Recent studies, such as Sivertsen et al. [33], Manber et al. [34], Espie et al. [35] and Harris et al. [36] have highlighted the actigraphy potential to assess the change in sleep patterns in response to cognitive behavioural therapy conducted in patients with insomnia. It is appreciated an improvement in the subjective perception of these patients regarding their sleep pattern.

In this context, actigraphy has also often been used to evaluate the effects of pharmacological interventions for sleep problems [8,37]. Actigraphy has proved to be sensitive enough to detect secondary changes to such interventions. So, in different studies, the effects of temazepam in patients with insomnia have been evaluated [38]. Also the effects of melatonin and zopiclone have been tested in patients with inadequate sleep patterns [39]. In this research line, an interesting study about the effect of melatonin in patients with cystic fibrosis was conducted by De Castro-Silva et al. [40] and was published in the Journal of Pineal Research in 2010. In this study, 20 patients with cystic fibrosis were randomized to receive placebo or melatonin for 21 days. They were monitored with actigraphy 6 days before starting treatment and on the third day of the same. It was showing an improvement in the efficiency and sleep duration.

Use of actigraphy in pediatric population

Based on all that has been explained before, we deduce that actigraphy can be a method particularly valid in children, because the fact that the information provided by the parents as the only source of information can limit the accuracy of the knowledge that we have about children sleep [41]. According to the increasing use of actigraphy in this knowledge area, a significant increase in the number of studies conducted on actigraphy in children is observed (Figure 1). We can emphasize the fact that the number of published studies in 2010 is similar to the total of published studies between 1991 and 2001.

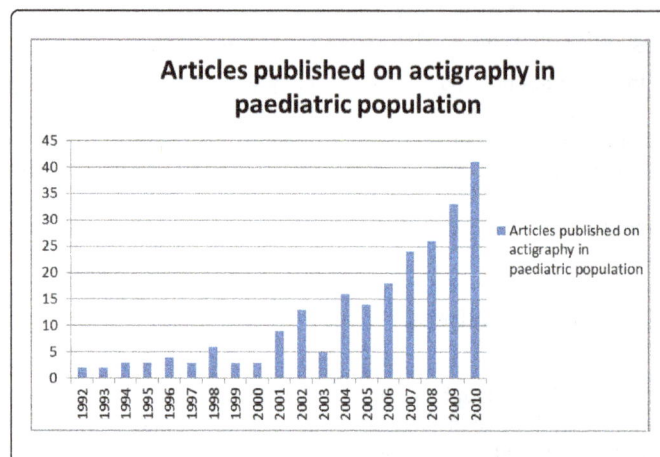

In 2007 the American Academy of Sleep Medicine established that "Actigraphy is indicated for delineating sleep patterns, and to document treatment responses in normal infants and children (in whom traditional sleep monitoring by polysomnography can be difficult to perform and/or interpret), and in special paediatric populations" [42]. Despite this recommendation, nowadays there is not standardized practices regarding collection parameters and scoring actigraphic signals, so we want to make some recommendations as to the paediatric population is concerned.

As regards the choice of actigraph, we must consider the type of device (warranty, battery, maintenance, software program associated and support service), and if it fits in size, weight and comfort with the age the child population of the study [41].

Regarding study design, we need to take into account how the actigraph will be delivered and collected, as well as the time required for data collection. The actigraph usually requires to be placed a minimum of 7 nights [43], and even sometimes 2 weeks if the detected differences between weekdays and weekend are of interest. In addition, variables to be evaluated should be selected a priori, deciding who will fill out sleep diary (parent, child ...), the frequency with which sleep diary will be completed and the format of a diary (paper, electronic, phone call ...) [41].

In terms of managing data, sleep diary should be used to reduce the frequency of artefacts (movements of device, prolonged periods of low activity, periods of activity that should be recognized as sleep or nighttime awakenings movements that may be due to bed sharing, and any cause of atypical sleep as an intercurrent disease, fever ...) [41]; on the other hand, it is also necessary to select the scoring algorithms and the threshold level for awakening depending on the kind of study population and previously published studies [41]. Authors should include in their research articles not just the way they handled the data, but also the missing data and rules of coding and processing of data [41].

In this context, Meltzer et al. [41] proposed a list of data to be recorded in this research area using actigraphy in paediatric population (Table 1). Their study was published in 2012 in Sleep Medicine Reviews.

Device information:
-The name of the device, the model, the name and the location of the manufacturer
-The placement of the device
-The measured epoch length, the mode of data collection, the use of the event marker, and the algorithm or wake sensitivity threshold
-Justification for the algorithm that is chosen
-The type and version of software used
-Some information of sensitivity and specificity
Sleep diary:
-Type of sleep diary used (paper, electronic, telephone call)
-The person who completed sleep diary (parent, child)
-Frequency of diary completion (at bedtime only, morning and evening)
Data collection and processing (including missing data):
-Number of nights of data collection
-Number of weekday and weekend nights (if relevant)
-Methods used to identify and handle artifact
-Number of lost data due to technical failure, participant non-adherence, artifact
Data variables:
-Clear definition of the variables, including ones automatically calculated by manufacturer scoring programs (sleep bouts, wake bouts, motionless sleep or immobile time, circadian parameters)
-Clear definition of the scoring rules used, using common/standardized names

Table 1: Standard offer of information to including in the literature of investigation of the paediatric dream with actigraphy.

Discussion

Despite what some clinicians may think, the available evidence suggests that drugs for attention-deficit and hyperactivity disorder (ADHD) are just one of the possible causes of sleep problems associated with it. Children with ADHD exhibit significantly more sleep disorders compared with their controls regardless of the medication used. We can include among these disorders: bedtime resistance, sleep-onset difficulties, and night awakenings, difficulties with morning awakenings, sleep-disordered breathing, and daytime sleepiness [44]. Several studies suggest that sleep disorders affect more than 50% of children affected by ADHD. In our article we briefly describe the major sleep disorders and their association with ADHD in order to get an idea of the importance of this relationship.

A literature review of 2005 [45] concluded that up to 44% of patients with ADHD suffered from restless legs syndrome (RLS) or similar symptoms, and 26% of subjects with RLS had symptoms of ADHD . Although data are probably overestimated, and causality of this association is not well defined, from a clinical point of view the RLS may exacerbate ADHD symptoms. In addition, children with RLS can develop resistance to bedtime, since they associate this time with unpleasant sensations of RLS. Parents may interpret this refusal as an expression of their general oppositional behaviour [46], ignoring the sleep disturbance. On the other hand, ADHD may worsen symptoms of RLS, as proposed by Chervin et al [47] and Wagner et al [48]. Therefore, the RLS should be systematically investigated in children with ADHD or symptoms similar thereto.

Another sleep disturbance described in children with ADHD is periodic limb movements during sleep (PLMS). Huang et al. found

that 10.2% of patients with ADHD suffered from this disorder compared with 0% of controls [49]. This association was subsequently confirmed by Bruni et al. [50].

It has been reported that children with ADHD without medication and sleep-onset insomnia (SOI) exhibit a delay in the evening peak melatonin secretion [51], so it has been hypothesized that the sleep-onset insomnia in these children could be due to a circadian rhythm alteration [52]. This could contribute to bedtime resistance and discomfort symptoms during sleep, which may be erroneously considered as an expression of their general behaviour disorder [46]. Therefore, the rate of melatonin secretion should be studied in children with ADHD and sleep-onset insomnia and/or resistance to bedtime.

Excessive nocturnal motor activity (arms or legs) has been documented also by actigraphy in children with ADHD [52,53]. It was subsequently confirmed by an infrared camera [54], although this has not led to differences in polysomnographic recordings.

The relationship between sleep-disordered breathing (SDB) and ADHD is not well established [47]. Chervin states that the values of AHI (apnea-hypopnea index) obtained in children with ADHD (1 to 5), although not very high, they are suggestive of paediatric obstructive sleep apnea and require medical attention.

Moreover, we should not forget the impact that psychiatric comorbidity with ADHD (such as oppositional disorder, anxiety disorders, learning disorders, various behavioural disorders, tics and Tourette's syndrome [55]) and/or the treatments used for the same, may have on sleep disturbance as a causal factor to consider adding. This is demonstrated in a recent article published by Moreau et al. in 2013. They collected 41 children diagnosed with ADHD between 6 and 13 years, compared those without psychiatric comorbidity with those who showed it, and they observed a higher percentage of sleep disturbances in the latter [56].

It has also suggested that stimulant drugs used as treatment of ADHD can negatively influence on sleep, due to its "rebound" effect (intensification of the symptoms of ADHD when drug effect disappears). Results of different studies are opposing [56,57] and it seems that vulnerability to these negative effects can be probably related to individual factors such as Brown and McMullen said [58]. In this context it seems appropriate to quote an article published in 2014, consisting of a meta-analysis that included 393 patients with ADHD who were randomized to either methylphenidate versus placebo. They monitored data using actigraphy and they founded a significant reduction in total sleep time in patients who received methylphenidate [59].

Results

After all this, there is a clear need to investigate sleep disorders in all children referred for consultation for possible ADHD, as an appropriate management of sleep problems in these children may improve both quality of life and their families. Moreover, more studies are considered necessary to investigate this association, and where actigraphy acquires an important role as a primary screening test.

The main conclusions that can be deduced from this review are:

• Sleep disorders have become one of the emerging problems in childhood, reaching a prevalence of 15 to 20%, with a course that tends to be stable with the child's age.

- The ADHD and sleep disorders association is increasingly recognized. Although its genesis is multifactorial and still not fully clear, has great potential impact on the prognosis and quality of life of these patients and their families.

- The actigraphy is now a valid and reliable method to assess sleep, which correlates well with PSG in the normal population and in specific populations. Its application in paediatric population allows us to study sleep-wake patterns over long periods with great stability in their measurements and avoiding the difficulties of polysomnographic studies in children.

- Using actigraphs in patients with ADHD who report sleep problems as a method of screening and initial evaluation of these alterations could reconsider the management and treatment of these children, with a positive influence in their prognosis.

References

1. Working Group on Clinical Practice Guide to Sleep Disorders in Children and Adolescents in Primary Care (2011) Clinical Practice Guide of Sleep Disorders in Children and Adolescents in Primary Care. Quality Plan for the National Health System of the Ministry of Health, Social Policy and Equality. Unit Health Technology Assessment Agency Lain Entralgo; Clinical Practice Guides in the NHS: UETS No 2009/8

2. Owens JA, Witmans M (2004) Sleep problems. Curr Probl Pediatr Adolesc Health Care 34: 154-179.

3. Kohyama J (1998) Sleep as a window on the developing brain. Curr Probl Pediatr 28: 69-92.

4. Jenni OG, Borbély AA, Achermann P (2004) Development of the nocturnal sleep electroencephalogram in human infants. Am J Physiol Regul Integr Comp Physiol 286: R528-538.

5. Anders T, Sadeh A, Appareddy V (1995) Normal sleep in neonates and children. In: R Ferber and M Kryger (Edn) Principles and Practice of Sleep Medicine in the Child. WB Saunders Co., Philadelphia: 7-18.

6. So K, Adamson TM, Horne RS (2007) The use of actigraphy for assessment of the development of sleep/wake patterns in infants during the first 12 months of life. J Sleep Res 16: 181-187.

7. Sadeh A (2011) The role and validity of actigraphy in sleep medicine: An update. Sleep Medicine Reviews 15: 259-267.

8. Sadeh A, Hauri PJ, Kripke DF, Lavie P (1995) The role of actigraphy in the evaluation of sleep disorders. Sleep 18: 288-302.

9. Sadeh A, Acebo C (2002) The role of actigraphy in sleep medicine. Sleep Med Rev 6: 113-124.

10. Polanczyk G, de Lima MS, Horta BL, Biederman J, Rohde LA (2007) The worldwide prevalence of ADHD: a systematic review and metaregression analysis. Am J Psychiatry 164: 942-948.

11. Corkum P, Tannock R, Moldofsky H (1998) Sleep disturbances in children with attention-deficit/hyperactivity disorder. J Am Acad Child Adolesc Psychiatry 37: 637-646.

12. Owens JA (2005) The ADHD and sleep conundrum: a review. J Dev Behav Pediatr 26: 312-322.

13. Insana SP, Gozal D, Montgomery-Downs HE (2010) Invalidity of one actigraphy brand for identifying sleep and wake among infants. Sleep Med 11: 191-196.

14. Sitnick SL, Goodlin-Jones BL, Anders TF (2008) The use of actigraphy to study sleep disorders in preschoolers: some concerns about detection of nighttime awakenings. Sleep 31: 395-401.

15. de Souza L, Benedito-Silva AA, Pires ML, Poyares D, Tufik S, et al. (2003) Further validation of actigraphy for sleep studies. Sleep 26: 81-85.

16. Tryon WW (2004) Issues of validity in actigraphic sleep assessment. Sleep 27: 158-165.

17. Gnidovec B, Neubauer D, Zidar J (2002) Actigraphic assessment of sleep-wake rhythm during the first 6 months of life. Clin Neurophysiol 113: 1815-1821.

18. Hyde M, O'Driscoll DM, Binette S, Galang C, Tan SK, et al. (2007) Validation of actigraphy for determining sleep and wake in children with sleep disordered breathing. J Sleep Res 16: 213-216.

19. Laakso ML, Leinonen L, Lindblom N, Joutsiniemi SL, Kaski M (2004) Wrist actigraphy in estimation of sleep and wake in intellectually disabled subjects with motor handicaps. Sleep Med 5: 541-550.

20. Holley S, Hill CM, Stevenson J (2010) A comparison of actigraphy and parental report of sleep habits in typically developing children aged 6 to 11 years. Behav Sleep Med 8: 16-27.

21. Sadeh A, Dahl RE, Shahar G, Rosenblat-Stein S (2009) Sleep and the transition to adolescence: a longitudinal study. Sleep 32: 1602-1609.

22. Sazonov E, Sazonova N, Schuckers S, Neuman M; CHIME Study Group (2004) Activity-based sleep-wake identification in infants. Physiol Meas 25: 1291-1304.

23. Enomoto M, Endo T, Suenaga K, Miura N, Nakano Y et al. (2009) Newly developed waist actigraphy and its sleep/wake scoring algorithm. Sleep Biol Rhythms 7: 17-22.

24. Chae KY, Kripke DF, Poceta JS, Shadan F, Jamil SM, et al. (2009) Evaluation of immobility time for sleep latency in actigraphy. Sleep Med 10: 621-625.

25. Lichstein KL, Stone KC, Donaldson J, Nau SD, Soeffing JP, et al. (2006) Actigraphy validation with insomnia. Sleep 29: 232-239.

26. Buysse DJ, Cheng Y, Germain A, Moul DE, Franzen PL, et al. (2010) Night-to-night sleep variability in older adults with and without chronic insomnia. Sleep Med 11: 56-64.

27. Sforza E, Zamagni M, Petiav C, Krieger J (1999) Actigraphy and leg movements during sleep: a validation study. J Clin Neurophysiol 16: 154-160.

28. Sforza E, Johannes M, Claudio B (2005) The PAM-RL ambulatory device for detection of periodic leg movements: a validation study. Sleep Med 6: 407-413.

29. Montgomery-Downs HE, Crabtree VM, Gozal D (2005) Actigraphic recordings in quantification of periodic leg movements during sleep in children. Sleep Med 6: 325-332.

30. Elbaz M, Roue GM, Lofaso F, Quera Salva MA (2002) Utility of actigraphy in the diagnosis of obstructive sleep apnea. Sleep 25: 527-531.

31. Gagnadoux F, Nguyen XL, Rakotonanahary D, Vidal S, Fleury B (2004) Wrist-actigraphic estimation of sleep time under nCPAP treatment in sleep apnoea patients. Eur Respir J 23: 891-895.

32. Middelkoop HA, Lammers GJ, Van Hilten BJ, Ruwhof C, Pijl H, et al. (1995) Circadian distribution of motor activity and immobility in narcolepsy: assessment with continuous motor activity monitoring. Psychophysiology 32: 286-291.

33. Sivertsen B, Omvik S, Havik OE, Pallesen S, Bjorvatn B, et al. (2006) A comparison of actigraphy and polysomnography in older adults treated for chronic primary insomnia. Sleep 29: 1353-1358.

34. Manber R, Edinger JD, Gress JL, San Pedro-Salcedo MG, Kuo TF, et al. (2008) Cognitive behavioral therapy for insomnia enhances depression outcome in patients with comorbid major depressive disorder and insomnia. Sleep 31: 489-495.

35. Espie CA, MacMahon KM, Kelly HL, Broomfield NM, Douglas NJ, et al. (2007) Randomized clinical effectiveness trial of nurse-administered small-group cognitive behavior therapy for persistent insomnia in general practice. Sleep 30: 574-584.

36. Harris J, Lack L, Wright H, Gradisar M, Brooks A (2007) Intensive Sleep Retraining treatment for chronic primary insomnia: a preliminary investigation. J Sleep Res 16: 276-284.

37. Stanley N (2003) Actigraphy in human psychopharmacology: a review. Hum Psychopharmacol 18: 39-49.

38. Wilson SJ, Rich AS, Rich NC, Potokar J, Nutt DJ (2004) Evaluation of actigraphy and automated telephoned questionnaires to assess hypnotic effects in insomnia. Int Clin Psychopharmacol 19: 77-84.

39. Paul MA, Gray G, Sardana TM, Pigeau RA (2004) Melatonin and zopiclone as facilitators of early circadian sleep in operational air transport crews. Aviat Space Environ Med 75: 439-443.

40. de Castro-Silva C, de Bruin VMS, Cunha GMA, Nunes DM, Medeiros CAM et al. (2010) Melatonin improves sleep and reduces nitrite in the exhaled breath condensate in cystic fibrosis - a randomized, double-blind placebocontrolled study. J Pineal Res 48: 65-71.

41. Meltzer LJ, Montgomery-Downs HE, Insana SP, Walsh CM (2012) Use of actigraphy for assessment in pediatric sleep research. Sleep Med Rev 16: 463-475.

42. Morgenthaler T, Alessi C, Friedman L, Owens J, Kapur V, et al. (2007) Practice parameters for the use of actigraphy in the assessment of sleep and sleep disorders: an update for 2007. Sleep 30: 519-529.

43. Acebo C, Sadeh A, Seifer R, Tzischinsky O, Wolfson AR, et al. (1999) Estimating sleep patterns with activity monitoring in children and adolescents: how many nights are necessary for reliable measures? Sleep 22: 95-103.

44. Konofal E, Lecendreux M, Cortese S (2010) Sleep and ADHD. Sleep Med 11: 652-658.

45. Cortese S, Konofal E, Lecendreux M, Arnulf I, Mouren MC, et al. (2005) Restless legs syndrome and attention-deficit/hyperactivity disorder: a review of the literature. Sleep 28: 1007-1013.

46. Cortese S, Lecendreux M, Mouren MC, Konofal E (2006) ADHD and insomnia. J Am Acad Child Adolesc Psychiatry 45: 384-385.

47. Chervin RD, Archbold KH, Dillon JE, Pituch KJ, Panahi P, et al. (2002) Associations between symptoms of inattention, hyperactivity, restless legs, and periodic leg movements. Sleep 25: 213-218.

48. Wagner ML, Walters AS, Fisher BC (2004) Symptoms of attention-deficit/hyperactivity disorder in adults with restless legs syndrome. Sleep 27: 1499-1504.

49. Huang YS, Chen NH, Li HY, Wu YY, Chao CC, et al. (2004) Sleep disorders in Taiwanese children with attention deficit/hyperactivity disorder. J Sleep Res 13: 269-277.

50. Bruni O, Ferri R, Verrillo E, Miano S (2006) New approaches to the study of leg movements during sleep in ADHD children. In: Proceedings of the 20th meeting of the Associated Sleep Societies Sleep 29: 259.

51. Van der Heijden KB, Smits MG, Van Someren EJ, Gunning WB (2005) Idiopathic chronic sleep onset insomnia in attention-deficit/hyperactivity disorder: a circadian rhythm sleep disorder. Chronobiol Int 22: 559-570.

52. Corkum P, Tannock R, Moldofsky H, Hogg-Johnson S, Humphries T (2001) Actigraphy and parental ratings of sleep in children with attention-deficit/hyperactivity disorder (ADHD). Sleep 24: 303-312.

53. Porrino LJ, Rapoport JL, Behar D, Ismond DR, Bunney Jr WE (1983) A naturalistic assessment of the motor activity of hyperactive boys. II. Stimulant drug effects. Arch Gen Psychiatry 40: 688–693.

54. Konofal E, Lecendreux M, Bouvard MP, Mouren-Simeoni MC (2001) High levels of nocturnal activity in children with attention-deficit hyperactivity disorder: a video analysis. Psychiatry Clin Neurosci 55: 97-103.

55. Pliszka S; AACAP Work Group on Quality Issues (2007) Practice parameter for the assessment and treatment of children and adolescents with attention-deficit/hyperactivity disorder. J Am Acad Child Adolesc Psychiatry 46: 894-921.

56. Moreau V, Rouleau N, Morin CM (2014) Sleep of children with attention deficit hyperactivity disorder: actigraphic and parental reports. Behav Sleep Med 12: 69-83.

57. Corkum P, Moldofsky H, Hogg-Johnson S, Humphries T, Tannock R (1999) Sleep problems in children with attention-deficit/hyperactivity disorder: impact of subtype, comorbidity, and stimulant medication. J Am Acad Child Adolesc Psychiatry 38: 1285-1293.

58. Brown TE, McMullen WJ Jr (2001) Attention deficit disorders and sleep/arousal disturbance. Ann N Y Acad Sci 931: 271-286.

59. De Crescenzo F, Armando M, Mazzone L, Ciliberto M, Sciannamea M, et al. (2014) The use of actigraphy in the monitoring of methylphenidate versus placebo in ADHD: a meta-analysis. Atten Defic Hyperact Disord 6: 49-58.

40

The Endothelial Cell Secretome as a Factor of Endothelium Reparation: The Role of Microparticles

Alexander E Berezin*

Consultant of Therapeutic Unit, Private Hospital "Vita-Center", Zaporozhye, Ukraine

***Corresponding author:** Alexander E Berezin, MD, PhD, Consultant of Therapeutic Unit, Private Hospital "Vita-Center" and Consultant of Therapeutic Unit, Department of Internal Medicine, Medical University, Zaporozhye, Ukraine; E-mail: dr_berezin@mail.ru

Abstract

The secretome is considered a combination of factors produced by cells due to abundant spectrum of autocrine/paracrine triggers. All these actively synthetizing and secreting factors include proteins, adhesion and intercellular signal molecules, peptides, lipids, free DNAs, microRNAs, and microparticles (MPs). The components of secretome mutually may interact and thereby modify the MPs' structure and functionality. As a result, communicative ability of endothelial cell-derived MPs may sufficiently impaire. Subsequently, cross talk between some components of secretome might modulate delivering cargos of MPs and their regenerative and proliferative capabilities via intercellular signaling networks. The aim of the review is to discuss the effect of various components of secretome on MP-dependent effects on endothelium.

Keywords: Endothelium; Endothelial cells; Secretome; Reparation; Microparticles

Introduction

For last decade, elevated circulating level of microparticles (MPs) produced by various types of blood cells have been defined in the patients with established cardiovascular (CV) disease, as well as in individuals at higher risk of CV events and diseases [1-4]. There is suggestive evidence that a number of circulating endothelial cell-derived MPs might be a clinically useful biomarker that pretty accurate predicts CV complications in general populations and patients with known CV disease [5-7]. Although an origin of endothelial cell-derived MPs from activated or apoptotic cells is crucial for realizing tissue repair, degenerative processes modulation, immune mediation, and directly/indirectly vascular injury [8], there are several controversies regarding an involvement of MPs in pathogenesis of CV disease [9-11]. The first controversy affects the pathophysiological properties of MPs. Indeed, the MPs secreted by activated endothelial cells may contribute to tissue reparation, restore endothelial function, mediate progenitor cell mobbing and differentiation, whereas apoptotic MPs are able directly injury endothelial cells and via a transfer of several proteins, active molecules, chromatin compounds including microRNAs and DNAs, regulate inflammation, coagulation, and immune response [12]. The next controversy relates a different presentation of endothelial cell-derived MPs in plasma of healthy individuals and changing of their numbers in various CV diseases and CV risks. Interestingly, circulating number of MPs originated from apoptotic endothelial cells increases in patients with CV risk factors, after newly CV events and in individuals with established CV disease. However, the ability of activated endothelial cells to active secret MPs progressively decreases depending on CV risk presentation, i.e., diabetes mellitus, abdominal obesity, insulin resistance, renal disease, and is due co-existing endothelial disintegrity [13-15]. Unfortunately, although there is strong association between circulating number of activated endothelial cell-derived MPs and CV risk, elevated level of apoptotic endothelial cell-derived MPs appears to be much more accurate predictive biomarker relating to CV death and CV diseases progression [16]. Another controversy is that the endothelial cell-derived MPs are constitutive biomarker of endothelial dysfunction playing a pivotal role in inflammation, vascular injury, angiogenesis, and thrombosis. However, the circulating number of endothelial cell-derived MPs predicts CV manifestation and progression regardless a severity of endothelial dysfunction. In fact, the imbalance between number of circulating endothelial cell-derived MPs distinguished their origin (activated or apoptotic endothelial cells) can be applied as more promising routine tests to improve CV risk prediction [17,18]. Whether "impaired phenotype" of endothelial cell-derived MPs as a causality factor contributed the vascular "competence" in CV disease is a predominantly pre-existing phenomenon associated with genetic/epigenetic performances or is resulting in various metabolic and age-dependent factors is not clear. Probably, variable effect of endothelial cell-derived MPs might relate to particularities of the triggers, which induced cell mechanisms of synthesis and secretion of secretome. The aim of the review is to discuss the effect of various components of secretome on MP-dependent effects on endothelium.

Secretome: definition and components

The variable spectrum of paracrine factors secreted by cells due to specific and non-specific triggers with exerted biological effects on target cells is determined by secretome. By now, the secretome is considered a collection of factors consisting of transmembrane proteins and other components actively secreted by cells into the extracellular space. All these synthetizing and secreting factors include proteins, adhesion and intercellular signal molecules, peptides, lipids, free DNAs, microRNAs, and extracellular vesicles (i.e., exosomes and MPs). A significant portion (roughly 20%) of the human secretome consists of secretory proteins incorporated into microvesicles.

Definition of microparticles

MPs are large and very variable on their shapes and dimensions (predominantly 100-1000 nm) heterogeneous sub-population of extracellular vesicles (EVs), which are shedding from plasma membranes of parent cells in response to cell' activation, injury, and/or apoptosis [19]. EVs contain cell-specific collections of proteins, glycoproteins, lipids, nucleic acids and other molecules, which are non-specific for EVs. Depending on their origin EVs are graduated to follow subsets, i.e., the exosomes (30-100 nm in diameter), the microvesicles (50-1000 nm in diameter), ectosomes (100-350 nm in diameter), small-size MPs (<50 nm in diameter) known as membrane particles and apoptotic bodies (1-5 μm in diameter). The exosomes are formed by inward budding of the endosomal membrane and are released on the exocytosis of multivesicular bodies known as late endosomes, whereas the microvesicles are attributed via budding from plasma membranes [20,21].

MPs are released by cellular vesiculation and fission of the membrane of cells. Under normal physiological condition a phospholipid bilayer of plasma membrane of cells represented phosphatidylserine and phosphatidylethanoalamine in inner leaflets, whereas phosphatidylcholine and sphingomyelin represent in the external leaflets. The asymmetrical distribution of phospholipids in the plasma membrane is supported by activity of three major intracellular ATP-dependent enzyme systems, i.e., flippase, floppase, and scramblase. Because aminophospholipids are negatively charged, but phospholipids exhibit neutral charge, the main role of intracellular enzyme systems is supporting electrochemical gradient. Both flippase and floppase belong to family of ATP-dependent phospholipid translocases [22].

The flippase translocates phosphatidylserine and phosphatidylethanoalamine from the external leaflets to the inner one. The floppase transports phospholipids in the opposite direction. Finally, scramblase being to Ca^{2+} dependent enzyme system exhibits unspecifically ability of moving of phospholipids between both leaflets of plasma membrane [23].

Importantly, disappearing of the asymmetrical phospholipid distribution in the bilayer of the cell membrane is considered a clue for vesiculation and forming of MPs. Indeed, both processes of apoptosis or cell activation are required asymmetry in phospholipid distribution that leads to cytoskeleton modifications, membrane budding and MPs release. The mechanisms of vesiculation affect genome and may mediate by some triggers including inflammation, while in some cases there is a spontaneous release of MPs from stable cells or due to injury from necrotic cells or from mechanically damaged cells. Particularly, the MPs are released in both constitutive and controlled manners, regulated by intercellular Ca^{2+} and Rab-GTP-ases and activation of μ-calpain. μ-Calpain is a Ca^{2+}-dependent cytosolic enzyme belong to protease, which cleaves talin and α-actin, leading to decreased binding of integrins to the cytoskeleton and a reduction in cell adhesion and integrity [24].

Recently MPs are considered a cargo for various molecules. Indeed, MPs carry proteins, RNA, micro-RNA, and DNA fragments from their cells of origin to other parts of the body via blood and other body fluids. Within last decade it has become to know that MPs would act as information transfer for target cells. However, the difference between innate mechanisms affected the release of MPs from stable cells, activated cells or apoptotic cells is yet not fully investigated and requires more studies.

Endothelial cell-derived microparticles

Endothelial cells release phenotypically and quantitatively distinct MP populations due to two main mechanisms, i.e., cell activation and apoptosis. As a result, MPs are sufficiently distinguished one another in their ability to present some antigens [19] and intravesicle components, i.e. matrix metalloproteinases (MMP)-2, MMP-9, MT1-MMP, chromatin, active molecules (heat shock proteins), some hormones (angiotensin II), growth factors (transforming factor-beta) [24-27]. It is suggested that the epigenetic modification of the parent cells might directly regulatory impact on functionality of secreted MPs and their ability to influence various biological effects [28]. Indeed, the endothelial cell-derived MPs isolated from the serum of patients with diabetes mellitus, chronic kidney disease, heart failure and atherosclerosis are defective in ability to induce vascular relaxation, maturation of progenitor cells and endothelium repair [29-32]. As factors contributing in the response of the target cells after stimulation MPs could be pointed inflammatory cytokines (tumor necrosis factor-alpha, interleukin: IL-4, IL-17), glucose, advanced glycation end-products, uremic toxins, free DNA, products of lipid peroxidation [33]. Nonetheless, hypoxia-modified endothelial cell-derived MPs are able to carry reactive oxygen species and thereby may impair target cells by promoting apoptosis and oxidative stress [34]. One cannot be excluded the role of metabolomics-regulated microenvironments of target cells as a causative factor modifying the response after MPs' cooperation [35,36]. It has been postulated that activation of p^{53} subunit, Akt/GSK-3beta and JAK2/STAT3 signaling pathways are involved in the regulation of MPs' synthesis and that these molecular targets are under close control of various metabolites and intermediates, as well as epigenetics' mechanisms [37-40]. Thus, secretome of endothelial cells including metabolites, proteins, intermediates, DNAs/reactive oxygen radicals, active molecules, may probably modify and even alter a communicative ability of MPs secreted by endothelial cells [41-44].

Relation between secretome and endothelial cell functionality

Endothelial cell-derived MPs are not only delivery of intra-vesicular cargo and information, but they may directly modulate vascular function via autocrine and paracrine effects through surface interaction of the target cells, and cellular fusion [45]. Subsequently, in vitro investigation has shown that the MPs and other fractions of secretome might mutually influence one another [9]. The final result of the interrelation may be shaping brand new biological components with irradiative abilities toward target cells [46,47]. Finally, it has been suggested that enhancing of the target cell mobility and differentiation through MP production could be impaired, inverted or even sufficiently changed [48]. Indeed, secretome of apoptotic peripheral blood cells may induce cytoprotection effect instead expected worsening tissue remodeling in animal model of acute myocardial infarction [49-51]. Additionally, this effect is probably due to the activation of pro-survival signalling cascades in the cardiomyocytes and the increase of homing of regenerative cells through stimulation of metabolically modified MPs. Additionally, in clinical settings angiogenic early outgrowth endothelial progenitor cells have been reported to contribute to endothelial regeneration and to limit neointima formation after vascular injury through cooperation with metabolically modified MPs [52].

Thus, there is a large body of evidence regarding being of modifying effect of secretome components on MPs' ability for tissue regeneration or injury. Moreover, regenerative potency of apoptotic cell secretome was even higher than those in activated cells. However, new phenomenon opens serious perspective to clinical implementation of MPs as not just diagnostic tool with predictive possibilities, but as transfer system with therapeutic potencies [43,54].

Whether endothelial cell-derived MPs are capable to induce variable effects on target cells depending on proteomic of MPs or functional nature of secretome is not fully understood [55]. In fact, cross talk between some components of secretome including MPs might modulate delivering cargos of MPs through involving the intercellular signalling networks and thereby modify their regenerative and proliferative capabilities. Future investigations are requires to define the role of secretome in MPs' ability to produce different biological effects regarding endothelial repair, while recent studies have suggested the predominantly role of MPs' origin in this matter.

Conclusion

The endothelial cells secretome has most commonly investigated in pre-clinical settings as a source of regulating factors that influence target cells. However, the interaction between different components of secretome leads to modification of the MPs' structure and functionality. It has been hypothesized that endothelial regeneration is under tight control of autocrine and paracrine mechanisms affecting not just parent endothelial cells, but also secretome of them. The matter of metabolic modification of one is uncertain and requires more investigations in future.

References

1. Thulin Å, Christersson C, Alfredsson J, Siegbahn A (2016) Circulating cell-derived microparticles as biomarkers in cardiovascular disease. Biomark Med 10: 1009-1022.

2. Berezin AE, Kremzer AA, Martovitskaya YV, Berezina TA, Gromenko EA (2016) Pattern of endothelial progenitor cells and apoptotic endothelial cell-derived microparticles in chronic heart failure patients with preserved and reduced left ventricular ejection fraction. E Bio Medicine 4: 86-94.

3. Berezin AE, Kremzer AA, Berezina TA, Martovitskaya YV (2015) Pattern of circulating microparticles in chronic heart failure patients with metabolic syndrome: Relevance to neurohumoral and inflammatory activation. BBA Clin 4: 69-75.

4. Berezin AE, Kremzer AA, Cammarota G, Zulli A, Petrovic D, et al. (2016) Circulating endothelial-derived apoptotic microparticles and insulin resistance in non-diabetic patients with chronic heart failure. Clin Chem Lab Med 54: 1259-1267.

5. Berezin AE, Kremzer AA, Berezina TA, Martovitskaya YV (2016) The Pattern of circulating microparticles in patients with diabetes mellitus with asymptomatic atherosclerosis. Acta Clin Belg 71: 38-45.

6. Berezin AE, Kremzer AA, Martovitskaya YV, Samura TA, Berezina TA, et al. (2015) The utility of biomarker risk prediction score in patients with chronic heart failure. Int J Clin Exp Med 8: 18255-18264.

7. Berezin AE, Kremzer AA, Martovitskaya YV, Samura TA, Berezina TA (2014) The predictive role of circulating microparticles in patients with chronic heart failure. BBA Clin 3: 18-24.

8. Berezin AE (2015) Impaired Phenotype of Circulating Endothelial-Derived Microparticles: Novel Marker of Cardiovascular Risk. J Cardiol Ther (Hong Kong) 2: 273-278.

9. Beer L, Mildner M, Gyöngyösi M, Ankersmit HJ (2016) Peripheral blood mononuclear cell secretome for tissue repair. Apoptosis 21: 1336-1353.

10. Jeske WP, Walenga JM, Menapace B, Schwartz J, Bakhos M (2016) Blood cell microparticles as biomarkers of hemostatic abnormalities in patients with implanted cardiac assist devices. Biomark Med 10: 1095-1104.

11. Baron M, Boulanger CM, Staels B, Tailleux A (2012) Cell-derived microparticles in atherosclerosis: biomarkers and targets for pharmacological modulation? J Cell Mol Med 16: 1365-1376.

12. Berezin A, Zulli A, Kerrigan S, Petrovic D, Kruzliak P (2015) Predictive role of circulating endothelial-derived microparticles in cardiovascular diseases. Clin Biochem 48: 562-568.

13. Amabile N, Gurin AP, Leroyer A, Mallat Z, Nguyen C, et al. (2005) Circulating endothelial microparticles are associated with vascular dysfunction in patients with end-stage renal failure. J Am Soc Nephrol 16: 3381-3388.

14. Pirro M, Schillaci G, Bagaglia F, Menecali C, Paltriccia R, et al. (2008) Microparticles derived from endothelial progenitor cells in patients at different cardiovascular risk. Atherosclerosis 197: 757-767.

15. Yue WS, Lau KK, Siu CW, Wang M, Yan GH, et al. (2011) Impact of glycemic control on circulating endothelial progenitor cells and arterial stiffness in patients with type 2 diabetes mellitus. Cardiovasc Diabetol 10: 113.

16. Berezin A (2016) The Clinical Utility of Circulating Microparticles' Measurement in Heart Failure Patients. J Vasc Med Surg 4: 275-284.

17. Berezin AE (2016) Impaired Immune Phenotype of Endothelial Cell-derived Micro Particles: The Missing Link between Diabetes-related States and Risk of Cardiovascular Complications? J Data Mining Genom Proteom 7: 195.

18. Nozaki T, Sugiyama S, Koga H, Sugamura K, Ohba K, et al. (2009) Significance of a multiple biomarkers strategy including endothelial dysfunction to improve risk stratification for cardiovascular events in patients at high risk for coronary heart disease. J Am Coll Cardiol 54: 601-608.

19. Ullal AJ, Pisetsky DS, Reich C (2010) Use of SYTO 13, a fluorescent dye binding nucleic acids, for the detection of microparticles in in vitro systems. Cytometry A 77: 294-301.

20. Cocucci E, Meldolesi J (2015) Ectosomes and exosomes: shedding the confusion between extracellular vesicles. Trends Cell Biol 25: 364-372.

21. Colombo M, Raposo G, Théry C (2014) Biogenesis, secretion, and intercellular interactions of exosomes and other extracellular vesicles. Annu Rev Cell Dev Biol 30: 255-289.

22. Piccin A, Murphy WG, Smith OP (2007) Circulating microparticles: pathophysiology and clinical implications. Blood Rev 21: 157-171.

23. Tesselaar ME, Romijn FP, Van DL, Prins FA, Bertina RM, et al. (2007) Microparticle-associated tissue factor activity: a link between cancer and thrombosis? J Thromb Haemost 5: 520-527.

24. Simak J, Gelderman MP (2006) Cell membrane microparticles in blood and blood products: potentially pathogenic agents and diagnostic markers. Transfus Med Rev 20: 1-26.

25. Reich C, Pisetsky DS (2009) The content of DNA and RNA in microparticles released by Jurkat and HL-60 cells undergoing in vitro apoptosis. Exp Cell Res 315: 760-768.

26. Horstman LL, Jy W, Jimenez JJ, Ahn YS (2004) Endothelial microparticles as markers of endothelial dysfunction. Front Biosci 9: 1118-1135.

27. Mayr M, Grainger D, Mayr U, Leroyer AS, Leseche G, et al. (2009) Proteomics, metabolomics, and immunomics on microparticles derived from human atherosclerotic plaques. Circ Cardiovasc Genet. 2: 379-388.

28. Mause SF, Weber C (2010) Microparticles: protagonists of a novel communication network for intercellular information exchange. Circ Res 107: 1047-1057.

29. Helmke A, von Vietinghoff S (2016) Extracellular vesicles as mediators of vascular inflammation in kidney disease. World J Nephrol 5: 125-138.

30. Lu Y, Li L, Yan H, Su Q, Huang J (2013) Endothelial microparticles exert differential effects on functions of Th1 in patients with acute coronary syndrome. Int J Cardiol 168: 5396-5404.

31. Angelot F, Seillès E, Biichlé S, Berda Y, Gaugler B, et al. (2009) Endothelial cell-derived microparticles induce plasmacytoid dendritic cell maturation: potential implications in inflammatory diseases. Haematologica. 94: 1502-1512.

32. Carpintero R, Gruaz L, Brandt KJ, Scanu A, Faille D, et al. (2010) HDL interfere with the binding of T cell microparticles to human monocytes to inhibit pro-inflammatory cytokine production. PLoS One 5: e11869.

33. Scanu A, Molnarfi N, Brandt KJ, Gruaz L, Dayer JM, et al. (2008) Stimulated T cells generate microparticles, which mimic cellular contact activation of human monocytes: differential regulation of pro- and anti-inflammatory cytokine production by high-density lipoproteins. J Leukoc Biol 83: 921-927.

34. Zhang Q, Shang M, Zhang M, Wang Y, Chen Y, et al. (2016) Microvesicles derived from hypoxia/reoxygenation-treated human umbilical vein endothelial cells promote apoptosis and oxidative stress in H9c2 cardiomyocytes. BMC Cell Biol 17: 25.

35. Nomura S, Tandon NN, Nakamura T, Cone J, Fukuhara S, et al. (2001) High-shear-stress-induced activation of platelets and microparticles enhances expression of cell adhesion molecules in THP-1 and endothelial cells. Atherosclerosis 158: 277-287.

36. Boulanger CM, Scoazec A, Ebrahimian T, Henry P, Mathieu E, et al. (2001) Circulating microparticles from patients with myocardial infarction cause endothelial dysfunction. Circulation 104: 2649-2652.

37. Song JQ, Teng X, Cai Y, Tang CS, Qi YF (2009) Activation of Akt/GSK-3beta signaling pathway is involved in intermedin(1–53) protection against myocardial apoptosis induced by ischemia/reperfusion. Apoptosis 14: 1299-1307.

38. Jiang X, Guo CX, Zeng XJ, Li HH, Chen BX, et al. (2015) A soluble receptor for advanced glycation end-products inhibits myocardial apoptosis induced by ischemia/reperfusion via the JAK2/STAT3 pathway. Apoptosis 20: 1033-1047.

39. Ou ZJ, Chang FJ, Luo D, Liao XL, Wang ZP, et al. (2011) Endothelium-derived microparticles inhibit angiogenesis in the heart and enhance the inhibitory effects of hypercholesterolemia on angiogenesis. Am J Physiol Endocrinol Metab 300: E661-E668.

40. Deregibus MC, Cantaluppi V, Calogero R, Lo Iacono M, Tetta C, et al. Endothelial progenitor cell derived microvesicles activate an angiogenic program in endothelial cells by a horizontal transfer of mRNA. Blood 110: 2440-2448.

41. Eckers A, Haendeler J (2015) Endothelial cells in health and disease. Antioxid Redox Signal. 22: 1209-1211.

42. Radecke CE, Warrick AE, Singh GD, Rogers JH, Simon SI, et al. (2014) Coronary artery endothelial cells and microparticles increase expression of VCAM-1 in myocardial infarction. Thromb Haemost 113: 605-616.

43. Arderiu G, Peña E, Badimon L (2015) Angiogenic Microvascular Endothelial Cells Release Microparticles Rich in Tissue Factor That Promotes Postischemic Collateral Vessel Formation. Arterioscler Thromb Vasc Biol 35: 348-357.

44. Zhang J, Ren J, Chen H, Geng Q (2014) Inflammation induced-endothelial cells release angiogenesis associated-microRNAs into circulation by microparticles. Chin Med J (Engl) 127: 2212-2217.

45. Curtis AM, Edelberg J, Jonas R, Rogers WT, Moore JS, et al. (2013) Endothelial microparticles: sophisticated vesicles modulating vascular function. Vasc Med 18: 204-214.

46. Mukherjee P, Mani S (2013) Methodologies to decipher the cell secretome. Biochim Biophys Acta 1834: 2226-2232.

47. Ankersmit HJ, Hoetzenecker K, Dietl W, Soleiman A, Horvat R, et al. (2009) Irradiated cultured apoptotic peripheral blood mononuclear cells regenerate infarcted myocardium. Eur J Clin Invest 39: 445-456.

48. Makridakis M, Roubelakis MG, Vlahou A (2013) Stem cells: insights into the secretome. Biochim Biophys Acta 1834: 2380-2384.

49. Lichtenauer M, Mildner M, Hoetzenecker K, Zimmermann M, Podesser BK, et al. (2011) Secretome of apoptotic peripheral blood cells (APOSEC) confers cytoprotection to cardiomyocytes and inhibits tissue remodelling after acute myocardial infarction: a preclinical study. Basic Res Cardiol 106: 1283-1297.

50. Lichtenauer M, Mildner M, Baumgartner A, Hasun M, Werba G, et al. (2011) Intravenous and intramyocardial injection of apoptotic white blood cell suspensions prevents ventricular remodelling by increasing elastin expression in cardiac scar tissue after myocardial infarction. Basic Res Cardiol 106: 645-655.

51. Lichtenauer M, Mildner M, Werba G, Beer L, Hoetzenecker K, et al. (2012) Anti-thymocyte globulin induces neoangiogenesis and preserves cardiac function after experimental myocardial infarction. PLoS One 7: e52101.

52. Mause SF, Ritzel E, Liehn EA, Hristov M, Bidzhekov K, et al. (2010) Platelet microparticles enhance the vasoregenerative potential of angiogenic early outgrowth cells after vascular injury. Circulation 122: 495-506.

53. Vlassov AV, Magdaleno S, Setterquist R, Conrad R (2012) Exosomes: current knowledge of their composition, biological functions, and diagnostic and therapeutic potentials. Biochim Biophys Acta 1820: 940-948.

54. Ankrum JA, Miranda OR, Ng KS, Sarkar D, Xu C, et al. (2014) Engineering cells with intracellular agent-loaded microparticles to control cell phenotype. Nat Protoc 9: 233-245.

55. Le Bihan MC, Bigot A, Jensen SS, Dennis JL, Rogowska-Wrzesinska A, et al. (2012) In-depth analysis of the secretome identifies three major independent secretory pathways in differentiating human myoblasts. J Proteomics. 77: 344-56.

41

White Coat Hypertension is a Pioneer Sign of Metabolic Syndrome

Mehmet Rami Helvaci[1*] **and Ali Ozcan**[2]

[1]*Professor of Internal Medicine, Medical Faculty of the Mustafa Kemal University, Hatay, Turkey*

[2]*Professor of Biochemistry, Medical Faculty of the Mustafa Kemal University, Hatay, Turkey*

[*]**Corresponding author:** Mehmet Rami Helvaci, Professor of Internal Medicine, Medical Faculty of the Mustafa Kemal University, 31100, Serinyol, Antakya, Hatay, Turkey; E-mail: mramihelvaci@hotmail.com

Abstract

Metabolic syndrome is an accelerated systemic atherosclerotic process terminating with obesity, hypertension, diabetes mellitus, peripheric artery disease, chronic renal disease, chronic obstructive pulmonary disease, cirrhosis, coronary heart disease, stroke, and eventually early aging and death. It shows itself with some reversible components including smoking, overweight, hyperbetalipoproteinemia, hypertriglyceridemia, dyslipidemia, impaired fasting glucose, impaired glucose tolerance, and white coat hypertension (WCH). The terminal consequences are probably due to the smoking and excess weight induced chronic inflammatory process on the endothelial system for a long period of time. WCH is a pioneer sign of the accelerated systemic atherosclerotic process that can be detected easily, and treated by preventing weight gain.

Keywords: White coat hypertension; Metabolic syndrome; Atherosclerosis

Introduction

A causative relationship between excess weight and systemic atherosclerosis is known for many years under the title of metabolic syndrome [1,2]. The syndrome is characterized by a low-grade chronic inflammatory process probably initiated in early life, and can be slowed down with appropriate nonpharmaceutical approaches including lifestyle changes, diet, and exercise [3,4]. But probably the syndrome cannot be prevented completely, since aging alone may be one of the significant facilitator factor of the systemic atherosclerotic process. The metabolic syndrome may contain early reversible indicators such as white coat hypertension (WCH), impaired fasting glucose (IFG), impaired glucose tolerance (IGT), hypertriglyceridemia, hyperbetalipoproteinemia, dyslipidemia, overweight, and smoking for the development of irreversible diseases including obesity, hypertension (HT), type 2 diabetes mellitus (DM), peripheric artery disease (PAD), coronary heart disease (CHD), chronic obstructive pulmonary disease (COPD), cirrhosis, chronic renal disease (CRD), stroke, and eventually early aging and death [5]. In another word, the syndrome induced systemic atherosclerosis is probably the leading cause of death for both sexes all over the world. For example, prevalences of hypertriglyceridemia, hyperbetalipoproteinemia, dyslipidemia, IGT, and WCH had a parallel fashion to excess weight by increasing until the seventh decade of life and decreasing afterwards (p<0.05 nearly in all steps) in a previous study [6]. On the other hand, prevalences of HT, DM, and CHD always continued to increase without any decrease by decades (p<0.05 nearly in all steps) indicating their irreversible natures [6]. After development of one of the terminal consequences, the nonpharmaceutical approaches will provide little benefit to prevent development of the others probably due to cumulative effects of the risk factors on the endothelial system for a long period of time [7,8]. According to our opinion, obesity should be included among the terminal consequences of the syndrome since after development of obesity; pharmaceutical and nonpharmaceutical approaches will provide little benefit either to heal obesity or to prevent its complications.

Excess weight probably initiates to a chronic and low-grade inflammatory process on many systems, especially on the endothelial system, and risk of death from all causes including cardiovascular diseases and cancers increases parallel to the range of moderate to severe weight excess in all age groups [9]. The effects of weight on blood pressure (BP) were also shown previously that the prevalence of normotension (NT) was significantly higher in the underweight (80.3%) than the normal weight (64.0%) and overweight cases (31.5%, p<0.05 for both) and 55.1% of cases with HT had obesity against 26.6% of cases with NT (p<0.001) in another study [10,11]. So the dominant underlying causative factor of the metabolic syndrome appears as an already existing excess weight or a trend towards excess weight, which is probably the main cause of insulin resistance, dyslipidemia, IFG, IGT, and WCH [4]. Even prevention of the accelerating trend of weight with diet or exercise, even in the absence of a prominent weight loss, will probably result with resolution of many reversible indicators of the syndrome [12-14]. But according to our opinion, limitation of excess weight as an excess fat tissue in and around abdomen under the heading of abdominal obesity is meaningless, instead it should be defined as overweight or obesity via body mass index (BMI), since adipocytes function as an endocrine organ that produces a variety of cytokines and hormones in anywhere of the body [4]. The resulting hyperactivity of sympathetic nervous system and renin-angiotensin-aldosterone system is probably associated with insulin resistance, elevated BP, and chronic endothelial inflammation. Similarly, the Adult Treatment Panel III reported that although some people classified as overweight with a large muscular mass, most of them also have excess fat tissue, and excess weight does not only predispose to CHD, stroke, and several other atherosclerotic consequences, it also has a high burden of other CHD risk factors including dyslipidemia, DM, and HT [15].

Elevated BP increases risks of major cardiovascular events including renal failure, myocardial infarction, stroke, and cardiovascular death.

But diagnosis and management of HT is complicated by the fact that BP varies greatly, depending on physical and mental stresses. Furthermore, the elderly people tend to have an abnormal circadian rhythm and a normally higher systolic BP than younger individuals. In addition, in the doctor's office in particular, measurements are often too high which is called as WCH. WCH is defined as office BP of ≥ 140/90 mmHg for systolic and/or diastolic but home BP of <135/85 mmHg for both. According to our experience, there are many people using antihypertensive medication, which has been initiated just after a single office measurement, but actually being normotensive. A practicable and inexpensive supplementary method to avoid inaccurate results is home blood pressure measurement (HBPM). This approach may enable numerous measurements to be obtained, which can more accurately reflect the real situation than one off-measurement in the physician's office. Since HBPM is easily accepted by patients, it is reasonable to recommend taking several measurements. For example, HBPM (mean of three to 38 measurements) was a better predictor of total mortality than office measurements at screening in the Ohasama study [16]. The authors have used a schedule for HBPM with a single morning measurement, and advised taking as many measurements as possible (preferably more than 14) for the best prediction of stroke risk. Additionally, recent HT guidelines propose HBPM as an important means to evaluate the response to antihypertensive treatment, to improve compliance with therapy, and most importantly, as an alternative to 24 hour ambulatory blood pressure measurement (ABPM) to confirm or refute the WCH [17]. HBPM is useful not only for diagnosis of HT but also for its management including choice and titration of antihypertensive drugs. A minimal antihypertensive effect and duration of action of antihypertensives can be determined by HBPM. The duration of action of drugs is established by the comparison of the antihypertensive effect in the morning with that in the evening. Appropriateness of HBPM to guide antihypertensive treatment was only tested in one large-scale randomized trial: the THOP (Treatment of Hypertension Based on Home or Office Blood Pressure) trial, in which it was shown that antihypertensive treatments based on home instead of office BP measurements led to a less intensive drug treatment, but also to less BP control with no difference in general well-being and left ventricular mass [18]. In another study, both HBPM and ABPM appeared to be appropriate methods for detection of masked hypertension (MHT) [19]. Similarly, we could not detect any significant difference for diagnosis of WCH and MHT between HBPM and ABPM and it was observed on ABPM that the white coat effect was initiated by leaving home to come to hospital [20]. Additionally, HBPM can provide a greater number of readings and, when automatic devices are used, an absence of observer bias. It may also reduce the number of doctor visits. Patients can use this method several times by themselves in a year without requiring any ambulatory device. It is also a less expensive method of BP monitoring. Furthermore, self-measurement can also reveal therapeutic effects more reliably and has a greater predictive value for organic damage. So HBPM should be the preferred method for the diagnosis of MHT and HT against office measurements and ABPM due to its simplicity and effectiveness, and should be applied to all people above the age of 40 years once a year due to high prevalence of HT and MHT in this age group.

There are various reports about the prognostic significance of WCH in the literature. In a 7.4 year follow-up study, there was no evidence that WCH exhibited a clearly higher risk for the development cardiovascular events [21]. In another study, complication risks of

WCH were not found as different from NT [22]. On the other hand, the intima-media thickness and cross-sectional area of the carotid artery were found to be similar in patients with WCH and HT, and significantly higher than patients with NT, and the authors concluded that there is target organ damage in WCH, and WCH should not be considered as an innocent trait [23]. It was reported in the Ohasama study that WCH is a risk factor for the development of home HT [16]. In an 8-year follow-up study again, 46.9% of cases with WCH and 22.2% of cases with NT progressed to HT [24]. Similarly, plasma homocysteine levels were higher, and left ventricle mass index was greater in WCH compared to NT groups (p<0.001 for both) [23]. It was reported in the literature that WCH is associated with some features of the metabolic syndrome and more than 85% of cases with the syndrome have elevated BP levels in another study [4,25]. On the other hand, we observed very high prevalences of WCH even in early decades, 23.2% in the third and 24.2% in the fourth decades of life [6]. The very high prevalences of WCH in society were also shown by some other studies [26,27]. When we compared the NT, WCH, and HT groups in another study prevalence of all health problems including obesity, IGT, DM, and CHD had significant progressions from the NT towards the WCH and HT groups, and the WCH group was found as a progression step in between [28]. But as an interesting result, the prevalence of dyslipidemia was the highest in the WCH group, and it was 41.6% among them versus 19.6% of NT (p<0.001) and 35.5% of HT groups' (p<0.05) [28]. Similar results indicating the higher prevalence of dyslipidemia in WCH cases were also observed in another study against to another study indicating serum trigliseride and cholesterol levels did not differ significantly between NT, WCH, and HT cases in men in the literature [29,30]. The relatively lower prevalence of dyslipidemia in HT group may be explained by the already increased adipose tissue per taken fat in HT cases, since prevalence of obesity was significantly higher in HT against WCH groups (p<0.01) [28]. So the detected higher prevalence of WCH even in early decades, despite the lower prevalence of excess weight in these age groups, may show a trend of getting weight and its terminal consequences. Probably all of the associations are closely related with the metabolic syndrome since WCH and dyslipidemia may be two initial signs of the syndrome. On the other hand, we accept WCH as a different entity from borderline/mild HT due to the completely normal HBPM and ABPM values in WCH cases, whereas they are abnormal in mild HT cases [20].

According to our experience, there are many patients not using any antihypertensive medication, which has been evaluated just after a single office BP measurement, but actually they have MHT. Prevalence of WCH and MHT increased with aging in a previous study [15]. Whereas we observed an increased prevalence of MHT by aging, too, but the prevalence of WCH increased until the fourth decade and then began to decrease, and was lowered to 8% in the eighth decade, whereas it was higher than 40% in the third, fourth, and fifth decades of life [20]. We detected prevalence of MHT as lower than 5% until the seventh decade of life and it was 7% in seventh and 16% in the eighth decades [20]. Its rate never exceeded 25% of all HT cases [20]. As an opposite finding to us, MHT was detected as common as WCH, and masking was correlated with male sex and young age, thus suggesting a causal relationship with greater daytime physical activity [31]. Whereas according to our results, WCH is a much frequent phenomenon than MHT until the eighth decade, and MHT is mainly detected in elders [20]. Additionally, MHT showed an equal sexual distribution in our study [20]. As a parallel finding to us, the prevalence of WCH was found to be 5% between the ages of 65 and 70 years in another study [32]. But in the same study, the white coat effect was found to be more marked for systolic than diastolic BP, and the study was concluded as previously observed higher BPs seen in the elders may be explained by the greater white coat effect. Whereas, diastolic white coat effect was observed in 64%, diastolic and systolic in 33%, and systolic alone only in 2% of the WCH cases by us [20]. According to our opinion, due to the very high prevalence of WCH even in early decades and sexual distribution differences between WCH and HT cases, WCH should be thought as a response of the body against various stresses including weight gain.

Smoking alone may be one of the major underlying causes of the systemic atherosclerotic process, and even cancers [33,34]. Its atherosclerotic effect is the most obvious in Buerger's disease. It is an inflammatory disease characterized by obliterative changes in small and medium-sized arteries and veins, and it has never been documented in nonsmokers. Although the well-known strong atherosclerotic effects of smoking, some studies reported that smoking in humans and nicotine administration in animals are associated with a decrease of body weight [35]. Evidence revealed an increased energy expenditure while smoking both on rest and light physical activity [36], and nicotine supplied by patch after smoking cessation decreased caloric intake in a dose-related manner [37]. According to an animal study, nicotine may lengthen intermeal time, and decreases amount of meal eaten [38]. Additionally, body weight seems to be the highest in former, the lowest in current, and medium in never smokers [39]. Smoking may be associated with post cessation weight gain, but evidence suggests that risk of weight gain is the highest during the first year after quitting and declines over the years [40]. Similarly, although the CHD were detected with similar prevalence in both sexes in the previous study prevalence of smoking and COPD were higher in males against the higher prevalence of BMI and its terminal consequences including HT and DM in females [33]. This result may indicate both the weight decreasing and strong atherosclerotic effects of smoking. Similarly, the incidence of a myocardial infarction is increased sixfold in women and threefold in men who smoke at least 20 cigarettes per day compared to the never smoked cases [41]. Similar to the previous study the proportion of smokers is consistently higher in men in the literature [33,34]. So smoking is probably a powerful atherosclerotic factor with some suppressor effects on appetite. But smoking may also show the weakness of volition to control eating in the metabolic syndrome, so it may indicate additional risk of excess weight and its consequences. Similarly, prevalence of HT, DM, and smoking were the highest in the highest triglyceride having group as a significant indicator of the metabolic syndrome [8].

Conclusion

As a conclusion, metabolic syndrome is an accelerated systemic atherosclerotic process terminating with obesity, HT, DM, PAD, CRD, COPD, cirrhosis, CHD, stroke, and eventually early aging and death. It shows itself with some reversible components including smoking, overweight, hyper-betalipoproteinemia, hypertriglyceridemia, dyslipidemia, IFG, IGT, and WCH. The terminal consequences are probably due to the smoking and excess weight induced chronic inflammatory process on the endothelial system for a long period of time. WCH is a pioneer sign of the accelerated systemic atherosclerotic process that can be detected easily, and treated by preventing weight gain.

References

1. Eckel RH, Grundy SM, Zimmet PZ (2005) The metabolic syndrome. Lancet 365: 1415-1428.

2. Grundy SM, Brewer HB Jr, Cleeman JI, Smith SC Jr, Lenfant C (2004) Definition of metabolic syndrome: Report of the National Heart, Lung, and Blood Institute/American Heart Association conference on scientific issues related to definition. Circulation 109: 433-438.

3. Tonkin AM (2006) The metabolic syndrome(s)? Curr Atheroscler Rep 6: 165-166.

4. Franklin SS, Barboza MG, Pio JR, Wong ND (2006) Blood pressure categories, hypertensive subtypes, and the metabolic syndrome. J Hypertens 24: 2009-2016.

5. Helvaci MR, Kaya H, Gundogdu M (2012) Gender differences in coronary heart disease in Turkey. Pak J Med Sci 28: 40-44.

6. Helvaci MR, Kaya H, Gundogdu M (2012) White coat hypertension may be an initial sign of metabolic syndrome. Acta Med Indones 44: 222-227.

7. Helvaci MR, Kaya H, Sevinc A, Camci C (2009) Body weight and white coat hypertension. Pak J Med Sci 25: 6: 916-921.

8. Helvaci MR, Kaya H, Gundogdu M (2010) Association of increased triglyceride levels in metabolic syndrome with coronary artery disease. Pak J Med Sci 26: 667-672.

9. Calle EE, Thun MJ, Petrelli JM, Rodriguez C, Heath CW Jr (1999) Body-mass index and mortality in a prospective cohort of U.S. adults. N Engl J Med 341: 1097-1105.

10. Helvaci MR, Ozcura F, Kaya H, Yalcin A (2007) Funduscopic examination has limited benefit for management of hypertension. Int Heart J 48: 187-194.

11. Helvaci MR, Kaya H, Yalcin A, Kuvandik G (2007) Prevalence of white coat hypertension in underweight and overweight subjects. Int Heart J 48: 605-613.

12. Azadbakht L, Mirmiran P, Esmaillzadeh A, Azizi T, Azizi F (2005) Beneficial effects of a Dietary Approaches to Stop Hypertension eating plan on features of the metabolic syndrome. Diabetes Care 28: 2823-2831.

13. Volek JS, Feinman RD (2005) Carbohydrate restriction improves the features of Metabolic Syndrome. Metabolic Syndrome may be defined by the response to carbohydrate restriction. Nutr Metab (Lond) 2: 31.

14. Helvaci MR, Kaya H, Borazan A, Ozer C, Seyhanli M, et al. (2008) Metformin and parameters of physical health. Intern Med 47: 697-703.

15. (2002) Third Report of the National Cholesterol Education Program (NCEP) Expert Panel on Detection, Evaluation, and Treatment of High Blood Cholesterol in Adults (Adult Treatment Panel III) final report. Circulation 106: 3143-3421.

16. Ohkubo T, Asayama K, Kikuya M, Metoki H, Hoshi H, et al. (2004) How many times should blood pressure be measured at home for better prediction of stroke risk? Ten-year follow-up results from the Ohasama study. J Hypertens 22: 1099-1104.

17. Chobanian AV, Bakris GL, Black HR, Cushman WC, Green LA, et al. (2003) The Seventh Report of the Joint National Committee on Prevention, Detection, Evaluation, and Treatment of High Blood Pressure: the JNC 7 report. JAMA 289: 2560-2572.

18. Hond ED, Celis H, Fagard R, Keary L, Leeman M, et al. (2003) THOP investigators. Self-measured versus ambulatory blood pressure in the diagnosis of hypertension. J Hypertens 21: 717-722.

19. Stergiou GS, Salgami EV, Tzamouranis DG, Roussias LG (2005) Masked hypertension assessed by ambulatory blood pressure versus home blood pressure monitoring: is it the same phenomenon? Am J Hypertens 18: 772-778.

20. Helvaci MR, Seyhanli M (2006) What a high prevalence of white coat hypertension in society! Intern Med 45: 671-674.

21. Polonia JJ, Gama GM, Silva JA, Amaral C, Martins LR, et al. (2005) Sequential follow-up clinic and ambulatory blood pressure evaluation in a low risk population of white-coat hypertensive patients and in normotensives. Blood Press Monit 10: 57-64.

22. Fagard RH, Van Den Broeke C, De Cort P (2005) Prognostic significance of blood pressure measured in the office, at home and during ambulatory monitoring in older patients in general practice. J Hum Hypertens 19: 801-807.

23. Nakashima T, Yamano S, Sasaki R, Minami S, Doi K, et al. (2004) White-coat hypertension contributes to the presence of carotid arteriosclerosis. Hypertens Res 27: 739-745.

24. Ugajin T, Hozawa A, Ohkubo T, Asayama K, Kikuya M, et al. (2005) White-coat hypertension as a risk factor for the development of home hypertension: the Ohasama study. Arch Intern Med 165: 1541-1546.

25. Mule G, Nardi E, Cottone S, Cusimano P, Incalcaterra F, et al. (2007) Metabolic syndrome in subjects with white-coat hypertension: impact on left ventricular structure and function. J Hum Hypertens 21: 854-860.

26. Hozawa A, Ohkubo T, Kikuya M, Yamaguchi J, Ohmori K, et al. (2002) Blood pressure control assessed by home, ambulatory and conventional blood pressure measurements in the Japanese general population: the Ohasama study. Hypertens Res 25: 57-63.

27. Celis H, Fagard RH (2004) White-coat hypertension: a clinical review. Eur J Intern Med 15: 348-357.

28. Helvaci MR, Kaya H, Duru M, Yalcin A (2008) What is the relationship between white coat hypertension and dyslipidemia? Int Heart J 49: 87-93.

29. Helvaci MR, Kaya H, Seyhanli M, Cosar E (2007) White coat hypertension is associated with a greater all-cause mortality. J Health Sci 53: 156-160.

30. Bjorklund K, Lind L, Vessby B, Andrén B, Lithell H (2002) Different metabolic predictors of white-coat and sustained hypertension over a 20-year follow-up period: a population-based study of elderly men. Circulation 106: 63-68.

31. O'Brien E, Asmar R, Beilin L, Imai Y, Mallion JM, et al. (2003) European Society of Hypertension recommendations for conventional, ambulatory and home blood pressure measurement. J Hypertens 21: 82-848.

32. Hunt KJ, Resendez RG, Williams K, Haffner SM, Stern MP (2004) National Cholesterol Education Program versus World Health Organization metabolic syndrome in relation to all-cause and cardiovascular mortality in the San Antonio Heart Study. Circulation 110: 1251-1257.

33. Helvaci MR, Aydin Y, Gundogdu M (2012) Smoking induced atherosclerosis in cancers. HealthMED 6: 3744-3749.

34. Fodor JG, Tzerovska R, Dorner T, Rieder A (2004) Do we diagnose and treat coronary heart disease differently in men and women? Wien Med Wochenschr 154: 423-425.

35. Grunberg NE, Greenwood MR, Collins F, Epstein LH, Hatsukami D, et al. (1992) National working conference on smoking and body weight. Task Force 1: Mechanisms relevant to the relations between cigarette smoking and body weight. Health Psychol 11: 4-9.

36. Walker JF, Collins LC, Rowell PP, Goldsmith LJ, Moffatt RJ, et al. (1999) The effect of smoking on energy expenditure and plasma catecholamine and nicotine levels during light physical activity. Nicotine Tob Res 1: 365-370.

37. Hughes JR, Hatsukami DK (1997) Effects of three doses of transdermal nicotine on post-cessation eating, hunger and weight. J Subst Abuse 9: 151-159.

38. Miyata G, Meguid MM, Varma M, Fetissov SO, Kim HJ (2001) Nicotine alters the usual reciprocity between meal size and meal number in female rat. Physiol Behav 74: 169-176.

39. Laaksonen M, Rahkonen O, Prattala R (1998) Smoking status and relative weight by educational level in Finland, 1978-1995. Prev Med 27: 431-437.

40. Froom P, Melamed S, Benbassat J (1998) Smoking cessation and weight gain. J Fam Pract 46: 460-464.

41. Prescott E, Hippe M, Schnohr P, Hein HO, Vestbo J (1998) Smoking and risk of myocardial infarction in women and men: longitudinal population study. BMJ 316: 1043-1047.

Permissions

All chapters in this book were first published in JMS, by OMICS International; hereby published with permission under the Creative Commons Attribution License or equivalent. Every chapter published in this book has been scrutinized by our experts. Their significance has been extensively debated. The topics covered herein carry significant findings which will fuel the growth of the discipline. They may even be implemented as practical applications or may be referred to as a beginning point for another development.

The contributors of this book come from diverse backgrounds, making this book a truly international effort. This book will bring forth new frontiers with its revolutionizing research information and detailed analysis of the nascent developments around the world.

We would like to thank all the contributing authors for lending their expertise to make the book truly unique. They have played a crucial role in the development of this book. Without their invaluable contributions this book wouldn't have been possible. They have made vital efforts to compile up to date information on the varied aspects of this subject to make this book a valuable addition to the collection of many professionals and students.

This book was conceptualized with the vision of imparting up-to-date information and advanced data in this field. To ensure the same, a matchless editorial board was set up. Every individual on the board went through rigorous rounds of assessment to prove their worth. After which they invested a large part of their time researching and compiling the most relevant data for our readers.

The editorial board has been involved in producing this book since its inception. They have spent rigorous hours researching and exploring the diverse topics which have resulted in the successful publishing of this book. They have passed on their knowledge of decades through this book. To expedite this challenging task, the publisher supported the team at every step. A small team of assistant editors was also appointed to further simplify the editing procedure and attain best results for the readers.

Apart from the editorial board, the designing team has also invested a significant amount of their time in understanding the subject and creating the most relevant covers. They scrutinized every image to scout for the most suitable representation of the subject and create an appropriate cover for the book.

The publishing team has been an ardent support to the editorial, designing and production team. Their endless efforts to recruit the best for this project, has resulted in the accomplishment of this book. They are a veteran in the field of academics and their pool of knowledge is as vast as their experience in printing. Their expertise and guidance has proved useful at every step. Their uncompromising quality standards have made this book an exceptional effort. Their encouragement from time to time has been an inspiration for everyone.

The publisher and the editorial board hope that this book will prove to be a valuable piece of knowledge for researchers, students, practitioners and scholars across the globe.

List of Contributors

Frank Comhaire
Department of Endocrinology, Ghent University Hospital, Belgium

Unyime Sunday Jasper
Department of physiotherapy, Plateau State Specialist Hospital, Jos, Nigeria

Djuma Lukonga
Faculty of Medicine, University of Kinshasa, DR Congo

Jean-Robert Rissassy Makulo, Augustin Luzayadio Longo, Tresor Monsere, Ernest Kiswaya Sumaili and Francois Bompeka Lepira
Faculty of Medicine, University of Kinshasa, DR Congo
Nephrology Unit, Department of Internal Medicine, University Clinics of Kinshasa, University of Kinshasa, DR Congo

Jean De Dieu Manyebwa and Hippolyte Nanituma Situakibanza
Faculty of Medicine, University of Kinshasa, DR Congo
Infectious Diseases Unit, Department of Internal Medicine, University Clinics of Kinshasa, University of Kinshasa, DR Congo

Jean Bosco Lasi Kasiam
Faculty of Medicine, University of Kinshasa, DR Congo
Endocrinology and Metabolic Diseases Unit, Department of Internal Medicine, University Clinics of Kinshasa, University of Kinshasa, DR Congo

Roger Mwimba Mbungu
Faculty of Medicine, University of Kinshasa, DR Congo
Department of Gynecology and Obstetrics, University Clinics of Kinshasa, University of Kinshasa, DR Congo

Jean-Marie Ntumba Kayembe
Faculty of Medicine, University of Kinshasa, DR Congo
Pneumology Unit, Department of Internal Medicine, University Clinics of Kinshasa, University of Kinshasa, DR Congo

Derar Refaat
Department of Theriogenology, Faculty of Veterinary Medicine, Assiut University, Assiut, Egypt

Hamdoun
Department of Animal and Poultry Production, Faculty of Agriculture, Sohag University, Sohag, Egypt

Giasuddin ASM
Medical Research Unit (MRU), MHWT, Dhaka-1230, Bangladesh

Khadija Akther Jhuma, Md Abdul Mobin Choudhury and Mujibul Haq AM
Medical College for Women and Hospital, Dhaka-1230, Bangladesh

Rajat Choudhuri, Sandeep Kr. Kar, Dhiman Adhikari and Sabyasachi Sinha
Department of Anaesthesiology and Department of Cardiac Anaesthesiology, Institute of Post Graduate Medical Education &Research, Kolkata, India

Ayesha Farooq, Sufian Sorathia and Hamid Feiz
Aventura Hospital and Medical Center, Aventura, USA

Sameer Shaharyar
Aventura Hospital and Medical Center, Aventura, USA
Center for Prevention and Wellness Research, Baptist Health South Florida, Miami, FL 33139, USA

Lara Roberson
Center for Prevention and Wellness Research, Baptist Health South Florida, Miami, FL 33139, USA

Jiaqiang Zhou, Jiahua Wu, Fang Wu and Hong Li
Department of Endocrinology, Sir Run Run Shaw Hospital, Zhejiang University School of Medicine, Hangzhou, 310016, China

Fengqin Dong and Zhe Zhang
Department of Endocrinology, The First Affiliated Hospital, Zhejiang University School of Medicine, Hangzhou, 310003, China

Spagnuolo MI, Liguoro I and Guarino A
Department of Translation Science of Medicine University, Federico II, Naples, Italy

Ryoma Michishita
Laboratory of Exercise Physiology, Faculty of Health and Sports Science, Fukuoka University, Fukuoka, Japan

Hiroaki Tanaka, Yasuki Higaki and Akira Kiyonaga
Laboratory of Exercise Physiology, Faculty of Health and Sports Science, Fukuoka University, Fukuoka, Japan
Institute for Physical Activity, Fukuoka University, Fukuoka, Japan

Takuro Matsuda
Institute for Physical Activity, Fukuoka University, Fukuoka, Japan

Department of Physical Medicine and Rehabilitation, Fukuoka University Hospital, Fukuoka, Japan

Hideaki Kumahara
Faculty of Nutritional Sciences, Nakamura Gakuen University, Fukuoka, Japan

Makoto Ayabe
Faculty of Computer Science and Systems Engineering, Okayama Prefectural University, Okayama, Japan

Takuro Tobina
Faculty of Nursing and Nutrition, Laboratory of Exercise Physiology, University of Nagasaki, Nagasaki, Japan

Eiichi Yoshimura
Department of Food and Health Science, Prefectural University of Kumamoto, Kumamoto, Japan

Lesmana CRA
Department of Internal Medicine, Hepatology Division, Cipto Mangunkusumo Hospital, Digestive Disease and GI Oncology Center, Medistra Hospital, Jakarta, Indonesia

Arun Raghavan, Nanditha Arun, Snehalatha Chamukuttan, Priscilla Susairaj, Vijaya Lakshminarayanan and Ramachandran Ambady
India Diabetes Research Foundation and Dr. A. Ramachandran's Diabetes Hospitals, Chennai, India

Cem Aygun
Department of Gastroenterology and Hepatology, Istanbul Medipol University, Istanbul, Turkey

Claudia Tosti, Valentina Cappelli and Vincenzo De Leo
Obstetrics and Gynecology, Department of Molecular and Developmental Medicine, University of Siena, Policlinico "Santa Maria alle Scotte", Viale Bracci, 53100 Siena, Italy

Andrea Romani
Department of Physiology and Biophysics, Case Western Reserve University, USA

Chesinta Voma
Department of Physiology and Biophysics, Case Western Reserve University, USA
Department of Clinical Chemistry, Cleveland State University, USA

Zienab Etwebi and Danial Amir Soltani
Department of Clinical Chemistry, Cleveland State University, USA

Colleen Croniger
Department of Nutrition, Case Western Reserve University, USA

Micaela Gliozzi, Ross Walker and Vincenzo Mollace
Institute of Research for Food Safety and Health (IRC-FSH), University of Catanzaro "Magna Graecia", Catanzaro, Italy

Francisco Herlânio Costa Carvalho, Helvécio Neves Feitosa, Julio Cesar Garcia de Alencar, Lívia Rocha de Miranda Pinto and Francisco Edson de Lucena Feitosa
Federal University of Ceará, Department of Public Health, St Prof. Costa Mendes, 1608 – 5th Floor, Rodolfo Teófilo, Fortaleza, Ceará, Brazil

Ana Ciléia Pinto Teixeira Henriques
Federal University of Ceará, Department of Public Health, St Prof. Costa Mendes, 1608 – 5th Floor, Rodolfo Teófilo, Fortaleza, Ceará, Brazil
Metropolitan College of Grande Fortaleza, Assis Chateaubriand Maternity Teaching Hospital, Federal University of Ceará, Brazil

Samsad Jahan
Department of Gynaecology and Obstetrics, BIRDEM, Dhaka, Bangladesh

Chaudhury Meshkat Ahmed
Department of Cardiology, BSMMU, Dhaka, Bangladesh

Samira Humaira Habib
Health Economics Unit, BADAS, Dhaka, Bangladesh

Akter Jahan
Govt Homeopathic College, Dhaka, Bangladesh

Farzana Sharmin
Department of Obstetrics and Gynecology, BIHS, Dhaka, Bangladesh

Md Sakandar Hyet Khan
Red Crescent Hospital, Cox's Bazar, Bangladesh

Manisha Banarjee
Department of Gynecology and Obstetrics, Dhaka Medical College Hospital, Dhaka, Bangladesh

Keerthi Kupsal, Saraswati Mudigonda and Surekha Rani Hanumanth
Department of Genetics, University College of Science, Osmania University, Telangana, Hyderabad-500007, India

Nyayapathi VBK Sai and Krishnaveni Neelala
Department of Cardiology, South Central Railway Hospital, Lallaguda-500013, Secunderabad, India

Assi Milwidsky, Itzhak Shapira, Sivan Letourneau-Shesaf, Sharon Greenberg, Shlomo Berliner and OriRogowski
Department of Medicine "C" and "E", of the Tel Aviv Sourasky Medical Center, Affiliated to the Sackler Faculty of Medicine, Tel Aviv University, Tel Aviv, Israel

Arie Steinvil
Department of Cardiology, of the Tel Aviv Sourasky Medical Center, Affiliated to the Sackler Faculty of Medicine, Tel Aviv University, Tel Aviv, Israel

Rona Limor
Department of Laboratory, of the Tel Aviv Sourasky Medical Center, Affiliated to the Sackler Faculty of Medicine, Tel Aviv University, Tel Aviv, Israel

Long NM, Burns TA, Volpi Lagreca G, Alende M and Duckett SK
Department of Animal and Veterinary Sciences, Clemson University, Clemson, SC 29634, USA

Fitsum Girma Tadesse
Department of Medical Microbiology, Radboud Institute for Molecular Life Sciences, Route 268, Geert Grooteplein 26-28, Nijmegen 6525 GA, Netherlands

Yesehak Worku
Department of Biochemistry, College of Medicine, Addis Ababa University, Addis Ababa, Ethiopia

Yeweyenhareg Feleke
Department of Internal Medicine, Faculty of Medicine, Addis Ababa University, Addis Ababa, Ethiopia

Tarek H. El-Metwally
Faculty of Medicine, Assiut University, Assiut, POB: 71526, Egypt

Bahaa Kornah, Hesham Safwat, Tharwat Abdel Ghany and Mohamed Abdel-AAl
Al-Azhar University, Cairo, Egypt
Manshet El bakey Hospital, Alazhar University, Cairo, Egypt

Ankita Bohra and Bhateja S
P.G Oral Medicine and Radiology Department, Vyas Dental College and Hospital, Jodhpur, India

Fikru Tafese, Beyene Wondafirash, Sintayehu Fekadu, Garumma Tolu and Gugsa Nemarra
Department of Health Service Management, School of Public Health, Jimma University, Jimma, Ethiopia

Elias Teferi
Department of Public health, College of Medicine and Health Sciences, Ambo University, Addis Ambo, Ethiopia

Seyed Rafie Arefhosseini
Department of food technology, Faculty of Nutrition sciences, Tabriz University of Medical sciences, Tabriz, Iran

Mehrangiz Ebrahimi-Mamaeghani
Nutrition Research center, Faculty of Nutrition sciences, Tabriz University of Medical sciences, Tabriz, Iran

Somayeh Mohammadi
Department of Nutrition, Faculty of Nutrition sciences, Tabriz University of Medical Sciences, Tabriz, Iran

Nilesh Kumar J Patel, Deepak Asti, Nikhil Nalluri, Hafiz Khan, Ritesh Kanotra, Pandya Bhavi, James Lafferty and Jeffrey Rothman
Staten Island University Hospital, Staten Island, New York, USA

Sushruth Edla
St Vincent Charity Medical Center, Cleveland, Ohio, USA

Sohil Golwala
American University of The Caribbean, Sint Maarten, Corel Gables, Florida, USA

Achint Patel, Shantanu Solanki and Shilp Kumar Arora
Icahn School of Medicine at Mount Sinai, New York, USA

Abhishek Deshmukh
University of Arkansas, Little Rock, UALR, USA

Nilay Patel, Apurva O Badheka and Laurent Legault
Pediatric Endocrinology Department, McGill University, the Montreal Children's Hospital, 2300 Rue Tupper, Montreal, H3H 1P3, Canada
Pediatric Endocrinology Department, Hôpital Maisonneuve-Rosemont, 5415 Boulevard de l' Assomption, Montréal, QC H1T 2M4, Canada

Reem AL Khalifah
Pediatric Endocrinology Department, McGill University, the Montreal Children's Hospital, 2300 Rue Tupper, Montreal, H3H 1P3, Canada
Pediatric Department, King Saud University, Riyadh, Saudi Arabia

Marc Girard
Radiology Department, Hôpital Maisonneuve-Rosemont, 5415 Boulevard de l' Assomption, Montréal, QC H1T 2M4, Canada

Abdoulaye Diané, Geoffrey W Payne and Sarah L Gray
Northern Medical Program, University of Northern British Columbia, Prince George, Canada

Anand CR, Sandeep Saxena, Khushboo Srivastav, Poonam Kishore and Shashi K Bhaskar
Department of Ophthalmology, King George's Medical University, Lucknow, India

Arvind Misra
Department of Medicine, King George's Medical University, Lucknow, India

Shankar M Natu
Department of Pathology, King George's Medical University, Lucknow, India

Abbas A Mahdi
Department of Biochemistry, King George's Medical University, Lucknow, India

Vinay K Khanna
Indian Institute of Toxicology and Research, Lucknow, India

Mette Viftrup-Lund, Melina Gade and Finn F Lauszus
Department of Gynecology and Obstetrics, Herning Hospital, Denmark

Brian Miller
School of Sport Science and Wellness Education, The University of Akron, Akron, OH, USA
Health Education and Promotion, School of Health Sciences, Kent State University, Kent, OH, USA

Mark Fridline
Department of Statistics, The University of Akron, Akron, OH, USA

Kazuhiko Nishimura, Hideaki Katuyama, Hiroshi Nakagawa and SaburoMatuo
Laboratory of Bioenvironmental Sciences, Course of Veterinary Science, Graduate School of Life and Environmental Sciences, Osaka Prefecture University, Osaka, Japan

Rodhan Khthir and Felyn Luz Espina
Marshall university-school of medicine, Huntington, West Virginia, USA

Mehmet Rami Helvaci
Department of Internal Medicine, Medical Faculty of Mustafa Kemal University, Antakya, Turkey

Ramazan Davran
Department of Radiology, Medical Faculty of Mustafa Kemal University, Antakya, Turkey

Akin Aydogan, Seckin Akkucuk, Mustafa Ugu and Cem Oruc
Department of General Surgery, Medical Faculty of the Mustafa Kemal University, Antakya, Turkey

Pejcic Ana and Minic Ivan
Department of Periodontology and Oral Medicine, University of Nis, Serbia

Mirkovic Dimitrije
Private Practice – "Smile-Dent", Nis, Serbia

Stojanovic Mariola
Institute for Public Health, University of Nis, Serbia

Markolf Hanefeld and Frank Pistrosch
GWT-TUD GmbH, Study center Prof. Hanefeld, Dresden, Germany

Jan Schulze
Saxonian Chamber of Physicians, Dresden, Germany

Ulrike Rothe
Health Sciences/Public Health, Faculty of Medicine, TU Dresden, Germany

Sambhu D Varma
Department of Ophthalmology and Visual Sciences, University of Maryland School of Medicine, Baltimore, USA
Department of Biochemistry and Molecular Biology, University of Maryland School of Medicine, Baltimore, USA

Kavita R Hegde
Department of Ophthalmology and Visual Sciences, University of Maryland School of Medicine, Baltimore, USA
Department of Natural Sciences, Coppin State University, Baltimore, USA

Checa-Ros Ana
School of Medicine of Granada, San Cecilio University Hospital, Spain
Department of Pediatrics, University of Granada, San Cecilio Hospital, Spain

Vargas-Pérez M, Molina-Carballo A, Uberos-Fernández J and Muñoz-Hoyos A
Department of Pediatrics, University of Granada, San Cecilio Hospital, Spain

Muñoz-Gallego A
Department of Language and Computer Science, University of Málaga, Spain

Alexander E Berezin
Consultant of Therapeutic Unit, Private Hospital "Vita-Center", Zaporozhye, Ukraine

Mehmet Rami Helvaci
Professor of Internal Medicine, Medical Faculty of the
Mustafa Kemal University, Hatay, Turkey

Ali Ozcan
Professor of Biochemistry, Medical Faculty of the
Mustafa Kemal University, Hatay, Turkey

Index

www.ingramcontent.com/pod-product-compliance
Lightning Source LLC
Chambersburg PA
CBHW080249230326
41458CB00097B/4181